# Occupational and Environmental Reproductive Hazards:

## A GUIDE FOR CLINICIANS

# Occupational and Environmental Reproductive Hazards:

## A GUIDE FOR CLINICIANS

Edited by

MAUREEN PAUL, M.D., M.P.H.

**Assistant Professor**

**Departments of Obstetrics and Gynecology and Family
and Community Medicine
(Occupational Health Program)
University of Massachusetts Medical Center
Worcester, Massachusetts**

**Illustrated by**

PETER ROSENBLATT, M.D.

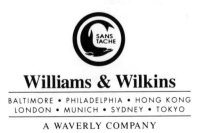

**Williams & Wilkins**

BALTIMORE • PHILADELPHIA • HONG KONG
LONDON • MUNICH • SYDNEY • TOKYO

A WAVERLY COMPANY

*Editor:* Charles W. Mitchell
*Project Manager:* Raymond E. Reter
*Copy Editor:* Shelley Potler
*Designer:* Karen S. Klinedinst
*Illustration Planner:* Wayne Hubbel

Accurate indications, adverse reactions, and dosage schedules for drugs are provided in this book, but it is possible that they may change. The reader is urged to review the package information data of the manufacturers of the medications mentioned.

*Printed in the United States of America*

Chapter reprints are available from the publisher.

**Library of Congress Cataloging-in-Publication Data**

Occupational and environmental reproductive hazards : a guide for clinicians / edited by
  Maureen Paul.
      p.     cm.
  Includes bibliographical references and index.
  ISBN 0-683-06801-6
  1. Reproductive toxicology.    I. Paul, Maureen.
  [DNLM: 1. Environmental Pollutants—adverse effects.
  2. Occupational Diseases.    3. Reproduction—drug effects.
  4. Teratogens—toxicity.    WQ 205 015]
  RA1224.2033    1992
  616.6′5071—dc20
  DNLM/DLC
  for Library of Congress                                          92-13719
                                                                       CIP


                                                        93   94   95   96
                                        2    3    4    5    6    7    8    9    10

This book is dedicated to the education of clinicians,

the reproductive health of all workers and citizens,

and to my daughter, Dillon.

# Preface

I will never forget my sense of bewilderment some 8 yr ago when, as a practicing obstetrician-gynecologist, a prenatal patient first handed me a stack of chemical data sheets and asked me to determine the safety of her job during pregnancy. She could not afford to leave her job, but she wanted information about her potential occupational risks and ways to minimize them. Thanks to my former chemistry classes, I at least vaguely recognized some of the ethyls, hexyls, and oxides on those mysterious data sheets. Beyond that, however, I knew little about the risks of these industrial chemicals or even where to turn for help.

This scenario may sound familiar to practitioners involved in reproductive or primary care medicine; for, despite the as yet poor integration of these issues into medical and nursing education, we are faced with a host of patient concerns ranging from use of hair dyes to video display terminals, from radon to pesticides, from lead to cytomegalovirus. If this is so, this book was written with you in mind. Its primary purpose is to provide clinicians with some answers to the most commonly asked questions about reproductive hazards and to offer an effective approach to addressing patient concerns.

"But why now?", you may ask. Surely many of these exposures are not new. We have all heard stories of the nightmarish working conditions at the turn of the century. For years, we have been aware of potential drug teratogenicity, the sterilizing effects of high-dose radiation therapy, and the sexual dysfunction induced by some antihypertensive medications. Why then are issues of occupational and environmental reproductive toxicology assuming more central focus in the lives of today's clinicians?

The answer to this question lies not in a single cataclysmic event but in a convergence of social, economic, scientific, and political forces that have emerged over many years. The post-World War II era ushered in technological advances that revolutionized industry and permeated every aspect of our lives. This transformation was accompanied by a virtual explosion of synthetic chemicals onto the U.S. market. By the 1980s, 4 million chemicals were identified; over 60,000 were in widespread commercial use in Western nations, with at least 1000 new chemicals introduced each year. Yet, due in part to their sheer numbers and inadequate premarket testing, little was known about the acute and chronic health effects of these industrial agents.

While the thalidomide tragedy of the late 1950s catalyzed research into the teratogenic effects of pharmaceuticals taken by women during pregnancy, it was not until the discovery of sterility among male workers exposed to the pesticide dibromochloropropane (DBCP) in the late 1970s that the reproductive effects of industrial chemicals received widespread attention. With this unfortunate event, the purview of toxicologists and epidemiologists widened from drugs to workplace and general environment exposures, from birth defects to a broad array of adverse developmental and reproductive outcomes, and from women to both sexes.

Indiscriminate use and careless disposal of these industrial chemicals eventually resulted in public outcry. The environmental movement was born in the hearts of citizens who watched buried toxic wastes bubble up from the soil in their community playgrounds and backyards and who wondered about the link between these exposures and their health or that of their families. In most cases that came under investigation, concerns about adverse pregnancy outcomes and childhood cancers were paramount. As more and more hazardous waste sites were discovered, a grassroots environmental movement swept the nation, demanding effective responses from industry, scientists, government, and the health care system.

At the same time, women were entering the U.S. workforce in unparalleled numbers. From 1970–1990, the proportion of women in the civilian labor force increased from 43% to 58%. These women were primarily employed in the burgeoning microelectronics industry and in the growing services sectors. Today, two-thirds of women of childbearing age are employed outside the home, earning incomes essential to their well-being. This demographic shift fueled concerns about reproductive health hazards in the new female-intensive industries and highlighted the need for adequate family care benefits, medical benefits, and parental leave.

Throughout the 1970s and 80s, public awareness about occupational and environmental hazards was also bolstered by the passage of abundant legislation aimed at curtailing environmental contamination and promoting health and safety in the workplace. The Occupational Safety and Health Act of 1970 established the mechanisms and agencies responsible for the promulgation and enforcement of occupational health and safety standards. Numerous other statutes addressed air pollutants, drinking water contaminants, transport and disposal of toxic chemicals, and the clean-up of hazardous waste sites. Of utmost importance was the passage of legislation in the 1980s giving workers and citizens, as well as the clinicians who cared for them, the "right to know" about toxic chemicals in their workplaces and communities.

In keeping with historic precedents, the issue of protection from reproductive hazards also raised the spectre of discrimination against women workers. In the late 1970s, the American Cyanamid Company in Willow Island, West Virginia, adopted a "fetal protection" policy that excluded all women of childbearing capacity from employment in certain hazardous areas of the plant. Some women workers underwent surgical sterilization to keep their jobs. Other companies soon followed suit, resulting in a decade-long battle between industry and labor and women's rights organizations over the fate of these exclusionary practices. This conflict recently culminated in a landmark Supreme Court decision (*United Automobile Workers v. Johnson Controls*) that rendered corporate "fetal protection" policies illegal under federal antidiscrimination statutes. In the aftermath of this decision, public health officials, labor advocates, and policymakers are grappling anew with the problem of reproductive hazards and with formulating solutions that are equitable and protective of both sexes. This initiative extends well beyond exclusionary corporate practices per se to examine the inadequacies of current occupational and environmental standards in protecting reproductive health as well as the options and remedies available to workers and citizens exposed to these hazards.

In the wake of these intense changes, the health care system has had a difficult time keeping pace with growing public demands for information about occupational and environmental hazards. With fewer than 1500 Board-certified occupational medicine physicians in the United States, most of whom are employed by industry, these issues are increasingly permeating the practices of primary health care providers who are generally still poorly prepared to address them. This problem was recently recognized in a series of reports by the Institute of Medicine (IOM). Acknowledging that primary providers cannot be expected to become experts in occupational and environmental medicine, the IOM urges that clinicians learn, at a minimum, how to take an initial screening history, how to identify patients at potential risk, and how to initiate appropriate consultations and referrals. To accomplish these objectives, the IOM reports promote the integration of occupational and environmental health issues into medical education curricula as well as the development of readily accessible clinical information and referral resources for primary providers.

It is my hope that this book will further the goals addressed by the IOM and will serve as an important resource for obstetricians-gynecologists and all primary health care providers involved in the promotion of reproductive health. Its pages reflect years of my own training and clinical experience with patients concerned about occupational and environmental reproductive risks, as well as the knowledge of many other experts who have been involved in this important public health arena.

The book is divided into four general sections. Section I provides important background information about the physiology of reproduction and development and where and how toxicants exert their effects. Section II provides a brief overview of toxicological and epidemiological research methods used to assess the effects of toxicants on reproduction and development. Section III concentrates on the clinical evaluation and management of patients and includes a general approach to clinical problems, specific case examples, and a discussion of important legal and policy issues. The final section of the book provides information on specific reproductive and developmental hazards including physical agents, biological agents, and various classes of chemicals. In addition to workplace toxicants, it addresses issues of community contamination, household hazards, and substance abuse.

I would like to extend my appreciation to the many people who made this book possible. First, I want to thank each and every author for the tremendous time and energy spent in writing chapters for the book. Without their expertise and dedication, this project would not have been realized. Second, I am deeply indebted to Marcia Bowles and Susan Wortman who worked tirelessly typing and putting the manuscripts into appropriate format. Finally, I want to thank the workers and citizens whose lives and experiences are the ultimate source of knowledge for this book.

*Maureen Paul, M.D., M.P.H.*

# Contributors

ANN ASCHENGRAU, D.Sc.
Assistant Professor of Public Health
Boston University School of Public Health
Boston, Massachusetts

ELIZABETH AVERILL, R.N., M.S.N.
Health Programs Director
Workplace Health Fund
Washington, D.C.

DAVID BELLINGER, Ph.D., M.Sc.
Assistant Professor of Neurology
Harvard Medical School
Neuroepidemiology Unit
Children's Hospital
Boston, Massachusetts

JOAN E. BERTIN, J.D.
Associate Director
Women's Rights Project
American Civil Liberties Union
New York, New York

MITCHELL BESSER, M.D., M.P.H.
Department of Obstetrics and Gynecology
Brigham and Women's Hospital
Boston, Massachusetts

ROBERT L. BRENT, M.D., Ph.D.
Louis and Bess Stein Professor of Pediatrics
Chairman, Department of Pediatrics
Jefferson Medical College
Philadelphia, Pennsylvania

GRETA R. BUNIN, Ph.D.
Assistant Professor of Pediatrics
Department of Oncology
Children's Hospital
Philadelphia, Pennsylvania

H. WESTLEY CLARK, M.D., J.D., M.P.H.
Assistant Clinical Professor
Department of Psychiatry
University of California, San Francisco
Chief, Substance Abuse Special Populations
Department of Veterans Affairs Medical
  Center
Community Liaison and Public Policy
  Component
San Francisco Treatment Research Unit
University of California, San Francisco
San Francisco, California

ALAN G. FANTEL, Ph.D.
Research Professor
Department of Pediatrics
University of Washington School of
  Medicine
Seattle, Washington

GLADYS FRIEDLER, Ph.D.
Science Scholar
The Mary Ingraham Bunting Institute
Radcliffe College
Cambridge, Massachusetts

HOWARD HU, M.D., M.P.H., Sc.D.
Associate Professor of Medicine
Channing Laboratory
Harvard Medical School
Occupational Health Program
Department of Environmental Health
Harvard School of Public Health
Boston, Massachusetts


BARBARA JANTAUSCH, M.D.
Assistant Professor of Pediatrics
George Washington University Medical
    Center
Children's National Medical Center
Washington, D.C.


JAMES S. KESNER, Ph.D.
Research Biologist
Functional Toxicology Section
National Institute for Occupational Safety and
    Health
Cincinnati, Ohio


MARIAN C. MARBURY, Sc.D.
Environmental Epidemiologist
Section of Chronic Disease and Environmental
    Epidemiology
Minnesota Department of Health
Minneapolis, Minnesota


DONALD R. MATTISON, M.D.
Dean
Graduate School of Public Health
Professor of Environmental & Occupational
    Health and Obstetrics and Gynecology
University of Pittsburgh
Pittsburgh, Pennsylvania

MELISSA McDIARMID, M.D., M.P.H.
Assistant Professor
Environmental Health Sciences
The Johns Hopkins School of Hygiene and
    Public Health
Baltimore, Maryland
Office of Occupational Medicine
Occupational Safety and Health
    Administration
United States Department of Labor
Washington, D.C.


M. JANE MEADOWS, Ph.D.
Science Department
Hall High School
Little Rock, Arkansas


MARVIN MEISTRICH, Ph.D.
Professor and Biophysicist
Department of Experimental Radiotherapy
M.D. Anderson Cancer Center
Houston, Texas


RICHARD K. MILLER, Ph.D.
Professor of Ob/Gyn and Toxicology
Director, Division of Research
Department of Obstetrics and Gynecology
University of Rochester School of Medicine
    and Dentistry
Rochester, New York


PHILIP E. MIRKES, Ph.D.
Research Professor
Department of Pediatrics
University of Washington School of Medicine
Seattle, Washington


MARION MOSES, M.D.
President
Pesticide Education Center
San Francisco, California

KENNETH L. NOLLER, M.D.
Professor and Chairman
Department of Obstetrics and Gynecology
University of Massachusetts Medical School
Worcester, Massachusetts

DAVID OZONOFF, M.D., M.P.H.
Professor and Chief
Environmental Health Section
Boston University School of Public Health
Boston, Massachusetts

MAUREEN PAUL, M.D., M.P.H.
Assistant Professor
Departments of Obstetrics and Gynecology
  and Family and Community Medicine
  (Occupational Health Program)
Director, Occupational and Environmental
  Reproductive Hazards Center
University of Massachusetts Medical Center
Worcester, Massachusetts

DAVID PLOWCHALK, PH.D.
Research Toxicologist
E.I. Dupont deNemours and Company
Haskell Laboratory for Toxicological and
  Industrial Medicine
Newark, Delaware

PETER ROSE, M.D.
Associate Professor
Department of Obstetrics and Gynecology
Chair, Division of Gynecologic Oncology
University of Massachusetts Medical School
Worcester, Massachusetts

STEVEN M. SCHRADER, PH.D.
Chief, Functional Toxicology Section
Experimental Toxicology Branch
Division of Biomedical and Behavioral Science
National Institute for Occupational Safety and
  Health
Cincinnati, Ohio

SHERRY G. SELEVAN, PH.D.
Reproductive Epidemiologist
United States Environmental Protection
  Agency
Washington, D.C.

JOHN L. SEVER, M.D., PH.D.
Professor of Pediatrics, Obstetrics and
  Gynecology, Microbiology, and
  Immunology
Children's National Medical Center
George Washington University Medical
  Center
Washington, D.C.

THOMAS H. SHEPARD, M.D.
Professor
Department of Pediatrics
University of Washington School of Medicine
Seattle, Washington

TERESA SILVAGGIO, M.D., M.P.H.
Graduate Student
Graduate School of Public Health
University of Pittsburgh
Pittsburgh, Pennsylvania

EMIL SMITH, PH.D.
Associate Professor
Department of Pharmacology
University of Massachusetts Medical School
Worcester, Massachusetts

YORAM SOROKIN, M.D.
Associate Professor
Director of Labor and Delivery
Department of Obstetrics and Gynecology
Division of Maternal Fetal Medicine
Wayne State University School of Medicine
Detroit, Michigan

MERYLE WEINSTEIN, B.A.
Community Liaison and Public Policy
Component
San Francisco Treatment Research
Unit
University of California, San Francisco
San Francisco, California

LAURA S. WELCH, M.D.
Associate Professor of Medicine
Director, Division of Occupational and
Environmental Medicine
George Washington University School of
Medicine
Washington, D.C.

ELISABETH A. WERBY, J.D.
Special Projects Attorney
Women's Rights Project
American Civil Liberties Union
New York, New York

MARY S. WOLFF, Ph.D.
Associate Professor
Department of Community Medicine
Mt. Sinai School of Medicine
New York, New York

PETER K. WORKING, Ph.D.
Director of Pharmacology/Toxicology
Liposome Technology Incorporated
Menlo Park, California

# Contents

Preface / vii    Contributors / xi

**I**

·····································································

# Basic Principles

# Male Reproductive Toxicology[a]

## STEVEN M. SCHRADER, JAMES S. KESNER

In 1775, an English physician named Percival Pott reported a high incidence of scrotal cancer among chimney sweeps. This observation led to protective regulations in the form of bathing requirements for these workers (1). This response represents one of the earliest occupational health interventions involving the male reproductive system. While male reproductive toxicology remained of interest in the intervening 200 years, this area of occupational medicine was not established until 1977 when Whorton and associates reported the effects of the nematocide, dibromochloropropane (DBCP), on male workers (2). In this case, the animal toxicologists had done their job. In 1961, it had been reported that DBCP reduced testicular weights in rodents (3). Unfortunately, this report went essentially unnoticed until workers became infertile and, in some cases, sterile due to occupational exposure to the pesticide.

Toxicants can attack the male reproductive system at one of several sites or at multiple sites, as illustrated in Figure 1.1. Primary targets include the neuroendocrine system, the testes, post-testicular sites including the accessory sex glands, and sexual function.

The endocrine system, in concert with the nervous system, coordinates function of the various components of the reproductive axis. The testes produce the sperm; yet other processes important for normal fertility, including maturation of the sperm and addition of seminal excretions, occur after the sperm leave the testes. Finally, libido and the associated erection and ejaculation are requisite for normal, unaided male reproductive performance.

With thousands of chemicals in use in the workplace and with new ones added each year, most agents have not been thoroughly tested for male reproductive toxicity. This chapter, however, provides basic information on the known targets of male reproductive toxicants and the methods available to detect adverse effects at early stages.

## NEUROENDOCRINE SYSTEM

A detailed description of the reproductive neuroendocrine axis is beyond the scope of this chapter and has been reviewed elsewhere (4–6). The following overview of this axis provides a basis for discussing sites of toxicological insult.

[a]This chapter was prepared by Drs. Schrader and Kesner as part of their official duties at the National Institute for Occupational Safety and Health. Therefore, copyright is not claimed on this chapter.

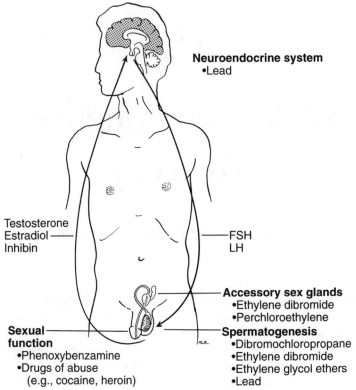

**Figure 1.1.** Toxicants can act at multiple sites to disrupt normal functioning of the male reproductive system. Primary targets include the *neuroendocrine system*, the *testes*, the *accessory sex glands*, and *sexual function*. Examples of toxicants that act at these various sites are provided.

The reproductive neuroendocrine axis of the male involves principally the central nervous system (CNS), the anterior pituitary gland, and the testes. Inputs from the CNS and from the periphery are integrated by the hypothalamus, which directly regulates gonadotropin secretion by the anterior pituitary gland. The gonadotropins, in turn, act primarily upon the Leydig cells within the interstitium and Sertoli and germ cells within the seminiferous tubules to regulate spermatogenesis and hormone production by the testes.

## Hypothalamic-Pituitary Axis

The hypothalamus secretes the neurohormone, gonadotropin-releasing hormone (GnRH), into the hypophyseal portal vasculature for transport to the anterior pituitary gland. The pulsatile secretion of this decapeptide causes the concomitant release of luteinizing hormone (LH) and, with lesser synchrony and one-fifth the potency, of follicle-stimulating hormone (FSH) (6). Substantial evidence supports the existence of a separate FSH-releasing hormone, although none has yet been isolated (7).

Both LH and FSH are glycoprotein dimers comprised of a common $\alpha$- and specificity-imparting $\beta$-protein subunits. These hormones are secreted by the anterior pituitary gland into the circulation. LH acts directly upon the Leydig cells to stimulate synthesis and release of testosterone, whereas FSH stimulates aromatization of testosterone to estradiol by the Sertoli cell. (The testes contribute only 10–30% of the circulating estradiol in the male; the remainder is derived from peripheral aromatization of androgens (8)). Gonadotropic stimulation causes the release of these steroid hormones into the spermatic vein.

Gonadotropin secretion is, in turn, checked by testosterone and estradiol through negative feedback mechanisms (Fig. 1.1). Testosterone regulates hypothalamic GnRH secretion, primarily by reducing the pulse frequency of LH release. Estradiol, on the other hand, acts upon the pituitary gland to reduce the magnitude of gonadotropin release. Through these endocrine feedback loops, testicular function in general, and testosterone secretion specifically, are maintained at a relatively steady state.

## Pituitary-Testicular Axis

Both LH and FSH are necessary for normal spermatogenesis. LH induces high intratesticular concentrations of testosterone. Pituitary FSH and testosterone from the Leydig cells act upon the Sertoli cells within the seminiferous tubule epithelium to initiate spermatogenesis. Sperm production persists after removing either LH (and presumably the high intratesticular testosterone concentrations) or FSH, but it is quantitatively reduced. FSH is required to initiate spermatogenesis at puberty and, to a lesser extent, to reinitiate spermatogenesis that has been arrested (5, 9).

The hormonal synergism that serves to maintain spermatogenesis may entail recruitment by FSH of differentiated spermatogonia to enter meiosis, while testosterone controls specific, subsequent stages of spermatogenesis. FSH and testosterone may also act upon the Sertoli cell to stimulate production of one or more paracrine factors that affect the number of Leydig cells and their testosterone production (9). Testosterone and FSH stimulate protein synthesis by Sertoli cells, including synthesis of androgen-binding protein (ABP), while FSH alone stimulates synthesis of aromatase and inhibin. ABP is secreted primarily into the seminiferous tubular fluid and is transported to the proximal portion of the caput epididymis, possibly serving as a local carrier of androgens (6). Aromatase catalyzes the conversion of testosterone to estradiol in the Sertoli cells and in other peripheral tissues.

Inhibin is a glycoprotein consisting of two dissimilar, disulfide-linked subunits, α and β. Although inhibin preferentially inhibits FSH release, it may also attenuate LH release in the presence of GnRH stimulation (10). FSH and LH stimulate inhibin release with approximately equal potency (11). Interestingly, inhibin is secreted into the spermatic vein as pulses that are synchronous with those of testosterone (12). This observation probably does not reflect direct actions of LH or testosterone on Sertoli cell activity, but rather effects of other Leydig cell products secreted either into the interstitial spaces or the circulation.

Prolactin, which is also secreted by the anterior pituitary gland, acts synergistically with LH and testosterone to promote male reproductive function. Prolactin binds to specific receptors on the Leydig cell and increases the amount of androgen-receptor complex within the nucleus of androgen-responsive tissues (13). Hyperprolactinemia is associated with reductions of testicular and prostate size, semen volume, and circulating concentrations of LH and testosterone (14). Hyperprolactinemia has also been associated with impotence, apparently independent of altering testosterone secretion (15).

## Assessment Methods

Overt clinical manifestations of toxic exposure targeting the reproductive neuroendocrine system most commonly reflect alterations in androgen-dependent biological processes. During the physical examination, modifications in any of the following traits may indicate that androgen production has been affected: (a) nitrogen retention and muscular development; (b) maintenance of the external genitalia and accessory sexual organs; (c) maintenance of the enlarged larynx and thickened vocal cords responsible for the male voice; (d) beard, axillary, and pubic hair growth and temporal hair recession and balding; (e) libido and sexual performance; (f) organ-specific proteins in tissues (e.g., liver, kidneys, salivary glands); and (g) aggressive behavior (6).

A number of hormonal assays are available to assess the reproductive endocrine status of males who present with evidence of hypogonadism or who are exposed to potential reproductive toxicants. The endocrine profile currently used by the National Institute for Occupational Safety and Health (NIOSH) to evaluate working populations exposed to potential reproductive toxicants includes measurement of LH, FSH, testosterone, and prolactin in appropriate body fluids. With minor methodological modifications, the same profile can be used for clinical purposes.

FSH and LH are generally decreased in conditions that directly affect hypothalamo-pituitary function and are often increased with primary testicular toxicity, due to loss of feedback inhibition by the sex steroid hormones. Measurement of prolactin levels is important in patients exposed to drugs or chemicals that induce hyperprolactinemia or in men who present with impotence or evidence of a CNS tumor (16). Estradiol assays are also indicated in males with gynecomastia.

Because the circulating profile of LH is pulsatile, serial blood samples are the best way to estimate the status of this hormone for the individual. Pooled results of three samples collected at 20-min intervals provide a reasonable estimate of mean concentration (16). Alternatively, an integral of the pulsatile LH secretion rate can be obtained by measuring this gonadotropin in urine.

FSH levels in blood are not as variable as those for LH; this is attributable, in part, to the longer circulating half-life of FSH. Thus, analysis of a single blood sample from an individual provides a more reliable estimate of FSH than LH. For the sake of convenience, FSH can also be measured in urine. Gonadotropins and other protein hormones are not exuded into the saliva.

Prolactin secretion is variable and affected by several factors including a circadian rhythm (17), eating (18), and physical and psychological stress (19). These variables should be controlled whenever possible. Prolactin has not been found in saliva, nor are specific immunoassays presently available for measuring intact or fragmented prolactin in urine.

Approximately 2% of circulating testosterone is free; the remainder is bound to sex hormone-binding globulin (SHBG), albumin, and other serum proteins. The free circulating testosterone is the active component and, therefore, provides a more accurate marker of physiologically available testosterone than does total testosterone when SHBG concentration or binding is altered (16). (SHBG and ABP are very similar, yet distinct, glycoprotein dimers. While ABP is produced by the testes and is primarily restricted therein, SHBG is of unknown origin and circulates peripherally (20)).

Circulating testosterone levels, like those for LH, fluctuate considerably over time. Estimates of free and total testosterone can be determined in single blood samples, but are greatly improved by assaying multiple blood samples and pooling the results. Alternatively, a single measurement of a testosterone metabolite in urine (e.g., androsterone, etiocholanolone, or testosterone glucuronide) provides a convenient index of total testosterone (6). Quantifying testosterone in saliva affords a convenient alternative to blood sampling while providing a measure of the unbound, biologically active component of circulating testosterone (21).

Estimates of serum estradiol levels based on a single sample are acceptable but are markedly improved by analyzing two or three samples collected at 20-min intervals (22). Relative to testosterone, estradiol has lower affinity for SHBG, but significantly greater binding to serum albumin (23). As with testosterone, only 2–3% of circulating estradiol is unbound to serum proteins. While measuring this unbound fraction may be a more biologically relevant measure than total estradiol, the minute quantities of free estradiol ($\leq 1$ pg/ml) challenge the sensitivity limits of existing routine immunoassays. For this same reason, salivary estradiol measurements are also impractical (21). An integral of total estradiol secretion into the blood can be estimated by measuring a metabolite of estradiol in urine, estrone-3-glucuronide (24).

Some toxicants alter hepatic metabolism of sex steroid hormones and may affect the concentration of steroid hormone metabolites in urine. Lead, for example, reduces the amount of sulphated steroids excreted into the urine (25).

Serial blood sampling is obviously impractical for population-based studies. In these cases, a single blood sample can be used to estimate LH, FSH, testosterone, and prolactin levels. Blood levels for both gonadotropins become elevated during sleep as the male enters puberty, while testosterone levels maintain this diurnal pattern through adulthood in men (26). Thus, biological samples should be collected at approximately the same time of day to avoid variations due to diurnal secretory patterns.

## Examples of Toxicant Effects

Lead is a classic example of a toxicant that affects the neuroendocrine system. In one study, occupational exposure of males to lead for 1–5 yr reduced serum levels of free and total testosterone and elevated SHBG and LH concentrations in the circulation (27). These results are consistent with the notion that lead acts at the testis to reduce testosterone production, leading to increased production of SHBG (28) and LH. Lesser exposures to lead affected sperm count in the absence of detectable hormonal disturbances (29).

Male workers involved in the manufacture of DBCP had elevated serum levels of LH and FSH and reduced sperm count and fertility. Apparently, these effects are sequelae to DBCP actions upon the Leydig cells, resulting in altered androgen production or action (30).

Compounds may also exert toxicity by virtue of structural similarity to reproductive steroid hormones (30). By binding to the respective endocrine receptor, toxicants may act as hormonal agonists or antagonists to disrupt biological responses. For example, dichlorodiphenyltrichloroethane (DDT) and its meta-bolites exhibit steroidal properties and may alter male reproductive function by interfering with steroidal hormone functions. Xenobiotics such as polychlorinated biphenyls (PCBs), polybrominated biphenyls, and organochlorine pesticides may also interfere with male reproductive function by exerting estrogenic agonist/antagonist activity (30).

## SPERM PRODUCTION, MATURATION, AND TRANSPORT

Spermatogenesis and spermiogenesis are the cytological processes that result in the formation of mature spermatozoa from stem cells. As shown in Figure 1.2, these processes take place in the seminiferous tubules of the sexually mature male. Sperm motility and fertilizing capacity are acquired during transit through the epididymis and vas deferens. A brief overview of sperm production and post-testicular events is presented in this section; extensive reviews can be found elsewhere (31–33).

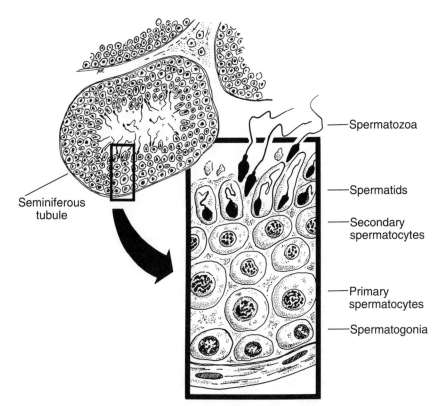

**Figure 1.2.** Spermatogenesis and spermiogenesis occur within the seminiferous epithelium of the testes.

Seminiferous tubule

Spermatozoa

Spermatids

Secondary spermatocytes

Primary spermatocytes

Spermatogonia

## Spermatogenesis and Spermiogenesis

Unlike the female who receives a fixed endowment of germ cells prenatally, males produce millions of sperm daily in a cyclical, constantly renewing process of cell division. Three major elements comprise sperm cell production: (*a*) mitotic proliferation; (*b*) meiotic division; and (*c*) morphological transformation. In humans, the total duration of spermatogenesis is approximately 74 days (Fig. 1.3).

The seminiferous tubules in the human are 30–70 cm long and 150–300 μm in diameter (34). The basic germ (stem) cells for spermatogenesis are the spermatogonia, which are positioned along the basement membrane of the seminiferous tubules. Spermatogonia are classified as Types A and B. Subclassifications of Type A spermatogonia include Type Ad (dark stain), Type Ap (pale stain), Type Ac (cloudy stain, intermediate to Ad and Ap), and Type Al (elongated shape) (35).

Paniagua et al. (35) have described the function of each subclass of Type A spermatogonia. Type Ad spermatogonia serve as the immediate precursors and divide mitotically to yield Type Al cells. Mitotic division of Type Al cells gives rise to both Type Ad and Type Ap cells. The production of the Ad spermatogonia serves to replenish the supply of precursors, while Type Ap spermatogonia undergo another mitotic division to produce Type Ac spermatogonia. Successive mitotic divisions transform the Type Ac spermatogonia to Type B spermatogonia and then to primary spermatocytes. At this point, the spermatocyte is classified as a resting (preleptotene) spermatocyte.

This series of mitotic divisions increases the number of cells entering meiosis. The resting primary spermatocytes migrate through tight junctions formed by the Sertoli cells to the luminal side of this testis barrier. At this point, DNA synthesis is complete except, possibly, for DNA repair in late zygotene or early pachytene stages of meiosis (36).

Meiosis commences once the primary spermatocytes encounter the lumen of the seminiferous tubule. The primary spermatocytes are activated from the preleptotene stage and differentiate sequentially into leptotene, zygotene, pachytene, and diplotene spermatocytes. During the leptotene stage, the chromatin condenses and becomes filamentous; the homologous chromosomes then move together during the zygotene stage. During the pachytene stage, the chromosome pairs shorten and condense further, the nuclear and cytoplasmic volumes increase, and RNA synthesis accelerates. Chromosomal autosomes may "cross over" during the pachytene stage. The diplotene stage is characterized by continued condensation of the chromosomes and separation of the chromosomal pairs. The nuclear membrane breaks down, and microtubular spindles attach to the chromosomal pairs, causing them to separate. At this point, the first meiotic division is complete and two pseudodiploid secondary

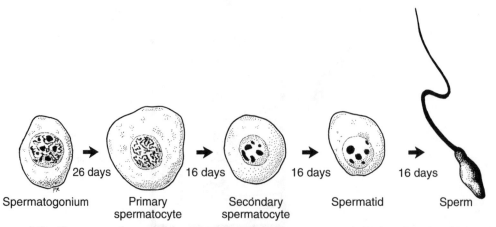

| Spermatogonium | Primary spermatocyte | Secondary spermatocyte | Spermatid | Sperm |

26 days → 16 days → 16 days → 16 days

**Figure 1.3.** The process of spermatogenesis in humans requires approximately 74 days. Data based on Heller CG, Clermont Y. Kinetics of the germinal epithelium in man. Rec Prog Horm Res 1964;20:545–575.

spermatocytes are formed. The secondary spermatocytes undergo the second meiotic division to yield equal numbers of spermatids bearing X- and Y-chromosomes.

Spermiogenesis consists of the ensuing morphological transformation of spermatids to spermatozoa. The DNA and nuclear proteins condense, forming a tight complex that then migrates toward the cell membrane. The golgi form lysosomal granules that coalesce into a proacrosomal granule. This granule also migrates, becomes interposed between the nucleus and the cell membrane, and flattens to form the acrosome. Centrioles move to the "caudal" side of the nucleus to form the axoneme, the axial filament complex that will become the sperm tail. Mitochondria migrate to the anterior portion of this filamentous element to form the midpiece region. The cytoplasm is sequestered into a droplet that forms at the neck of the sperm and moves down the newly formed tail. This process removes the remaining cellular components from the spermatid.

When spermiogenesis is complete, the sperm cell is released by the Sertoli cell into the seminiferous tubule lumen by a process referred to as spermiation. These sperm migrate along the tubule to the rete testis and into the head of the epididymis.

## Post-testicular Events

When the sperm leave the seminiferous tubules, they are immature, incapable of fertilization, and unable to swim. The environments and changes the sperm cells undergo until leaving the urethra are described below.

### EPIDIDYMIS

Spermatozoa released into the lumen of the seminiferous tubule are suspended in fluid produced primarily by the Sertoli cells. Sperm are concentrated within this fluid and flow continuously from the seminiferous tubules, through the ionic milieu within the rete testis, through the vasa efferentia, and into the epididymis (Fig. 1.4). The epididymis is a single, highly coiled tube (5–6 m long) in which sperm spend 12–21 days.

Within the epididymis, the nature of the suspension fluid changes, and sperm acquire progressive motility and fertilizing capacity. The epididymis absorbs components from the fluid (including ABP and other secretions from the Sertoli cells), thereby concentrating the

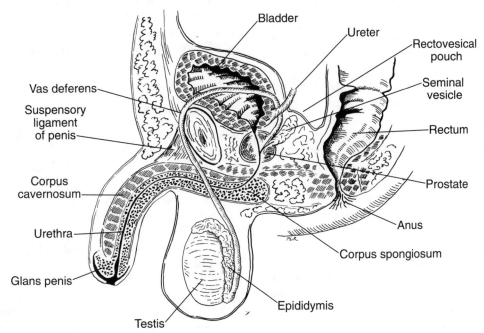

**Figure 1.4.** The male reproductive organs: lateral view.

spermatozoa. The epididymis also contributes secretions to the suspension fluid, including glycerylphosphorylcholine (GPC) and carnitine. Sperm morphology continues to transform in the epididymis. The cytoplasmic droplet is shed, and the sperm nucleus further condenses.

## VAS DEFERENS AND AMPULLA

The vas deferens is approximately 45 cm long and connects the tail of the epididymis with the urethra (Fig 1.4). At the fundus of the bladder, the vas deferens enlarges and forms the ampulla. The vas deferens plays a minor role in secreting seminal plasma fluids. While the epididymis is the principal storage reservoir for sperm until ejaculation, about 30% of the sperm in an ejaculate comes from the vas deferens. Frequent ejaculation accelerates passage of sperm through the epididymis and may increase the number of immature (infertile) sperm in the ejaculate (35).

## ACCESSORY SEX GLANDS

Once within the vas deferens, the sperm are transported by the muscular contractions of ejaculation rather than flow of fluid. During ejaculation, fluids are forcibly expelled from the accessory sex glands, giving rise to the seminal plasma. Seminal plasma is not essential for fertilization. Thus, the artificial insemination of sperm collected from the epididymides results in conception. On the other hand, seminal plasma contributes importantly to the normal coitus-fertilization scenario. Seminal plasma serves as a vehicle for sperm transport, a buffer from the hostile acidic vaginal environment, and an initial energy source for the sperm. Cervical mucus prevents passage of seminal plasma into the uterus. Some constituents of seminal plasma, however, are carried to the site of fertilization by adhering to the sperm membrane.

The accessory glands do not expel their secretions at the same time. Rather, the bulbourethral (Cowper's) glands first extrude a clear fluid, followed by the prostatic secretions, the sperm-concentrated fluids from the epididymides and ampulla of the vas deferens, and

finally, the largest fraction comes primarily from the seminal vesicles. Thus, seminal plasma is not a homogeneous fluid.

## Bulbourethral Glands

The bulbourethral glands are paired and are round and lobular in shape. These glands secrete about 0.1 ml of fluid rich in mucoproteins that lubricate the distal urethra.

## Prostate Gland

The prostate gland is comprised of two lateral lobes and one median lobe. It is a structural extension of the urinary bladder and consists of smooth muscle encapsulating fibrous glandular tissue. Prostatic fluid is clear, has a pH of about 6.5, and contributes 0.5 ml to the average ejaculate. Prostatic fluid contains high concentrations of citric acid, acid phosphatase, calcium, zinc, spermine, amylase, and inositol.

## Seminal Vesicles

The seminal vesicles are two distinct lobular pouches that are 5–10 cm long. The seminal vesicles contribute approximately 2.5 ml to the average ejaculate. The pH of this fluid ranges from neutrality to slightly alkaline. The vesicular fluid contains high concentrations of potassium, phosphorylcholine, fructose, prostaglandins, substrates for coagulation, and most of the proteins within the seminal plasma.

## Assessment Methods

### SEMEN ANALYSIS

Semen analysis is the most common method used to determine the effects of a toxicant on sperm production. The various indices that are routinely measured in the assessment of occupational exposure are presented in Table 1.1. Sperm count and sperm morphology provide indices of the integrity of spermatogenesis and spermiogenesis. Thus, the number of sperm in the ejaculate is directly correlated with the number of germ cells per gram of testis (37), while abnormal morphology is probably the result of defective spermiogenesis. Alterations in sperm motility or viability suggest post-testicular effects.

**Table 1.1.**
**Semen Profile for Assessing Reproductive Toxicant Effects**

Sperm concentration
Sperm viability
  Vital stain
  Hypo-osmotic swelling
Sperm motility
  Percent motile
  Curvilinear velocity
  Straight-line velocity
  Linearity
  Lateral head amplitude
  Beat cross frequency
Sperm size and shape
  Morphology
  Morphometry
Semen parameters
  pH
  Volume
  Marker chemicals from glands
  Toxicant or metabolite concentrations

## Methodological Considerations

The semen sample is collected by masturbation after a set time of abstinence (usually 2 days) and delivered to the laboratory within 1 hr of ejaculation. In the clinical setting, semen samples can often be collected at the health care facility. The various fractions of semen can be collected by a technique known as split ejaculate (38). This procedure exploits the fact that distinct, sequential muscular contractions are responsible for ejaculation of the various semen fractions. If sperm fractions are to be studied, clinicians ask that two fractions be collected. The first fraction contains the majority of the sperm and the sperm with highest motility, while the second consists of secretions from the seminal vesicles.

The initial evaluation of the specimen is conducted when the sample arrives at the laboratory and consists of recording the temperature, turbidity, color, liquefaction time, volume, osmolality, and pH of the semen. Video recordings are useful for motility assessments and sperm counts.

Sperm concentration and motility characteristics should be measured in a chamber at least 10 μm deep for the sperm to move freely in all planes.

Measurements of sperm motility and velocity are conducted using a microscope stage warmed to 37°C. An attempt to record 100 motile sperm per sample is desirable if one is interested in the distribution of velocity measurements, but 50 motile sperm will suffice if means are to be compared. If the videotapes are being used to calculate the percent motility, one should avoid "hunting" for motile sperm. All fields examined or searched should be included in the calculations. Therefore, recording a certain number of arbitrary fields is advised. If a computer-assisted sperm analysis (CASA) system is employed for motility and velocity estimates, the number of sperm per field must be reduced with iso-osmotic buffer to minimize cell collisions.

Sperm morphology should be estimated on air-dried, stained semen smears. Variations in sperm size and shape are not distinct, but rather represent a continuum. This presents a challenge within, and especially among, laboratories to establish a repeatable system for morphological classification. With recent advances in computerized image analyses, several methods of sperm morphometry have been introduced (39–42). These morphometric analysis systems provide objective assessments of individual sperm head size and shape. Comparisons of measurements between different analysis systems should be avoided. Sperm morphometry is now routinely used as part of the assessment of reproductive hazards to the male worker (43).

Sperm viability can be determined by two methods: eosin Y stain exclusion (44) and hypo-osmotic swelling (HOS assay)(45). These techniques test for the structural and functional integrity of the cell membrane, respectively (46).

Biochemical analysis of seminal plasma provides insights into the function of the accessory sex glands. Specific chemicals serve as markers for each gland. For example, the epididymis is represented by GPC, the seminal vesicles by fructose, and the prostate gland by zinc. This type of analysis provides only gross information on glandular function and little or no information on other secretory constituents. Measuring semen pH and osmolality provide additional general information on the nature of seminal plasma.

Seminal plasma can also be analyzed for the presence of a toxicant or its metabolites. Heavy metals have been detected in seminal plasma using atomic absorption spectrophotometry (47), while halogenated hydrocarbons have been measured in seminal fluid by gas chromatography after extraction (48) or protein-limiting filtration.

## Interpretation of Semen Analysis

The proper interpretation of a semen analysis is critical. It is important not to overemphasize the normal/abnormal ranges, overinterpret a single semen analysis, or unduly weigh the importance of one variable over another. Fertility assessment is further complicated by the many variables that determine the reproductive status of the prospective mate.

The historical data in the literature can be confusing. Studies may report sperm counts in terms of "normal" means and ranges, "fertile" means and ranges, or control population mean and range. Generally, reports from proven fertile men indicate an average sperm count of approximately 100 million, while studies of populations not selected for fertility status report lower means of approximately 50–80 million. Each laboratory must establish its own "normal" or "fertile" range for comparison. Some basic guidelines have been published by the World Health Organization (49).

It is generally believed that there is a fecundity curve for each semen characteristic, rather than a magical threshold below which conception does not occur (Fig. 1.5). For example, while oligospermia is commonly defined as a sperm count below 20 million/ml, successful conception can occur at lower counts. At the same time, at values below 20 million/ml, the probability of conception decreases steadily with reductions in sperm count (50). For some men, even a modest toxicant-induced reduction in sperm count could bring them into the oligospermic range, thereby decreasing the likelihood of successful impregnation.

Another issue in conducting semen analysis is the reliability of a single semen sample for representing an individual's true semen quality. Data from a recent study of unexposed workers lend insight into this issue (51). In this study, sperm count had a high within-subject

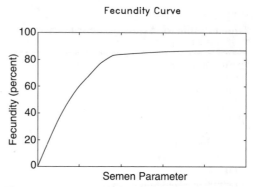

**Figure 1.5.** This fecundity curve illustrates the relationship between changes in a sperm parameter such as sperm count and male fecundity (a measure of the ability of the male to fertilize a female). This model suggests that decreased male fecundity may be a nonthreshold phenomenon, i.e., as the sperm parameter decreases, the chance of successful conception decreases.

coefficient of variation, i.e., a single sample sperm count was not very representative of the true mean concentration based on multiple samples over time. However, intraclass correlation was high, indicating that men with high counts generally tended to stay high and vice versa. The percentage of motile sperm also had poor precision, and its repeatability was poorer than that for sperm count. The percentage of sperm with normal morphology was both precise and quite stable over time.

Various semen parameters measure different aspects of the reproductive potential. No single variable is a measure of fecundity. Thus, a semen sample with 100 million sperm with 10% motility is probably no better than a semen sample with 10 million sperm with 100% motility.

## PROMISING NEW METHODS

Promising new methods are being evaluated for assessing the effects of toxicants on the male reproductive system. The sperm penetration assay (SPA), also known as the zona free hamster egg penetration assay, provides information on sperm function. To perform this assay, sperm are capacitated and then incubated with hamster eggs with the zona pellucida removed. The frequency of sperm penetration is then calculated. This procedure has been used in the clinical setting and is quite routine in several laboratories (52).

The DNA stability assay may provide information regarding genetic damage to sperm. To perform the assay, the sperm DNA is stressed thermally or chemically and then stained with acridine orange. Double-stranded DNA stains green, while single-stranded DNA stains red. Animals exposed to known mutagens have an increase in single-stranded DNA (53, 54), indicating an increase in genetic damage. The fertility rate of bulls is correlated with the percentage of double-stranded DNA (55). A recent report indicates that the DNA stability assay is highly repeatable between ejaculates from the same man (56). At present, this procedure has been developed in only a few laboratories. Methods to evaluate DNA adducts and DNA probes are on the horizon. DNA adducts, the complex formed between a toxicant or its metabolites and the sperm nucleotide, may be carried in the sperm chromatin to the site of fertilization. New methods for labeling nucleotides may permit the detection of these adducts in ejaculated sperm. DNA probes are monoclonal antibodies to distinct modifications of the DNA molecule (57) and may allow for the detection of subtle changes in the DNA code.

## Toxicant Effects

Toxicants can disrupt spermatogenesis at several points. The stage(s) of spermatogenesis targeted by a toxicant determines both the time required for clinical expression of the injury and the prospects for recovery. Due to irreversibility, the most damaging toxicants are those that kill or genetically alter (beyond repair mechanisms) Type A spermatogonia or Sertoli cells.

Animal studies have been useful to determine the stage at which a toxicant attacks the spermatogenic process. Sampling occurs after short-term exposure to a toxicant. By knowing the duration required for each spermatogenic stage, one can extrapolate to estimate the affected stage. For example, exposure of male rats to 2-methoxyethanol resulted in reduced fertility after 4 weeks (58). This evidence, corroborated by histological examination, indicates that the target of toxicity is the spermatocyte (59). Semen analyses of serial ejaculates of men inadvertently exposed to potential toxicants for a short time may provide similar useful information.

Exposure to DBCP reduced sperm concentration in human ejaculates from a median of 79 million cells/ml in unexposed men to 46 million cells/ml in exposed workers (60). Long after removal from exposure, workers with reduced sperm counts experienced partial recovery, while men who had been azoospermic remained sterile (61). Testicular biopsy revealed that the target of DBCP was the spermatogonia, substantiating the severity of the effect seen with stem cell injury.

Genetic damage is difficult to detect in human sperm. Laboratory animal studies using the dominant lethal assay (62) indicate that paternal exposure can produce early pregnancy loss. In humans, an association between paternal occupational exposures and spontaneous abortion has been suggested for agents such as anesthetic gases, organic solvents, and metallurgic factory exposures (63, 64). While human data are still limited, such findings indicate a need for methods to detect genetic damage in human sperm. The issue of paternally mediated developmental effects is further discussed in Chapter 5.

A toxicant or its metabolite may act directly on accessory sex glands to alter the quality or quantity of their secretions. Alternatively, the toxicant may enter the seminal plasma (65) and affect the sperm, be absorbed through the vaginal mucosa after intercourse, or be carried to the site of fertilization on the sperm membrane and affect the ova or conceptus.

Ethylene dibromide (EDB) is one example of a toxicant that exerts post-testicular effects. Short-term exposure to the toxicant reduced sperm velocity and semen volume (66). Chronic exposure decreased sperm motility and viability, decreased seminal fructose levels, and increased semen pH (66). An EDB metabolite was present within the semen of some exposed workers (48). Other potential toxicants that have been detected in semen include lead, cadmium, hexachlorobenzene, hexachlorocyclohexane, dieldrin, and PCBs (47).

## SEXUAL FUNCTION

Human sexual function refers to the integrated activities of the testes and secondary sex glands, the endocrine control systems, and the CNS-based behavioral and psychological components of reproduction. A brief overview follows. If more detail is desired, several reviews are available (67–69).

Erection, ejaculation, and orgasm are three distinct, independent physiological and psychodynamic events that normally occur concurrently in men.

## Erection

Erection results from the engorgement of blood within the corpora cavernosa of the penis. Parasympathetic stimulation induces dilation of the penile arterioles and closure of the venous valves to cause accumulation of blood within the cavernosa. Two independent mechanisms may induce erection. A sacral reflex arc triggers erections induced by tactile stimulation of the genitalia. Nontactile, erotic stimuli stimulate several regions of the brain including the thalamic nuclei, the rhinencephalon, and the limbic structures. These neural signals are mediated by the autonomic nervous system (69).

Impotence, the failure to achieve and/or maintain an erection, may have either a psychogenic or organic etiology. Organic impotence is characterized by reduced ability to achieve an erection at any time, whether awake or asleep. In most cases, psychologically impotent men can experience spontaneous erections during rapid eye movement (REM) sleep (69). To differentiate between the two etiologies, devices can be worn on the penis to detect changes associated with nocturnal erections including penile circumference, pulsatile blood flow, volume, or axial rigidity (the resistance of the penis to buckling when a known weight is applied to the glans penis).

Priapism is a condition in which an erection occurs without sexual arousal and without resolution after ejaculation. This condition appears to reflect an autonomic nervous system imbalance resulting in inappropriate arteriole dilation without subsequent venous drainage.

## Ejaculation and Orgasm

Ejaculation involves emission of seminal components into the urethra and the pulsatile ejec-

tion of the semen from the urethra. The sensation that typically accompanies ejaculation is orgasm. Emission of seminal components from the seminal vesicles, prostate gland, and vas deferens into the prostatic urethra is controlled by reflex activity from the thoracolumbar sympathetic neural network. Parasympathetic innervation controls the pulsatile contractions of bulbocavernosus and ischiocavernosus muscles that orchestrate to eject the semen rhythmically from the urethra. Contraction of muscles generates afferent signals that are transmitted to the cerebral cortex, generally eliciting the sensory experience of orgasm (67). Thus, emission of seminal components to the urethra can be blocked with α-adrenoceptive antagonists without blocking the sensations of ejection and orgasm, even though there will be little or no semen ejaculated.

## Libido

Loss of interest in sexual activity may also be of either psychogenic or organic origin. Most organic causes are associated with endocrine imbalances of testosterone and/or prolactin.

## Assessment Methods

Assessment of occupationally induced sexual dysfunction is difficult, inasmuch as it usually relies on the testimony of the worker. This testimony may be confounded by the bias of the individual to guard his masculine image or to attribute a pre-existing libido problem to exposures at work.

Burris et al. (70) recently reported application of a monitor for assessing erection at home. This method may provide a convenient means by which to evaluate erectile function of exposed workers.

Assessment of ejaculate volume can provide information on the integrity of the emission phase of ejaculation. This measurement also reflects the secretory capacities of the accessory sex glands. Thus, a semen sample of reduced volume, but with a normal ratio of marker chemicals, supports a diagnosis of an emission phase defect.

## Toxicant Effects

Few reliable data are available on toxicant-induced effects on sexual function. Drugs have been shown to affect each of the three stages of male sexual function (71), indicating the potential for occupational exposures to exert similar effects. Antidepressants, testosterone antagonists, and stimulants of prolactin reduce libido in men. Antihypertensive drugs that act on the sympathetic nervous system induce impotence in some men, but paradoxically, priapism in others. Phenoxybenzamine, an α-adrenoceptive antagonist, has been used clinically to block seminal emission, but not orgasm (72). Anticholinergic effects of some antidepressant drugs permit seminal emission, while blocking seminal ejection and orgasm.

Recreational drugs also affect sexual function (71). Ethanol can reduce impotence while enhancing libido. Cocaine, heroin, and high doses of cannabinoids reduce libido. Opiates also delay or impair ejaculation.

## SUMMARY

Toxicants can attack the male reproductive system at several sites. As summarized in Table 1.2, an arsenal of laboratory assessment procedures is available for detecting the effects of toxicants at many of these sites. While most of the methodologies were originally developed and validated for the clinical assessment of infertility, they have also proven useful in the evaluation of cohorts of exposed men in population-based studies.

## REFERENCES

1. Sherman IW, Sherman VG. Biology: a human approach. New York: Oxford University Press, 1979:153–154.
2. Whorton D, Krauss RM, Marshall S, Milby TH. Infertility in male pesticide workers. Lancet 1977;2:1259–1260.
3. Torkelson TR, Sadek SE, Rowe VK. Toxicologic investigations of 1,2-dibromo-3-chloropropane. Toxicol Appl Pharmacol 1961;3:545–559.
4. Fink G. Gonadotropin secretion and its control. In: Knobil E, Neill JD, eds. The physiology of reproduction. New York: Raven Press Ltd, 1988:1349–1377.
5. Matsumoto AM. Hormonal control of human spermatogenesis. In: Burger H, deKretser D, eds. The testis. 2nd ed. New York: Raven Press Ltd, 1989:181–196.
6. Bardin CW. Pituitary-testicular axis. In: Yen SSC, Jaffe RB, eds. Reproductive endocrinology. Philadelphia: WB Saunders Co., 1986:177–199.
7. Culler MD, Negro-Vilar A. Evidence that pulsatile follicle-stimulating hormone secretion is independent of endogenous luteinizing hormone-releasing hormone. Endocrinology 1986;118:609–612.
8. Longcope C, Sato K, McKay C, Horton R. Aromatization by splanchnic tissue in men. J Clin Endocrinol Metab 1984;58:1089–1093.
9. Sharpe RM. Follicle-stimulating hormone and spermatogenesis in the adult male. J Endocrinol 1989;121:405–407.
10. Kotsugi F, Winters SJ, Keeping HS, Attardi B, Oshima H, Troen P. Effects of inhibin from primate Sertoli cells on follicle-stimulating hormone and luteinizing hormone release by perifused rat pituitary cells. Endocrinology 1988;122:2796–2802.
11. McLachlan RL, Matsumoto AM, Burger HG, de Kretser DM, Bremner WJ. Relative roles of follicle-stimulating hormone and luteinizing hormone in the control of inhibin secretion in normal men. J Clin Invest 1988;82:880–884.

**Table 1.2.**
**Assessment of Reproductive Function**[a]

| Assessment Method | Endocrine System | Testes | Post-testicular | Sexual Function |
|---|---|---|---|---|
| FSH | X | | | |
| LH | X | | | |
| Testosterone | X | | | |
| Prolactin | X | | | |
| Sperm count | | X | | |
| Sperm morphology and morphometry | | X | | |
| Sperm viability: Vital stain and HOS | | | X | |
| Sperm motility: % motile and velocity | | ? | X | |
| Semen biochemistry | | | X | |
| Semen pH | | | X | |
| Sperm penetration assay | | X | X | |
| Nocturnal penile measurements | | | | X |
| Personal history | | | | X |

a FSH = follicle-stimulating hormone; LH = luteinizing hormone; HOS = hypo-osmotic swelling assay.

12. Winters SJ. Inhibin is released together with testosterone by the human testis. J Clin Endocrinol Metabol 1990;70:548–550.

13. Baker HWG, Worgul TJ, Santen RJ, Jefferson LS, Bardin CW. Effect of prolactin on nuclear androgens in perifused male accessory sex organs. In: Troen P, Nankin H, eds. The testis in normal and infertile men. New York: Raven Press Ltd, 1977:379–385.

14. Segal S, Yaffe H, Laufer N, Ben-David M. Male hyperprolactinemia: effects on fertility. Fertil Steril 1979;32:556–561.

15. Thorner MO, Edwards CRW, Hanker JP, Abraham G, Besser GM. Prolactin and gonadotropin interaction in the male. In: Troen P, Nankin H, eds. The testis in normal and infertile men. New York: Raven Press Ltd, 1977:351–366.

16. Sokol RZ. Endocrine evaluations in the assessment of male reproductive hazards. Repro Toxicol 1988;2:217–222.

17. Sassin JF, Frantz AG, Weitzman ED, Kapen S. Human prolactin: 24-hour pattern with increased release during sleep. Science 1972;177:1205–1207.

18. Ishizuka B, Quigley ME, Yen SSC. Pituitary hormone release in response to food ingestion: evidence for neuroendocrine signals from gut to brain. J Clin Endocrinol Metab 1983;57:1111–1116.

19. Frantz AG, Kleinberg DL, Noel GL. Studies on prolactin in man. Rec Prog Horm Res 1972;28:527–590.

20. Danzo BJ, Bell BW, Black JH. Human testosterone-binding globulin is a dimer composed of two identical protomers that are differentially glycosylated. Endocrinology 1989;124:2809–2817.

21. Raid-Fahmy D, Read GF, Walker RF, Griffiths K. Steroids in saliva for assessing endocrine function. Endocrinol Rev 1982;3:367–395.

22. Winters SJ, Troen P. Testosterone and estradiol are co-secreted episodically by the human testis. J Clin Invest 1986;78:870–873.

23. Lipsett MB. Steroid hormones. In: Yen SSC, Jaffe RB, eds. Reproductive endocrinology. Philadelphia: WB Saunders Co, 1986:140–153.

24. Wright K, Collins DC, Musey PI, Preedy JKR. Direct radioimmunoassay of specific urinary estrogen glucosiduronates in normal men and non-pregnant women. Steroids 1978;31:407–426.

25. Apostoli P, Romeo L, Peroni E, et al. Steroid hormone sulphation in lead workers. Br J Ind Med 1989;46:204–208.

26. Plant TM. Puberty in primates. In: Knobil E, Neill JD, eds. The physiology of reproduction. New York: Raven Press Ltd, 1988:1763–1788.

27. Rodamilans M, Osaba MJ Mtz, To-Figueras J, et al. Lead toxicity on endocrine testicular function in an occupationally exposed population. Hum Toxicol 1988;7:125–128.

28. Plymate SR, Leonard JM, Paulsen CA, Fariss BL, Karpas AE. Sex hormone-binding globulin changes with androgen replacement. J Clin Endocrinol Metab 1983;57:645–648.

29. Assennato G, Paci C, Baser ME, et al. Sperm count suppression without endocrine dysfunction in lead-exposed men. Arch Environ Health 1986;41:387–390.

30. Mattison DR, Plowchalk DR, Meadows MJ, Al-Juburi AZ, Gandy J, Malek A. Reproductive toxicity: male and female reproductive systems as targets for chemical injury. Med Clin North Am 1990;74:391–411.

31. Setchell BP, Pilsworth LM. The functions of the testes of vertebrate and invertebrate animals. In: Burger H, de Kretser D, eds. The testis. 2nd ed. New York: Raven Press Ltd, 1989:1–66.

32. de Kretser DM, Kerr JB. The cytology of the testis. In: Knobil E, Neill JD, eds. The physiology of reproduction. New York: Raven Press Ltd, 1988:837–932.

33. Waller DP, Nikurs AR. Review of the physiology and biochemistry of the male reproductive tract. J Am Coll Toxicol 1986;5:209–223.

34. Zaneveld LJD. The biology of human spermatozoa. Obstet Gynecol Ann 1978;7:15–40.

35. Paniagua R, Codesal J, Nistal M, Rodriguez MC, Santamaria L. Quantification of cell types throughout the cycle of the human seminiferous epithelium and their DNA content. Anat Embryol 1987;176:225–230.

36. Johnson MH, Everitt BJ. Essential reproduction. 3rd ed. Oxford: Blackwell Scientific Publications, 1980.

37. Zukerman Z, Rodriguez-Rigau LJ, Weiss DB, Chowdhury AK, Smith KD, Steinberger E. Quantitative analysis of the seminiferous epithelium in human testicular biopsies, and the relation of spermatogenesis to sperm density. Fertil Steril 1978;30:448–455.

38. Marmar JI, Praiss DE, Debenedictis TJ. Statistical comparisons of the parameters of semen analysis of whole semen verses the fractions of the split ejaculate. Fertil Steril 1978;39:439–443.

39. Katz DF, Overstreet JW, Pelprey RJ. Integrated assessment of the motility, morphology, and morphometry of human spermatozoa. INSERM 1981;103:97–100.

40. Schrader SM, Turner TW, Hardin BD, Niemeier RW, Burg JR. Morphometric analysis of human spermatozoa. J Androl 1984;5:22.

41. Jagoe RJ, Washbrook NP, Hudson EA. Morphometry of spermatozoa using semiautomatic image analysis. J Clin Pathol 1986;39:1347–1352.

42. Moruzzi JF, Wyrobek AJ, Mayall BH, Gledhill BL. Quantification and classification of human sperm morphology by computer assisted image analysis. Fertil Steril 1988;50:142–152.

43. Schrader SM, Ratcliffe JM, Turner TW, Hornung RW. The use of new field methods of semen analysis in the study of occupational hazards to reproduction: the example of ethylene dibromide. J Occup Med 1987;29:963–966.

44. Eliasson R, Treichl L. Supravital staining of human spermatozoa. Fertil Steril 1971;22:134–137.

45. Jeyendran RS, Van den Ven HH, Perez-Pelaez M, Crabo BG, Zaneveld LJD. Development of an assay to assess the functional integrity of the human sperm membrane and its relationship to other semen characteristics. J Reprod Fertil 1984;70:219–228.

46. Schrader SM, Platek SM, Zaneveld LJD, Perez-Pelaez M, Jeyendran RS. Sperm viability: a comparison of analytical methods. Andrologia 1986;18:530–538.

47. Stachel B, Dougherty RC, Lahl U, Schlosser M, Zeschmar B. Toxic environmental chemicals in human semen: analytical method and case studies. Andrologia 1989;21:282–291.

48. Zikarge A. Cross-sectional study of ethylene dibromide-induced alterations of seminal plasma biochemistry as a function of post-testicular toxicity with relationships to some indices of semen analysis and endocrine profile [Dissertation]. Houston: University of Texas Health Science Center, 1986.

49. Belsey MA, Moghissi KS, Eliasson A, Paulsen CA, Gallegos AJ, Prasal MRN. Laboratory manual for the examination of human semen and semen cervical mucus interaction. Singapore: Press Concern, 1980.

50. Meistrich ML, Brown CC. Estimation of the increased risk of human infertility from alterations in semen characteristics. Fertil Steril 1983;40:220–230.

51. Schrader SM, Turner TW, Breitenstein MJ, Simon SD. Longitudinal study of semen quality of unexposed workers. Reprod Toxicol 1988;2:183–190.

52. Rogers BJ. Use of SPA in assessing toxic effects on male fertilizing potential. Reprod Toxicol 1988;2:233–240.

53. Evenson DP, Baer RK, Jost LK, Gesch RW. Toxicity of thiotepa on mouse spermatogenesis as determined by dual-parameter flow cytometry. Toxicol Appl Pharmacol 1986;82:151–163.

54. Evenson DP, Janca FC, Jost LK, Baer RK, Karabinus DS. Flow cytometric analysis of effects of 1,3-dinitrobenzene. J Toxicol Environ Health 1989;28:81–98.

55. Ballachey BE, Hohenboken WD, Evenson DP. Heterogeneity of sperm nuclear chromatin structure and its relationship to bull fertility. Biol Reprod 1987;36:915–925.

56. Evenson DP, Jost L, Baer R, Turner T, Schrader S. Longitudinal study of semen quality of unexposed workers: individuality of DNA denaturation patterns in human sperm. Reprod Toxicol 1991;5:115–125.

57. Hecht NB. Detecting the effects of toxic agents on spermatogenesis using DNA probes. Environ Health Prospect 1987;74:31–40.

58. Chapin RE, Dutton SL, Ross MD, Lamb JC IV. Effects of ethylene glycol monomethyl ether (EGME) on mating performance and epididymal sperm parameters in F344 rats. Fundam Appl Toxicol 1985;5:182–189.

59. Chapin RE, Dutton SL, Ross MD, Sumrell BM, Lamb JC IV. The effects of ethylene glycol monomethyl ether on testicular histology of F344 rats. J Androl 1984;5:369–380.

60. Whorton D, Milby TH, Krauss RM, Stubbs HA. Testicular function in DBCP exposed pesticide workers. J Occup Med 1979;21:161–166.

61. Eaton M, Schenker M, Wharton D, Sanurels S, Perkins C, Overstreet J. Seven year follow-up of workers exposed to 1,2-dibromo-3-chloropropane. J Occup Med 1986;28:1145–1150.

62. Ehling UH, Machemer L, Buselmaier W, et al. Standard protocol for the dominant lethal test on male mice. Arch Toxicol 1978;39:173–185.

63. Schrag S, Dixon R. Occupational exposures associated with male reproductive function. Ann Rev Pharmacol Toxicol 1985;25:567–592.

64. Taskinen H, Anttila A, Lindbohm M-L, Sallmen M, Hemminki K. Spontaneous abortions and congenital malformations among the wives of men occupationally exposed to organic solvents. Scand J Work Environ Health 1989;15:345–353.

65. Mann T, Lutwak-Mann C. Passage of chemicals into human and animal semen: mechanisms and significance. CRC Crit Rev Toxicol 1982;11:1–14.

66. Schrader SM, Turner TW, Ratcliffe JM. The effects of ethylene dibromide on semen quality: a comparison of short term and chronic exposure. Reprod Toxicol 1988;2:191–198.

67. deGroat WC, Booth AM. Physiology of male sexual function. Ann Intern Med 1980;92:329–331.

68. Thomas AJ Jr. Ejaculatory dysfunction. Fertil Steril 1983;39:445–454.

69. Krane RJ, Goldstein I, de Tejada IS. Impotence. N Engl J Med 1989;321:1648–1659.

70. Burris AS, Banks SM, Sherins RJ. Quantitative assessment of nocturnal penile tumescence and rigidity in normal men using a home monitor. J Androl 1989;10:492–497.

71. Fabro S. Drugs and male sexual function. Reprod Toxicol, A Medical Letter 1985;4:1–4.

72. Shilon M, Paz GF, Homonnai ZT. The use of phenoxybenzamine treatment in premature ejaculation. Fertil Steril 1984;42:659–661.

# 2

# Female Reproductive Toxicology

DAVID PLOWCHALK, M. JANE MEADOWS, DONALD R. MATTISON

Normal reproductive function in the female requires integration of the hypothalamic-pituitary-ovarian axis (HPOA) and proper functioning of each of its components. Interference at any level by a xenobiotic may ultimately impair normal ovarian processes such as oogenesis, folliculogenesis, follicle function, ovulation, luteinization, and corpus luteum function. Clinically, disruption of the HPOA may manifest as amenorrhea, menstrual irregularity, or reduced fertility. The following section briefly reviews some basic mechanisms of action of reproductive toxicants and then discusses some of the sites of chemical injury to the HPOA that will ultimately disrupt female reproductive function.

## MECHANISMS OF ACTION OF REPRODUCTIVE TOXICANTS

### Direct-acting Reproductive Toxicants

Reproductive toxicants can be classified as either direct- or indirect-acting toxicants based on their mechanism of action (1). Direct-acting reproductive toxicants elicit their effects by virtue of their inherent chemical reactivity or through structural similarity to endogenous compounds.

## CHEMICAL REACTIVITY

Compounds that fall into this category are toxic due to their inherent chemical reactivity, i.e.,

they react with and damage important cellular macromolecules or organelles, thereby disrupting processes essential for the integrity of the reproductive system (Table 2.1). For example, the inherent electrophilic reactivity of alkylating agents allows them to interact with nucleophilic sites of important cellular components (DNA, RNA, proteins/enzymes). A number of metals such as lead, mercury, and cadmium are also thought to be reproductive toxicants because of their chemical reactivity (2).

## STRUCTURAL SIMILARITY

These compounds exert their toxic effects through their similarity to biologically important molecules. They can imitate the action of endogenous molecules or are similar enough to compete for the receptors of an endogenous compound (Table 2.2). Moreover, they are capable of triggering inappropriate responses or blocking normal responses in the target cell or organ. These compounds are generally agonists or antagonists of endogenous hormones. One of the best examples of compounds that act via their structural similarity are oral contraceptives (estrogen and progestin analogs) that interfere with normal ovarian function by suppressing gonadotropin secretion. Other examples include polychlorinated biphenyls (PCBs), polybrominated biphenyls (PBBs), and organo-

**Table 2.1.**
**Direct-acting Reproductive Toxicants (Chemical Reactivity)**

| Compound | Effect | Site | Mechanism | Reference |
|---|---|---|---|---|
| Alkylating agents | Altered menses<br>Amenorrhea | Ovary | Follicle toxicity | 18 |
| Lead | Abnormal menses<br>Ovarian atrophy<br>Decreased fertility | Hypothalamus?<br>Pituitary?<br>Ovary? | Decreased FSH<br>Decreased<br>  progesterone | 19–21 |
| Mercury | Abnormal menses | Hypothalamus?<br>Ovary | Follicle toxicity<br>Granulosa cell<br>  proliferation | 2 |
| Cadmium | Follicular atresia<br>Persistent diestrus | Ovary<br>Pituitary<br>Hypothalamus | Vascular toxicity<br>Direct toxicity | 2 |

**Table 2.2.**
**Direct-acting Reproductive Toxicants (Structural Similarity)**

| Compound | Effect | Site | Mechanism | Reference |
|---|---|---|---|---|
| Oral contraceptives | Altered menses | Hypothalamus<br>Pituitary | Altered FSH, LH<br>  release | 27 |
| Azathioprine | Reduced follicle<br>  numbers | Ovary<br>Oogenesis | Purine analog | 28 |
| Halogenated<br>hydrocarbons<br>  Chlordecone<br>  DDT[a]<br>  2,4-D[b]<br>  Lindane<br>  Toxaphene<br>  Hexachlor | Sterility<br>Altered menses<br>Infertility<br>Amenorrhea<br>Hypermenorrhea | Hypothalamus?<br>Pituitary? | Estrogen agonists | 3–5 |

[a]Dichlorodiphenyltrichloroethane
[b]2,4-dichlorophenoxyacetic acid

chlorine pesticides, many of which are estrogen agonists (3–5).

## Indirect-acting Reproductive Toxicants

Indirect-acting toxicants act to alter reproductive function either after metabolic activation to an active species or by altering normal endocrine homeostasis.

### METABOLISM

In the process of removing a xenobiotic from the body, pathways that normally detoxify chemicals may generate a number of metabolites that are more reactive than the parent compound (Table 2.3). These metabolites may then interact by the mechanisms that were mentioned above for direct-acting compounds. For example, cyclophosphamide is an indirect acting toxicant, requiring metabolic activation by cytochrome P-450 monooxygenase enzymes before it can generate chemically reactive metabolites (6). Some of these metabolites are responsible for several different types of female reproductive toxicity including ovarian and uterine toxicity (7–9). Similarly, polycyclic aromatic hydrocarbons (PAH) are also dependent on microsomal enzymes for their bioactivation to highly potent metabolites capable of destroying ovarian follicles (10).

### ENDOCRINE HOMEOSTASIS

This category includes compounds that alter the pattern of release or circulating levels of steroid hormones important in reproduction by affecting steroid production, secretion, or clearance (Table 2.4). Altered circulating levels

**Table 2.3.**
**Indirect-acting Reproductive Toxicants (Metabolic Activation)**

| Compound | Effect | Site | Mechanism | Reference |
|---|---|---|---|---|
| Cytoxan | Amenorrhea<br>Premature ovarian failure | Ovary | Follicle destruction | 6–9 |
| Polycyclic aromatic hydro-carbons | Impaired fertility? | Ovary<br>Liver | Follicle destruction<br>Enzyme induction | 10, 22–25 |
| Cigarette smoke | Altered menses<br>Impaired fertility<br>Reduced age at menopause | Ovary | Follicle destruction<br>Blocked ovulation | 26 |
| DDT[a] metabolites | Altered steroid metabolism | Liver | Enzyme induction | 5 |

[a]Dichlorodiphenyltrichloroethane

**Table 2.4.**
**Indirect-acting Reproductive Toxicants (Disrupted Homeostasis)**

| Compound | Effect | Site | Mechanism | Reference |
|---|---|---|---|---|
| Halogenated hydro-carbons | | | | |
| DDT[a] | Abnormal menses | Hypothalamus?<br>Pituitary? | FSH<br>LH | 3, 5, 11 |
| PCBs, PBBs[b] | Abnormal menses | Hypothalamus?<br>Pituitary?<br>Liver | FSH<br>LH<br>Enzyme induction | 4 |
| Barbiturates | Increased steroid clearance | Liver | Enzyme induction | 12 |

[a]Dichlorodiphenyltrichloroethane
[b]Polychlorinated and polybrominated biphenyls

of steroids can disrupt the feedback loops of the HPOA that control the normal ovarian cycle. Examples of these compounds include barbiturates, PAH, PCBs, PBBs, dichloro-diphenyltrichloroethane (DDT), and other insecticides known to induce enzyme systems selectively (3–5, 11, 12).

## TARGET SITES FOR CHEMICAL INJURY IN THE FEMALE REPRODUCTIVE SYSTEM

### Hypothalamus

The hypothalamus has permissive control of the menstrual cycle through the pulsatile release of gonadotropin-releasing hormone (GnRH) at a critical frequency and concentration. The release of GnRH is an intrinsic property of the hypothalamus; however, it is modulated by both stimulatory and inhibitory actions of extrahypothalamic factors (e.g., neurotransmitters, progesterone). Once released into the hypophyseal portal system, GnRH acts at the anterior pituitary to initiate the synthesis, storage, and secretion of the gonadotropins, follicle-stimulating hormone (FSH) and luteinizing hormone (LH). Deviations in the pattern of GnRH release can seriously alter normal pituitary secretion of gonadotropins (13–15). Experimental disruption of the hypothalamus or the communication pathways to the anterior pituitary results in gonadal atrophy and amenorrhea (13–15).

A chemical might disrupt the reproductive function of the hypothalamus by altering the frequency or amplitude of GnRH pulses. The processes susceptible to chemical injury are those involved in the synthesis and secretion of GnRH, i.e., transcription or translation, packaging or axonal transport, and secretory mechanisms. Altered frequency or amplitude of the GnRH pulses could also result from disruptions in stimulatory or inhibitory pathways that regulate the release of GnRH. Catecholamines, dopamine, serotonin, GABA (γ-aminobu-tyric acid), and endorphins all have some potential for altering the release of GnRH. Therefore, xenobiotics that are agonists or antagonists of these compounds have the potential ability to modify GnRH release, thus interfering with communication with the pituitary.

## Anterior Pituitary

FSH, LH, and prolactin are three protein hormones secreted by the anterior pituitary that are essential for normal reproductive capacity. They play a critical role in maintaining the ovarian cycle, governing follicle recruitment and maturation, steroidogenesis, completion of ova maturation, ovulation, and luteinization. Precise control of the reproductive cycle is accomplished by the anterior pituitary in response to positive and negative feedback signals from the ovary. The appropriate release of FSH and LH during the cycle controls events of normal follicular development, and in their absence, amenorrhea and gonadal atrophy ensue.

The gonadotropins play a critical role in initiating changes in the morphology and steroidal microenvironments of ovarian follicles through the stimulation of steroid production and induction of receptor populations. Timely and adequate release of these gonadotropins is also essential for ovulatory events and a functional luteal phase. Toxicant-induced alterations in the synthesis, storage, or secretion of gonadotropins would seriously disrupt reproductive capacity. Steroid receptor agonists and antagonists might initiate an inappropriate release of gonadotropins from the pituitary, thereby disrupting the ovarian cycle. Xenobiotics might also interfere with normal feedback dynamics of ovarian steroids or other ovarian factors. Chemicals that alter endocrine homeostasis would induce steroid metabolizing enzymes, thus reducing steroid half-life and the circulating level of steroids at the pituitary.

## Ovary

As the basic reproductive unit of the ovary, the follicle maintains the delicate hormonal environment necessary to support the growth and maturation of an oocyte. This complex process is known as folliculogenesis and involves both intra- and extra-ovarian regulation. There are numerous morphological and biochemical changes occurring as a follicle progresses from a primordial follicle to a Graafian follicle, and each stage of follicular growth exhibits unique patterns of gonadotropin sensitivity, steroid production, and feedback pathways. These characteristics infer that a number of potential sites are available for xenobiotic interaction. Also, there are different follicle populations within the ovary that allow for differential follicle toxicity. The patterns of infertility induced by a chemical agent would be dependent upon the follicle type affected. For example, toxicity to primordial follicles would not produce immediate signs of infertility, but would ultimately lead to a shortened reproductive life span. On the other hand, toxicity to the antral or preovulatory follicles would result in an immediate loss of reproductive function.

The follicle complex is composed of three basic components: (*a*) granulosa cells, (*b*) thecal cells, and (*c*) the oocyte. Each of these components has characteristics that may make it uniquely susceptible to chemical injury.

## GRANULOSA CELLS

As a component of the follicle, and as the supporting cell for oocytes, granulosa cells have several sites of vulnerability to damage or chemical injury (Table 2.5). These sites include FSH and LH receptors and processes involved in steroid production and cell proliferation. Gonadotropin receptors are essential for the integration of hormonal signals from the central nervous system and other locations by the granulosa cells. Chemicals that are gonadotropin antagonists, damage the gonadotropin receptors, or uncouple the receptor from other molecules essential for action will clearly have an adverse effect on granulosa cell function. For example, a toxicant that is a gonadotropin antagonist and acts by blocking access to the receptor will clearly impair FSH-stimulated estrogen synthesis during the follicular phase of the cycle.

Several groups have explored methodology for screening xenobiotics for granulosa cell toxicity in vitro by measuring effects on progesterone production by porcine granulosa cells in

**Table 2.5.**
**Granulosa Cells As Targets for Chemical Injury**

| Site of Action | Mechanism of Action (Outcome) |
|---|---|
| FSH and LH receptors | Decreased receptor population |
| | Competition for receptor |
| | Uncoupling of receptor to secondary messenger |
| |    (Decreased estradiol production) |
| |    (Accumulation of androgens → atresia) |
| |    (Inadequate luteinization) |
| |    (Decreased progesterone production) |
| |    (Luteal phase defects) |
| Steroid production | Altered estrogen production |
| |   Inhibits or depresses aromatase activity |
| |     (Excessive follicular androgens → atresia) |
| |   Inadequate source of androgens |
| |     (Decreased estrogen → altered follicle growth) |
| | Altered progesterone production |
| |   Inhibition of enzymes responsible for biosynthesis of progesterone from cholesterol |
| |   Inadequate luteinization of granulosa cells |
| |     (Decreased progesterone → inhibition of FSH surge) |
| |     (Decreased progesterone → luteal phase defect) |
| Cell proliferation | General cytotoxicity |
| | Mitotic inhibitors |
| | Reduced production of growth factors |
| |   (Follicular atresia?) |

culture (16). Estradiol suppression of progesterone production by granulosa cells has been demonstrated in this system and utilized as a verification of granulosa cell responsiveness. The pesticide o,p-DDT and its p,p-DDT isomer produced dramatic suppression of progesterone production, apparently with potencies equivalent to that of estradiol. In contrast, the pesticides—malathion, parathion, and dieldrin—and the fungicide—hexachlorobenzene—were without effect. Similar studies have also explored the effect of benzo(α)pyrene (BP) and some selected metabolites on granulosa cell function. They have also demonstrated that certain metabolites produce granulosa cell toxicity, while others have no effect on granulosa cell function (17). The attractiveness of isolated systems like this is their economy and ease of use; however, since granulosa cells represent only one component of the reproductive system, lack of toxicity from a xenobiotic does not imply lack of reproductive hazard.

## THECAL CELLS

Thecal cells provide the androgenic precursors for estrogens synthesized by the granulosa cells (Table 2.6). Thecal cells are believed to be recruited from ovarian stroma cells during follicle formation and growth. Recruitment may involve stromal cell proliferation as well as migration to regions around the follicle. Clearly, xenobiotics that impair cell proliferation, migration, and communication will impact on thecal cell function. In addition, alterations in thecal cell androgen production are expected to have a significant effect on follicle function. Excess production of androgens by thecal cells may lead to follicle atresia, while impaired androgen production may lead to decreased estrogen synthesis by granulosa cells. At the present time, little is known about thecal cell vulnerability to xenobiotics.

## OOCYTES

There are data that clearly demonstrate that oocytes in both humans and experimental animals are damaged or destroyed by xenobiotics. Sites of action for chemical injury include processes integral to oocyte maturation and meiotic cell division (Table 2.7). Alkylating agents have been shown to destroy oocytes in both humans and experimental animals (18). Lead

**Table 2.6.**
**Thecal Cells As Targets for Chemical Injury**

| Site of Action | Mechanism of Action (Outcome) |
|---|---|
| LH receptors | Decreased receptor population |
| | Competition for receptor |
| | Uncoupling of receptor to secondary messenger |
| |    (Decreased androgen biosynthesis) |
| |    (Insufficient substrate for granulosa cells) |
| |    (Altered follicular growth) |
| Steroid production | Inhibition of enzymes responsible for the biosynthesis of androgens from cholesterol |
| |    (Altered androstenedione and testosterone levels) |
| |    (Insufficient substrate for granulosa cells) |
| Cell proliferation | Disrupted migration of stroma to form thecal cell layer |
| | General cytotoxicity |
| | Mitotic inhibitors |
| | Reduced production of growth factors |

**Table 2.7.**
**Oocytes As Targets for Chemical Injury**

| Site of Action | Mechanism of Action (Outcome) |
|---|---|
| Oocyte maturation | Disrupted communication between oocyte and granulosa cells of the corona radiata |
| |    (Loss of proper biochemical signals for maturation) |
| | Interference with synthesis and secretion of the zona pellucida proteins |
| |    (Abnormal sperm receptor content → nonviable ovum) |
| | General cytotoxicity to cellular processes |
| |    (Oocyte death) |
| Meiotic maturation | Damage to oocyte DNA |
| | Disrupted communication with granulosa cells |
| | Interference with mechanisms that control germinal vesicle breakdown |
| |    (Untimely meiotic divisions) |

has also been observed to produce ovarian toxicity characterized by follicular atresia in rodents and nonhuman primates (19–21). Other metals, including mercury and cadmium, have also been shown to produce ovarian damage that may be mediated through oocyte toxicity (2).

We have conducted a series of experiments to define the ovarian toxicity of the PAH, BP (22–25). Following intraperitoneal treatment with BP, murine oocytes were destroyed in a time-, strain-, species- and dose-dependent fashion. Subsequent experiments revealed BP to be an indirect-acting ovarian toxicant. To produce murine ovarian toxicity, BP must be metabolized by one or more pathways to a reactive product responsible for oocyte destruction. Intraperitoneal treatment suggests that one metabolic pathway for production of an ovotoxic product is via oxidation at the 7,8 position. Intraovarian injection experiments

suggest that the ultimate ovotoxic product is a 7,8-dihydrodiol-9,10-epoxide. PAHs, including BP, are important constituents of cigarette smoke. Experimental data regarding the ovarian toxicity of PAH assume particular interest in light of human studies suggesting an inverse, dose-dependent effect of cigarette smoking on age at menopause (26).

## CONCLUSIONS

The female reproductive system is a complex system that requires precisely regulated local and circulating hormones for proper functioning. Multiple sites are available for disruption of reproduction in the female. Unfortunately, few data are currently available addressing the actual vulnerability of female reproduction to xenobiotics. When experiments have been conducted, impairment of reproduction or reproductive processes has been demonstrated for many chemicals. Careful attention to the design of animal experiments focusing on the vulnerable processes in female reproduction and broadening our knowledge of the impact of chemicals on female reproductive function are essential for the development of public health strategies that protect reproductive health.

## REFERENCES

1. Mattison DR, Thomford PJ. Mechanisms of action of reproductive toxicants. In: Working P, ed. Toxicology of the male and female reproductive systems. New York: Hemisphere Publishing Corp, 1989:101–129.
2. Mattison DR. Ovarian toxicity: effects on sexual maturation, reproduction and menopause. In: Clarkson TW, Nordberg GF, Sager PR, eds. Reproductive and developmental toxicity of metals. New York: Plenum Press, 1983:317–342.
3. Bitman J, Cecil HC. Estrogenic activity of DDT analogs and polychlorinated biphenyls. J Agric Food Chem 1970;18:1108–1112.
4. Kimbrough RD. The toxicity of polychlorinated polycyclic compounds and related chemicals. Crit Rev Toxicol 1974;4:2:445–489.
5. Kupfer D. Effects of pesticides and related compounds on steroid metabolism and function. Crit Rev Toxicol 19754;4:83–124.
6. Shiromizu K, Thorgeirsson SS, Mattison DR. Effect of cyclophosphamide on oocyte and follicle number in Sprague-Dawley rats, C57BL/6N and DBA/2N mice. Pediatr Pharmacol 1984;4:213–221.
7. Plowchalk DR, Mattison DR. Phosphoramide mustard is responsible for the ovarian toxicity of cyclophosphamide. Toxicol Appl Pharmacol 1991;107:472–481.
8. Mattison DR, Plowchalk DR. Assessment of cyclophosphamide-induced uterine toxicity. Reprod Toxicol, in press.
9. Plowchalk DR, Mattison DR. Structural and functional changes in the C57BL/6N mouse ovary following cyclophosphamide treatment. Reprod Toxicol, in press.
10. Takizawa K, Yagi H, Jerina DM, Mattison DR. Murine strain differences in ovotoxicity following intraovarian injection with benzo($\alpha$)pyrene, ($+$)-(7R,8S)-oxide,($-$)-(7R,8R)-dihydrodiol, or ($+$)-(7R,8S)-diol-(9S,10R)-epoxide-2. Cancer Res 1984;44:2571–2576.
11. Welch RM, Levin W, Kuntzman R, Jacobson M, Conney AH. Effect of halogenated hydrocarbon insecticides on the metabolism and uterotropic action of estrogens in rats and mice. Toxicol Appl Pharmacol 1971;19:234–236.
12. Aronson JK, Grahame-Smith DG. Clinical pharmacology: adverse drug interactions. Br Med J 1981;282:288–291.
13. Baker TG. The control of oogenesis in mammals. In: Migley AR, Sadler WA, eds. Ovarian follicular development and function. New York: Raven Press, 1979:353–364.
14. Fink G. Gonadotropin secretion and its control. In: Knobil E, Neill JD, eds. The physiology of reproduction. New York: Raven Press, 1988:1349–1377.
15. diZerega G, Hodgen GD. Folliculogenesis in the primate ovarian cycle. Endocr Rev 1981;2:27–49.
16. Haney AF, Hughes SF, Hughes CL Jr. Screening of potential reproductive toxicants by use of porcine granulosa cell cultures. Toxicology 1984;30:227–241.
17. Miller MM, Weitzman G, London S, Mattison DR. Unpublished observations on the effect of BP and BP metabolites on granulosa cells in vitro. Soc Gynecol Invest, in preparation.
18. Barber HRK. The effect of cancer and its therapy upon fertility. Int J Fertil 1981;26:250–259.
19. Petrusz P, Weaver CM, Grant LD, Mushak P, Krigman MR. Lead poisoning and reproduction: effects on pituitary and serum gonadotropins in neonatal rats. Environ Res 1979;19:383–391.
20. Vermande-VanEck GJ, Meigs JW. Changes in the ovary of the rhesus monkey after chronic lead intoxication. Fertil Steril 1960;11:223–234.
21. Wide M. Interference of lead with implantation in the mouse: effect of exogenous estradiol and progesterone. Teratology 1980;21:187–191.
22. Mattison DR, Shiromizu K, Nightingale MS. Oocyte destruction by polycyclic aromatic hydrocarbons. Am J Ind Med 1983;4:191–202.
23. Mattison DR, Thorgeirsson SS. Ovarian aryl hydrocarbon hydroxylase activity and primordial oocyte toxicity of polycyclic aromatic hydrocarbons in mice. Cancer Res 1979;39:3471–3475.
24. Shiromizu K, Mattison DR. The effect of intraovarian injection of benzo($\alpha$)pyrene on primordial oocyte number and ovarian aryl hydrocarbon [benzo($\alpha$)pyrene] hydroxylase activity. Toxicol Appl Pharmacol 1984;76:18–25.
25. Takizawa K, Yagi H, Jerina DM, Mattison DR. Experimental ovarian toxicity following intraovarian injection of benzo($\alpha$)pyrene or its metabolites in mice and rats. In: Dixon RL, ed. Reproductive toxicology. New York: Raven Press, 1985:69–93.
26. Mattison DR. The effects of smoking on reproduction from gametogenesis to implantation. Environ Res 1982;28:410–433.
27. Harrington JM, Stein GF, Rivera RO, deMorales AV. Occupational hazards of formulating contraceptives: a survey of plant employees. Arch Environ Health 1978;33:12–15.
28. Reimers TJ, Sluss PM, Goodwin J, Seidel GE. Bigeneration effects of 6-mercaptopurine on reproduction in mice. Biol Reprod 1980;22:367–375.

**3**

............................................................

# Comparative Approach to Toxicokinetics

TERESA SILVAGGIO, DONALD R. MATTISON

Men and women differ in many ways, including physiological factors that impact on toxicokinetics. These differences need to be delineated to protect all workers from potentially hazardous workplace environments. In this chapter, pertinent physiological and toxicokinetic functions in pregnant women are compared to those of men and nonpregnant women, where data allow. This approach provides a means of exploring how differences in these factors contribute to variations in exposures, target tissue doses, and responses to chemicals. Physiological parameters important in toxicokinetics include: body weight, body composition, surface area, blood volumes, organ and tissue volumes, basal metabolism, cardiac output, minute ventilation, alveolar ventilation, respiratory frequency, total lung capacity, vital capacity, functional residual capacity, gastrointestinal function, renal function, hematological parameters, and vascular bed volumes.

Complex alterations in pulmonary, cardiovascular, renal, gastrointestinal, and hepatic function occur during pregnancy (Table 3.1). These physiological changes can alter toxicokinetic factors and affect the response of the pregnant woman and fetus to certain chemicals (1–5). Toxicokinetics quantitates absorption, distribution, metabolism, and excretion of chemicals. Different toxicokinetic models have been employed to describe the effects of physi-

ological adaptations during pregnancy on the kinetics of xenobiotics in the maternal organism (2, 4–6). By correlating the external dose of a chemical with its concentration at the target tissue and observing the effect, better estimations of allowable exposure limits for all employees can be determined.

## ABSORPTION

Absorption is the process by which xenobiotics cross body membranes and enter into the bloodstream (7). The gastrointestinal tract is an important route by which toxicants are absorbed in the nonoccupational setting. In the workplace, inhalation and absorption through the skin are major routes. For each of these routes of absorption, diffusion, described by Fick's Law, is the primary transport mechanism. The equation describing Fick's Law is:

$$J = \frac{D \times K}{L} dC$$

where $J$ is the flux of the xenobiotic per unit area of barrier (skin, lung, gastrointestinal mucosa), $D$ is the diffusion coefficient of the agent through the barrier, $K$ is the partition coefficient of the agent, $dC$ is the concentration gradient across the barrier, and $L$ is the thickness of the barrier.

**Table 3.1.**
**Physiological and Toxicokinetic Changes During Pregnancy[a]**

| Parameter | Physiological Change | Toxicokinetic Change |
| --- | --- | --- |
| Absorption | | |
|   Gastric emptying time | Increased | Absorption increased |
|   Intestinal motility | Decreased | Absorption increased |
|   Pulmonary function | Increased | Pulmonary exposure increased |
|   Cardiac output | Increased | Absorption increased |
|   Blood flow to skin | Increased | Absorption increased |
|   Dermal hydration | Increased | Absorption $\pm$ |
| Distribution | | |
|   Plasma volume | Increased | Concentration decreased |
|   Total body water | Increased | Concentration decreased |
|   Plasma proteins | Decreased | Concentration $\pm$ |
|   Body fat | Increased | Concentration decreased |
|   Cardiac output | Increased | Rate of distribution increased |
| Metabolism | | |
|   Hepatic metabolism | $\pm$ | Metabolism $\pm$ |
|   Extrahepatic metabolism | $\pm$ | Metabolism $\pm$ |
|   Plasma proteins | Decreased | Metabolism $\pm$ |
| Excretion | | |
|   Renal blood flow | Increased | Increased renal elimination |
|   Glomerular filtration rate | Increased | Increased renal elimination |
|   Pulmonary function | Increased | Increased pulmonary elimination |
|   Plasma proteins | Decreased | Elimination $\pm$ |

[a]Modified from Mattison DR, Blann E, Malek A. Physiological alterations during pregnancy: impact on toxicokinetics. Fundam Appl Toxicol 1991;16:215.

## Gastrointestinal Absorption

Absorption can take place at different sites along the gastrointestinal tract. Lipid solubility, pH, and ionization are all important factors in determining the absorption of a chemical. The nonionized form of a chemical is the most lipid soluble and, hence, may diffuse across membranes more readily. The pH of the stomach and intestine differ and can affect solubility and absorption of xenobiotics and chemicals depending on transit and residence time in each area of the gastrointestinal tract.

Data presented in Geigy's Scientific Tables (8, 9), which represent the combined results of several studies, indicate that the pH of gastric juice is more acidic in males than females (1.92 vs. 2.59) (10), and basal and maximal flow of gastric juice and acid secretion is higher in men than women (11). Gastric acid secretion in pregnant women is reduced by over 30% compared to nonpregnant women (12). A decline in gastric secretion may lead to increases in pH of

the gastrointestinal tract, resulting in decreased absorption of weak acids and increased absorption of weak bases.

Reduced intestinal motility may increase the overall absorption of a chemical, whereas increased motility tends to decrease absorption (13). In the pregnant woman, intestinal motility is decreased and gastric emptying time is increased (1). As a result, toxicants will have a longer residence time in the stomach and the small intestine. If the xenobiotic is absorbed through the small intestine, increased residence time in the stomach may delay the time to peak concentration in the maternal compartment. Moreover, the xenobiotic may be metabolized or degraded in the stomach, so that increased residence time will decrease the amount available for absorption. If the ingested xenobiotic moves through the stomach unaltered, the longer time in the small intestine may increase the fraction absorbed. For example, if only 25% of a xenobiotic is absorbed during passage through the small intestine in the nonpregnant woman and reduced intestinal motility in the pregnant woman increases the fraction absorbed to 50%, the concentration of the xenobiotic will be increased during pregnancy. If the absorbed xenobiotic is then distributed to susceptible target tissues, one could predict a greater toxic effect.

## Transdermal Absorption

The extent of absorption of toxicants by the skin in occupational settings is an important determinant of systemic effects. Transdermal absorption occurs most commonly through the epidermis which is separated from the dermis and subdermal tissue by a basement membrane. The epidermis, an avascular tissue, is composed of five layers: stratum corneum, stratum lucidem, stratum granulosum, stratum spinosum, and stratum basale. The environment of the lower layers is essentially aqueous, while the densely packed cornified cells of the stratum corneum form a lipid-rich protective barrier. Transdermal absorption of a chemical thus requires diffusion through a lipid-rich environment followed by diffusion through an aqueous environment (3). Chemicals may also be metabolized in the dermal tissue layers. In addition, these layers may form a reservoir for the toxicant, allowing absorption into the circulation long after exposure.

The rate of transdermal absorption of water-soluble xenobiotics or chemicals is generally determined by the rate of transport across the stratum corneum. For lipid-soluble agents, the rate of absorption is generally determined by the partitioning between the lipid-rich stratum corneum and the aqueous environment of the epidermis. This can be estimated by the partition coefficient of the xenobiotic between water and octanol. Other factors affecting rates of transdermal absorption include molecular weight, use of a solvent carrier, surface area available for absorption, physical integrity of the epidermis, hydration state of the stratum corneum, site of application of exposure, occlusion, and temperature.

As the molecular weight of the toxicant decreases, the rate of diffusion through the skin is increased. Similarly, according to Fick's law of diffusion, as the surface area of the epidermis exposed to the chemical increases, the amount transferred per unit time increases. Because the total body surface area is greater for males, the rate of transdermal absorption from a given exposure should also be greater, assuming all other factors are equal (Table 3.2).

According to Fick's law, as the thickness of the barrier decreases, the flux across the barrier increases. Differences in thickness of the epidermis, in particular, the stratum corneum, can therefore impact on transdermal absorption. Damaging the stratum corneum—either by injury or by stripping away layers of cornified epithelial cells with adhesive tape—also increases the rate of absorption. There are some variations in epidermal thickness between males and females depending on the location. In the arms and fingers, the epidermis is slightly thicker in males (14), which may have some impact on transdermal absorption in the workplace.

Increasing the hydration state of the stratum corneum increases transdermal absorption of many polar molecules. While sex-specific dif-

**Table 3.2.**
**Anatomic Parameters for Men, Nonpregnant Women, and Pregnant Women**

| Parameter | Adult Male[a] | Adult Female[a] | Reference Adult Male[b] | Reference Adult Female[b] | Pregnant Female[c] |
|---|---|---|---|---|---|
| Body weight (kg) | $71.7 \pm 10$ | $56.7 \pm 8.6$ | 70 | 58 | 62.5[d] |
| Body length (cm) | $174.5 \pm 6.6$ | $62.2 \pm 6.1$ | 170 | 160 | 160 |
| Body surface area (cm$^2$) | | | 18,000 | 16,000 | 16,500[e] |

[a]Values in this column are reported as mean ± SD and derived from data from Stoudt et al. (42, 43) as cited in International Commission on Radiological Protection (ICRP) no. 23. Report of the task group on reference man (44), pp. 13, 15.
[b]International Commission on Radiological Protection (ICRP) no. 23. Report of the task group on reference man (44), pp. 13, 15.
[c]Pregnant female at 40 weeks' gestation.
[d]Hytten and Chamberlain (1) and Hytten and Leitch (19).
[e]Derived from a nomogram for assessment of the surface area of adults as a function of weight and length, which appeared in Documenta Geigy, Scientific tables, 7th ed, 1970, Supplement.

**Table 3.3.**
**Body Composition Parameters for Men, Nonpregnant Women, and Pregnant Women[a]**

| Parameter | Adult Male[b] | Adult Female[b] | Reference Adult Male[c] | Reference Adult Female[c] | Pregnant Female at Term |
|---|---|---|---|---|---|
| Total body water | 60% TBW (43.2 L) | 55% TBW (31.4 L) | 600 ml/kg TBW (42.0 L) | 500 ml/kg TBW (29.0 L) | 33.0 L[d] |
| Extracellular water | 15% TBW (10.8 L) | 15% TBW (8.6 L) | 260 ml/kg TBW (18.2 L) | 200 ml/kg TBW (11.6 L) | 15.0 L[d] |
| Intracellular water | 45% TBW (32.4 L) | 40% TBW (22.8 L) | 340 ml/kg TBW (23.8 L) | 300 ml/kg TBW (17.4 L) | 18.75 L[e] |
| Total blood volume | | | 5200 ml | 3900 ml | 5250 ml[f] |
| Plasma volume | | | 3000 ml | 2500 ml | 3750 ml[d] |
| RBC volume | | | 2200 ml | 1350 ml | 3600 ml[f] |

[a]TBW = total body weight, RBC = red blood cell.
[b]From Diem K, ed. Documenta Geigy, Scientific tables (8).
[c]From International Commission on Radiological Protection (ICRP), no. 23. Report of the task group on reference man (44), pp. 29–36.
[d]Modified from Mattison DR. Physiological variations in pharmacokinetics during pregnancy. In: Fabro S, Scialli AR, eds. Drug and chemical action in pregnancy. New York: Marcel Dekker, 1986:48.
[e]Estimate using 300 ml/kg TBW value from reference [c] above for a pregnant female weighing 62.5kg at 40 weeks' gestation.
[f]Hytten FE, Leitch I. The physiology of human pregnancy. Oxford: Blackwell, 1971:26.

ferences in the hydration status of the epidermis have not been investigated, inferences may be made from data on the extracellular and intracellular body water content in males and females. Total body water, intracellular body water, and extracellular body water are all increased in males. Values are also greater in pregnant women than nonpregnant women, but still less than in males (Table 3.3). Pregnant females and males may thus have altered transdermal absorption of certain toxicants based on the hydration state of the stratum corneum.

Blood flow to the skin may also affect transdermal absorption of toxicants. According to data from Williams and Legett (15), the percentage of cardiac output to the skin (5%) and blood perfusion rate to the skin (120 ml/kg/min) do not differ for males and females. However, there are substantial changes in blood flow to different regions of the skin during pregnancy. Blood flow to the hand increases approximately six-fold during pregnancy (16), and blood flow to the foot doubles. At the same time, there are only small increases in blood flow to the forearm and leg. These alterations in dermal blood flow during pregnancy may have a significant impact on transdermal absorption of xenobiotics.

## Pulmonary Absorption

Pulmonary volumes and respiratory flow rates are important toxicokinetic parameters, espe-

cially when the route of exposure is via inhalation, an important route of exposure in occupational settings. Absorption, metabolism, and excretion may all be related to pulmonary function. Gender differences in pulmonary function can alter the toxicokinetics of certain chemicals. Lung volumes correlate with total body weight and surface area; therefore, one would expect higher volumes in men compared to women (Table 3.4). Total lung capacity (TLC), functional residual capacity (FRC), vital capacity (VC), and dead space volume (VD) are all higher in men than in women.

Pulmonary function also changes during pregnancy (Table 3.4). Although the respiratory rate is unaltered, the tidal volume (TV) is increased by 39% from 487 to 678 ml/min. Increases in minute ventilation parallel increases in tidal volume. As a result, the amount of inhaled toxicants may be significantly greater during pregnancy. The increases in tidal and minute volumes also suggest an increase in pulmonary distribution and alveolar mixing of gases, lessening the time to reach alveolar steady state. Gas transfer, however, appears to be decreased due to interstitial changes in the lungs during pregnancy. For example, the pulmonary diffusion capacity of carbon monoxide is reduced from 26.5 to 22.5/min/mm Hg (17).

During an 8-hr exposure in the workplace, the largest pulmonary dose would be delivered to the pregnant woman (Table 3.5). The threshold limit value for arsenic is 0.2 mg/m$^3$.

**Table 3.4.**
**Lung Capacities and Volumes in Men, Nonpregnant Women, and Pregnant Women[a]**

| | Total Body Height (cm) | Total Body Weight (kg) | Total Body Surface Area (m²) | TLC[b] (L) | FRC[b] (L) | VC[b] (L) | VD[b] (ml) | TV[b] (ml/min) | V[b] (L/min) | RR[b] (br/min) | Volume of Air Exchanged in 8 hr Resting (L) |
|---|---|---|---|---|---|---|---|---|---|---|---|
| Men | 175 | 70 | 1.8 | 5.6 | 3.1 | 4.3 | 160 | 750 | 7.5 | 15 | 3600 |
| Nonpregnant women | 163 | 58 | 1.6 | 5.0[c] | 2.8[c] | 3.3 | 130 | 487[c] | 6.0 | 15 | 2900 |
| Pregnant women | 163 | 62.5 | 1.65 | 4.7[c] | 2.3[c] | 3.3[c] | | 678[c] | 10.5[c] | 16 | 5000 |

[a]Data adapted from International Commission on Radiological Protection (ICRP). Report of the task group on reference man. ICRP publication 23. New York: Pergamon Press, 1975:344–347.
[b]TLC = total lung capacity (amount of gas contained in the lung at the end of a maximal inspiration); FRC = functional residual capacity (volume of gas remaining in the lungs at the resting expiratory level); VC = vital capacity (maximal volume of gas that can be expelled from the lungs by forceful effort after a maximal inspiration); VD = dead space volume; TV = tidal volume (volume of gas inspired or expired during each respiratory cycle); V = minute ventilation; RR = respiratory rate (breaths per minute).
[c]Data derived from deSwiet M. The respiratory system. In: Hytten FE, Chamberlain G, eds. Clinical physiology in obstetrics. Oxford: Blackwell, 1980:79–100.

**Table 3.5.**
**Effect of Pregnancy on Pulmonary Dose of Selected Xenobiotics[a]**

| Compound | Recommended Exposure Limit[b] (mg/m³) | Pulmonary Dose[c] (mg) | | |
|---|---|---|---|---|
| | | Men | Nonpregnant Women | Pregnant Women |
| Arsenic | 0.2 | 0.72 | 0.58 | 1.00 |
| Benzene | 32 | 115 | 93 | 160 |
| Ethylene oxide | 1.8 | 6.5 | 5.2 | 9 |

[a]Modified from Mattison, DR. Physiologic variations in pharmacokinetics during pregnancy. In: Fabro S, Scialli AR, eds. Drug and chemical action in pregnancy. New York: Marcel Dekker, 1986:90.
[b]Threshold Limit Values 1991–1992, American Conference of Governmental Industrial Hygienists (45).
[c]Pulmonary dose refers to the amount of xenobiotic delivered to the lung in an 8-hr period when the level of exposure is at the recommended exposure limit. Pulmonary parameters used in calculation of pulmonary dose taken from Table 3.4.

During an 8-hr work exposure at that level, the male would inhale 0.72 mg, the nonpregnant female would inhale 0.58 mg, and the pregnant female would inhale 1.00 mg. Similar results are noted for benzene and ethylene oxide. A study of Swedish workers in the ceramics industry by Gerhardsson and Ahlmark (18) suggests that women are more vulnerable to silicosis than men. The prediagnosis duration of exposure to dust was significantly shorter for the women than for the men (20.5 ± 8.6 yr vs. 28 ± 10.1 yr, p<.001), and the progression of lesions demonstrated roentgenographically was more pronounced in women.

During exercise, both TV and respiratory frequency are increased, resulting in increased minute volume. By inference, these changes during exercise are comparable with changes due to exertion in the workplace (Table 3.6). The trend of increased values in males vs. females is noted for both the resting and various activity levels. Data on minute ventilation ranges associated with various activity levels in pregnant women are scarce. Hytten and Leitch (19) report the results of Widlund (20) in which no differences were noted in the relative increase in minute volume between pregnant and nonpregnant women after exercise. One may assume, however, that the increases in respiratory parameters during gestation will be amplified in the pregnant woman who is exercising or whose job requires physical exertion. Pernoll et al. (21) determined that oxygen consumption increased during pregnancy under standard exercise conditions. Respiratory function was increased in both the resting and exercising pregnant state compared to nonpregnant values. There may be increases in absorption and distribution of inhaled toxicants resulting from these increases in respiratory parameters during gestation.

### Cardiac Output

Cardiac output (CO) and regional distribution of flow are two important parameters that will

**Table 3.6.**
**Minute Ventilation Means (Ranges) by Sex and Activity Level**

| | | Ventilation (liters/min) | | | |
|---|---|---|---|---|---|
| Subject | Weight (kg) | Resting | Light | Moderate | Heavy |
| Male[a] | 70.0 | 12.2 | 13.8 | 40.9 | 80.0 |
| | | (2.3–18.8) | (2.3–27.6) | (14.4–78.0) | (34.6–183.4) |
| Nonpregnant female[a] | 65.4 | 5.7 | 8.1 | 26.5 | 47.9 |
| | | (4.2–11.66) | (4.2–29.4) | (20.7–34.2) | (23.4–114.8) |
| Pregnant female[b] | 81.8 | 7.1 | 10.1 | 33.1 | 60.0 |

[a]Adapted from U.S. Environmental Protection Agency (EPA), Exposure Assessment Group. Exposure factors handbook. Washington, DC: U.S. EPA, 1989:3–14.
[b]These are estimated values derived by assuming that body weight increases 25% during gestation and that a proportionate increase in minute ventilation occurs.

impact on toxicokinetics, especially absorption. CO is most commonly standardized with respect to body parameters and reported as the cardiac index (CI), defined by the equation:

$$CI = CO \text{ (liters/min)}/BSA \text{ (m}^2\text{)}$$

where *BSA* is the body surface area. When standardized for BSA, CI is nearly identical for both sexes from ages 18–44 yr (22).

CO increases approximately 50% during pregnancy (16). This increase occurs by the end of the first trimester and remains elevated over the remainder of pregnancy. The increase in CO is accomplished by an increase in both stroke volume and heart rate. Supine CO, however, decreases toward the end of pregnancy to values that approximate the nonpregnant supine CO. This decrease is due to reduction in venous return secondary to occlusion of the inferior vena cava by the gravid uterus (22).

Distribution of CO, or regional blood flow, can impact on toxicokinetics. Williams and Legett (15) have proposed reference values for resting blood flow to organs and tissues for typical 35-yr-old males and females. Significant differences occur for resting blood flow as a percentage of CO to skeletal muscle (greater for men) and adipose tissue (greater for women). These differences may reflect gender-based differences in the percentage of total body mass represented by each tissue (15).

During pregnancy, increased CO leads to an increase in uterine blood flow that approximates 150 ml/kg/min at term (23, 24). This value is comparable to uterine blood flows determined in experimental animals. Blood flow to the skin and kidney is also increased during gestation. Renal blood flow is increased by

approximately 50% very early in pregnancy. No significant changes are reported in cerebral or hepatic blood flows; however, there is a paucity of information regarding regional blood flow changes during pregnancy (25).

## DISTRIBUTION

Distribution is the process by which a xenobiotic is translocated from sites of absorption or metabolism to tissues and organs throughout the body. The rate of distribution is determined by regional blood flow, diffusion of the chemical through the cell membranes of the target tissues, and the chemical's affinity for different tissues (7). Toxicants vary in their distribution. Some readily cross cell membranes and are distributed throughout the body, while others that do not cross have a limited distribution and may remain within the vascular compartment. Lipid-soluble xenobiotics may accumulate in fat, while other agents concentrate in certain tissues because of protein binding. In the storage form, the chemical will usually not exert its toxic effect (7) but is also not available for elimination.

The one-compartment model has been employed to examine the toxicokinetic characteristics of xenobiotics in both nonpregnant and pregnant individuals (2, 3, 5). However, many xenobiotics require more complicated models to characterize absorption, distribution, metabolism, and elimination accurately. In this model, the chemical distributes instantaneously through the apparent volume of distribution. As the chemical is eliminated, generally with an exponential decay, the concentration in the plasma decreases, with plasma and tissue concentrations in equilibrium. The apparent volume of distribution ($V_d$) is a theoretical volume that is defined by the equation:

$$V_d = D/C_0$$

where $V_d$ is the volume of the distribution, $D$ is the dose of chemical administered, and $C_0$ is the concentration in the plasma at time zero. The total amount of chemical in the body (represented by $D$) is the body burden (7). The apparent $V_d$ is integral in determining the body burden of a xenobiotic. According to the above equation, the amount of chemical in the body is equal to the product of $V_d \times C$, the concentration of the chemical in plasma. Chemicals that are bound to plasma proteins are confined to the vascular compartment and are not available to target tissues. The high plasma concentration is reflected in a small $V_d$. Chemicals with high affinity for specific tissues concentrate in the tissues and not in the plasma, resulting in a very large $V_d$. Chemicals with large $V_d$ are usually eliminated slowly.

Body composition parameters (Table 3.3) are important toxicokinetically, especially in regard to $V_d$. Sex-specific differences in these parameters may account for differences in concentration of a xenobiotic and result in varying responses. Total body water (TBW), extracellular water (ECW), intracellular water (ICW), total blood volume (TBV), plasma volume (PV), and RBC volume (RBCV) are greater for men than nonpregnant women. Therefore, if an average male and an average female are exposed to the same dose of a water-soluble xenobiotic, the greater TBW, PV, ECW, and ICW will increase the $V_d$ and, thus, decrease the concentration of the xenobiotic in the male.

During pregnancy, changes in body weight, plasma proteins, plasma volume, extracellular fluid volume, total body water, and body fat may alter xenobiotic distribution (1–5). In the average female, weight increases from 50 kg at the start of pregnancy to approximately 63 kg at 40 weeks. Total body water increases from 25 liters in the nonpregnant female to 33 liters at term, but remains less than the reference adult male at 42 liters. Maternal extracellular fluid volume increases from 11 liters in the nonpregnant female to 15 liters over the course of pregnancy, compared to 18.2 liters in the adult reference male. Plasma volume increases from 2.5 liters in the nonpregnant female to 3.8 liters in the pregnant female at term, greater than the 3 liters in the reference adult male. These volume measurements in the pregnant female exceed all nonpregnant female values and also exceed total blood volume, plasma volume, and RBC volume values for the adult male. These differences may be important, especially for xenobiotics distributed into plasma. For example, the lowest initial xenobiotic concentration may be in the pregnant female at 40 weeks' gestation.

In many toxicokinetic models, maternal $V_d$ increases continuously during gestation; however, it does not increase for all xenobiotics. At times, it is inferred that an increase in $V_d$ has occurred because of an observed decrease in plasma concentration. However, other factors such as an increase in the rate of elimination, decrease in a binding protein, or a decrease in the rate of absorption may also reduce serum xenobiotic concentrations.

Decreases in plasma-binding proteins, such as albumin, may increase the amount of free xenobiotic or chemical available for extravascular distribution, for delivery to target tissues, and for elimination. Differences in the availability of, or affinity for, protein-binding sites may also affect the concentration of a xenobiotic. Studies assessing variations in serum binding of xenobiotics between men and women were not identified during the preparation of this chapter.

Total protein and serum albumin concentrations do not significantly differ between males and nonpregnant females (26). With advancing age, total protein concentrations decrease earlier in women than in men (9). Total protein content of serum decreases in pregnancy, primarily due to a decrease in albumin (27). It falls over the first trimester and plateaus during midpregnancy at a level that is almost 1 g/100 ml below nonpregnant female values. By 37–40 weeks of gestation, albumin concentration is approximately 0.8 g/100 ml lower than nonpregnant female values.

Body fat composition also impacts on toxicokinetics. The body can be divided into fat-containing and fat-free tissues. Body fat can be further categorized into "essential" and "nonessential" fat. Essential fat is composed of lipid constituents of cells and constitutes about 2–5% of the lean body mass (28). Nonessential fat is excess storage fat that is contained in adipose tissue. Increases in body fat composition may lead to a greater body burden of lipid-soluble xenobiotic.

Body fat as a percentage of total body weight is higher in women than in men and increases by age in both sexes (29). The total body fat for an adult reference male is 13.5 kg. Maternal body fat increases by about 25%, from 16.5 kg in the nonpregnant female to 19.8 kg at 40 weeks' gestation (2, 30). The larger proportion of body fat in women and increase in body fat in pregnant women may increase the body burden of lipid-soluble, slowly metabolized toxicants, especially during gestation.

## METABOLISM

Metabolism is a major factor in determining response to xenobiotics. Biotransformation includes all of the biochemical processes involved in changing a chemical into a secondary product with greater or lesser toxicity than the parent compound. These processes usually enhance the water solubility of the xenobiotic, facilitating excretion in urine or feces. Biotransformation occurs predominantly in the liver, but there are also extrahepatic sites of metabolism such as the lung, kidney, intestinal tract, and skin. Biotransformation can also occur in the placenta and in fetal tissues.

Many factors impact on the rate of biotransformation of xenobiotics. Factors that affect uptake of xenobiotics by target tissues are also important in metabolism, since the toxicant must reach cellular sites of biotransformation. Thus, lipid solubility, protein binding, dose, and route of exposure all affect the rate of biotransformation. In addition, individuals show large variation in metabolism of xenobiotics. However, data regarding the rates of metabolism of toxicants for males as well as nonpregnant and pregnant females are scarce. In humans, sex-dependent differences in biotransformation have been observed for a few specific xenobiotics such as nicotine, acetylsalicylic acid, and heparin (31).

Metabolism of xenobiotics or chemicals may be estimated by basal metabolic rates (BMR).

Brozek and Grande, cited in Kinney et al. (32), and Geigy, Scientific Tables (9) determined that hepatic metabolism, which is predominantly responsible for biotransformation of many chemicals, contributes 25% to the BMR. Differences in BMRs may suggest variations in hepatic metabolism and toxicant biotransformation. BMR is affected by factors such as sex, age, height, body composition, and hormonal balance (33, 34). Standard BMRs have been derived for men and women ages 18–40 years (35). For all ages, men have a higher BMR than women.

BMR incorporates a number of cellular functions from different cell types. Because the metabolism of adipose tissue differs from that of muscle tissue, some of the differences between men and women are attributed to body composition (36). Cunningham (37) reviewed multiple studies and concluded that the lower BMR per unit BSA is actually the reflection of a reduction of lean body mass in women due to a smaller skeletal muscle component. BMR rises during gestation secondary to increased oxygen consumption by many different organs (17). The organs responsible for increased oxygen consumption early in pregnancy are predominantly the heart (increased CO) and kidney (increased renal sodium reabsorption). At term, however, the fetus, placenta, and uterus account for a substantial portion of the increase in oxygen consumption. Therefore, during pregnancy, the contribution to BMR from different organs differs from that of males and nonpregnant females.

The altered hormonal milieu of pregnancy is associated with changes in hepatic and extrahepatic xenobiotic metabolism (2, 38, 39). Changes in hepatic metabolism can have an impact on the first-pass effect of xenobiotics given orally in pregnancy. The first-pass effect describes the phenomenon whereby the chemical is biotransformed by either the gastrointestinal tract, liver, or lung and eliminated before entering the bloodstream (7). Metabolism by the fetus and placenta may alter the maternal level of a toxicant or its metabolites and may also influence fetal or placental xenobiotic toxicity. Gillette (40) evaluated the impact of fetal metabolism on maternal and fetal xenobiotic levels. He suggests that, for a lipid-soluble xenobiotic rapidly transferred across the placenta, fetal metabolism has only a small effect on maternal concentrations but may lower fetal levels by one-half. If the xenobiotic is slowly transported to the fetus, metabolism in fetal tissues may have an even greater impact on fetal concentration.

## ELIMINATION

Xenobiotics are generally eliminated from the body by renal, hepatic, or pulmonary routes. Toxicants may also be excreted via bodily secretions such as sweat, tears, and milk (7). Biotransformation of lipid-soluble agents must occur before excretion via the kidneys or bile. Lipophilic chemicals that are poorly metabolized may be excreted predominantly in breast milk.

Renal function is important for elimination. Chemicals can be excreted into the urine through glomerular filtration, passive diffusion, and active secretion. Increases in renal blood flow and glomerular filtration will increase the elimination rate of xenobiotics cleared by the kidneys. When standardized for BSA, renal blood flow, glomerular filtration, tubular secretion, and tubular reabsorption are all larger in men than in nonpregnant women (1). During gestation, changes in renal blood flow, glomerular filtration rates, hepatic blood flow, bile flow, and pulmonary function may alter maternal elimination of a xenobiotic. Maternal renal plasma flow increases from 500–700 ml/min/1.73 $m^2$, a 1.44-fold increase over the nonpregnant female value and a 1.1-fold increase over the male value. Glomerular filtration also increases during pregnancy. At the beginning of gestation, glomerular filtration is approximately 100 ml/min/1.73 $m^2$. By 20 weeks' gestation, the glomerular filtration rate has increased to approximately 150 ml/min/1.73 $m^2$, a 1.5-fold increase over the nonpregnant female value and a 1.2-fold increase over the male value (41).

$V_d$ and elimination rates interact to affect the concentration of a toxicant in the maternal organism. For a particular toxicant, the combined effect of increased $V_d$ and increased rate of elimination may substantially decrease the area under the concentration-versus-time curve. Consider a xenobiotic whose $V_d$ increases proportional to maternal weight during pregnancy and whose rate of elimination also increases during pregnancy proportional to pulmonary or renal excretion. The increased $V_d$ decreases the initial concentration of xenobiotic in maternal plasma, while the increase in the elimination rate constant increases the rate at which the xenobiotic is cleared from the body. This example suggests that, for some xenobiotics, maternal tolerance may actually increase during pregnancy as compared to the nonpregnant female and male. However, increased renal clearance during pregnancy may, by increasing the dose of xenobiotic delivered, increase toxicity to the maternal urinary tract. There also may be a toxicant whose $V_d$ increases but whose rate of elimination decreases. In this case, the same exposure to a pregnant female and nonpregnant individual may cause a higher concentration and greater toxicity in the pregnant woman.

There is a paucity of data regarding the impact of changes in pulmonary and hepatic function on elimination. Pulmonary function changes significantly during pregnancy (Table 3.4). As a result of the increase in minute volume, the amount of inhaled toxicants significantly increases during pregnancy. One can assume that these same increases in pulmonary function during pregnancy may also increase pulmonary elimination. However, it is unknown whether these postulated increases in pulmonary elimination are sufficient to override the increase in pulmonary absorption.

Little is known about differences in hepatic function between men, nonpregnant women, and pregnant women. Liver function tests are generally the same for these groups, although excretion of bromosulfophthalein is slowed during pregnancy, which may be due to delayed hepatic excretion (38). This delay in excretion may also affect the hepatic and biliary excretion of toxicants, but experimental and clinical data are lacking.

Predicting the effect of pregnancy on rate of elimination is not as straightforward as predicting the changes in $V_d$. For xenobiotics excreted predominantly by renal mechanisms, there appears to be an increase in the rate of elimination during pregnancy. For xenobiotics cleared by hepatic metabolism, two separate patterns of change during pregnancy have emerged. For some xenobiotics (e.g., phenytoin), pregnancy appears to increase clearance, whereas for others (e.g., meperidine), pregnancy appears to decrease clearance. The message contained in these observations is that toxicokinetics does differ between men and women and should be expected to change during pregnancy. It is essential, therefore to characterize toxicokinetics in all workers to identify the susceptible populations and institute appropriate exposure guidelines to prevent chemically induced disease.

## CONCLUSION

There are significant differences in physiological parameters between men and nonpregnant women that may impact on toxicokinetic factors such as absorption, distribution, metabolism, and elimination. In addition, there are substantial physiological and body composition changes that occur during pregnancy. These physiological adaptations are thought to be necessary for the success of the pregnancy and for fetal growth and development. However, these changes may also alter the toxicokinetics of substances encountered in the workplace.

Physiological and toxicokinetic factors must be considered in determining allowable exposure limits for men, nonpregnant women, and pregnant women and in establishing guidelines to protect reproductive and developmental health. With the increased number of women of reproductive age in the workplace, many of whom will want to continue working during pregnancy, it is important to define the effect of physiological adaptations on the amount and concentration of xenobiotics in the maternal and fetal compartments. Any method of quantitative risk assessment must consider these physiological differences between and among the groups. Data on physiological, toxicokinetic, and metabolic parameters for both sexes needs to be developed more extensively. Once the data are broadly available, it will be possible to institute quantitative risk assessment based on physiological and toxicokinetic differences. This databased approach will act to protect all workers and increase their access to all worksites.

References

1. Hytten FE, Chamberlain G, eds. Clinical physiology in obstetrics. Oxford: Blackwell, 1980.
2. Mattison DR. Physiological variations in pharmacokinetics during pregnancy. In: Fabro S, Scialli AR, eds. Drug and chemical action in pregnancy. New York: Marcel Dekker, 1986:37–102.
3. Mattison DR. Transdermal drug absorption during pregnancy. Clin Obstet Gynecol 1990;33:718–727.
4. Mattison DR, Blann E, Malek A. Physiological alterations during pregnancy: impact on toxicokinetics. Fundam Appl Toxicol 1991;16:215–218.
5. Mattison DR, Malek A, Cistola C. Physiological adaptations to pregnancy: impact on pharmacokinetics. In: Yaffe A, ed. Pediatric pharmacology: therapeutic principles in practice. 2nd ed. Philadelphia: WB Saunders, 1992:81–96.
6. Fisher JW, Whittaker TA, Taylor DH, Clewell HJ III, Andersen ME. Physiologically based pharmacokinetic modeling of the lactating rat and nursing pup: a multiroute exposure model for trichloroethylene. Toxicol Appl Pharmacol 1990;102:497–513.
7. Klaassen DC. Distribution, excretion, and absorption of toxicants. In: Klaassen CD, Amdur MO, Doull J, eds. Casarett and Doull's toxicology. New York: MacMillan Publishers, 1986:33–63.
8. Diem K, ed. Documenta Geigy, Scientific tables. 6th ed. Basel: JR Geigy S.A., 1962:538.
9. Lentner C, ed. Geigy, Scientific tables, vol 1 & 3. 8th ed. Basel: CIBA-Geigy Limited, 1981.
10. Dotevall G. Gastric secretion of acid in diabetes mellitus during basal conditions and after maximal histamine stimulation. Acta Med Scand 1961;170:59–69. Cited in Geigy, Scientific tables, 1981:125.
11. Feifel G, Lorenz W, Heimann A. Bestimmung der basalen und maximal stimulierten. Magensaftsekrection Kretische Untersuchunger zur Durchfuhrung, Auswertung und Benrteilung von Majensellretistesten Klin Wochenschr 1972;50:413–422. Cited in Geigy, Scientific tables 1981:124.
12. Murray FA, Erskin JP, Fielding J. Gastric secretion in pregnancy. Br J Obstet Gynaecol 1957;64:373. Cited in: Hytten FE, Chamberlain G, eds. Clinical physiology in obstetrics. Oxford: Blackwell, 1980:147–162.
13. Levine RR. Factors affecting gastrointestinal absorption of drugs. Am J Dig Dis 1970;15:171–188. Cited in: Klaassen CD, Amdur MO, Doull J, eds. Casarett and Doull's toxicology. New York: Macmillan Publishers, 1986:55.
14. Southwood WFW. The thickness of the skin. Plast Reconstr Surg 1955;15:423–429. Cited in: International Commission on Radiological Protection (ICRP). Report of the task group on reference man. ICRP publication no. 23. New York: Pergamon Press, 1975:49.
15. Williams LR, Legett RW. Reference values for resting blood flow to organs of man. Clin Phys Meas 1989;10:187–217.
16. deSwiet M. The cardiovascular system. In: Hytten FE, Chamberlain G, eds. Clinical physiology in obstetrics. Oxford: Blackwell, 1980:289–327.
17. deSwiet M. The respiratory system. In: Hytten FE,

Chamberlain G, eds. Clinical physiology in obstetrics. Oxford: Blackwell, 1980:79–100.

18. Gerhardsson L, Ahlmark A. Silicosis in women. Experience from the Swedish pneumoconiosis register. J Occup Med 1985;27:347–350.

19. Hytten FE, Leitch I. The physiology of human pregnancy. Oxford: Blackwell, 1971.

20. Widlund G. The cardio-pulmonal function during pregnancy. Acta Obstet Gynecol Scand 1945;25(Suppl I):1–125. Cited in: Hytten FE, Leitch I, eds. The physiology of human pregnancy. Oxford: Blackwell, 1971:129.

21. Pernoll ML, Metcalf J, Schleuber TL, Welch JE, Matsomato J. Oxygen consumption at rest and during exercise in pregnancy. Respir Physiol 1975;25:285–293.

22. Williams LR. Reference values for total blood volume and cardiac output in humans. Personal communication, 1991.

23. Moawad AH, Lindheimer MD, eds. Uterine and placental blood flow. New York: Masson, 1982:19–199.

24. Metcalf J, Stock MK, Banon DH. Maternal physiology during gestation. In: Knobil E, Neill J, eds. The physiology of reproduction. New York: Raven Press, 1988:2145–2176.

25. Brinkman CR. Biologic adaptation to pregnancy. In: Maternal fetal medicine: principles and practice. 2nd ed. Philadelphia: WB Saunders, 1989:734–745.

26. Keating FR, Jones JD, Elveback LR, Randall RV. The relation of age and sex to distribution of values in healthy adults of serum calcium inorganic phosphorus, magnesium, alkaline phosphatase, total protein, albumin, and blood urea. J Lab Clin Med 1969;73:825–834.

27. Hytten FE. Nutrition. In: Hytten FE, Chamberlain G, eds. Clinical physiology in obstetrics. Oxford: Blackwell, 1980:163–187.

28. Benke AR. Role of fat in gross body composition and configuration. In: Rubahl K, Issekutz D, eds. Fetus and tissue. New York: McGraw-Hill, 1964:285–313.

29. Young CM, Blandin J, Tensuan R, Fryer HH. Body composition studies of "older" women, thirty to seventy years of age. Ann NY Acad Sci 1963;110:589–607. Cited in: International Commission on Radiological Protection (ICRP). Report of the task group on reference man. ICRP publication no. 23. New York: Pergamon Press, 1975:42.

30. Hytten FE. Weight gain in pregnancy. In: Hytten FE, Chamberlain G, eds. Clinical physiology in obstetrics. Oxford: Blackwell, 1980:3–42.

31. Sipes IG, Gandolfi AJ. Biotransformation of toxicants. In: Klaassen CD, Amdur MO, Doull J, eds. Casarett and Doull's toxicology. New York: Macmillan Publishers, 1986:64–98.

32. Brozek J, Grande F, Anderson JT, Keys A. Densitometric analysis of body composition: revision of some quantitative assumptions. Ann NY Acad Sci 1963;110:113–140. Cited in Geigy, Scientific tables, 1981:228–230.

33. Tata JR. Basal metabolic rate and thyroid hormones. Advances Metab Disord 1964;1:153–189. Cited in Geigy Scientific Tables, 1981:228.

34. Swift RW, Fisher KH. In: Beston, McHenry, eds. Nutrition. New York: Academic Press, 1964;181. Cited in Geigy Scientific Tables, 1981:228.

35. Dubois EF. Basal energy metabolism at various ages; man. In: Altman PL, Dittmer, DS, eds. Metabolism. Bethesda: Fed Am Soc Exp Biol, 1968:345.

36. Ljunggren H. Sex differences in body composition. In: Brozek J, ed. Human body composition: approaches and applications. Oxford: Pergamon Press, 1963:129–135.

37. Cunningham JJ. Body composition and resting metabolic rate: the myth of feminine metabolism. Am J Clin Nutr 1982;36:721–726.

38. Lewis PJ. Drug metabolism. In: Hytten FE, Chamberlain G, eds. Clinical physiology in obstetrics. Oxford: Blackwell, 1980:271–282.

39. Lewis PJ. Clinical pharmacology in obstetrics. Boston: Wright PSG, 1983.

40. Gillette JR. Factors that affect drug concentrations in maternal plasma. In: Wilson JD, Fraser FC, eds. Handbook of teratology, vol. 3. New York: Plenum Press, 1977:35–71.

41. Davison JM. The urinary system. In: Hytten FE, Chamberlain G, eds. Clinical physiology in obstetrics. Oxford: Blackwell, 1980:289–327.

42. Stoudt H, Damon A, McFarland RA. Heights and weights of white Americans. Human Biol 1960; 32:331–341.

43. Stoudt HW, Damon A, McFarland R, Roberts J. Weight, height and selected body dimensions of adults, United States, 1960–62. Vital and health statistics. Data from the National Health Survey, U.S. Department of Health, Education and Welfare, National Center for Health Statistics, series 11, no. 8. Washington, DC: U.S. Government Printing Office, 1965.

44. Snyder WS (Chairman), Cook MJ, Karhausen R, Kowells GP, Nisset ES, Tipton IH. Report of the task group on reference man. International Commission on Radiological Protection (ICRP) Publication no. 23. New York: Pergamon Press, 1975:1–418.

45. American Conference of Governmental Industrial Hygienists. 1991–1992 Threshold limit values of chemical substances and physical agents and biological exposure indices. American Conference of Governmental Industrial Hygienists, 1991.

## SUGGESTED DATA RESOURCES

1. American College of Obstetricians and Gynecologists. Guidelines on pregnancy and work. NIOSH research project, U.S. Department of Health, Education and Welfare, Contract no. 210-76-0159, Rockville, MD, 1977.

2. American Conference of Governmental Industrial Hygienists. 1991–1992 Threshold limit values of chemical substances and physical agents and biological exposure indices. American Conference of Governmental Industrial Hygienists, 1991.

3. Lentner C, ed. Geigy scientific tables, vol 1&3. 8th ed. Basel: CIBA-Geigy Limited, 1981.

4. Stoudt HW, Damon A, McFarland R, Roberts J. Weight, height and selected body dimensions of adults, United States, 1960–62. Vital and health statistics. Data from the National Health Survey, U.S. Department of Health, Edu-

cation and Welfare, National Center for Health Statistics, series 11, no. 8. Washington, DC: U.S. Government Printing Office, 1965.

5. Synder WS (Chairman), Cook MJ, Karhausen R, Kowells GP, Nisset ES, Tipton IH. Report of the task group on reference man. International Commission on Radiological Protection (ICRP) Publication no. 23, New York: Pergamon Press, 1975:1–418.

6. U.S. Environmental Protection Agency (EPA). Exposure Assessment Group, Office of Health and Environmental Assessment. Exposure factors handbook. EPA/60018–89/043. Washington, DC: U.S. EPA, 1989:313–14.

# 4

········································

# Developmental Toxicology: Prenatal Period

THOMAS H. SHEPARD, ALAN G. FANTEL, PHILIP E. MIRKES

This chapter provides a basic understanding of the area of developmental toxicology, with emphasis on the prenatal period. Developmental toxicity is any form of adverse outcome that originates from exposures before conception, during pregnancy, or throughout childhood and adolescence. Outcomes such as low birthweight or retarded osseous or behavioral development are potentially reversible with time, while congenital defects represent permanent alterations in morphology or function in offspring. A developmental toxicant may be a chemical, drug, infectious agent, physical agent, or maternal condition. Teratology is the branch of science that deals specifically with the causes, mechanisms, manifestations, and prevention of congenital defects. A congenital defect has its genesis during embryonic or fetal development and consists of a major or minor deviation from normal morphology or function. It may include chromosome imbalances, molecular or genetic changes, as well as structural defects. A congenital anomaly is a defect that can be identified visually.

Development begins with the *embryonic* period, which extends from fertilization until completion of major organogenesis (Fig. 4.1). The embryonic period is divided into 23 Streeter's stages. The preimplantation stage includes the first 6–7 days after fertilization. In the human, the end of the embryonic period is 55–60 days from fertilization and is characterized by a crown to rump length of 33 mm and the appearance of bone and external characteristics specific to the species. The *fetal* period extends from the end of embryonic period until birth. The *neonatal* period usually consists of the first 4 weeks after birth, while *infancy* extends until 2 yr of age.

Clinical manifestations of developmental toxicity can differ in type, frequency, and severity among individuals. Many developmental endpoints are interrelated, and their expression depends on the properties of the agent, dose and timing of exposure, genetic susceptibility, and other factors. Figure 4.2, for example, illustrates the dose relationships for embryofetal toxicity, teratogenicity, and maternal toxicity for three types of teratogenic agents. In this chapter, the mechanisms of developmental toxicity and factors influencing response to developmental toxicants are explored, with emphasis on two important endpoints, congenital defects and fetal loss.

## MECHANISMS OF DEVELOPMENTAL TOXICITY

The ultimate goal of research in developmental toxicology/teratology is to prevent negative outcomes of human reproduction such as spontaneous abortion, stillbirth, prematurity, and congenital defects. This goal presents scientists

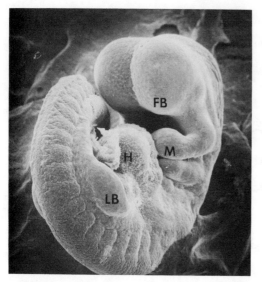

**Figure 4.1.** Scanning electron microscopic picture of embryo during organogenesis. *LB*: upper limb bud; *M*: mandibular arch; *H*: heart; *FB*: forebrain. Rat, day 11; original magnification × 40.

As originally proposed by Wilson (1), the term "mechanism" is defined as the "early, if not the first, event(s) . . . in a series of events intervening between a cause and an effect." Other investigators have used the term to mean some or all events in the pathogenesis that begins with the initial insult and culminates in developmental toxicity. This latter definition reflects the realization that developmental toxicants rarely, if ever, interact with only one cellular target. In most instances, toxic agents interact with multiple targets; identifying the first event, much less the first event that initiates the developmental pathogenesis, can rarely be accomplished unambiguously. In this section, we define mechanisms in the less restrictive sense of any or all of the events initiated by a developmental toxicant, realizing that there is also value in elucidating the first event. A general scheme for reproductive mechanisms is shown in Figure 4.3.

with an exciting, yet extremely difficult, challenge. In this section, we address one aspect of the attempt to meet this challenge, i.e., to understand the mechanisms by which negative reproductive outcomes are produced.

## Genetic Mechanisms

### MUTATION

Approximately 20–30% of all human birth defects arise from gene mutations entering the zygote from the male or female germ cell.

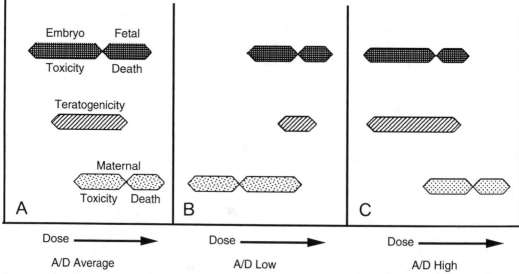

**Figure 4.2.** Theoretic diagrams of dose ranges for embryofetal toxicity, teratogenicity, and maternal toxicity. *A* represents a commonly seen association with embryofetal toxicity appearing at low doses followed by teratogenicity and, finally, maternal toxicity. The adult to developmental ratio (*A/D*) would be average (e.g., retinoids). *B* represents an agent that would kill the mother, and no teratogenicity would be found (e.g., cyanide). *C* represents the most concerning situation from a teratological perspective, where the embryofetal toxicity and teratogenicity dose ranges are much lower than the maternal range. This results in a *high A/D* ratio (e.g., thalidomide).

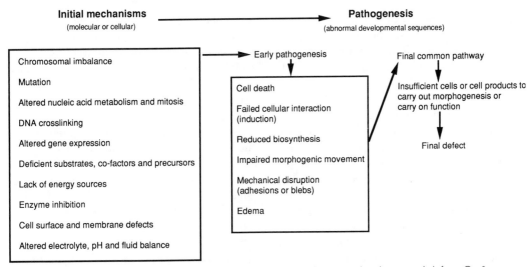

**Figure 4.3.** Diagram of the elements in successive stages leading to a developmental defect. One or more initial basic changes leads to early pathogenesis and then to a final pathway that is often characterized by reduction in cell number or products. Modified from Wilson JG. Environment and birth defects. New York: Academic Press, 1973:25.

Gene mutations may be single base pair substitutions, the loss (deletion) or addition (insertion) of one or more base pairs, or larger submicroscopic changes involving more extensive deletions or duplications. These mutations can be induced experimentally by a variety of chemical and physical agents to which humans are frequently exposed, and a large number of mutations in animals and humans are associated with abnormal developmental outcomes. These lines of evidence highlight the importance of DNA as a cellular target, and gene mutation as the initiating event (mechanism in the strict sense), in developmental toxicity. Although some germ cell mutations incorporated into a developing zygote can undoubtedly produce structural and/or functional defects, it remains unclear whether mutations induced at later stages of development, when the embryo contains many cells, can elicit such effects. Further knowledge will require the application of improved molecular methods to elucidate the whole chain of events (mechanisms in the wider sense) that begins with induction of a mutation and culminates in developmental toxicity.

### CHROMOSOMAL DEFECTS

It is now well established that chromosomal defects are associated with developmental toxicity, particularly with pregnancy loss or con-genital mental retardation in liveborns. These abnormalities range from the addition (e.g., trisomy 21) or deletion (e.g., Turner syndrome, 45,X) of whole chromosomes to deletions of parts of chromosomes (e.g., Cat-Cry syndrome, 5p deletion). While the majority of chromosomal defects are lethal to the developing organism, a variety of syndromes characterized by mild to severe alterations in essentially all organ systems can be seen in surviving infants. The initiating event in the production of these chromosomal defects is rarely known. However, factors such as advanced maternal age, ionizing radiation, some chemicals, and certain viruses are known to be associated with chromosomal defects (2).

### Cellular Mechanisms

### ALTERED CELL-CELL INTERACTIONS

Normal development requires the complex interaction of a variety of cellular factors including, but not limited to, morphogens, growth factors, extracellular matrix molecules (e.g., laminin), cell adhesion molecules, and gap junctions. These factors have in common the demonstrated or proposed property of facilitating cell-cell interactions known to be essential for normal embryonic and fetal development. Any interference in the normal function of these factors could be the initiating event in subsequent pathogenesis induced by a developmental toxicant. Although no agents have been identified that specifically interact with factors involved in cell communication, several lines of evidence provide support for this mechanism of developmental toxicity. First, research has now demonstrated that gap junctions are abundant throughout development and play a role in cell-cell communication (3). These data provide a basis for postulating that gap junctions are potential targets for developmental toxicants. Using antibodies to gap junctional proteins, one research group demonstrated that these antibodies block cell-cell communication in early frog embryos. Moreover, abnormal development and structural defects occurred in tissues derived from cells whose communication was blocked by these gap junctional antibodies. Welsch et al. (3) found that several animal teratogens including retinoic acid, diphenylhydantoin, warfarin, and several monoalkyl ethers of ethylene glycol disrupted gap junctional communication between cultured V79 cells. Two nonteratogens, saccharin and L-ascorbic acid, produced no effect on gap junctional communication. Additional work in this area is warranted.

A second area of promising research involves cell adhesion molecules (CAMs). CAMs are large cell surface glycoproteins that are responsible for certain types of cell-cell interactions during development. Edelman (4) has demonstrated that CAMs change in amount (prevalence modulation), position or distribution (polarity modulation), or in molecular structure (chemical modulation) during development. Recent experiments reveal that antibodies to specific CAMs can block their function and lead to altered morphology. The levels of one particular CAM (N-CAM) are elevated in human embryos with neural tube defects. What is not known at this time is whether specific teratogens can affect the function of CAMs. Nonetheless, accumulated evidence indicates that CAMs represent an important potential target for developmental toxicants.

## CELL MOVEMENTS

Many aspects of normal embryogenesis are known or postulated to require embryonic cell movement from one region of the developing organism to another. Examples include migration of primary mesoderm between ectoderm and endoderm, migration of neural crest cells, and movement of germ cell progenitors from extraembryonic sites to the gonadal ridges. Neural crest derivatives contribute to the development of skin (primarily pigment cells), the sensory and autonomic nervous systems, skeletal and connective tissues, and the endocrine system. Perturbations in any factor related to cell migration would be expected to have profound effects on development.

## CELL DEATH

Although normal embryogenesis requires rapid cell division and the production of millions of cells for tissue and organ formation, cell death is also common and necessary for the normal development of many organs. The observation that cell death always occurs in a reproducible spatiotemporal fashion led early investigators to label this phenomenon as "programmed cell death" (PCD). It is well known that many, if not all, teratogens induce episodes of cell death in tissues or organs. Recently, Sulik et al. (5) postulated that some teratogens, e.g., ethanol and retinoic acid, exert their teratogenic effects by expanding areas of normal PCD. Although some teratogens may exert their action via this mechanism, it is unclear why some cells not normally destined to die are killed by teratogens, while their neighbors are not. The series of steps involved in the process of cell death are also not well understood. Recent evidence indicates that cell death genes exist and that protein synthesis is required for cell death. These exciting findings must be extended to the field of developmental toxicology if the role of cell death in abnormal development is to be clarified.

## Biochemical Mechanisms

### ALTERED BIOSYNTHESIS

Normal embryogenesis requires the coordinated synthesis of three major classes of macromolecules: DNA, RNA, and proteins. Research aimed at determining the importance of these macromolecules as targets for developmental toxicity has a rich history; only a brief and selective summary of this work is possible here. Reviews by Ritter (6) and Skalko (7) are available for more extensive discussions of this topic.

Agents that inhibit DNA synthesis have long been recognized as potent teratogens in laboratory animals and, in some cases, humans. Many of these agents, such as hydroxyurea, cytosine arabinoside (ara-C), and cyclophosphamide (CP), are also potent antitumor agents due to their cytotoxicity. Work in our laboratory over the past 10 yr has focused on the mechanism by which CP exerts its teratogenic effects in rat embryos. CP itself is nonteratogenic and requires activation via cytochrome P-450 enzymes to exert its teratogenic action. The embryotoxic metabolites generated from this activation process are phosphoramide mustard (PM) and acrolein (AC). These two metabolites produce their embryotoxic effects by intercalating with different macromolecular targets. PM achieves its effects by cross-linking DNA, while AC interacts with proteins (although the specific proteins have not been identified). While PM exerts its embryotoxicity by affecting the DNA of the embryo, AC mediates its action through the extraembryonic yolk sac (8).

Our research has also shown that CP induces an episode of cell death in the exposed embryo. Like other teratogens that cause cell death, CP-induced cell lethality is not random. Some tissues such as those of the developing heart are completely resistant to the cytotoxic effects of CP, whereas the tissues of the developing central nervous system (CNS) are sensitive. Understanding the molecular basis of this differential sensitivity may provide insights into the more general question of why some cells within a tissue die in response to a teratogenic exposure, while other cells do not. To date, our research has eliminated several possible explanations for the observed differential sensitivity such as differential uptake of the drug, variable binding of activated CP to macromolecules, and differential detoxification of CP intermediates. We have discovered that the type of DNA damage induced by CP is different in heart tissue compared with neuroepithelial tissue. CP induces significantly higher levels of DNA-DNA cross-links in cells of the neuroepithe-

lium compared with the levels induced in cardiac cells. In addition, we have indirect evidence that the repair capabilities of DNA differ in the two tissues. Our research, together with that of others, provides one of the more detailed pictures of how a teratogen exerts its effects. Through these investigations, we are beginning to understand the mechanisms by which toxicants initiate the pathogenesis that culminates in overt developmental aberrations.

Much less is known about the roles played by RNA and proteins in developmental toxicity. Clearly, transcription and translation are essential cellular events, suggesting that RNA and proteins are also potential targets for developmental toxicants. Inhibitors of RNA and protein synthesis have been tested to determine if they can induce developmental toxicity. In general, the results of these studies have been relatively uninformative. Actinomycin, an inhibitor of RNA synthesis, has been shown to produce developmental toxicity; however, efforts to understand the underlying mechanisms have provided little specific information. Inhibitors of protein synthesis, such as cycloheximide and puromycin, are, at best, weakly teratogenic. Overall, research in this area has languished in recent years. This is probably because inhibitors of RNA and protein synthesis lack any degree of specificity, a key parameter necessary for inducing developmental toxicity, particularly birth defects. A more promising approach might focus on the effects of developmental toxicants on specific gene sequences and their protein products.

## ALTERED GENE EXPRESSION

It is well known that different tissues in the adult body express specific sets of proteins that, at one level, define a particular tissue or organ. Although many details are missing, this differential gene expression arises as a complex series of events during embryogenesis. Normal development requires a precise program of gene activation (and inactivation), and disruption of this program should lead to adverse effects. The abnormal development of embryos with specific gene mutations or transgenic inserts illustrates this point. Whether developmental toxicants can exert their adverse effects by altering the pattern of gene expression is an open question; however, recent research described below indicates that altered gene expression can have profound effects on development.

Homeobox-containing genes were initially discovered as genes that play important roles in the control of morphogenesis and pattern formation in Drosophila. More recently, homologs of these Drosophila genes have also been isolated from mammals as so-called Hox genes. Although the role of these genes in mammalian development is as yet unknown, it is assumed that they influence morphogenesis and pattern formation. Recent work by Peter Gruss and his colleagues (9) provides initial support for this assumption. These investigators constructed a hybrid homeobox gene (Hox 1.1) by removing the normal promoter region of this gene and replacing it with the promoter region of the β-actin gene. This hybrid construct was then inserted into the pronucleus of a fertilized egg to produce transgenic offspring. Because actin gene expression normally occurs in all cells of the developing embryo, the presence of the hybrid construct in the transgenic embryos led to expression of Hox 1.1 in all cells of the embryo, i.e., ectopic expression. Normally, Hox 1.1 is expressed at specific stages of development (maximal expression on day 12) and in a specific spatial pattern (neural tube, spinal ganglia, and sclerotomes). The intriguing finding was that transgenic offspring, in which ectopic expression of Hox 1.1 occurred, exhibited birth defects characterized by cleft palate, fused eyelids, open eyes, and nonfused pinna. Thus, abnormal expression of a gene is correlated with abnormal embryogenesis. In addition, the spectrum of defects observed in these transgenic animals mirrors that observed in experimental animals exposed in utero to retinoic acid as well as the human syndrome known as the first and second arch syndrome (Goldenhar's). Although speculative, these observations suggest that the mechanism inducing retinoic acid embryopathy and Goldenhar's syndrome may involve abnormal expression of homeobox genes. These research approaches hold great promise in our attempts to understand normal development and mechanisms by which teratogens interfere with critical developmental events.

## ALTERED ENERGY METABOLISM

Embryogenesis is a time of rapid cell proliferation and growth, both of which require uninterrupted high levels of energy (adenosine triphosphate or ATP). As outlined by Wilson (1), there are four main pathways by which ATP levels can be adversely modulated by teratogens: (*a*) inadequate glucose stores; (*b*) interference with glycolysis; (*c*) interference with the citric acid cycle; and (*d*) impairment of the terminal electron transport system. If different populations of cells within the embryo have different energy requirements, altered energy metabolism would be expected to produce abnormal embryonic development. This has been elegantly demonstrated by the work of Mackler and Shepard (10) regarding the relationship of oxidative energy metabolism and achondroplasia. Their research has shown that, in both the achondroplastic mutant in rabbits (ac/ac) and in some forms of human achondroplasia, a partial defect in terminal electron transport exists. They postulate that this oxidative defect is selectively expressed in the oxygen-poor cartilaginous growth plates, resulting in reduced cell division and tissue growth and, ultimately, in the characteristic shortening of the long bones.

These results indicate that mutations affecting energy metabolism can produce profound developmental defects. In addition, a fairly extensive literature demonstrates that agents capable of interfering with energy metabolism (e.g., riboflavin deficiencies and 6-aminonicotinamide) are potent developmental toxicants. Although a precise cause and effect relationship has been difficult to demonstrate in these studies, the findings emphasize the need for continued research.

## ALTERED ELECTROLYTE AND FLUID BALANCE

During normal embryogenesis, critical fluid-filled spaces develop including the ventricles of the brain, the cardiovascular space, as well as extraembryonic compartments (amnion, allantois, and yolk sac). Grabowski (11) has reviewed the literature and postulated that regulation of these fluid-filled spaces is essential for normal embryogenesis. He has also presented a mechanistic pathway involving alterations in fluid balance and abnormal development termed the "edema syndrome." Using hypoxia as the initiating agent, Grabowski has shown that one of the early changes induced by oxygen deprivation is hypoosmolarity in the extraembryonic compartments. This hypoosmolarity promotes an inrush of fluids leading to hypervolemia and increased blood pressure, which, in turn, produce edema, hematomas, and blisters in a variety of tissues. Tissue disruption then leads to abnormal embryogenesis. In addition to hypoxia, agents such as trypan blue, hypertonic solutions, and adrenal cortical hormones induce a similar syndrome. Moreover, many teratogens, especially those studied in vitro, have been reported to cause edema in the exposed embryo. Thus, osmolar imbalance may be a mechanism of toxicity common to a wide variety of developmental toxicants.

## ALTERED pH

Intracellular pH is known to control or to be associated with a variety of functions critical for normal development such as proliferation, differentiation, protein synthesis, contraction, gap junctional conductance, cytoskeletal protein interactions, and glycolysis (12). Over the past 7 yr, Scott et al. (13) have shown that certain teratogens decrease intracellular pH in target cells, inducing either intra- or extracellular acidosis. Among these agents, acetazolamide is the best studied. Regulation of intracellular pH as a potential mechanism of developmental toxicity is particularly intriguing, since many teratogens are weak acids (e.g., valproic acid) or induce acidosis (e.g., alcohol, diabetes mellitus, phenylketonuria).

## PATHOLOGICAL MANIFESTATIONS

Pathological mechanisms in the embryo and/or fetus differ in many ways from those in adults. The usual inflammatory process is absent, and the conceptus mounts very little immunological response, especially during the earlier periods. Dead cells are phagocytized without scar formation, resulting in absence or diminution of the affected organ. In addition, cell death itself is essential to normal morphogenesis of embryonic organs and occurs in a planned,

orderly fashion. For instance, cell death between the digits allows for their separation; in its absence, webbing between the fingers can result. During both early and late fetal development, various deformations can arise because of oligohydramnios and positional restrictions. Clubbed foot, for example, is sometimes associated with restricted space in the uterus.

## MANIFESTATIONS OF DEVELOPMENTAL TOXICITY

### Congenital Defects

#### FREQUENCY AND IMPORTANCE

Congenital defects are the number one cause of death in infants (14). Two to three percent of newborns have a major anomaly requiring medical attention (15, 16). Certain minor anomalies such as cleft uvula, preauricular tags, or minor hypospadias are found as often as 1% each in carefully examined individuals. After the end of the first year, an additional 5% of defects are detected. This group may include aneuploidy (0.5% of newborns), mental retardation (approximately 3% of school-aged children), and certain defects of the renal and cardiac systems.

Table 4.1 gives some examples of rates of congenital defects at different stages of human development. Embryos and fetuses that spontaneously die in utero have a rate of congenital anomalies of about 20%; by natural and unknown causes, about 60% of malformed conceptuses are lost (17). Up to 40% of early spontaneous abortions may have aneuploidy. The congenital defect rate in stillbirths and prematures is intermediate to that of the embryo and the newborn (18). These differences in observed rates at various stages of development can seriously impact on interpretation of human epidemiological studies of reproductive outcomes.

Our knowledge about the causes and prevention of congenital defects is limited. About 20% of congenital defects are associated with gene mutations and another 5% are associated with chromosomal aberrations. Less than 10% of the remaining anomalies are known to be due to teratogenic agents. Although slightly over one-half of the approximate 2000 agents

**Table 4.1.**
**Defect Rates per 1000 at Different Stages of Development[a]**

| | Spontaneous Abortuses | Elective Termination | Stillborn and Premature | Newborns |
|---|---|---|---|---|
| Neutral tube defects | 13.8 | 2.4 | 4.4 | 0.3–0.9 |
| Cleft palate | 1.3 | 1.1 | 1–4 | 1.0–2.7 |
| Cleft lip/palate | 6.9 | 3.2 | 8 | 0.4 |
| Cyclopia | 2.7 | 2.1 | | 0 |
| Polydactyly | 2.7 | 2.8 | | 0.5–1.4 |
| Sirenomelia and caudal regression | 4.2 | | | 0 |
| Amniotic bands | 4.2 | | | 0.03 |
| Turner's syndrome | 90 | | | 0.05 |
| Total anomaly rate | 200 | | 90–140 | 20–30 |
| Chromosome aneuploidy | 300–600 | 28 | 50 | 5 |

[a]Data derived from Shepard TH, Fantel AG, Fitzsimmon J. Congenital defect rates among spontaneous abortuses: twenty years of monitoring. Teratology 1989;39:325–331; Fantel AG, Shepard TH. Morphological analysis of spontaneous abortuses. In: Bennett MJ, Edmonds DK, eds. Spontaneous and recurrent abortion. Oxford: Blackwell Publications, 1987:8–28.

tested in laboratory animals are teratogenic, only about 30 have been shown to be teratogenic in humans (19, 20). Known and suspected human teratogens are listed in the Appendix at end of the chapter. However, the majority of the 90,000 chemicals in widespread commercial use have not been adequately tested for developmental toxicity.

The disproportionate identification of animal teratogens is due to use of higher doses, larger number of exposed fetuses, and other methodological factors unique to experimental systems. Most teratologists accept the principle that any agent can be shown to be teratogenic in an animal provided enough is given at the sensitive time in development (Karnofsky's principle).

## PRINCIPLES OF TERATOGENESIS

In this section, we consider determinants of the types, severity, and incidences of abnormalities that may result from exposure of the gravida to embryotoxicants. In particular, the consequences of such exposures are strongly conditioned by inherent characteristics of the exposed subject, as well as by those of the agent. Other important factors include dose, timing, and route of exposure. The complexity of these factors and their interactions have limited the development of accepted risk assessment models in teratology. Further progress requires commitment to basic studies in mechanistic teratology (1, 21).

## Agents

A wide range of agents is capable of inducing malformations in animals. These agents include insufficient or excessive endogenous compounds, medications, industrial chemicals, environmental contaminants, physical conditions, and infectious agents. There is a broad spectrum of embryotoxic effects that can be induced by specific agents or classes of agents; studies in experimental animals have generated descriptions of malformation patterns associated with more than 2000 substances (20, 22, 23). As mentioned earlier, only approximately 1% of these agents has been definitively associated with malformations in humans.

Teratogenic agents can be classified on a conceptual spectrum that ranges from general to specific. A *general* teratogen is theoretically capable of damaging any organ or tissue exposed during a sensitive stage in development. Although it is likely that no "pure" general teratogen in fact exists, the closest example might be X-irradiation, which is capable of inducing a broad range of defects, depending on the time in gestation when exposure occurs. Figure 4.4 presents the differing results of exposure of pregnant rats to 100 rad of X-irradiation at different times in gestation. Although irradiation clearly has a broad range of developmental targets, atomic bomb data from Hiroshima and Nagasaki indicate the extreme sensitivity of regions of the CNS and temporal sensitivity of the first trimester. Sensitivity of a

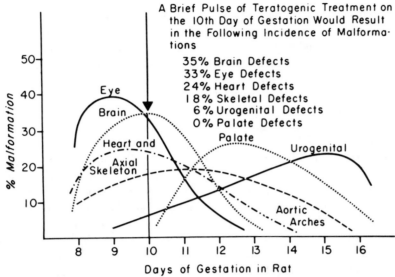

**Figure 4.4.** Group of curves representing the susceptibility of particular organs and organ systems in rat embryos to irradiation given on different days of gestation. If the agent were applied on day 10, a syndrome would result involving the organs, the curves of which are intersected by the vertical line, with percentages of incidence corresponding to the points at which the curves were crossed. Shifting the time of treatment from day 10 to another day would alter the composition of the syndrome both qualitatively and quantitatively. Modified from Wilson JG. Environment and birth defects. New York: Academic Press, 1973:19.

tissue may result from differences in mitotic rates, oxygenation, rates of cytotoxic repair, concentrations of cytoprotective compounds, or other metabolic specifics.

Radioiodine and other goitrogenic compounds represent examples from the *specific* end of the teratogenic spectrum. The spatial and temporal specificity of these compounds derive from the capacity of the developing thyroid to collect and to store iodine after 70 days of gestation; alteration in growth of the thyroid is the major malformation induced. Significantly, agents that have frequently associated "index" malformations often also exert other, less constant (or perhaps less obvious) effects. For example, although phocomelia was the most common feature of the thalidomide embryopathy, many other abnormalities were repeatedly observed. Specific agents often induce "syndromes" of effects seen in a variety of organs and tissues; but, because the developmental sensitivities of individual tissues vary widely, the complete range of teratogenic features is infrequently observed in a single individual. This factor clearly acts to complicate risk assessment in teratology. Participation of a qualified dysmorphologist in clinical assess-

ment and epidemiological studies of malformations is important for accurate classification.

## Timing

Organogenesis is recognized as the period during which embryos are maximally sensitive to the teratogenic activity of toxic agents. This sensitive period in rodents is approximately 1 week, while in humans it lasts approximately 40 days. Because terminal differentiation of cells is incomplete before organogenesis, exposures very early in gestation tend to have a dichotomous outcome, inducing lethality at high doses or permitting systemic repair to occur at low doses. Exceptions may exist, however. Several recent reports indicate that preimplantation exposure to certain organic toxicants may have teratogenic consequences in experimental animals. The most common feature of exposure to developmental toxicants during the later fetal period is size reduction of the fetus and/or its organs.

Perhaps because of its long period of differentiation and development, the teratogenic sensitivity of the CNS may extend even beyond parturition. Nevertheless, its maximal sensitivity occurs during first-trimester organogenesis in humans. Teratogenicity studies of individuals irradiated at Hiroshima and Nagasaki, those exposed to severe famine in the Netherlands during the Second World War, and studies involving high-dose ethanol consumption (fetal alcohol syndrome) all confirm the heightened teratogenic vulnerability of the brain during the first trimester.

Because there are major differences in the developmental time tables for specific embryonic structures, the precise timing of exposure during organogenesis is a key determinant of outcome of exposure. As shown in Figure 4.4, temporal windows of sensitivity to irradiation differ for individual organs in the rat, and teratogenic sensitivity appears to be at its peak early in organogenesis. An obvious corollary of these observations is that the number of systems damaged by a teratogenic insult increases with the total time of exposure.

## Dose

As in other areas of toxicology, documentation of embryotoxicity requires that the incidence of teratogenicity increase with the dose administered. In the absence of a statistically significant dose-response relationship, it is not possible to distinguish a true from a fortuitous association. The limited number of humans affected by teratogens prevents finding a dose-response. In experimental animal models, virtually all teratogenic dose-response curves display a threshold. Doses just below the threshold are considered to be at the "no-observed-adverse-effect level" (NOAEL). Although the basis of this threshold is often unclear, it is believed that the induction of permanent malformations may require a minimal number of cellular "hits" before the repair capacity of the embryo is exceeded. This concept generally separates teratology from the fields of mutagenesis and carcinogenesis, where a single hit is postulated to be causative. A thoughtful discussion of the threshold question has been published (24).

Virtually any agent represents a potential teratogen. The so-called principle of Karnofsky states that any agent will display teratogenic activity at some dose at the appropriate time in

some animal. This includes many exposures that are intuitively innocuous (water, salt) or that have been shown by epidemiological study to be nonteratogenic in humans. Unlike most other subdisciplines of toxicology, developmental toxicology involves multiple distinct targets—prospective mother, father (in the case of germ cell mutation), and conceptus(es). For prenatal exposures, effects on the pregnant woman and conceptus are often related in complex ways, and toxicity data from both must be considered in the evaluation of experimental data and their application to teratogenicity screening (Fig. 4.2). There is a wide potential range in the ratios between maternal and embryonic toxicity for agents. The ratio between adult and developmental toxicity (A/D ratio) serves as an estimate of the relative embryotoxicity.

Animal testing is generally performed at doses up to those that exceed maternally toxic levels. These doses may greatly exceed actual or anticipated human exposure levels. Clearly, agents such as thalidomide that display high A/D ratios represent the greatest threats to human embryonic development. However, certain therapeutic agents, such as the retinoids used to treat cystic acne, are employed at or near levels that are toxic to the mother. These too may pose grave risks to the embryo.

## Route

The route of exposure is another determinant of the embryotoxic action of an agent. For example, thalidomide is an effective teratogen when administered by the oral route, but not when administered intraperitoneally. When testing is carried out for regulatory purposes, it is important to employ the route closest to that of actual or anticipated human exposure. Thus, drugs given orally are generally tested by gastric intubation; parenteral compounds are administered to experimental animals by subcutaneous, intraperitoneal, or intravenous routes, as appropriate. Since inhalation represents the most common route of exposure in the industrial setting, exposures by inhalation are important to consider but very costly to perform.

Although the contribution of route as a determinant of teratogenic outcome is poorly understood, the following features may be involved: (a) agents administered orally may be hydrolyzed in the stomach or not absorbed; (b) agents administered subcutaneously may be slowly absorbed, limiting peak blood concentrations that can reach the conceptus; (c) the route of administration of an agent is an important determinant of its sites and rates of biotransformation, pharmacokinetics, and elimination. Many teratogens must be bioactivated by the mother or conceptus to be active.

## Species/Strain

The forms, frequencies, and severity of abnormalities induced by individual embryotoxicants are strongly dependent on the genetic and phenotypic backgrounds of the pregnant woman and conceptus(es). The teratogenic responses of several animal strains to a number of agents have been summarized (23). Most human teratogens are active in experimental animals. Any of the factors discussed above may be involved in the differential responses of different animals. For example, pathways of drug metabolism in different strains or species may result in exposure of embryos to different metabolites (agents). Temporal differences in lengths of gestation or organogenetic events may result in differing periods of exposure to toxicants. As noted previously, test doses may greatly exceed human exposures, and differences in maternal and embryonic drug metabolism, elimination, and sensitivity may modulate exposure to potent embryotoxicants. Apparent species differences may also result from exposures via different routes. For example, human exposure routes may be impractical in experimental animals as is frequently the case with drugs of abuse. Differences in placental membranes, as well as placental transport and biotransformation, may modulate embryonic exposures. Genetic background and differences in developmental processes may also be important. Suffice it to say that the features discussed here represent only a small sample and that their complex interactions are likely to be found at the heart of species and strain specificity.

A practical extension of this subject (pharmacogenetics) is to detect human genetic dimorphisms in metabolic activity among individuals exposed to certain toxicants. It is possible that genetic subgroups can be identified and shown to be more susceptible to the teratogenic action of certain agents. For example, the anticonvulsant medication, phenytoin, is metabolized to reactive epoxide intermediates. Genetic differences have been identified in the activity of epoxide hydrolase, the enzyme that detoxifies these reactive metabolites, and may influence fetal susceptibility to the teratogenic effects of this agent (25). Similarly, recent evidence suggests that the risk for alcohol-related birth defects may be affected by genetic variability in polymorphisms for alcohol dehydrogenases, the rate-limiting enzymes in ethanol metabolism (26). A greater understanding of pharmacogenetics could lead to important preventive measures.

## Fetal Loss

During the prenatal period, the human conceptus faces severe selective pressures; loss rates are high, particularly during the early weeks following conception. When determined by maternal interview, the spontaneous abortion rate is commonly placed at around 15%; but more careful ascertainment of pregnancies following the first missed menstrual period increases the figure to nearly 25%. Data from a number of sources now indicate that even this figure is considerably below the actual rate, because the majority of loss occurs before pregnancies are clinically identified. When these studies are considered, the total rate of loss of human conceptuses approaches 50%.

These higher estimates of loss are based on data from several different types of studies. First, a direct examination of the uterine contents of pregnant women undergoing hysterectomy before the first missed menstrual period found that well over 50% of specimens showed embryonic and trophoblastic abnormalities incompatible with intrauterine survival (27). Second, the Boues and their colleagues performed careful analysis of karyotype in spontaneous abortion (28). Employing some simple assumptions regarding the absence of expected (and complementary) karyotypes, they concluded that the majority of embryos with deviant karyotypes aborted before implantation and clinical recognition of pregnancy. Combining ascertained with "silent" loss, they calculated a rate of embryonic loss of 50%. Finally, recent studies have utilized sensitive radioimmunoassays of human chorionic gonadotropin (HCG) to detect pregnancy during the first 2 weeks after implantation. This research has documented a total rate of pregnancy wastage of approximately 40% (29). This figure would likely be increased if pregnancy could be documented in the first week before implantation and differentiation of the trophoblast. Clearly any study of spontaneous abortions among workers must take these variations under consideration.

The reasons for the high incidence of pregnancy loss in humans remain largely unknown. Studies reveal considerable heterogeneity among abortus specimens; some have chromosomal and morphological abnormalities, whereas others are apparently normal. As indicated in Table 4.1, aneuploidy is common among human abortuses, and over 90% of chromosomal aberrations are lethal in utero. On the other hand, among late embryonic specimens, it is estimated that only 8% of chromosomally normal and 2–3% of karyotypically and morphologically normal conceptions miscarry (30). Moreover, most aneuploid specimens abort during the first 4–6 weeks of pregnancy, while loss of normal conceptuses is more common later in gestation (31, 32). We believe that selective pressure against aneuploidy is relatively relaxed in humans. In contrast to most other mammals, there is no obligate breeding season in humans, permitting successful delivery and infant rearing throughout the year. The absence of temporal constraints on reproduction should permit early prenatal losses to be replaced, minimizing compromise of fitness.

In general, sources of pregnancy wastage can be categorized into intrinsic abnormalities of the conceptus (e.g., gene mutations, chromosomal anomalies) and environmental factors (including the immediate uterine environment, maternal conditions, or external exposures), acting alone or in concert. Intrinsic defects may be either maternal or paternal in origin, arising in the germ cells before conception or at the time of fertilization. For example, advanced maternal age and X-irradiation are associated with aneuploid conceptions. In approximately 5% of recurrent abortion cases, balanced translocations are found in one parent. To date, few environmental factors have been definitively linked to spontaneous abortion. Some postulated risk factors are listed in Table 4.2 (33, 34).

With the exception of a few factors such as parental age, several lines of evidence suggest that the role of environmental factors is most notable among chromosomally normal conceptions. First, analyses of fetal loss among geographically disparate populations at various time intervals reveal remarkable consistency in the proportions of specific chromosomal aberrations at miscarriage. While rates of chromosomally normal loss are similar in the first trimester across studies, frequencies differ markedly for the second trimester, suggesting an influence of environmental factors (32). Second, in a large case-control study involving karyotypes of over 1000 spontaneous abortion specimens, parental occupation was not significantly associated with chromosomally abnormal abortion (35, 36). On the other hand, a few environmental factors such as maternal cigarette smoking (30) and fever during pregnancy (37) were associated with increased loss of karyotypically normal fetuses. Finally, the frequency of occurrence of any single chromosomal aberration is exceedingly small compared to the rate of chromosomally normal losses. From an epidemiological perspective, exposures that increase the incidence of a specific anomaly would have little effect on the overall observed miscarriage rate, while those affecting loss of chromosomally normal conceptions would be much more readily detectable (30).

Studies examining the karyotypic, morphological, and histological characteristics of spontaneous abortion specimens are essential to an understanding of the mechanisms by which intrinsic factors and exposure to environmental agents result in fetal wastage. In all epidemiological investigations of malformations, it is also important to consider that the dose-response curves of many teratogens include an embryolethal segment at the high end. This fact can obscure the interpretation of developmental dose-response relationships by removing malformed infants from the observation at the higher dose ranges (38).

**Table 4.2.**
**Some Possible Environmental Risk Factors for Spontaneous Abortion**[a]

| Factor(s) | Comment |
|---|---|
| Parental age | Advanced maternal age associated with increase in trisomic and chromosomally normal abortions |
| Socioeconomic status | Increased risk of chromosomally normal abortion among socially disadvantaged populations; results may be confounded by differences in ethnicity, patterns of medical care utilization, environmental exposures, etc. |
| Previous abortion | Conflicting evidence regarding role of multiple, prior, induced abortions; may depend on method of termination; prior spontaneous losses increase risk of recurrence; repeat losses to the same woman tend to be chromosomally normal |
| Immunological factors | Increased risk of chromosomally normal losses; important etiological factor in recurrent abortion |
| Hormonal factors | Luteal phase defects implicated in recurrent abortion; in utero diethylstilbestrol (DES) exposure associated with increased risk of spontaneous loss; no increased loss rate among users of oral contraceptives |
| Chronic diseases | Risk in diabetics relates to degree of glucose control; some studies show increased loss rates among untreated epileptics, others do not; systemic lupus erythematosus associated with increased risk; role of thyroid diseases remains unclear |
| Anatomic abnormalities | Uterine anomalies associated with increased risk of chromosomally normal loss; cervical incompetence increases risk of mid trimester abortion; risk factors include prior cervical surgery (dilatation & curettage, amputation, conization), DES exposure, parity |
| Maternal fever | Increased risk of chromosomally normal abortion; difficult to separate role of fever from infection itself |
| Cigarette smoking | Modest dose-related effect on risk for chromosomally normal abortion; in one study, increased risk found only in socially disadvantaged women |
| Alcohol | Dose-related increase in risk of chromosomally normal loss; in one study, effect noted only in socially disadvantaged women |
| Irradiation | Possible association with aneuploid abortion (triploidy, possibly trisomy) |

[a]Modified from Kline J, Stein Z, Susser M. Conception to birth: epidemiology of prenatal development. New York: Oxford University Press, 1989:123.

## SUMMARY

This chapter has presented an overview of developmental toxicity, with particular emphasis on teratogenicity and fetal loss. Developmental toxicity, however, encompasses a broad range of adverse outcomes that result from deleterious exposures in the preconception period, throughout gestation, and postnatally until sexual maturation. We are only beginning to understand the varied and complex molecular mechanisms by which developmental toxicants exert their effects. This chapter highlights research areas that are currently receiving attention as well as those that are receiving less attention, but which previous work indicates are important. In so doing, we hope to encourage others to embark upon research careers that will provide some of the missing information concerning mechanisms of developmental toxicity. This knowledge is essential if we are ever to predict and prevent the action of environmental agents hazardous to human development.

## REFERENCES

1. Wilson JG. Current status of teratology—general principles and mechanisms derived from animal studies. In: Wilson JG, Fraser FC, eds. Handbook of teratology, Vol. 1. New York: Plenum Press, 1977:47–74.
2. Hsu LYF, Hirschorn K. Numerical and structural chromosome anomalies. In: Wilson JG, Fraser FC, eds. Handbook of teratology, Vol II. New York: Plenum Press, 1977:41–49.
3. Welsch F, Stedman DB, Carson JL. Teratogen interference with cell interactions: cell-to-cell channel disruption as a potential mechanism of abnormal development. In: Welsch F, ed. Approaches to elucidate mechanisms in teratogenesis. Washington, DC: Hemisphere Publishing Corporation, 1987:233–254.
4. Edelman GM. Morphoregulatory molecules. Biochemistry 1988;27:3533–3354.

5. Sulik KK, Cook CS, Webster WS. Teratogens and craniofacial malformations: relationships to cell death. Development 1988;213–231.

6. Ritter EJ. Altered biosynthesis. In: Wilson JG, Fraser FC, eds. Handbook of teratology, Vol. 2. New York: Plenum Press, 1977:99–106.

7. Skalko RG. Cellular adhesions in teratogenesis. In: Persaud TVN, Chundley AE, Skalko RG, eds. Basic concepts in teratology. New York: Alan R. Liss, 1985:103–118.

8. Mirkes PE. Cyclophosphamide teratogenesis: a review. Teratog Carcinog Mutag 1985;5:75–88.

9. Balling R, Mutler G, Gruss P, Kessel M. Craniofacial abnormalities induced by ectopic expression of the homeobox gene Hox 1.1 in transgenic mice. Cell 1989;58:337–347.

10. Mackler B, Shepard TH. Human achondroplasia: defective mitochondrial oxidative energy metabolism may produce the pathophysiology. Teratology 1989;40:571–582.

11. Grabowski C. Altered electrolyte and fluid balance. In: Wilson JG, Fraser FC, eds. Handbook of teratology, Vol. 2. New York: Plenum Press, 1977:153–170.

12. Nuccitali R, Deamer D. Intracellular pH: its measurement, regulation and utilization in cellular functions. New York: Alan R. Liss, 1982.

13. Scott WJ, Duggon CA, Schreiner CM, Collins MD. Reduction of embryonic intracellular pH: a potential mechanism of acetazolamide-induced limb malformations. Toxicol Appl Pharmacol 1990;103:238–254.

14. Centers for Disease Control. Contribution of birth defects to infant mortality: United States, 1986. MMWR 1989;38:633–635.

15. McIntosh R, Merritt KK, Richards MR, Samuels MN, Bellows MS. The incidence of congenital malformations: a study of 5964 pregnancies. Pediatrics 1954;14:505–522.

16. Holmes LB. Congenital anomalies. In: Oski FA, ed. Principles and practice of pediatrics. Philadelphia: JB Lippincott, 1990:258–261.

17. Shepard TH, Fantel AG, Fitzsimmons J. Congenital defect rates among spontaneous abortuses: twenty years of monitoring. Teratology 1989;39:325–331.

18. Shepard TH, Fantel AG. Embryonic and early fetus loss. Clin Perinatol 1979; 6:219–243.

19. Shepard TH. Human teratogenicity. In: Barness L, ed. Advances in pediatrics. Chicago: Year Book Medical Publishers, 1986:33:225–268.

20. Shepard TH. A catalog of teratogenic agents. 6th ed. Baltimore: Johns Hopkins Press, 1989.

21. Juchau MR, ed. The biochemical basis of chemical teratogenesis. New York: Elsevier-North-Holland, 1981.

22. Schardein JL. Chemically induced birth defects. New York: Marcel Dekker, 1985.

23. Jelovsek FR, Mattison DR, Chen JC. Prediction of risk for human developmental toxicity: how important are animal studies for hazard identification? Obstet Gynecol 1989;74:624–636.

24. Gaylor DW, Sheehan DM, Young JF, Mattison DR. The threshold dose question in teratogenesis. Teratology 1988;8:389–391.

25. Beuhler BA, Delimont D, von Vaes M, Finnell RH. Prenatal prediction of risk of the fetal hydantoin syndrome. N Engl J Med 1990;322:1567–1572.

26. Sokol RJ, Smith J, Erhart CB, et al. A genetic basis for alcohol-related birth defects (ARBD). Alcohol 1989;13:343–348.

27. Hertig AT, Rock J, Adams EC, Menkin MC. Thirty-four fertilized human ova, good, bad, and indifferent, recovered from 210 women of known fertility. Pediatrics 1959;23:202–211.

28. Boue J, Boue A, Lazar P. Retrospective and prospective epidemiological studies of 1500 karyotyped human abortuses. Teratology 1975;12:11–26.

29. Wilcox AJ, Wernberg CR, O'Conner JG, et al. Incidence of early loss of pregnancy. N Engl J Med 1988;319:189–194.

30. Kline J, Stein Z, Susser M. Conception to birth: epidemiology of prenatal development. New York: Oxford University Press, 1989.

31. Fantel AG, Shepard TH. Morphological analysis of spontaneous abortuses. In: Bennett MJ, Edmonds DK, eds. Spontaneous and recurrent abortion. Oxford: Blackwell Publications, 1987:8–28.

32. Kline J, Stein Z. Epidemiology of chromosomal anomalies in spontaneous abortion: prevalence, manifestations and determinants. In Bennett MJ, Edmonds DK, eds. Spontaneous and recurrent abortion. Oxford: Blackwell Publications, 1987:29–50.

33. Faulk WP, Hunt JS. Human trophoblast antigens. Immunol Allerg 1990;10:27–47.

34. Bennett MJ, Edmonds DK, eds. Spontaneous and recurrent abortion. Oxford: Blackwell Scientific Publications, 1987.

35. Hatch M, Kline J, Stein Z, Warburton D. Male risk factors for spontaneous abortion [Abstract]. Am J Epidemiol 1984;120:499–500.

36. Silverman J, Kline J, Hutzler M, Stein Z, Warburton D. Maternal employment characteristics and the chromosomal characteristics of spontaneously aborted conceptions. J Occup Med 1985;27:427–438.

37. Kline J, Stein Z, Susser M, Warburton D. Fever during pregnancy and spontaneous abortion. Am J Epidemiol 1985;121:832–842.

38. Selevan SG, Lemasters GK. The dose-response fallacy in human reproductive studies of toxic exposures. J Occup Med 1987;29:451–454.

# Human Teratogens

## KNOWN TERATOGENIC AGENTS

Ionizing Radiation
    Atomic weapons
    Radioiodine
    Therapeutic
Infections
    Cytomegalovirus (CMV)
    Herpes virus hominis ? I and II
    Parvovirus B-19 (Erthema infectiosum)
    Rubella virus
    Syphilis
    Toxoplasmosis
    Venezuelan equine encephalitis virus
Metabolic Imbalance
    Alcoholism
    Endemic cretinism
    Diabetes
    Folic acid deficiency
    Hyperthermia
    Phenylketonuria
    Rheumatic disease and congenital heart
      block
    Virilizing tumors
Drugs and Environmental Chemicals
    Aminopterin and methylaminopterin
    Androgenic hormones
    Busulfan
    Captropril; Enalapril and renal damage
    Chlorobiphenyls
    Cocaine
    Coumarin anticoagulants
    Cyclophosphamide
    Diethylstilbestrol
    Diphenylhydantoin and trimethadione
    Etretinate
    Lithium
    Methimazole and scalp defects
    Mercury, organic

    Penicillamine
    Tetracyclines
    Thalidomide
    Trimethadione
    13-cis-retinoic acid (isotreninoin and Ac-
      cutane)
    Valproic acid

## POSSIBLE TERATOGENS

    Binge drinking
    Carbamazepine
    Cigarette smoking
    Disulfiram
    High Vitamin A
    Lead
    Primidone
    Streptomycin
    Toluene abuse
    Varicella virus
    Zinc deficiency

## UNLIKELY TERATOGENS

    Agent Orange
    Anesthetics
    Aspartame
    Aspirin (but aspirin in the second half of
      pregnancy may increase cerebral hem-
      orrhage during delivery)
    Bendectin (antinauseants)
    Birth control pills
    Marijuana, lysergic acid diethylamide
      (LSD)
    Metronidazole
    Oral contraceptives
    Rubella vaccine
    Spermicides
    Video display screens

# 5

·······························································

# Developmental Toxicology: Male-mediated Effects

Despite historical references to male-mediated effects on progeny that date from antiquity, studies of adverse influences on pregnancy have dealt almost exclusively with maternal variables. Both Carthage and Sparta had laws prohibiting the use of alcohol by newlyweds, and Robert Burton's *Anatomy of Melancholy*, published in 1621, cited Gellius: "If a drunken man get a child it will never likely have a good brain." The harmful effects of parental drinking were of grave concern during England's gin epidemic of the 1700s (1). By the early 20th century, these concerns were paralleled by medical interest in the effects of alcohol on offspring. Systematic reports linking reproductive effects to an industrial chemical were first published in the late 19th century and addressed lead toxicity. High rates of infertility, spontaneous abortions, stillbirths, neonatal deaths, macrocephaly, and convulsions in offspring were recorded in lead-working communities in many parts of Europe (2). Women were banned from work in the heavy lead trades, although the reports suggested that both males and females were adversely affected.

Human reproduction is intermittent in nature and characterized by low rates of conception, so that large study populations are often needed to detect significant effects of xenobiotic exposure. As a result, a variety of agents may impair reproduction but remain unde-

tected (3, 4). In addition, both partners may be exposed to a toxicant, compounding the challenge of assessing the comparative role of male and female variables.

Most discoveries in human reproductive biology are based upon earlier investigations in animals; this is due both to ethical constraints imposed on human studies and to the difficulties in controlling genetic, environmental, and exposure factors. Despite these limitations, past history indicates that it is usually the "rediscovery" of a reproductive hazard through human tragedy that directs appropriate attention to the problem (5), as illustrated by the history of reproductive studies in the 20 yr preceding the thalidomide epidemic of 1961. Despite the considerable body of evidence from animal research indicating that the mammalian placenta was not impervious to toxicants, it was not until the thalidomide tragedy that it became generally acknowledged that a variety of agents could cross the human placenta and affect the developing organism. Had thalidomide not produced obvious structural malformations, but resulted instead in more subtle alterations in postnatal development or behavior, there might still be a reluctance to acknowledge human placental transport of toxicants or the direct effect of environmental agents, such as radiation or viruses, upon the conceptus. Similarly, the identification of the nematocide dibromochloropropane (DBCP) as a reproductive toxicant in the human male was preceded by findings several years earlier of its adverse effects on animal reproduction (6).

The thalidomide tragedy resulted in active study of the sequelae of maternal exposure during pregnancy for the fetus and neonate. Yet reports of male-mediated effects on reproductive outcome were given little credence before the 1977 report of infertility in males exposed to DBCP (7). Epidemiological and animal research has since identified a number of drugs and other xenobiotic agents that may adversely affect the reproductive process in males and that are associated with adverse pregnancy outcome in their unexposed wives (8, 9). Nonetheless, there appears to be a reluctance to accept the accumulating evidence of paternally mediated effects on progeny outcome. This may be due, in part, to the difficulty in postulating mechanisms for paternal transmission, but possible cultural or other non-scientific rationale or skepticism cannot be dismissed (10).

## ASSESSMENT OF REPRODUCTIVE INJURY

To date, reproductive studies in the male have primarily explored the effects of toxic agents on fertility rather than on progeny. However, fertility assessments are limited by their insensitivity as measures of reproductive injury. Which of the most common measures of fertility (i.e., sperm concentration, motility, and morphology) best predict reproductive success or failure in humans is unknown, as is the relationship of various measures of sperm structure and function to reproductive outcome, should conception occur (4, 11, 12). In animal studies, gender-specific effects on fertility are usually not identified in single generation tests of reproduction; continuous breeding protocols, with cohabitation for 14 weeks and crossover matings between treated animals and untreated controls, are employed only if subfertility is evident (5). As a consequence, there is no information on male-mediated effects if fertility is unaffected. Improved test protocols are needed to assess the independent contribution of each parent to developmental outcome.

Evaluation of pregnancy outcome is required to assess the consequences of reproductive injury fully. Both human and animal studies should encompass not only measures of reproductive indices (e.g., pre- and postimplantation loss, spontaneous abortions, stillbirths, birthweight) and dysmorphology, but also evaluation of functional endpoints (e.g., behavioral, biochemical, neuroendocrine changes) throughout postnatal development. These measures frequently provide greater sensitivity in the detection of alterations induced by parental exposure than changes in genotoxic endpoints, such as dominant lethality or altered sperm morphology (13).

## AGENTS IN SEMEN

Xenobiotics can enter the fluids of the testis, epididymis, and male accessory organs and, ultimately, the semen. Catheterization and cannulation techniques have confirmed the presence of a wide range of exogenous agents at these several sites (14). By ligating the tubuli recti that lead from the testis to the epididymis, regional differences in semen composition can be identified. As demonstrated in animals, the many therapeutic and nontherapeutic chemicals identified in seminal fluid have the potential to impact reproductive outcome adversely (15, 16). Whether xenobiotic agents in seminal fluid can alter embryonic or fetal development postconception is unknown (17).

## MALE-MEDIATED EFFECTS ON DEVELOPMENTAL OUTCOME

As shown in Table 5.1, male-mediated effects on offspring have been demonstrated for a number of diverse agents used therapeutically, recreationally, and by accidental exposure in the workplace and environment. Effects observed in experimental animals include alterations in fetal and neonatal survival, growth, several behaviors, immunological competence, thermoregulation, responsivity to stress, and reproductive endocrinology. Effects in humans include an increase in spontaneous abortions, stillbirths, low birthweight, and an increased incidence of childhood malignancies (lymphomas, leukemias, neuroblastomas, brain and kidney tumors). Despite faulty design or inconclu-

**Table 5.1.**
**Some Agents With Reported Effects on Reproductive Outcome Following Paternal Exposure (Human/Infrahuman Species)[a]**

| Class | Agent | Effects[b] on Offspring | | | | | | | Reference |
|---|---|---|---|---|---|---|---|---|---|
| | | Death | BW | CM | Behav | CA | RE | Other | |
| Chemical | | | | | | | | | |
|   Therapeutic | Anesthetic gases | ±/− | +/+ | | o/+ | | | | 4, 33, 55–57 |
| | Cyclophospha-mide | o/+ | o/+ | o/+ | o/+ | o/+ | | o/+ | 25, 27–31, 58, 59 |
|   Recreational | Alcohol | o/− | +/± | −/− | o/+ | | o/+ | o/+ | 18–24, 60 |
| | Smoking | | | | | +/o | | | 41 |
| | Opiates | o/− | o/+ | | o/+ | | o/+ | o/+ | 4, 32, 48, 61, 62 |
|   Occupational | Agent Orange | ±/o | | ±/o | | | | | 63, 64 |
| | Lead | +/+ | o/+ | | o/+ | | | o/+ | 2, 34–36, 65 |
| | Fire smoke | | | +/o | | | | | 42, 43 |
| | Solvents, hydro-carbons | +/o | | | o/+ | +/o | | | 38–40, 50, 66 |
| Physical | Ionizing radia-tion | | | | o/+ | +/+ | | | 13, 44, 67 |
| | Electromag-netic fields | | | | | +/o | | | 46 |

[a]An overview of the spectrum of agents that have been reported to produce male-mediated alterations in fetal or postnatal development of offspring. Not intended to be inclusive.
[b]Death = spontaneous abortions, resorptions, or stillbirths; BW = reduced birthweight; CM = structural congenital malformations; Behav = behavioral alterations; CA = childhood cancer; RE = defects in reproductive endocrinology; Other = functional deficits (immunological, neurochemical, physiological; cross-generational); + = effect present; − = effect absent; o = not reported.

sive findings in some studies, there are sufficient valid and replicable data available in both the human and experimental literature to document the impact of the father on developmental outcome.

## Alcohol

The description in 1973 of the "fetal alcohol syndrome" led to extensive investigation into the effects of maternal consumption of alcohol during pregnancy on fetal and neonatal development. It was not accompanied by a similar concern for possible paternally mediated effects. Studies in the male have focused on genetic contributions to alcoholism or on alcohol-induced reproductive impairment, with little emphasis on the possible impact of the drug on offspring.

Recent studies suggest that paternal exposure to alcohol can influence subsequent outcome. Paternal exposure to ethanol, in the absence of maternal exposure, has been associated with alterations in growth, immunological competence, thermoregulation, behavior, and reproductive endocrinological parameters in rodent offspring (18–23). An association between paternal drinking and infant low birthweight has been noted in humans (24).

## Cyclophosphamide

Cyclophosphamide (CP), a cancer chemotherapeutic agent, is one of the most widely studied reproductive toxicants. The drug first gained attention in the late 1970s through several reports of decreased fertility in CP-treated male patients. In some cases, the drug-induced oligo- or azoospermia may have been irreversible and was accompanied by elevations in follicle-stimulating hormone (FSH) (25). No increase in spontaneous abortions or congenital abnormalities have been reported following paternal exposure, but systematic studies are lacking.

In animals, reduced testes weight, transient oligospermia, and a decrease in DNA synthesis in spermatogonia and RNA and protein synthesis in spermatids followed a single high dose of CP (26). In contrast, chronic low-dose exposure did not affect several measures of male reproductive function; no changes were observed in epididymal sperm counts, reproductive organ weights, or in serum testosterone or pituitary gonadotropins. Yet there were significant effects on pregnancy outcome including dose- and time-dependent increases in both pre- and postimplantation loss, increases in growth-retarded and malformed fetuses, and a marked depression of bone marrow (26–28).

In addition to effects on cell and organ systems, paternal exposure of rodents to CP resulted in significant delays in the appearance of standard neurobehavioral developmental landmarks and alterations in a variety of behaviors (29, 30). Learning deficits were reported in three successive generations ($F_3$) following paternal exposure ($F_0$) to low-dose CP, with a greater sensitivity of male progeny to CP-induced abnormalities (31). Both the apparent greater vulnerability of male progeny and cross-generational effects of male exposure have been observed after paternal exposure to other drugs (4, 22, 32, 33).

The detailed and varied profile of effects that have been recorded following paternal CP reflects extensive investigations on this agent. CP is known to suppress both meiosis and mitosis and might have been predicted to affect processes associated with cell replication and maturation during spermatogenesis. However, effects on developmental and behavioral parameters were apparent in the absence of detectable alterations in spermatogenesis and suggest that paternal effects can be variously expressed.

## Occupational and Environmental Agents

Paternal exposure to a number of occupational and environmental agents has been associated with adverse developmental outcomes in various studies. A few agents are briefly reviewed in this section; others, such as anesthetic gases and mercury, are addressed in other chapters of this book.

The literature on the effects of lead on reproduction primarily examines maternal exposure, although lead is a known abortifacient and spermicidal agent. There is convincing evidence that lead alters spermiogenesis and adversely affects fertility (34). Paternal exposure in rats results in a reduction of dendrites in hippocampal pyramidal cells and decrements in learning (35, 36). In a recent study of male workers, preconception blood lead levels greater than 30 μg/dl were associated with an increased risk of spontaneous abortion in their wives (37).

A seminal study examining paternal exposure and developmental outcome found an association between fathers' exposure to solvents or to employment in the aircraft industry and brain tumors in their children (38). Subsequently, many epidemiological studies have reported increases in childhood cancer after paternal exposure to various occupational agents (39). Associations have been observed between childhood brain cancer and paternal exposure to organic solvents in the chemical and petroleum industries and to paints. The latter are also associated with childhood leukemias. Exposure of male workers to organic solvents has also been reported to increase the risk of spontaneous abortion in their spouses (40).

A case-control study of prenatal exposure to parents' smoking and childhood cancer showed an association with father's smoking (in the absence of mother's smoking) and brain cancer, with an apparent greater risk for male children. Although interpretation of these findings is confounded by the possibility of passive exposure both in utero and after birth, the results suggest an independent male-mediated effect (41).

An exploratory case-control study of the risk of birth defects in children of male firefighters detected an increased incidence of septal heart defects, both ventricular and atrial (42). The study focused on structural malformations at birth, with no reported evaluation of possible malignancies. Given the potential reproductive toxicants present in fire smoke, an increase in offspring malignancies might be anticipated in this group barring appropriate precautionary measures to mitigate risk (43).

A six- to eight-fold increase in leukemia was found in children of fathers occupationally exposed to low-level radiation at England's Sellafield nuclear plant (44). This finding contrasts with the long-term studies of atomic bomb survivors that concluded that the risk of adverse reproductive outcome, including early cancer in offspring, was not significantly higher than for nonirradiated parents (45). However, epidemiological studies of genetic indicators are inherently difficult; although the risk may be small, there is no reason to believe that humans, unlike many other species, are exempt from radiation-induced genetic effects (45). Children of fathers exposed in the workplace to electromagnetic fields were also found to be at greater risk for neuroblastoma in early infancy (46).

## MECHANISMS

The etiology of male-mediated effects on developmental outcome is unknown. In animal studies, alterations have been observed after exposure during either pre- or postmeiotic stages of spermatogenesis or during epididymal transit or storage in the epididymal cauda. Thus, any plausible mechanism(s) for male-mediated effects must consider the timing and extent of exposure, as well as the nature of the particular chemical. Given the variety of agents that have been implicated and the wide spectrum of deficits that have been reported, it is unlikely that a single mechanism can adequately explain male-mediated changes. Effects of exogenous agents may result from direct exposure of germ cells at any stage of spermatogenesis or maturation. Alternatively, they may be the sequelae of indirect effects on the testis, epididymis, or accessory sex organs or involve complex interactions with the female at copulation and fertilization.

Induction of germinal mutations by radiation and chemical mutagens is well documented in animals; yet there is no firm evidence that any agent causes germinal mutations in humans, and monitoring for an increase in mutations has been unsuccessful (45, 47). It has been suggested that current methods are inadequate to detect heritable mutations in humans given the size of the exposed cohorts and that new approaches are needed (47). However, with known mutagens or carcinogens, it is reasonable to postulate genetic mechanisms to explain a paternal imprint.

Many of the male-mediated effects reported in the experimental literature involve nonmutagenic agents, and alternative mechanisms have been postulated. Paternal exposure may result in selection of a particular population of gametes for participation in the fertilization process (4). With agents that affect reproductive endocrinological parameters, the altered function of the father's hypothalamic-hypophyseal-gonadal (HPG) axis could participate in this process. The reported changes in HPG function of paternally exposed offspring offer further evidence of profound alterations in the reproductive axis (4, 23, 48). Xenobiotic-induced changes in sperm maturation during epididymal transport, in semen composition, or in sperm motility or metabolism could also affect the population of gametes available for fertilization (4, 9). Active participation of the female in sperm transport may also play a role in any selection process (49).

Male-mediated effects may involve some epigenetic phenomenon. Genomic imprinting may be involved in the genesis of some childhood cancers and has been postulated as a mechanism for the paternal induction of Wilms' tumor, associated with various occupational exposures of the male parent (50, 51). The mechanism of imprinting is thought to involve differential DNA methylation during gametogenesis or before formation of the zygote nucleus after fertilization (52). A related hypothesis focuses on chemically induced changes in the expression of cell surface receptor proteins which, by alterations in DNA, would permanently change cell phenotype (53). Similarly, as male and female pronuclei contribute differentially to the zygote (52), the formation of an adduct between the toxicant and one of the hundreds of proteins present on the sperm perinuclear matrix could potentially alter sperm function and subsequent development. Any epigenetic chromosomal modifications resulting from paternal exposure could also adversely impinge upon subsequent fetal development by affecting the placenta, as the paternal genome is essential for its development (52). In addition, toxicants present in semen could be absorbed through the vaginal epithelium, resulting in exposure of the embryo postconception and throughout pregnancy (17, 54).

## SUMMARY

There is sufficient evidence to suggest a significant role of the male in pregnancy outcome.

Research studies in both humans and animals document adverse developmental effects after paternal exposure to a wide variety of agents. As expected, reported effects vary with the type of agent, dose and duration of exposure, species, and other relevant variables. They frequently occur in the absence of detectable alterations in fertility or other commonly used indices of reproductive success. A wide spectrum of deficits in both prenatal and postnatal development of offspring has been reported including an increase in stillbirths and spontaneous abortions, fetal and neonatal growth retardation, childhood cancers, behavioral changes, altered reproductive function, and carryover of effects into a subsequent generation. There is no a priori reason to assume that male-mediated effects are limited to the agents studied to date. As research directed at paternal influences on the health of the fetus and neonate increases, the number of suspect agents will undoubtedly expand. The potential mechanism(s) for male-mediated effects have yet to be elucidated. However, the broad spectrum of changes reported to follow paternal exposures to several classes of toxicants warrants vigorous exploration of the role of paternal variables in developmental outcome.

## REFERENCES

1. Warner RH, Rosett HL. The effects of drinking on offspring. J Stud Alcohol 1975;36:1395–1420.
2. Rom WN. Effects of lead on the female and reproduction: a review. Mt Sinai J Med 1976;43:542–552.
3. Zenick H, Clegg ED. Assessment of male reproductive toxicity: a risk assessment approach. In: Hayes AW, ed. Principles and methods of toxicology. 2nd ed. New York: Raven Press, 1989:275–309.
4. Friedler G. Effects of limited paternal exposure to xenobiotic agents on the development of progeny. Neurobehav Toxicol Teratol 1985;7:739–743.
5. Lamb JC. Fundamentals of male reproductive toxicity testing. In: Lamb JC, Foster PMD, eds. Physiology and toxicology of male reproduction. New York: Academic Press, 1988:137–153.
6. Torkelson TR, Sadek SE, Rowe VK, et al. Toxicologic investigations of 1,2-dibromo-3-chloropropane. Toxicol Appl Pharmacol 1961;3:545–559.
7. Whorton D, Krauss KM, Marshall S, Milby TH. Infertility in male pesticide workers. Lancet 1977;2:1259–61.
8. Gunderson V, Sackett GP. Paternal effects on reproductive outcome and developmental risk. In: Lamb ME, Brown AL, eds. Advances in developmental psychology. Hillsdale, NJ: Lawrence Erlbaum Associates, 1982: 85–124.
9. Joffe JM, Soyka LF. Paternal drug exposure: effects on reproduction and progeny. Semin Perinatol 1981;6: 116–124.
10. Friedler G. The father and the fetus: facts and fallacies [Abstract]. Annual Meeting Program of American Association for the Advancement of Science, 1991:44.
11. Wyrobek AJ. Male biomarkers of abnormal reproductive outcome. Health Environ Digest 1990;4:1–4.
12. Mattison DR, Plowchalk DR, Meadows MJ, Al-Juburi AZ, Gandy J, Malek A. Reproductive toxicity: male and female reproductive systems as targets for chemical injury. Med Clin North Am 1990;74:391–411.
13. Lowery MC, Au WW, Adams PM, Whorton EB, Legator MS. Male-mediated behavioral abnormalities. Mutat Res 1990;229:213–229.
14. Mann T, Lutwak-Mann C. Passage of chemicals into human and animal semen: mechanisms and significance. Crit Rev Toxicol 1982;2:1–14.
15. Lutwak-Mann C. Observations on progeny of thalidomide-treated male rabbits. Br Med J 1964;1:1090–1091.
16. Hales BF, Smith S, Robaire B. Cyclophosphamide in the seminal fluid of treated males: transmission to females by mating and effect on progeny outcome. Toxicol Appl Pharmacol 1986;84:423–430.
17. Robaire B, Trasler JM, Hales BF. Consequences to the progeny of paternal drug exposure. In: Lobl JT, Hafez ESE, eds. Male fertility and its regulation. Reproductive health series. London: MTP Press, 1985:225–243.
18. Abel EL, Lee JA. Paternal alcohol exposure affects offspring behavior but not body or organ weights in mice. Alcohol Clin Exp Res 1988;12:349–355.
19. Abel EL, Tan SE. Effects of paternal alcohol consumption on pregnancy outcome in rats. Neurotoxicol Teratol 1988;10:187–192.
20. Berk RS, Montgomery IN, Hazlett LD, Abel EL. Paternal alcohol consumption: effects on ocular response and serum antibody response to Pseudomonas aeruginosa infection in offspring. Alcohol Clin Exp Res 1989;13:795–798.
21. Friedler G, Meadows M-E. Effects of paternal ethanol on ethanol-induced hypothermia in mouse offspring [Abstract]. Fed Proc 1987;46:538.
22. Friedler G. Effects of paternal exposure to alcohol and other drugs. Alcohol Health Res World (NIAAA) 1988;12:126–129.
23. Cicero TJ, Adams ML, O'Conner L, Nook B, Meyer ER, Wozniak D. Influence of chronic alcohol administration on representative indices of puberty and sexual maturation in male rats and the development of their progeny. J Pharm Exp Ther 1990;255:707–715.
24. Little RE, Sing CF. Father's drinking and infant birth weight: report of an association. Teratology 1987;36: 59–65.
25. Fairley KF, Barrie JU, Johnson W. Sterility and testicular atrophy related to cyclophosphamide therapy. Lancet 1972;1:568–569.
26. Trasler JM, Hales BF, Robaire B. Chronic low dose cyclophosphamide treatment of adult male rats: effect on fertility, pregnancy outcome and progeny. Biol Reprod 1986;34:275–283.
27. Trasler JM, Hales BF, Robaire B. Paternal cyclo-

phosphamide treatment of rats causes fetal loss and malformations without affecting fertility. Nature 1985;316:144–146.

28. Trasler JM, Hales BF, Robaire B. A time-course study of chronic paternal cyclophosphamide treatment in rats: effects on pregnancy outcome and the male reproductive and hematologic system. Biol Reprod 1987;37:317–326.

29. Adams PM, Fabricant JD, Legator MS. Cyclophosphamide-induced spermatogenic effects detected in the $F_1$ generation by behavioral testing. Science 1981;211: 80–82.

30. Fabricant JD, Legator MS, Adams PM. Post-meiotic cell mediation of behavior in progeny of male rats treated with cyclophosphamide. Mutat Res 1983;119:185–190.

31. Auroux M, Dulioust E, Selva J, Rince P. Cyclophosphamide in the $F_0$ male rat: physical and behavioral changes in three successive adult generations. Mutat Res 1990;229:189–200.

32. Joffe JM, Peruzovic M, Milkovic K. Progeny of male rats treated with methadone: physiological and behavioral effects. Mutat Res 1990;229:201–211.

33. Friedler G, Meadows M-E. Paternal exposure to nitrous oxide: effects on the development of offspring [Abstract]. Neurotoxicology 1986;7:365.

34. Lancranjan I, Popescu HI, Gavanescu O, Klepsch I, Serbanescu M. Reproductive ability of workmen occupationally exposed to lead. Arch Environ Health 1975;30:396–401.

35. Silbergeld EK, Akkerman M, Fowler BA, Albuquerque EX, Alkondon M. Lead: male-mediated effects on reproduction and neurodevelopment. Toxicology 1991;11:81.

36. Brady K, Herrera Y, Zenick H. Influence of parental lead exposure on subsequent learning ability of offspring. Pharmacol Biochem Behav 1975;3:561–565.

37. Lindbohm M-L, Salimen M, Anttila A, Taskinen H, Hemminki K. Paternal occupational lead exposure and spontaneous abortion. Scand J Work Environ Health 1991;17:95–103.

38. Peters JM, Preston-Martin S, Yu MC. Brain tumors in children and occupational exposure of parents. Science 1981;213:235–237.

39. Savitz DA, Chen J. Parental occupation and childhood cancer: review of epidemiologic studies. Environ Health Perspect 1990;88:325–337.

40. Taskinen H, Anttila A, Lindbohm ML, Sallman M, Hemminki K. Spontaneous abortion and congenital malformations among wives of men occupationally exposed to organic solvents. Scand J Work Environ Health 1989;15:345–352.

41. John EM, Savitz D, Sandler DP. Prenatal exposure to parents' smoking and childhood cancer. Am J Epidemiol 1991;133:123–132.

42. Olshan AF, Teschke K, Baird PA. Birth defects among offspring of firemen. Am J Epidemiol 1990;131: 312–321.

43. McDiarmid MA, Lees PSJ, Agnew J, Midzenski M, Duffy R. Reproductive hazards of fire fighting. II. Chemical hazards. Am J Ind Med 1991;19:447–472.

44. Gardner MJ, Snee MP, Hall AJ, Powell CA, Downes S, Terrell JD. Results of case-control study of leukaemia and lymphoma among young people near Sellafield nu-clear plant in West Cumbria. Br Med J 1990;300: 423–429.

45. Neel JV, Schull WJ, Awa AA, et al. The children of parents exposed to atomic bombs: estimates of the genetic doubling dose of radiation for humans. Am J Hum Genet 1990;46:1053–1072.

46. Spitz MR, Johnson CC. Neuroblastoma and paternal occupation. Am J Epidemiol 1985;121:924–929.

47. National Research Council. Biologic markers in reproductive toxicology. Washington, DC: National Academy Press, 1989:119–140.

48. Friedler G, Cicero TJ. Paternal pregestational opiate exposure in male mice: neuroendocrine deficits in their offspring. Res Communic Subst Abuse 1987;8:109–116.

49. Overstreet JW, Katz DF. Sperm transport and selection in the female genital tract. In: Johnson MH, ed. Development in mammals. New York: North Holland Pub Co, 1977:31–65.

50. Olshan AF, Breslow NE, Daling JR, et al. Wilms' tumor and paternal occupation. Cancer Res 1990;50:3212–3217.

51. Reik W, Surani MAH. Genomic imprinting and embryonal tumours. Nature 1989;338:112–113.

52. Norris ML, Barton SC, Surani MAH. The differential role of parental genomes in mammalian development. Oxford Rev Exp Biol 1990;12:225–244.

53. Campbell JH, Zimmermann EG. Automodulation of genes: a proposed mechanism for persisting effects of drugs and hormones in mammals. Neurobehav Toxicol Teratol 1982;4:435–439.

54. Benziger DP, Edelson J. Absorption from the vagina. Drug Metab Rev 1988;14:137–168.

55. Cohen EN, Brown BW, Bruce DL, et al. Occupational disease among operating room personnel. Anesthesiology 1974;41:321–340.

56. Cohen EN, Brown BW, Wu ML, et al. Occupational disease in dentistry and exposure to anesthetic gases. J Am Dent Assoc 1980;101:21–32.

57. Tannenbaum TN, Goldberg RJ. Exposure to anesthetic gases and reproductive outcome. J Occup Med 1985;27:659–668.

58. Hsu LL, Adams PM, Legator MS. Cyclophosphamide: effects of paternal exposure on the brain chemistry of the $F_1$ progeny. J Toxicol Environ Health 1987;21:471–48ŀ.

59. Jenkinson PC, Anderson D, Gangolli SD. Malformed foetuses and karyotype abnormalities in the offspring of cyclophosphamide and allyl alcohol-treated male rats. Mutat Res 1990;229:173–184.

60. Nelson BK, Brightwell WS, Mackensie-Taylor DR. Neurochemical, but not behavioral, deviations in the offspring of rats following prenatal or paternal inhalation exposure to ethanol. Neurotoxicol Teratol 1988;10: 15–22.

61. Friedler G, Wheeling HS. Behavioral effects in offspring of male mice injected with opioids prior to mating. Pharmacol Biochem Behav 1979;11:23–28.

62. Friedler G, Wurster-Hill D. Influence of morphine administration to male mice on their progeny. Proceedings Committee Problems Drug Dependence. Washington, DC: National Academy of Sciences, 1974:869–75.

63. Aschengrau A, Monson RR. Paternal military service in

Vietnam and the risk of late adverse pregnancy outcomes. Am J Public Health 1990;80:1218–1224.

64. Stellman SD, Stellman JM, Sommer JF Jr. Health and reproductive outcomes among American Legionnaires in relation to combat and herbicide exposure in Vietnam. Environ Res 1988;47:150–174.

65. Stowe HD, Goyer RA. The reproductive ability and progeny of $F_1$ lead-toxic rats. Fertil Steril 1971;22:755–760.

66. Lindbohm ML, Hemminki K, Bonhomme MG, et al. Effects of paternal occupational exposure on spontaneous abortions. Am J Public Health 1991;81:1029–1033.

67. Nomura T. Role of radiation-induced mutations in multi-generation carcinogenesis. In: International Agency for Research on Cancer (IARC). Perinatal and multigeneration carcinogenesis. Lyon, France: IARC, 1989: 375–387.

# 6

..............................................

# Lactation

MARY S. WOLFF

Counseling women regarding the many beneficial aspects of breastfeeding and managing patients who are infected or taking medications have long been integral components of postpartum care. Recently, environmental contamination has generated new concerns about the effects of xenobiotics in breast milk. This chapter reviews the anatomy and physiology of lactation and provides information about both the benefits of breastfeeding and the potentially harmful pollutants found in human milk.

## MAMMARY GLAND

### Anatomy

The milk-producing apparatus of the mammary gland is a tree-like system of lactiferous ducts whose branches increase in number as they radiate from the nipple (Fig. 6.1). During pregnancy and lactation, the distal branches develop into sac-like alveoli, the functional secretory units of the gland. Lining the alveoli are an inner layer of epithelial cells that synthesize milk and an outer layer of myoepithelial cells, involved in the muscular activity of milk ejection.

The mammary gland remains rudimentary before puberty. Rising estrogen levels at puberty stimulate growth of the duct system. With the onset of ovulation and progesterone production, alveolar buds develop within the mammary lobules. The extensive proliferation of milk-producing alveolar cells during pregnancy is promoted by dramatic increases in estrogen and progesterone, along with a concomitant rise in prolactin. During lactation, the area of the lobules is about five times that at puberty, and the number of alveolar buds per lobule increases, on average, from 11 to 180 (1).

## Milk Production

The secretory functions of the mammary gland occur within the mammary alveoli, which are present only during pregnancy and lactation. Rapid clearance of sex steroids at parturition allows prolactin and other hormones to initiate milk production in the alveolar epithelial cells. Milk is secreted into the lactiferous duct system, accumulating there until lactation occurs. Suckling stimulates release of oxytocin from the posterior pituitary, causing myoepithelial cell contractions that propel milk through the lactiferous ducts. Although prolactin levels decrease to pregestational levels by about 6 weeks postpartum, acute rises in prolactin with suckling allow for continued milk production (1).

Several functions of the alveolar epithelial cells are involved in milk production. Synthesis of lipids, lactose, casein, IgA, and other components occurs within these cells. In addition, a variety of important transport mechanisms regulate the composition of breast milk (Fig. 6.2).

Many nutrients in maternal blood enter the alveolar epithelial cell by passive diffusion across the rather porous basement membrane (2). Transport of chemicals and pharmacological agents may be passive (diffusion limited) or active (ionic or protein-bound). Entrance of neutral, nonionized compounds and nonion-

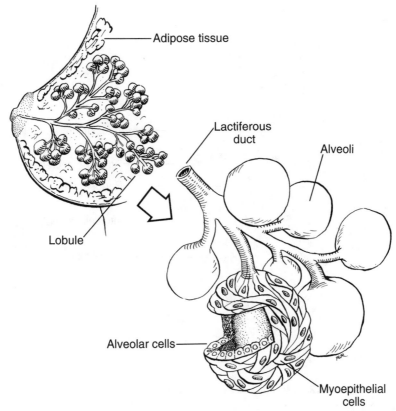

**Figure 6.1.** The mature mammary gland. The breast consists of 15–25 lobes emanating radially from the nipple. Each lobe is separated by connective tissue into smaller lobules. The main lactiferous duct within each lobe divides distally into smaller branches that terminate as alveolar buds in the lobules.

ized, protein-bound large molecules into the cell is facile via the lipid-rich membrane.

There are four means of transport from the cell into the alveolar space (Fig. 6.2) (3). Ions and water simply *permeate* across the membrane in the same way they entered. Immunoglobulins and other proteins from maternal plasma are transferred by *pinocytosis-exocytosis*. Proteins, sugar, and most milk nutrients are assembled within the cell's secretory vesicles and are transferred into the alveolar duct through *exocytosis*. *Apocrine secretion* of milk-fat globules occurs for triglycerides and other milk lipids synthesized within the cell.

In addition to migration through the alveolar cell, soluble nutrients and cells can travel directly to milk through the intercellular cleft between alveolar cells (*direct transfer*). These interstices gradually close over the duration of breastfeeding, which may explain the relative dearth of cells in breast milk later in lactation.

There is a gradual transition from colostrum to mature milk over the first few postpartum days, and milk composition continues to change as lactation progresses (4). Mature milk has less protein, more lactose and fat, and fewer cells than colostrum or transitional milk. Immunoglobulins also decrease as much as 10-fold during the first week of lactation.

## BENEFITS OF BREASTFEEDING

Human breast milk offers many advantages to infants. It is economical and provides psychological benefits to both mother and child. Human milk is digested and absorbed more easily than are substitutes. In sufficient quantity, breastfeeding alone provides optimal infant nutrition for at least 4–6 months. The volume early in lactation, 400–500 ml/day, grows to approximately 800 ml daily during full lactation. At 6 months of age, the infant may require

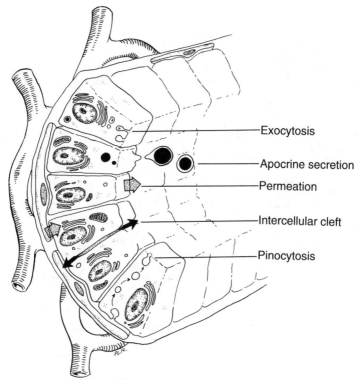

— Exocytosis

— Apocrine secretion

— Permeation

— Intercellular cleft

— Pinocytosis

**Figure 6.2.**   Mechanisms for transport of substances into breast milk.

additional nutrition, although the World Health Organization (WHO) suggests that this need may arise from the sequelae of infectious diseases rather than the insufficiency of breast milk (5). According to WHO, women must be severely malnourished to compromise the nutrition and volume of breast milk.

The main source of energy in milk is lipids, which are 98% triglycerides (3). The caloric content of breast milk (700 kcal/liter) is suited to the relatively slow growth of infants (6). Vitamins A, C, E, and K are higher in breast milk than in cows' milk, while vitamin D, riboflavin, and certain B vitamins are lower (7). Formula constituted from cows' milk or soya is fortified with vitamins and minerals under guidelines of WHO and the U.S. Food and Drug Administration (FDA). Some essential nutritive components are unique to human breast milk or exist in different forms or quantities than in cows' milk or formula (4, 6, 7). These differences may have important health implications (Table 6.1). Developmental benefits accrue from specific lipids, amino acids, and sugars in human milk that are particularly

well suited to brain and nervous system growth (4, 6). A number of infant illnesses can be prevented, at least in part, by breastfeeding. For example, allergic reactions induced by β-lactoglobulin in cows' milk are nonexistent in infants who are fed breast milk, which contains a different stereochemical form of the protein. Other conditions, such as gastrointestinal infections, Sudden Infant Death Syndrome, iron or calcium deficiencies, eczema, and obesity, are rare in breast-fed infants (4).

The immunological benefits of human milk are conferred by cellular components including macrophages, B and T lymphocytes, and leukocytes from the mother as well as by the soluble proteins IgA, lactoferrin, and interferon. IgA, a significant protective factor, is synthesized within the milk epithelial cells and differs from maternal IgA, suggesting that it may be engineered especially for infant protection. Cows' milk contains little IgA but greater amounts of IgG, which may also confer some immunological benefits. The processing and reconstitution of formula with protein and antibodies from cows' milk allow incorporation of some of these protective features into human milk substitutes (7).

The greatest immunological benefit of breastfeeding is the protection it provides against diarrhea (3). Breast milk is nutritionally sound and relatively free of pathogens. It promotes growth of protective lactobacilli in the gastrointestinal tract of infants. Immunoglobulins and other immune proteins provide protection from diarrhea (Table 6.1). Human milk contains maternal antibodies that may also defend against several intestinal pathogens (7, 8).

## CONTAMINANTS IN BREAST MILK

It is widely accepted that the benefits of breastfeeding far outweigh its potential disadvantages. This opinion is reflected in the recommendation by the Centers for Disease Control (CDC) that nursing mothers in Third World countries who are infected with human immunodeficiency virus (HIV) continue to breastfeed (9). Nevertheless, contaminants in breast milk may sometimes affect the course of lactation or infant health and development. In many instances, strategies to overcome these disadvantages can be undertaken. In rare cases of excessive contamination, it may be wise to avoid or temporarily to stop breastfeeding.

**Table 6.1.**
**Nutritive and Other Effects of Human Milk Components**[a]

| Milk Components | Effects |
| --- | --- |
| α-Lactoglobulin | Instead of β-lactoglobulin in cows' milk (most common infant allergin) |
| Lactoferrin | Immune, bacteriocidal, iron absorption |
| IgA | Anti-infection, antimicrobial |
| Lysozyme | Immune, antibacterial |
| Specific fatty acids | Brain development, antimicrobial |
| Lactose | Nonallergenic, improves iron absorption |
| Lymphocytes, macrophages | Immune |
| Cystine and taurine | Higher levels, conducive to neural development |

[a]Data from Blanc B. Biochemical aspects of human milk—comparison with bovine milk. World Rev Nutr Diet 1981;36:1–89; Packard VS. Human milk and infant formula. New York: Academic Press, 1982:269; Wolff MS. Occupationally derived chemicals in breast milk. Am J Ind Med 1983;4:259–286.

Formulae alternatives are not as strictly undesirable in more affluent countries as they are in less developed areas, where water impurity may be especially problematic.

Drugs and chemicals that affect the course of breastfeeding should be avoided or curtailed if possible. Drugs that can decrease lactation include L-dopa, ergots, androgens, pyridoxine, prostaglandins, bromocriptine, synthetic estrogens, and progesterone (2, 10). Dichloro-diphenyldichloroethane (DDE)—the primary residue of DDT in humans—has been associated with early weaning (11). This effect has been attributed to the estrogenic effects of DDT and its metabolites. Excessive use of alcohol and cigarettes may also impair lactation (2, 12).

The susceptibility of the neonate to the effects of xenobiotics and microbial exposures is attributable, in part, to poor immune competence and the immaturity of metabolic processes. Agents affecting the central nervous system (CNS) may be hazardous for infants because the brain continues to develop in the postnatal period (13). These substances include heavy metals, solvents, and many drugs.

Obviously, drugs that are present in sufficient doses in milk can have pharmacological effects in the infant. However, potential subtle or subclinical effects must also be kept in mind. For example, phenobarbital treatment for childhood seizures has recently been associated with cognitive deficits (14), suggesting that breast milk transmission may also be undesirable. Subtle developmental deficits have also been observed in children exposed transplacentally or through breast milk to low-level chemical contaminants such as lead or polychlorinated biphenyls (PCBs). Whereas reported neurological decrements are small, the public health implications of these findings may be significant, given the large numbers of children involved. In addition, multiple factors may interact (e.g., dietary deficiencies, alcohol, and lead exposure) to potentiate adverse health effects.

### Sources of Pollutants and Disposition in Milk

Exogenous chemicals in breast milk can arise from deliberate intake, as with drugs, alcohol, and smoking, or from unintentional environmental exposures to pollutants, as in the diet, water, dust, soil, or air. Occupational exposures are of particular concern due to their intensity. While xenobiotics absorbed by the mother can be found in breast milk, not all substances are equally well transmitted through the mammary system.

Milk concentration is ultimately limited by the maternal blood level of a substance, usually that found in the plasma. Disposition of chemicals in the mother's body may involve several compartments with different half-lives. Although many agents are rapidly eliminated, major proportions of some chemicals are sequestered into adipose tissue or bone. After exposure, maternal pharmacokinetics determine both the concentration and the duration of a chemical in the mother's blood. The proportion of a chemical transferred to milk is further dependent on its solubility and binding affinities, as well as on the properties of milk and maternal blood relative to a particular substance. As shown in Table 6.2, transfer is favored for neutral (nonionized), basic, low molecular weight, lipid-soluble compounds with minimal protein binding. Milk protein binding of drugs is usually lower than plasma binding, disfavoring milk transfer.

The term used to describe maternal absorption vs. infant availability is the milk-maternal plasma (M/P) ratio, which gives some indication of potential transfer to milk. However, milk and plasma levels vs. time are not always parallel, and an M/P ratio measured at a single time may under- or overestimate the total potential transfer from maternal blood to milk (Fig. 6.3). The use of infant dose as a percentage of maternal dose (Table 6.3) incorporates the M/P concept in a more comprehensive way, allowing projection of potential toxic or pharmacological effects in the child. For clinical purposes, the *concentration* of a chemical in milk can be used to indicate dangerous levels of exposure to the infant and the need for temporary cessation of nursing, while the *half-life* can help determine when to resume breastfeeding.

For reference, some typical milk half-lives for chemicals are given in Table 6.4. These clearance rates are more or less inversely related to M/P ratios (Table 6.3; Fig. 6.4). Lead, for example, has a long half-life in milk, but has a low M/P ratio. The long half-life represents mobilization of lead from bone stores.

Usually, chemical levels in milk are a function of both compartment storage and metabolic rate. Codeine has an M/P ratio similar to that of its metabolite, morphine; but codeine half-life in milk is approximately 2 hr, while morphine half-life is approximately 24 hr (15). The short codeine half-life is related to its rapid metabolism; the morphine persistence is related to fat solubility and slower metabolism.

For any single chemical, individual variation in milk concentration and half-life can be great, due to a number of physiological and anthropometric factors. Obesity tends to dilute concentration, while heightened blood flow enhances transfer to milk. Xenobiotic metabolism rates are affected by genetic variability and enzyme induction by other chemicals. Cigarette smoking, dietary composition, ingestion

**Table 6.2.**
**Characteristics of Chemicals and Drugs Favoring Distribution into Breast Milk[a]**

| | |
|---|---|
| Higher pKa | Basic drugs generally concentrate more in milk |
| Protein binding | Greater binding to milk protein (lower binding to plasma protein) favors milk; effect is usually a decrease in milk due to plasma protein binding |
| Low erythrocyte binding | Better transfer to milk |
| Low molecular weight | Easier passage through mammary alveolar membranes |
| Lipid solubility | Transport favored through lipid-rich membranes |
| Low ionizability | More membrane permeability, less binding impedance |
| Rapid blood flow | Rate of transfer to milk can keep pace with milk production |
| Permeability of mammary cell | More permeable early in lactation; both chemicals and cells penetrate the intercellular cleft by direct transfer |
| Metabolic rate | Slow metabolism favors prolonged half-life in milk |

[a]Data from Wilson JT. Drugs in breast milk. New York: ADIS Press, 1981; Wolff MS. Occupationally derived chemicals in breast milk. Am J Ind Med 1983;4:259–281.

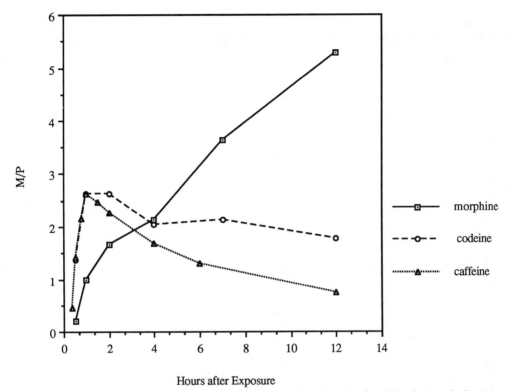

**Figure 6.3.** Variations in milk-plasma ratio (M/P) over time. Data from Findlay JWA, DeAngelis RL, Kearney MF, Welch RM, Findlay JM. Analgesic drugs in breast milk and plasma. Clin Pharmacol Ther 1981;29:625–633; Stavchansky S, Combs A, Sagraves R, Delgado M, Joshi A. Pharmacokinetics of caffeine in breast milk and plasma after single oral administration of caffeine to lactating mothers. Biopharm Drug Dispos 1988;9:285–299.

of charcoal-broiled beef, alcohol use, drug use, and environmental chemicals (e.g., DDT) can enhance enzyme levels by 2- to 60-fold (16). For example, the half-life of caffeine in breast milk varied among six women from 1–12 hr (17).

With persistent chemicals that are stored in bone or adipose tissue, the decline in milk concentrations corresponds to depletion of levels in the compartment where the chemical is sequestered. There may, in fact, be no metabolism of these substances. As illustrated in Figure 6.4, half-lives of halogenated hydrocarbons such as PCBs and DDT are disproportionally long relative to their M/P ratios. These residues are not metabolized and are fat-stored. Their M/P ratios reflect essentially a 1:1:1 equilibrium between the lipid compartments of adipose, plasma, and milk (18). For these types of chemicals, milk may be the most efficient, if not the only, means of elimination (19). Similar disparities between half-life and M/P ratio may be expected with chemicals that have extensive maternal plasma- or milk-binding properties.

## Exposures and Effects on Infants

The kinds of chemicals found in breast milk can be assigned to a few groups that will be discussed briefly, i.e., pharmaceutical drugs, naturally occurring dietary components, narcotics, pollutants derived from smoking, heavy metals, organic solvents, and persistent halogenated hydrocarbons including pesticides (Table 6.5). Detrimental cellular components, such as microbes, can also pass into breast milk. Radioactivity will not be discussed, but the unfortunate incident in Chernobyl in 1986 reminds us that milk is a fine conduit for radioactive fallout (20, 21).

### PHARMACEUTICAL DRUGS

Few drugs given to the mother escape transmission to milk. Exceptions include heparin, by

**Table 6.3.**
**Milk: Plasma (M/P) Ratios for Various Chemicals in Breast Milk[a]**

| Chemical (reference) | M/P | Infant Dose, as % Maternal Dose, Body Wt Adjusted[a] |
|---|---|---|
| Dicoumarol (12) | 0.02 | |
| Penicillin (12, 13) | 0.2 | <1 |
| Diazepam (13) | 0.2 | 2 |
| Lead (39) | 0.2 | |
| Salicylate (13) | 0.1–0.4 | 2 |
| (Aspirin) (2) | 0.6–1.0 | (7.5) |
| Lithium (13, 69) | 0.4 | 2 |
| Phenobarbital (12, 13, 70) | 0.3, 0.7 | 23–156 |
| Caffeine (12, 17) | 0.7–0.8 | 10 |
| Theophylline (13, 71) | 0.7–0.8 | 8–63 |
| Theobromine (13) | 0.7–0.8 | 20 |
| Cotinine[b] (30, 35) | 0.8 | 1–5 |
| Methadone (13, 25) | 0.8 | 0.5 |
| Mercury (50, 72) | 0.8–0.9 | |
| Ethanol (12, 13, 36) | 1 | 20 (4) |
| Codeine, morphine (13) | 2 | 7 |
| Pseudoephedrine (13) | 2.5 | 4 |
| Nicotine[b] (30, 35) | 2.9 | 1–5 |
| Erythromycin (12, 13) | 2.5–3.0 | 2 |
| Tetrachloroethylene (53) | ~3 | |
| DDE, PCBs, PBBs (19, 62, 73) | 3–10 | |
| Amphetamine (13) | 5 | 6 |
| Iodine[131] (12) | 65 | 8 (75) |
| Isoniazid (13) | >1 | 50 (11) |
| Thiouracil (12, 13) | 3 | 113 (75) |

[a]Values are from or derived from Atkinson HC, Begg EJ, Darlow BA. Drugs in human milk: clinical pharmacokinetic considerations. Clin Pharmacol 1988;14:217–240. Values in parentheses are from Vorherr H. Human lactation and breast feeding. In Larson BL, ed. Lactation: a comprehensive treatise, vol. IV. New York: Academic Press, 1978:182–269. Percents are adjusted for body weight of infant and mother, using 0.15 liters/kg/day infant "dose" and 60 kg maternal body weight. Atkinson et al. use the ratio of the areas under the pharmacokinetic curves for this estimate, rather than peak or average values. The resultant infant dose calculated may be somewhat lower than the peak M/P value, since milk and blood decline are not always parallel, but the estimate is more realistic in terms of estimating health effects or infant body burden. To calculate the approximate % infant dose not adjusted for body weight, divide by 15 (60 kg maternal body weight, 4 kg infant weight).
[b]1–5% includes cotinine; without cotinine, approximately 1%; estimated from references 30, 35 and data in Table 6.4.

**Table 6.4.**
**Approximate Half-lives of Chemicals in Breast Milk**

| Chemical (reference) | Half-life |
|---|---|
| Nicotine (35) | 1.5 hr |
| Cotinine | >4 hr |
| Codeine (15) | 2 hr |
| Salicylate | 2–6 hr |
| Ethanol (36) | 3 hr |
| Theophylline, theobromine, caffeine (17, 71) | 4–8 hr |
| Iodine (as MAA salt) (75) | 20 hr |
| Prednisolone (76) | 23 hr |
| Lead (45) | 13 weeks |
| PCBs, DDE, and similar substances (19, 40, 62) | 5–8 months |

virtue of its molecular weight, and warfarin, because of its binding properties (12). Information about pharmaceuticals in breast milk can be found in the *Physicians' Desk Reference* (22),

the American Academy of Pediatrics (AAP) guidelines (23), and other resources (2, 12, 13). Many reviews examine drugs within categories (sedatives, antihypertensives, etc.), so that some information can be deduced by analogy if no data are available on a specific drug. Consideration of chemical characteristics influencing distribution into breast milk (Table 6.2) can also be helpful. In addition to concise coverage of various classes of drugs with respect to pharmacology and presence in milk, the review by Peterson and Bowes (10) provides a useful guide to assessment of potential infant health effects.

In most clinical circumstances, the general approach to pharmaceutical use during lactation as described by the AAP (23) is appropriate. The AAP guidelines (Table 6.6) advise consideration of four basic questions: (*a*) Must the mother use a drug? (*b*) What is the safest

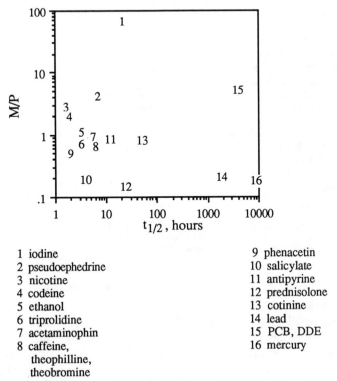

**Figure 6.4.**  Milk half-lives vs. milk-plasma (M/P) ratios. See Tables 6.3 and 6.4 for references.

| | |
|---|---|
| 1 iodine | 9 phenacetin |
| 2 pseudoephedrine | 10 salicylate |
| 3 nicotine | 11 antipyrine |
| 4 codeine | 12 prednisolone |
| 5 ethanol | 13 cotinine |
| 6 triprolidine | 14 lead |
| 7 acetaminophin | 15 PCB, DDE |
| 8 caffeine, | 16 mercury |
| theophilline, | |
| theobromine | |

**Table 6.5.**
**Some Chemical Contaminants of Human Milk: Estimated Levels in Developed Countries in the 1980s.**

| Chemical | Concentration in Breast Milk | Comments (reference) |
|---|---|---|
| Cadmium | 0.1–0.4 µg/liter | Higher with smoking (39, 41) |
| Lead | 20 µg/liter | Age of house, traffic (39, 41) |
| Fluoride | 10 µg/liter | Fluoridated water, 1 ppm (41) |
| Nicotine | 0–400 µg/liter | Including cotinine, only with smoking (32, 34) |
| Caffeine | 2–6 mg/liter | Equivalent of five cups coffee or caffeinated soft drinks (17) |
| PCBs, DDT, similar organo-chlorines | 2–100 µg/liter | Diet (19, 55, 77, 78) |
| Theobromine | 5 mg/liter | Chocolate (240 mg in 4 oz bar) (79) |
| Alcohol | 700 mg/liter | ½–2 hrs after 1.2 oz alcohol; blood alcohol 0.09% (36) |
| $Cs^{134} + Cs^{137}$ | 3 Bq/liter | Italy 3–9 months after Chernobyl (20, 21); ~2–3% natural background |

**Table 6.6.**
**Guidelines for Drugs in Breast Milk: American Academy of Pediatrics, 1989**[a]

Contraindicated
   Amphetamine, bromocriptine, cocaine, cyclophosphamide, cyclosporine, doxorubicin, ergotamine, heroin, lithium, marijuana, methotrexate, nicotine (smoking), phencyclidine (PCP), phenindione
Temporary cessation for clearance
   Radiopharmaceuticals (1–14 days)
Possible concern, effects on infants unknown
   Psychotropic drugs: antianxiety (benzodiazepines), antidepressant (including tricyclics), antipsychotics (including phenothiazines); chloramphenicol; metoclopramide K, metronidazole, tinidazole
Give to nursing mothers with caution, effects having been observed in infants
   Aspirin, clemastine, phenobarbital, primidone, sulfasalzaine
Usually compatible with breastfeeding[b]
   Anesthetics, anticoagulants, antiepileptics, antihistamines and decongestants, antihypertensives, anti-infective drugs, antithyroid drugs, cathartics, diuretics, hormones, muscle relaxants, stimulants, vitamins
Drugs indicated to be concentrated in milk
   Cimetidine, erythromycin, hydroxychloroquine, nadolol, pseudoephedrine, dyphylline, prazepam, metoclopramide, doxorubicin

[a]American Academy of Pediatrics, Committee on Drugs. Transfer of drugs and other chemicals into human milk. Pediatrics 1989;84:924–936.
[b]Drugs missing or listed as compatible that may be of questionable safety include the following (2, 13, 22, 74): alcohol, atropine, barbiturates, benadryl, bromide, caffeine, cimetidine, codeine, digoxin, diphenylhydantoin, erythromycin, estrogen, hydroxychlorquine, inderal, iodine, isoniazid, lindane, methadone, penicillin, prednisone, progesterone, reserpine, tetracycline, theophylline, thiouracil.

drug? (c) Should the infant be monitored? (d) Can the drug be taken at a time to minimize concentration in breast milk? These guidelines, however, are intended to protect the infant from major pharmacological reactions. A more conservative approach may be warranted in light of recent evidence linking some low-level chemical exposures with neurological deficits.

Several other general considerations apply to clinical evaluation of drugs in breast milk. As a rule, less than 1% of the maternal dose appears as the infant dose, even when adjusted for maternal and infant body weights (13). On the other hand, the infant's exposure may be longer; theophylline half-life is 30 hr in the infant, while it is less than 8 hr in the mother (12). In some cases, cumulative lower doses may become high enough to exert pharmacological effects. Medications with known M/P ratios greater than 1 require special attention. For drugs with short half-lives or those given in single (rather than multiple) doses, milk can be discarded during the affected interval. If possible, substitutes should be found for drugs with high M/P ratios and long half-lives.

## NATURAL DIETARY COMPONENTS

Lactating women should be aware of common substances in the diet that can affect the quality of milk. The methylxanthines can cause symptoms of irritability or can affect respiration in infants. Caffeine, theophylline, and theobromine (from chocolate) are members of this family. The pharmacokinetics in milk are similar for all three agents. Although the estimated infant dose is small, the infant half-life is long (30 hr for theophylline, 80 hr for caffeine) compared with adults (approximately 6 hr) (10). Therefore, the cumulative infant dose may be substantial.

Aflatoxin is a very toxic, carcinogenic mold product occurring on grains, including peanuts, and in human milk from Africa (7). Breast milk contamination with aflatoxin is not evident in developed countries.

## NARCOTICS

Little information is available on the effects of narcotics in breast milk. In the early literature, heroin withdrawal in the neonate was reported upon sudden weaning or delayed breastfeeding (24). Persistence of heroin in milk as the metabolite morphine can be inferred from the data on codeine.

The more recent literature has reported methadone and cocaine in breast milk. Methadone is transferred to mother's milk (25), although the infant dose is probably insignificant (less than 0.1 mg/day) (26). Its half-life is 8–10 hr. Cocaine and its metabolites persist in adults for more than 24 hr. This drug has been measured in both milk and infant urine over a period of 60 hr after use. During this time, the combined levels of cocaine and its hydrolysate in infant urine (200–1000 ng/ml) exceeded those in breast milk (0–400 ng/ml) (27).

## SMOKING AND ALCOHOL

Less than 20% of women in the U.S. and Canada now smoke while pregnant (28, 29). Approximately 40% of pregnant smokers quit during gestation. However, women who quit are almost exclusively those who smoke less than one pack per day, and many resume smoking later (29).

Maternal cigarette smoking has been associated with respiratory illness, acute toxicity, cardiotoxicity, and other reactions among newborns (28, 30, 31). Women who smoke may wean earlier (32). Passive smoke also affects the quality of breast milk and may have direct respiratory effects on children.

As a result of cigarette smoke exposure, cadmium, nicotine, and the nicotine metabolite, cotinine, are found in breast milk, as well as in maternal and infant blood (30, 33). Like other heavy metals, partition of cadmium to milk is poor (M/P approximately 0.1), but levels in maternal blood and milk are two to three times those of women who do not smoke.

Cigarette smoke is the only major source of nicotine and cotinine in milk and other human tissues. Levels in milk and in infants are proportional to the number of cigarettes smoked and to the degree of passive smoke exposure (28, 32, 34). Nicotine half-life in breast milk is less than 2 hr, as it is rapidly oxidized to cotinine (35). Cotinine is persistent (Table 6.4) and is detected at much higher levels than nicotine in milk and in infants (28, 30–34). While nontoxic, cotinine behavior in milk may reflect the presence of other adventitious components, such as polycyclic aromatic hydrocarbons, that could be similarly transferred via milk (29, 31).

Alcohol passes readily into breast milk, with an M/P ratio near 1, and has a milk half-life of approximately 3 hr. The metabolite acetaldehyde, which may be responsible for some of alcohol's toxic effects, is evidently not present in breast milk (36). Approximately 20% of the maternal dose is available to the infant, so that a maternal blood alcohol of 100 mg/dl (0.1%) corresponds to 5 mg/dl in the infant. This dose is insufficient to produce the usual acute effects of alcohol. In isolated cases, heavier drinking has been reported to cause infant intoxication and even the pseudo-Cushing syndrome seen among chronic alcoholics (12). Large amounts of alcohol may depress the milk ejection reflex and impair nursing.

Little information is available on breastfeeding and low-dose alcohol consumption by nursing women. In a recent report, infants whose mothers drank a beverage containing 0.3 gm ethanol per kg body weight immediately before breastfeeding consumed significantly less milk than unexposed infants (37). The dose administered in this study was insufficient to inhibit the milk ejection reflex but did alter the odor of milk and infant feeding behavior. Little et al. (38) reported that infants whose mothers consumed an average of one or more drinks daily while nursing had small, but statistically significant, decreases in motor development test scores at 1 yr of age. The mean scores of infants whose mothers consumed less than one drink daily did not differ from unexposed infants. Deficits in mental development were not noted in this study.

## HEAVY METALS

Lead, mercury, and cadmium are found in human milk. Cadmium in breast milk is derived from cigarette smoke and from the diet, but there are no reported adverse effects among infants. In the United Kingdom, formula has levels similar to those in human milk (39). Breast milk cadmium concentrations below 2 μg/liter have been observed in Finland, Sweden, and New Zealand, but studies from the United States and Europe show average levels of 2–40 μg/liter (40). Concentrations greater than 5 μg/liter could provide a substantial increment to infant dietary levels.

Levels of lead and mercury in breast milk are well below established exposure limits, but are sizeable when compared to other foodstuffs

**Table 6.7.**
**Lead in Breast Milk, Maternal Blood, and**
**Infant Blood (μg/dl)**

| Country (reference) | N | Maternal Milk | Maternal Blood | Cord Blood |
|---|---|---|---|---|
| Canada (41) | 210 | 0.055 | | |
| United Kingdom (39) | 28 | 1.9 | 10 | 9 |
| Malaysia (80) | 114 | 4.8 | 15 | 12 |
| United States (44) | 100/249 | 1.7 | | 7 |
|    [formula] | 73 | 2.3 | | |
| United States (81) | 39 | 0.3 | 12 | |
| WHO (world) (51) | 320 | 1.0[a] | | |

[a]Median of medians of six countries: Guatemala, Hungary, Nigeria, Philippines, Sweden, Zaire; range 0.3–1.7.

in the diet. Lead originates from a variety of environmental sources including paint and batteries. Levels in milk have been related to the age of a woman's house and to nearby traffic patterns (41). The latter source has become less important with the declining use of leaded gasoline.

Low-dose prenatal lead exposure has been associated with neurobehavioral deficits in children lasting at least until 2 yr of age (42). Postnatal exogenous exposures, such as ingestion of paint chips, can be responsible for mental decrements acquired later (43). Reported newborn cord blood lead levels are two to five times the concentrations found in milk (Table 6.7). Thus, the contribution of lead in breast milk to infant body burden is probably less important than prenatal and other postnatal exposures. However, calculating from normal levels (Table 6.7), lead from breast milk could easily double an infant's body burden within 1 month. This was not found for infants on diets low in lead (formula or breast milk with lead below 5 μg/kg/day or 25–40 μg/day); but at higher dietary lead levels (approximately 9 μg/kg/day or 61 μg/day), the blood lead levels of infants doubled within 2 months (44). Breastfed babies had slightly higher 6-month blood lead levels than did formula-fed infants (7.6 vs. 5.6 μg/dl). Levels in breast milk were fairly stable over the 6-month period, consistent with studies suggesting that lead is mobilized from maternal bone during lactation (45).

The rates of increase in lead body burden

due to milk intake may be slower than predicted for at least three reasons: (a) absorption through the gastrointestinal route is incomplete (approximately 30–50%) (46, 47); (b) infant body weight doubles within the first 5–6 months, diluting the lead concentration; (c) blood lead is an inexact measure of body burden, because lead is largely sequestered in bone. Thus, blood lead levels may remain constant even as infant body burden is increasing.

Mercury is present in the environment as inorganic and organic (mainly methyl) mercury. Methyl mercury exposure derives chiefly from contaminated fish. Mercury poisoning causes sensory-motor dysfunction and mental retardation in children after very high exposures either in utero or from breast milk (48). Lower level exposures may also be of concern because the developing human CNS is "remarkably sensitive" to methyl mercury (49).

Like lead, maternal and cord blood levels of mercury are approximately equivalent and are higher than those found in milk (18, 50, 51). Normal levels are 1–4 μg/liter in human milk. Binding of lead and mercury to red blood cells may facilitate placental passage but impede transfer to milk. Mercury levels in milk, at least theoretically, represent a substantial increment to neonatal body burden. (One day's milk at 3.1 μg/liter corresponds to about one-fourth of the body burden of an infant with 20 μg/liter in cord blood.) Chromium has also been reported in breast milk at average concentrations of 0.4 μg/liter, far below the allowable daily limit of 5–15 μg/kg/day (52).

## ORGANIC SOLVENTS

Organic solvents are absorbed mainly through the respiratory route and skin. The biological half-lives of solvents are typically short, in the range of several hours. Excretion occurs primarily through the lungs and through elimination of metabolites in the urine.

A few industrial solvents have been reported in breast milk. They are tetrachloroethylene (3–10 μg/liter), halothane (0.8–2.0 μg/liter), carbon disulfide (20–300 μg/liter), and dichloromethane (74 μg/liter) (18, 40). Solvents like tetrachloroethylene are lipid soluble and are slowly metabolized, so that their appearance in breast milk is not surprising. Solvents exert an anesthetic effect, although only at very high exposures unattainable from breast milk. In one report, neonatal jaundice was attributed to a nursing mother's exposure to tetrachloroethylene in a dry-cleaning facility (53).

## PESTICIDES AND PERSISTENT HALOGENATED HYDROCARBONS

The organochlorines, DDT and PCBs, are the prototypical environmental chemicals in breast milk. These organochlorine residues share chemical properties that result in accumulation in the environment—lipophilicity, resistance to metabolism, and low volatility. Environmental levels of pesticides such as DDE are now higher in undeveloped countries because of continued use, while PCBs are higher in industrialized nations (5, 54, 55). In the U.S., concentrations of DDT and PCBs in breast milk are approximately 50–100 ppb ($\mu$g/liter) (18, 40, 55). Other chlorinated hydrocarbon pesticides (dieldrin, lindane, hexachlorobenzene, heptachlor, chlordane, toxaphene, mirex) have also been reported in human milk worldwide at lower levels (1–5 ppb). Tetrachloro-p-dibenzo-p-diozin (dioxin, TCDD) and polychlorodibenzofurans (PCDFs) have been detected at extremely low concentrations (56). Chlordane was found in milk of women whose homes were treated for termites more than 2 yr earlier, at three times the level of milk from women in untreated homes (57).

Many of these organochlorines are pesticides that have entered the food chain. Pollution by PCBs is largely due to improper disposal or accidental spills from electrical capacitors and transformers. Polybrominated biphenyls (PBBs) appeared in human and cows' milk almost exclusively after a fire retardant was inadvertently mixed into livestock feed in Michigan in 1973–1974. Chlorinated dioxins and dibenzofurans, including TCDD, are byproducts of combustion and contaminants of wood preservatives, PCBs, and herbicides from the 2,4,5-tridichlorophenoxyacetic acid family.

In two environmental studies, prenatal exposure to PCBs was associated with small but significant sensory-motor effects in children through 2 yr of age. In one investigation, slightly impaired motor development was detected among children whose mothers had immediate postnatal breast milk PCB levels in the upper 95th percentile of the study group (58). The deficits were no longer apparent on retesting at ages 3–4 yr. In the other study, sensory deficits, as well as smaller gestational size, were seen among children with blood levels in approximately the top 25% who were observed until age 4 yr (59, 60). Exposure levels associated with neurological deficits were in the upper range for the studies, yet they are not excessively high: above 3 ppm in mother's milk (fat basis) and above 3 ng/ml in children's blood. Common occupational exposures result in levels 10–100 times higher (61). In both studies, effects were attributed to prenatal exposure. However, these results also sound a cautionary note for unduly exposing neonates postnatally.

Guidelines promulgated by WHO and the FDA are intended to protect human health for a lifetime of exposure. However, average levels of the most prominent organohalides in breast milk, DDE and PCB, exceed established allowable daily intakes (ADIs). The infant diet has other sources of organochlorine contaminants, but levels are generally well within the ADIs.

As other exposure sources decline, transfer of organochlorines from breast milk will probably be the most significant route of exposure for the child. A nursing infant doubles its natal body burden of organochlorines in approximately 3 months, and the child's blood level at this time begins to exceed its mother's (62, 63). Blood levels of PCBs among children have been clearly related to breastfeeding in studies by Japanese investigators (64), among occupationally exposed children, and by Jacobson et al. among children in Michigan (18, 65). Ironically, perhaps the only efficient route of elimination for an adult is through breast milk. The milk half-life for this family of chemicals is 6–24 months (19, 62).

## CELLULAR CONTAMINANTS

Detrimental cellular components such as microbes can pass into breast milk. The most recently reported, and perhaps most controversial, substance is HIV. Both the virus itself (66) and antibodies to HIV (67) have been reported in breast milk. The epidemiological evidence for HIV transmission through breast milk is limited. Although it is clear that nursing mothers can transmit the virus by some means, the contribution of nursing to infant risk is considered small compared with prenatal and natal exposures (9).

Cytomegalovirus (CMV) has been detected in human milk, and the epidemiological evidence strongly suggests that transmission to the infant occurs (68). CMV is more prevalent in early lactation, in keeping with the evidence that more cellular material is present at this time. Hepatitis B antigen, herpes simplex, and rubella have also been found or their transmission has been documented. These viral exposures do not appear to be very important routes of infant infection or of long-term immunity.

## SUMMARY AND CLINICAL RECOMMENDATIONS

It is important for clinicians to recognize and to promote the desirability of breastfeeding. Even short-term nursing can provide significant health and psychological benefits to the infant.

Low-level chemical contamination of breast milk has been found in surveys of urban populations in the U.S. and elsewhere, without reported overt toxicity. Recent investigations, however, suggest that low-level exposure to some neurotoxins may produce subtle cognitive deficits in infants exposed pre- or postnatally. Occasionally, environmental poisoning epidemics have resulted in significant breast milk contamination and adverse health effects in infants. Few data are available regarding the quality of breast milk among working women, although occupational exposures often occur at much higher levels than those found in the home or community. However, with rare exceptions, the presence of xenobiotics in human milk is not a reason to eschew or to terminate nursing.

Nevertheless, minimizing exposure to xenobiotics in breast milk is obviously desirable. The ability of infants to metabolize and excrete chemicals is poor, and the developing CNS may be particularly susceptible to adverse effects. Chemicals of most concern include those known to be highly toxic (e.g., lead) and persistent, fat-soluble agents (e.g., PCBs) that are excreted primarily through lactation and that bioaccumulate over an individual's life span.

Clinical assessment of patients involves a thorough occupational and environmental history to identify pertinent exposures. For persistent chemicals, even exposures in the remote past may have biological significance. Attention to drug use and chemical exposures before conception provides an optimal opportunity for preventive intervention through counseling and exposure abatement.

At times, patients will request a nonspecific chemical screen of their breast milk. This type of screening is neither cost-effective nor medically warranted; low-level contamination is ubiquitous and is neither a reason to curtail nor to terminate breastfeeding. If the history reveals significant exposure to one or more specific toxic and/or persistent chemicals, biological monitoring may be appropriate. Measurement of chemicals like lead and PCBs in human milk is expensive and requires access to specialized laboratories. In most instances, measurement of levels in maternal blood (preferably before the onset of lactation), with application of appropriate M/P ratios, can provide estimates of chemical concentrations in breast milk. As explained earlier, the concentration of a chemical in milk can be used to indicate excessive exposure to a toxicant, and the half-life can be used to determine how long to curtail breastfeeding. Milk can be pumped and discarded during this period to allow maintenance of lactation.

Approaches to optimizing milk quality can be actively and aggressively undertaken by a woman with the support of her health practitioner. The nursing mother is encouraged to minimize exposure to nonprescription medications, dietary methylxanthines, and recreational drugs. Therapeutic medications can be chosen with an eye to milk partition, as well as to the desired pharmacological effect on the mother. Excessive occupational exposures can often be reduced through workplace controls. Certainly the most effective approach involves preventive education and intervention before the onset of gestation.

*The insight of Walter Rogan on child development is very much appreciated. The able and diligent assistance of Steven Yuen in obtaining literature citations is gratefully acknowledged.*

## REFERENCES

1. Neville MC, Daniel CW, eds. The mammary gland: development, regulation, and function. New York: Plenum Press, 1987.

2. Vorherr H. Human lactation and breast feeding. In: Larson BL, ed. Lactation: a comprehensive treatise, Vol IV. New York: Academic Press, 1978:182–269.

3. Neville MC, Allen JC, Watters C. The mechanisms of milk secretion. In: Neville MC, Neifert MR, eds. Lactation: physiology, nutrition, and breast feeding. New York: Plenum Press, 1983:49–102.

4. Blanc B. Biochemical aspects of human milk—comparison with bovine milk. World Rev Nutr Diet 1981;36:1–89.

5. World Health Organization (WHO). The quantity and quality of breast milk. Geneva: WHO, 1985.

6. Casey CE, Hambidge KM. Nutritional aspects of human lactation. In: Neville MC, Neifert MR, eds. Lactation: physiology, nutrition, and breast feeding. New York: Plenum Press, 1983:199–240.

7. Packard VS. Human milk and infant formula. New York: Academic Press, 1982:269.

8. Neville MC, Neifert MR, ed. Lactation: physiology, nutrition, and breast feeding. New York: Plenum Press, 1983:456.

9. Oxtoby MJ. Human immunodeficiency virus and other viruses in human milk: placing the issues in broader prospective. Pediatr Infect Dis J 1988; 7:825–835.

10. Peterson RG, Bowes WA Jr. Drugs, toxins and environmental agents in breast milk. In: Neville MC, Neifert MR, eds. Lactation: physiology, nutrition, and breast feeding. New York: Plenum Press, 1983:367–403.

11. Rogan WJ, Gladen BC, McKinney JD, et al. Polychlorinated biphenyls (PCBs) and dichlorodiphenyldichloroethane (DDE) in human milk: effects on growth, morbidity, and duration of lactation. Am J Public Health 1987; 77:1294–1297.

12. Wilson JT. Drugs in breast milk. New York: ADIS Press, 1981.

13. Atkinson HC, Begg EJ, Darlow BA. Drugs in human milk-clinical pharmacokinetic considerations. Clin Pharmacol 1988;14:217–240.

14. Farwell JR, Young JL, Hirtz DG, Sulzbacher SI, Ellenberg JH, Nelson KB. Phenobarbital for febrile seizures—effects on intelligence and on seizure recurrence. N Engl J Med 1990; 322:364–369.

15. Findlay JWA, DeAngelis RL, Kearney MF, Welch RM, Findlay JM. Analgesic drugs in breast milk and plasma. Clin Pharmacol Ther 1981;29:625–633.

16. Conney AH. Induction of microsomal enzymes by foreign chemicals and carcinogenesis by PAH: GHA Clowes memorial lecture. Cancer Res 1982;42:4875–4917.

17. Stavchansky S, Combs A, Sagraves R, Delgado M, Joshi A. Pharmacokinetics of caffeine in breast milk and plasma after single oral administration of caffeine to lactating mothers. Biopharm Drug Dispos 1988;9:285–299.

18. Wolff MS. Occupationally derived chemicals in breast milk. Am J Ind Med 1983;4:259–281.

19. Rogan WJ, Gladen BC, McKinney JD, et al. Polychlorinated biphenyls (PCBs) and dichlorodiphenyldichloroethane (DDE) in human milk: effects of maternal factors and previous lactation. Am J Public Health 1986;76:172–177.

20. DiLallo D, Bertollini R, Campos Venuti G, Risica S, Perucci CA, Simula S. Radioactivity in breast milk in central Italy in the aftermath of Chernobyl. Acta Pediatr Scand 1987;76:530–531.

21. Gori G, Cama G, Guerresi E, et al. Radioactivity in breast milk and placentas during the year after Chernobyl. Am J Obstet Gynecol 1988;159:1232–1234.

22. Huff B, ed. Physicians' desk reference, 44th ed. Oradell, NJ: Medical Economics Co., Inc., 1990.

23. American Academy of Pediatrics, Committee on Drugs. Transfer of drugs and other chemicals into human milk. Pediatrics 1989;84:924–936.

24. Cobrinik RW, Hood RT, Chusxid E. The effect of maternal narcotic addiction on the newborn infant. Pediatr 1959;24:288–304.

25. Blinick G, Inturrisi CE, Jerez E, Wallach RC. Methadone assays in pregnant women and progeny. Am J Obstet Gynecol 1975;5:617–621.

26. Pond SM, Kreek MJ, Tong TG, Raghunath J, Benowitz NL. Altered methadone pharmacokinetics in methadone-maintained pregnant women. J Pharmacol Exp Ther 1985;233:1–6.

27. Chasnoff IJ, Lewis DE, Squires L. Cocaine intoxication in a breast-fed infant. Pediatrics 1987;80:836–838.

28. Labrecque M, Marcoux S, Weber JP, Fabia J, Ferron L. Feeding and urine cotinine values in babies whose mothers smoke. Pediatrics 1989;83:93–97.

29. Fingerhut LA, Kleinman JC, Kendrick JS. Smoking before, during, and after pregnancy. Am J Public Health 1990;80:541–544.

30. Luck W, Nau H. Nicotine and cotinine concentrations in serum and urine of infants exposed via passive smoking or milk from smoking mothers. J Pediatr 1985;107:816–820.

31. Woodward A, Grgurinovich N, Ryan P. Breast feeding and smoking hygiene: major influences on cotinine in urine of smokers' infants. J Epidemiol Community Health 1986;40:309–315.

32. Schwartz-Bickenbach D, Schulte-Hobein B, Abt S, Plum C, Nau H. Smoking and passive smoking during pregnancy and early infancy: effects on birth weight, lactation period, and cotinine concentrations in mother's milk and infant's urine. Toxicol Lett 1987;35:73–81.

33. Radisch B, Luck W, Nau H. Cadmium concentrations in milk and blood of smoking mothers. Toxicol Lett 1987;36:147–152.

34. Luck W, Nau H. Nicotine and cotinine concentrations in the milk of smoking mothers: influence of cigarette consumption and diurnal variation. Eur J Pediatr 1987;146:21–26.

35. Luck W, Nau H. Nicotine and cotinine concentrations in serum and milk of nursing mothers. Br J Clin Pharmacol 1984;18:9–15.

36. Kesaniemi Y. Ethanol and acetaldehyde in the milk and peripheral blood of lactating women after ethanol administration. J Obstet Gynecol Br Comm 1974;81:84–86.

37. Mennella JA, Beauchamp GK. The transfer of alcohol to

human milk: effects on flavor and the infant's behavior. N Engl J Med 1991;325:981–985.

38. Little RE, Anderson KW, Ervin CH, Worthington-Roberts B, Clarren SK. Maternal alcohol use during breast-feeding and infant mental and motor development at one year. N Engl J Med 1989;321:425–430.

39. Kovar IZ, Strehlow CD, Richmond J, Thompson MG. Perinatal lead and cadmium burden in a British urban population. Arch Dis Child 1984;59:36–39.

40. Jensen AA. Chemical contaminants in human milk. Residue Rev 1983;89:1–128.

41. Dabeka RW, Karpinski KF, McKenzie AD, Bajdik CD. Survey of lead, cadmium and fluoride in human milk and correlation of levels with environmental and food factors. Food Chem Toxicol 1986;24:913–921.

42. Bellinger D, Leviton A, Waternaux C, Needleman H, Rabinowitz M. Longitudinal analyses of prenatal and postnatal lead exposure and early cognitive development. N Engl J Med 1987;316:1037–1043.

43. Needleman HL, Bellinger D. The developmental consequences of childhood exposure to lead. Adv Clin Child Psychol 1984;7:195–220.

44. Rabinowitz M, Leviton A, Needleman H. Lead in milk and infant blood: a dose-response model. Arch Environ Health 1985;40:283–286.

45. Silbergeld EK. Lead in bone: implications for toxicology during pregnancy and lactation. Environ Health Perspect 1991;91:63–70.

46. Ziegler EE, Edwards BB, Jensen RL, Mahaffey KR, Fomon JS. Absorption and retention of lead by infants. Pediatrics 1978;12:29–34.

47. Ryu JE, Ziegler EE, Nelson SE, Fomon SJ. Dietary intake of lead and blood lead concentration in early infancy. Am J Dis Child 1983;137:886–891.

48. Bakir F, Damluji SF, Amin-Zaki L, et al. Methyl mercury poisoning in Iraq. Science 1973;181:230–241.

49. Clarkson TW, Nordberg GF, Sager PR. Reproductive and developmental toxicity of metals. Scand J Work Environ Health 1985;11:145–154.

50. Skerfving S. Mercury in women exposed to methylmercury through fish consumption and in their newborn babies and breast milk. Bull Environ Contam Toxicol 1988;41:475–482.

51. World Health Organization (WHO)/International Atomic Energy Agency (IAEA) collaborative study. Minor and trace elements in breast milk. Geneva: WHO, 1989; 19–66.

52. Kumpulainen J, Vuori E. Longitudinal study of chromium in human milk. Am J Clin Nutr 1980;33:2299–2302.

53. Bagnell PC, Ellenberger HA. Obstructive jaundice due to a chlorinated hydrocarbon in breast milk. Can Med J 1977;117:1047–1048.

54. Skaare JU, Tuveng JM, Sande HA. Organochlorine pesticides and polychlorinated biphenyls in maternal adipose tissue, blood, milk, and cord blood from mothers and their infants living in Norway. Arch Environ Contam Toxicol 1988;17:55–63.

55. Bush B, Snow J, Connor S, Koblintz R. Polychlorinated biphenyl congeners (PCBs), p,p'-DDE and hexachlorobenzene in human milk in three areas of upstate New York. Arch Environ Contam Toxicol 1985;14:443–450.

56. Jensen AA. Polychlorobiphenyls, polychlorodibenzo-p-dioxins and polychlorodibenzofurans in human milk, blood and adipose tissue. Sci Total Environ 1987;64:259–293.

57. Taguchi S, Yakushiji T. Influence of termite treatment in the home on the chlordane concentration in human milk. Arch Environ Contam Toxicol 1988;17:65–71.

58. Rogan WJ, Gladen BC, McKinney JD, et al. Neonatal effects of transplacental exposure to PCBs and DDE. J Pediatr 1986;109:335–341.

59. Jacobson SW, Fein G, Jacobson JL, Schwartz PM, Dowler JK. The effect of intrauterine PCB exposure on visual recognition memory. Child Dev 1985;56:853–860.

60. Fein G, Jacobson JL, Jacobson SL, Schwartz PM, Dowler JK. Prenatal exposure to polychlorinated biphenyls: effects on birth size and gestational age. J Pediatr 1984;105:315–320.

61. Wolff MS. Occupational exposure to polychlorinated biphenyls. Environ Health Perspect 1985;60:133–138.

62. Yakushiji T. Contamination, clearance, and transfer of PCB from human milk. Rev Environ Contam Toxicol 1988;101:139–164.

63. Mes J, Doyle JA, Adams BR, Davies DJ, Turton D. Polychlorinated biphenyls and organochlorine pesticides in milk and blood of Canadian women during lactation. Arch Environ Contam Toxicol 1984;13:217–223.

64. Yakushiji T, Watanabe I, Kuwabara K, et al. Postnatal transfer of PCBs from exposed mothers to their babies: influence of breast-feeding. Arch Environ Health 1984;39:368–375.

65. Jacobson JL, Humphrey HEB, Jacobson SW, Schantz SL, Mullin MD, Welch R. Determinants of polychlorinated biphenyls, polybrominated biphenyls, and dichlorodiphenyltrichloroethane in the sera of young children. Am J Public Health 1989;79:1401–1404.

66. Thiry L, Sprecher-Goldberger S, Jonckheer T, et al. Isolation of AIDS virus from cell-free breast milk of three health virus carriers. Lancet 1985;2:891–892.

67. VandePerre P, Hitimana D-G, Lepage P. Human immunodeficiency virus antibodies of IgG, IgA, and IgM subclasses in milk of seropositive mothers. J Pediatr 1988;113:1039–1040.

68. Pass RF. Transmission of viruses through human milk. In: Howell RR, Morriss FH Jr, Pickering LK, eds. Human milk in infant nutrition and health. Springfield, IL: Charles C Thomas, 1986.

69. Schou M, Amdisen A. Lithium and pregnancy. III. Lithium ingestion by children breast-fed by milk. Br Med J 1973;2:138.

70. Berlin CM. The excretion of drugs in human milk. In: Schwartz R, Yaffe S, eds. Drug and chemical risks to the fetus and newborn. New York: Alan R. Liss, 1980:115–127.

71. Yurchak AM, Jusko WJ. Theophylline secretion into breast milk. Pediatrics 1976;57:518–520.

72. Pitkin RM, Bahns JA, Filer LJ, Reynolds WA. Mercury in human maternal and cord blood, placenta, and milk. Proc Soc Exp Biol Med 1976;151:565–567.

73. Eyster JT, Humphrey HEB, Kimbrough RD. Partitioning of polybrominated biphenyls (PBBs) in serum, adipose

tissue, breast milk, placenta, cord blood, biliary fluid, and feces. Arch Environ Health 1983;38:47–53.

74. Riordan J, Riordan M. Drugs in breast milk. Am J Nurs 1984;84:328–332.

75. Wyburn JR. Human breast milk excretion of radionuclides following administration of radiopharmaceuticals. J Nucl Med 1973;14:115–17.

76. McKenzie SA, Selley JA, Agnew JE. Secretion of prednisolone into breast milk. Arch Dis Child 1975;50:894–896.

77. Mes J, Doyle JA, Adams BR, Davies DJ, Turton D. Polychlorinated biphenyls and organochlorine pesticides in milk and blood of Canadian women during lactation. Arch Environ Contam Toxicol 1984;13:217–223.

78. Nygren M, Rappe C, Lindstrom G, et al. Identification of 2,3,7,8-substituted polychlorinated dioxins and dibenzofurans in environmental and human samples. In: Rappe C, Choudharry G, Keith LH, eds. Chlorinated dioxins and dibenzofurans in perspective. Chelsea, MI: Lewis Publishers, Inc., 1986:15–34.

79. Resman BH, Blumenthal HP, Jusko WJ. Breast milk distribution of theobromine from chocolate. J Pediatr 1977;91:477–480.

80. Ong CN, Phoon WO, Law HY, Tye CY, Lim HH. Concentrations of lead in maternal blood, cord blood, and breast milk. Arch Dis Child 1985;60:756–759.

81. Rockway SW, Weber CW, Lei KY, Kemberling SR. Lead concentrations of milk, blood and hair in lactating women. Int Arch Occup Environ Health 1984;53:181–187.

# 7

Carcinogenesis

GRETA R. BUNIN, PETER G. ROSE, KENNETH L. NOLLER, EMIL SMITH[a]

## OVERVIEW

Whereas clinicians readily appreciate infertility and developmental abnormalities as legitimate reproductive endpoints, the link between the environment and reproductive system cancer may appear more obscure. There are, however, at least two reasons to broaden our understanding of reproductive hazards to include carcinogenesis: not only may environmental exposures be important in the etiology of reproductive tract tumors, but exposure to toxicants during the preconception period or pregnancy may contribute to later cancer development in offspring.

The capacity for chemical agents to induce cancer of the reproductive tract has been known for over 200 yr. In 1775, Percival Potts noted a high incidence of scrotal cancer among chimney sweeps in London. This description was the first reported association between an occupational exposure and a reproductive tract tumor. Since then, much has been learned about environmental risk factors for reproductive tract tumors, although the specific contribution of occupational exposures remains uncertain.

More recent scientific advances have turned attention to pre- and postconception mechanisms that influence cancer development, particularly in young people. Perhaps the most

fundamental of these was the recognition that mutagenic damage to germ or somatic cells represented an essential "initiating event" in carcinogenesis. The relatively short latency period for childhood cancers, approximately 40% of which occur before 4 yr of age, lent additional credence to mechanisms operative during the perinatal period. Soon, a genetic basis for some childhood cancers was established (e.g., retinoblastoma), and a number of congenital disorders were identified that had associated increased cancer risks (e.g., neurofibromatosis, Down syndrome). Finally, the discovery that diethylstilbestrol (DES) was a human transplacental carcinogen generated unprecedented experimental research related to prenatal chemical carcinogenesis.

The possibility of toxicant-induced carcinogenesis has obvious clinical relevance. Clusters of childhood cancer in contaminated communities such as Woburn, Massachusetts (Chapter 27) have resulted in untold emotional turmoil, considerable liability, and millions of dollars spent in research, control, and clean up. The DES experience has heightened the fear that some other presumably safe substance will have unforeseen adverse effects long after exposure. Unfortunately, these areas of research are still beset by methodological problems and considerable uncertainty. Although it is important that clinicians understand current knowledge in these fields, much more work is needed to answer definitively those questions posed by concerned workers and citizens.

This chapter considers cancer induction at

---

[a] Dr. Bunin contributed the section on "Parental Occupations and the Risk of Childhood Cancer"; Dr. Rose contributed the section on "Environmental and Occupational Risk Factors for Tumors of the Adult Reproductive Tract"; and Dr. Noller contributed the section on "Transplacental Carcinogenesis."

three levels. First, we review accumulated data regarding transplacental carcinogenesis following maternal exposure to carcinogenic chemicals. The second section discusses the relationships between parental occupation and childhood cancers, situations that may involve the initiation of cancer in the fetus or child during the reproductive process. Last, we consider tumors of the adult reproductive tract that may be related to later exposures to offending agents.

## TRANSPLACENTAL CARCINOGENESIS

In the April 22, 1971 issue of *The New England Journal of Medicine*, an article was published that caused widespread anguish among both patients and physicians, fostered thousands of drug-related liability claims, and changed forever the practice of obstetrics in the United States (1). Drs. Herbst, Ulfelder, and Poskanzer reported an association between in utero exposure to the synthetic nonsteroidal estrogen DES and the later development of clear cell adenocarcinoma of the vagina. Subsequent reports from other patient sources confirmed this association and, fortunately, suggested a relatively low risk of tumor occurrence (2, 3). While transplacental carcinogenesis had been documented in laboratory mammals and was considered to be possible in humans, this DES-cancer linkage remains our only clinical example of this phenomenon.

### Definition and Mechanisms

The term transplacental carcinogenesis implies that there is passage of a substance across the barriers of a mammalian placenta, and that this substance results in the initiation of a cancer that is expressed in the offspring at some time after the exposure. The carcinogen may be the parent compound itself or it may be a metabolite produced by maternal, placental, or fetal enzymatic reactions. Transplacental carcinogenesis is not usually used to describe direct invasion of the placenta and fetus by extension of a maternal neoplastic process. The most common example of this latter process in humans is melanoma.

Because many chemicals of low molecular weight are able to cross the placental membranes, the list of potential transplacental carcinogens is lengthy. In contrast to humans, nearly 40 chemicals have been identified as transplacental carcinogens in experimental animals (4).

Theoretically, there are many possible mechanisms of action of a transplacental carcinogen. Three of the more discussed are: (*a*) that the agent induces cancer directly by alteration of fetal DNA, causing a loss of control of cell growth; (*b*) that the substance alters the normal structure of the fetus (teratogenesis), making one or more tissues susceptible to carcinogenic exposures occurring later in life; and (*c*) that the agent modifies the fetal DNA that codes for a specific organ such that its susceptibility to later oncogenic exposures is increased. Establishing a mechanism of action for a specific agent becomes more complicated by introducing variables such as species differences, fetal sex, and varying postnatal exposures. Using DES as an example, tumorigenesis has been documented only for females, only after a period of at least several years (during which many exposures to other agents occur), and only in an organ system (the vagina and possibly cervix) that is embryologically unique, even among primates (5).

### Diethylstilbestrol

Twenty years have now passed since DES was first implicated in the etiology of clear cell cancer in young women whose mothers were treated with DES during pregnancy. While virtually all unbiased investigators accept the association, there is still no consensus regarding the mechanism of action.

DES is a teratogen. If given in adequate doses between approximately the 8th and 18th weeks of gestation, over one-third of resultant female offspring will have changes in the epithelial lining of the vagina (6). However, only about 1 in 1000 to 1 in 10,000 prenatally exposed women will develop cancer (7). Whether the cancer develops as a result of exposure of the atypical epithelium to an as yet unidentified agent or whether the epithelium itself is capable of spontaneous neoplastic change is unknown.

Because clear cell cancer usually occurs 17–22 yr after exposure to DES, vaginal exposure to many other agents has certainly occurred (e.g., douches, anti-infectives, tampons, semen). While the case-control investigative method employed by Herbst et al. clearly established an association between prenatal DES exposure and this tumor, many cofactors may be necessary to cause neoplasia. Indeed, because DES was used for many years as a growth stimulant in various farm animals, it is even possible that continuous, very low-dose exposure due to consumption of meat products is related to the occurrence of clear cell cancer.

If there is a positive aspect to the DES saga, it is that both physicians and patients have become more reluctant to prescribe or to consume medications during pregnancy. Additionally, pregnant women are now taking appropriate note of exposure to potentially harmful agents at work and in the home.

## PARENTAL OCCUPATION AND THE RISK OF CHILDHOOD CANCER

Interest in parental occupation as a possible risk factor for childhood cancer began with the observation by Fabia and Thuy (8) that children with cancer were more likely to have fathers employed in jobs with potential hydrocarbon exposure than children whose fathers were otherwise employed. The occupations classified as having potential hydrocarbon exposure were motor vehicle mechanics and service station attendants; machinists, miners, and lumbermen; and painters, dyers, and cleaners. The observed increase in risk was about twofold. Several subsequent studies attempted, but were generally unable, to replicate this finding (9–14). However, the new studies did observe associations between some of the hydrocarbon-exposed occupations and specific types of childhood cancers. More recently, researchers have conducted studies of single childhood cancers, as is appropriate for a group of diseases that are likely to have different etiologies.

### Basic Considerations

If occupational exposures of parents do increase the risk of cancer in children, the initiating event could occur before conception, during pregnancy, or after birth. Exposure of either parent before conception might result in a new germ cell mutation that confers increased cancer risk to the child. Current evidence suggests that most such germinal mutations are of paternal origin (15–17). During pregnancy, women might be exposed to toxicants at work that induce somatic mutations in the early embryo or that cross the placenta and affect the fetus. In addition, the father's work exposures during the pregnancy could harm the fetus if, for example, he brought substances into the home on his clothes. Postnatally, the child might be exposed to occupational substances through breast milk or via substances inadvertently brought home by either the mother or the father. This latter route of exposure has been documented in lead poisoning, berylliosis, chlordecone (Kepone) toxicity, and hyperestrogenism (18).

### Background

All of the studies investigating the relationship of paternal occupation to childhood cancer risk have used a case-control design. For most childhood cancers, the data are frustratingly inconsistent. It seems that for every report of an association with a particular occupation, there is another study with contradictory results. Methodological issues may explain some of the inconsistencies. For example, studies differ in whether exposures are inferred from job titles or self-reports by individuals. Both approaches have advantages and limitations. Self-reported exposure data allow for variation among jobs that have identical titles, while inferring exposures from job titles does not. However, when exposures are self-reported, parents of children with cancer and parents of healthy children may report their exposures differently. Differential reporting may produce spurious results if, for example, parents of children with cancer report exposures to pesticides that parents of healthy children do not report. Inferring exposures from job titles and industry codes minimizes the potential of this "recall bias."

Results of studies may also conflict because of differences in risk among age groups, countries, related occupations, and histological types. For example, the results of a study of leukemia in children who are less than 1 yr of age may conflict with a similar study in children who are less than 15 yr of age if the effect of the exposure is specific for a certain age range. Similarly, an exposure may increase the risk for some forms of the disease but not for others. In such cases, a study that included all types of leukemia would likely yield different results than one that focused on a single, relatively uncommon subtype. The varying occupational groupings used in different studies may also explain some of the discrepant results. Because of the limited number of parents in any single occupation, researchers have generally investigated groups of occupations with similar exposures. However, if only individuals in a single occupation are at risk, then larger groupings will obscure that risk. Results may also be inconsistent if individuals in the same occupations have different exposures or degrees of exposure in different countries.

## Leukemia

Vianna et al. (19) reported an approximate 2.5-fold increased risk of leukemia in infants whose fathers were occupationally exposed to motor vehicle exhaust fumes as drivers, motor vehicle mechanics, service station attendants, or railroad workers. In four other studies of individuals up to 15–20 yr of age, the odds ratios for similar occupational groupings were lower, ranging from 1.0–2.3 (10, 13, 14, 20). In two of the studies, at least one analysis of the motor vehicle-related category gave a statistically significant result (13, 14).

In some reports, parental exposure to paint was associated with childhood leukemia (21, 22). In a study of acute nonlymphocytic leukemia (ANLL), which accounts for approximately 15% of childhood leukemia, paternal employment as painter and maternal (but not paternal) self-reported paint exposure increased the risk (22). However, another study that investigated all leukemias and lymphomas found no association with the occupation of painter (23).

As employment in agriculture may increase the risk of leukemia in adults (24), this industry and its associated exposures (primarily pesticides) have been investigated in relation to childhood leukemia. A study of acute lymphocytic leukemia (ALL) that was performed in China observed an increased risk for mother's, but not father's, employment in agriculture

(25). However, no associations with parental employment in agriculture were observed in studies of ALL in the Netherlands (20) and in the U.S. (21).

In one U.S. study, ANLL was associated with both mother's and father's occupational exposure to pesticides (22). When both parents' exposures were considered simultaneously, only paternal exposure remained statistically significant. However, in the study of leukemia in China, the risk of ANLL was increased for mothers, but not for fathers, working in agriculture (25).

In two studies, one conducted in China and the other in the United States, associations were observed between ANLL and maternal employment in metal processing and refining (25). The risk was increased about 4.5-fold in both studies.

Recently, Gardner et al. (26) studied childhood leukemia near a nuclear waste reprocessing plant in the United Kingdom and noted an association with paternal employment at the plant. A dose-response relationship was observed between paternal radiation dose before the child's conception and the risk of leukemia. In the highest dose category, the odds ratio was 6–8, depending on the analysis. The authors' suggestion that radiation exposure at the plant caused leukemogenic germline mutations has been criticized on several grounds; however, these findings represent one of the few instances of a dose-response relationship of any exposure with childhood cancer.

Other exposures and industries of employment have been associated with childhood leukemia in single studies only: paternal employment in transportation equipment and machinery manufacturing (21); paternal exposure to solvents (22), including chlorinated solvents and methyl ethyl ketone (21), cutting oils (21), plastics (22), petroleum products (22), and lead (22); maternal employment in the personal service industry (beauty shops, domestic cleaning, laundries) (21), textile manufacturing (20), hydrocarbon-related occupations (20); and maternal exposure to sawdust (22).

## Brain Tumors

The first investigators to study parental occupation as a risk factor for childhood brain cancer observed a strong association with paternal employment in the aircraft industry (27) in children under 10 yr of age; however, two other studies found no association with the aircraft industry for children under 15 yr old (28, 29).

Three studies have reported an increased risk of childhood brain tumors with paternal exposure to paints (13, 27, 30), while three other studies have not (29, 31, 32). Thus, the data on paternal paint-related exposures and risk of childhood brain tumors are still inconclusive.

Brain cancer in children has been associated with paternal employment in agriculture in two studies (30, 31), but two other studies found no association with fathers who were farmers (8, 13).

Other parental occupations and industries have been reported as possible risk factors, but the data are very limited. In two studies, associations with paternal employment in the petroleum industry were reported, although neither was statistically significant (29, 33). Two studies have suggested an increased risk with paternal occupation as paper or pulp mill worker (11, 29). Two studies observed modest and statistically nonsignificant increases in risk associated with paternal electromagnetic field exposure (29, 33). Electrical assembling, installing, and repairing occupations were associated with increased risks in one study (31), but not in another (29). One group of researchers observed an association with paternal occupation of printer (29), but another group did not (31). Increased risks were also observed for fathers employed as chemical and drug salesmen (29), graphic arts workers (29), electricians (29), and metal-related workers (welders; plumbers; vehicle body workers; metal refining, processing, machining, working, fabrication, assembly, and repair workers) (28). Studies on paternal exposures to ionizing radiation have yielded inconclusive results (33, 34).

## Wilms' Tumor

The data on Wilms' tumors and parental occupation are more consistent than for leukemia and brain tumors. The four studies of Wilms' tumors reported associations with the following paternal occupations, respectively (35–38): (*a*)

occupations with potential exposure to lead (driver, motor vehicle mechanic, service station attendant, welder, solderer, metallurgist, scrap metal worker); (*b*) painter; (*c*) a grouping of welders, machinists, metal workers, and paper manufacturing workers; and (*d*) auto mechanics, auto body repairmen, and welders. In addition, three studies that investigated childhood cancers as a group presented results for Wilms' tumors separately (8, 11, 12). In one of these studies, an excess of mechanics, gas station attendants, and machinists was observed, although there were only 34 cases (11). The two other studies that analyzed Wilms' tumors together included only one machinist and no fathers with the other occupations of interest among 52 cases (8, 12). Considered in total, the data most strongly suggest that paternal occupation of welder may increase the risk of Wilms' tumor in children. The associations with employment as vehicle mechanic, gasoline station attendant, or painter are less strong, but deserve further investigation.

## Neuroblastoma

Three studies have investigated parental occupation and neuroblastoma. The first observed a statistically significant association with paternal exposure to aromatic and aliphatic hydrocarbons (39). The men included in this cluster were electricians, asbestos workers, electric and electronic workers, and printers. Further analysis also suggested an increased risk in jobs involving electromagnetic field exposure; however, two other studies did not confirm this finding (40, 41).

## Hepatoblastoma

In a study of hepatoblastoma, researchers observed significantly increased risks for both maternal and paternal occupational exposure to metals (22). For mothers, the metal exposures were commonly to welding and soldering fumes and most occurred daily, before and during pregnancy. For fathers, there was no difference in self-reported exposure to welding and soldering fumes, but more case than control fathers reported exposure to metal dusts and lead. Other findings included elevated risk for maternal exposure to paints or pigments and for maternal or paternal exposure to oil or coal products.

## Retinoblastoma

A study of retinoblastoma reported associations with metal-related jobs of fathers (42). Retinoblastoma may result from either germinal or somatic mutation, and the two forms can be largely distinguished by clinical characteristics (43). Retinoblastoma that likely resulted from new germinal mutations was associated with paternal occupation in primary metal manufacturing. The other, somatic form of retinoblastoma was associated with paternal employment as a welder, machinist, or metal worker.

## Conclusion

Although research on parental occupation and childhood cancer is in its infancy, there are some promising etiological clues. Exposure to metals has been associated with Wilms' tumor, ANLL, hepatoblastoma, retinoblastoma, and brain tumor. Increased risks of leukemia, ANLL, brain tumor, and Wilms' tumor have been observed in the offspring of individuals with occupational exposure to paints. Brain tumor and leukemia have been associated with employment in agriculture or exposure to pesticides. Future research may confirm or refute these clues. To date, most findings implicate work environments but provide little information about specific toxicants. For example, the concerning agent in metal-related jobs may not be a metal at all, but rather substances used with metals, such as solvents. In addition to epidemiological studies, laboratory investigations will be needed to help determine the timing of exposure that confers risk.

## ENVIRONMENTAL AND OCCUPATIONAL RISK FACTORS FOR TUMORS OF THE ADULT REPRODUCTIVE TRACT

Over the past 20 yr, a great deal of effort has been devoted to understanding the epidemiology of adult reproductive tract tumors. Recognition of environmental risk factors associated with reproductive neoplasms may help identify high-risk populations that should be more closely screened for these diseases. Ultimately,

if specific high-risk exposures can be avoided, the incidence of these tumors can be altered.

## Male Reproductive Tract Tumors

### PROSTATE CANCER

Prostate cancer is the most frequent cancer in men, occurring in 1 of 11 white males and 1 of 10 black males (44). The disease occurs primarily in men who are greater than 70 yr old and increases with age more than any other cancer.

Some studies, but not all, suggest that prostate cancer may be related to elevated testosterone levels (45). Studies have had conflicting results regarding the role of vasectomy as a risk factor (46–49). Dietary intake of animal fat is strongly associated with prostate cancer (50, 51). Consumption of vitamin A and its precursor β-carotene may decrease the risk (52). No association between smoking or alcohol, coffee, or tea consumption has been found for prostate cancer.

Although numerous studies of prostatic cancer and occupational exposure have been conducted, they have produced variable results. The Third National Cancer Survey found prostate cancer to be more common among ministers, plumbers, rubber workers, farmers, coal miners, and two types of retailers (53). More recently, Brownson et al. (54) reported elevated odds ratios for farmers, mechanics, sheet metal workers, and workers in several other manufacturing industries. Other studies have found conflicting results with respect to the risk among farmers. Ernster et al. (55) reported elevated odds ratios for four occupations: bookkeepers, shipping clerks, typesetters, and ship fitters. While no common carcinogen is obvious from these investigations, the elevated odds ratios suggest a possible environmental factor. The occupational exposure most often cited as a risk factor for prostatic cancer is exposure to cadmium; the reported relative risk (RR) ranges from 1.7–6.9 (56). No increased risk has been reported from radiation exposure.

### TESTES CANCER

Cancer of the testes is rare, accounting for only 1% of male cancers. However, there has been a dramatic increase in the disease in the last several decades. Testicular cancer, primarily of germ cell origin, is the most frequent malignancy for males 20–35 yr of age. The disease is less frequent in the black population and does not appear to be increasing.

Among reported risk factors for testicular cancer are low sperm count, fertility problems, and/or atrophic or cryptorchid testes (57, 58). The role of vasectomy is uncertain (59). Although estrogen use in pregnancy was suggested as a risk factor, subsequent studies of DES exposure have not confirmed the association (60).

Professional occupation is a risk factor for testicular cancer, but may be more a marker of social class than a causative association (61). Mills et al. (62) reported an association with farming as an occupation, but this finding was not substantiated by data in the Danish Cancer Registry (63). Other reported occupational risk factors are exposure to fertilizers (RR = 2.27), phenols (RR = 2.08), and smoke or fumes (RR = 2.83) (57). Mills et al. (62) also observed an increased risk of testicular cancer with exposure to oil and natural gas mining, but this was not confirmed by a population-based study from the New Mexico Tumor Registry (64).

Between 1982 and 1984, three workers from a leather tannery in Fulton County, New York, developed testicular cancer. A case-control study demonstrated that 5 of 10 testicular cancer patients in Fulton County were leather workers compared with 17 of 129 controls (65). The relative risk for testicular cancer among leather workers was 40.5 (95% CI 8.1–118.4). The suspected agent, dimethylformamide (DMF), had also recently been associated with testicular cancer. However, there are inconsistent findings regarding the association of DMF with testicular cancer in two other studies. As a result of these findings, DMF has been eliminated from many dyes and solvents. Methyl bromide has also been associated with testicular cancer (66).

Exposure of the testes to heat or trauma has been associated with testicular cancer in case-control studies but may reflect recall bias (67). No role for cigarette smoking, alcohol consumption, animal fat intake, or obesity has been identified (68). Testicular cancer has not been associated with x-rays below the waist (68) or with the use of electric blankets (69).

## PENILE CANCER

Cancer of the penis is extremely uncommon in industrialized societies. In contrast, the disease occurs commonly in Asia and Africa, where it accounts for 13% of all cancers. Greater than 90% of penile cancers are squamous and arise on the glans penis or prepuce.

Roles for smegma and phimosis have been postulated but remain uncertain. As in cervical cancer, human papilloma virus (HPV) types 16 and 18 have been identified in penile cancers and suggested as etiological agents (70), but sexual behavior has not been identified as a risk factor (71).

Cigarette smoking is positively associated with cancer of the penis in a dose-response fashion (71). In addition, the use of ultraviolet radiation with psoralens in the treatment of psoriasis has recently been implicated as a risk factor (72), while radiation used for diagnostic purposes has not. Although low socioeconomic class is associated with a three-fold risk of penile cancer, specific occupations have not been identified. There are also no known dietary or hormonal risk factors for the disease.

## SCROTAL CANCER

Scrotal cancer has been found commonly among metal workers (73) and in men exposed to mineral oils, pitch, and/or tar (74). The use of psoralens and ultraviolet radiation for the treatment of psoriasis is also associated with the disease (72). Roles for smoking or dietary or hormonal factors have not been identified. Interestingly, the incidence of cancer of the scrotum has been decreasing, probably as the result of improved worker protection (74).

## Female Reproductive Tract Tumors

### UTERINE CANCER

Uterine cancer is the most frequent gynecological cancer: 33,000 cases, but only 4000 deaths, are estimated for 1991 (44). The disease is usually diagnosed in its early stages, because most patients report quickly to their health care providers for abnormal vaginal bleeding.

Almost all cancers of the uterus arise from the glands of the endometrium and are carcinomas. The 3% arising from deeper uterine tissues are sarcomas. Most epidemiological studies have focused on endometrial carcinoma.

It is widely recognized that the development of endometrial carcinoma is associated with a variety of hyperestrogenic states, such as early menarche and late menopause (which lengthens total exposure of the endometrium to estrogen), obesity (because adipose tissue contains aromatose, an enzyme that converts adrenal androgens to estrone), polycystic ovarian disease (in which there is chronic anovulation and estrogen-mediated endometrial hyperstimulation), and the administration of estrogenic drugs (75–77). In addition, the occurrence of endometrial carcinoma is related to fat consumption (50, 78, 79), although the nature of the causal relationship is not yet clear.

The combination oral contraceptive agents currently available are progesterone dominant and confer protection from endometrial cancer (80). Interestingly, because cigarette smoking hydroxylates estrogen, it decreases the risk of endometrial carcinoma (81).

No associations between uterine cancer and occupation are known. Endometrial carcinoma has been reported after low-dose radiation to the pelvis; before 1950, this was a treatment for dysfunctional uterine bleeding, a practice that has since been discontinued. Endometrial carcinoma is not statistically increased following therapeutic doses of radiation (82). An association of uterine sarcoma with therapeutic radiation has been reported by some investigators; however, in the largest collaborative study to date, an increased risk was not evident (82).

## OVARIAN CANCER

Ovarian cancer is the most virulent of gynecological cancers, primarily because it is most often diagnosed in an advanced stage. In the U.S. alone, 20,500 cases and 12,400 deaths are estimated for 1991 (44). The worldwide incidence rates are highly variable. Because the disease is common in industrialized societies, it may result from some byproduct of industrialization. However, the highly industrialized nation of Japan has a very low incidence of the disease.

Incessant ovulation has been postulated as a risk factor for ovarian cancer, since the risk is decreased by either pregnancy or oral contraceptives (83) and is increased in patients with early menarche, late menopause, and regular menses (all signs of prolonged ovulation) (84). Walker et al. (85) reported an increased risk of ovarian germ cell tumors with DES or other maternal hormone use. There is apparently no association between epithelial ovarian tumors and use of noncontraceptive conjugated estrogens. Rates of ovarian cancer are positively correlated with fat consumption (50, 86, 87). In premenopausal patients, obesity is associated with serous and endometrioid tumors (88).

Two studies have related the incidence of ovarian cancer to coffee consumption (89, 90). However, these results are contradicted by the high incidence of ovarian cancer among vegetarians in Great Britain, despite a low per capita coffee consumption (91). Smoking or alcohol consumption has not been reported to increase the risk of ovarian cancer (89). A high intake of β-carotene has been reported to protect against ovarian cancer, even after correction for age, number of pregnancies, and body mass index (RR = 0.5) (92).

Since particulates of asbestos and talc were observed in sections of ovarian tumors (93), these materials have been carefully scrutinized. Newhouse (94) reported three deaths from ovarian cancer among women exposed to asbestos in industry, while only 0.6 were expected. Cramer et al. (95) reported an association of ovarian cancer with the use of talc. Both of these findings require confirmation.

Certain viral infections, including mumps and measles, have been reported to be associated with an increased incidence of ovarian cancer (96). However, Hartge et al. (97) found no association between a prior history of these diseases and ovarian cancer.

Some studies have found a small excess of ovarian cancers in patients exposed to ionizing radiation. A statistically significant increased risk of mortality from ovarian cancer was observed among atomic bomb survivors followed from 1950–1985. The relative risk of ovarian cancer death was increased approximately twofold among women exposed to 1 Gy (100 rad) compared with the nonexposed group (98).

Boice et al. (82) found no increase in ovarian cancer among 182,000 patients treated with radiation for cervical cancer.

## CERVICAL CANCER

Cancer of the cervix is the most frequent female cancer worldwide. Since the introduction of the Pap smear in 1943, there has been a dramatic decrease in the incidence and mortality of invasive cancer in screened populations. In the U.S., 13,500 cases with 6000 deaths are estimated for 1991 (44).

The importance of environmental influences on the development of cervical cancer was first recognized in 1842 when Rigoni-Stern noted the absence of cervical cancer in nuns. Since then, numerous investigations have focused on lifestyle and sexual practices as potential risk factors for the disease. Among the risk factors that have been identified are young age at first intercourse and multiple sexual partners (99, 100); prostitution; syphilis; herpes simplex virus (HSV)-2 infection (101, 102); and other sexually transmitted diseases including *Trichomonas vaginalis*, *Neisseria gonorrheae*, *Chlamydia*, cytomegalovirus, and condyloma acuminatum. All of these risk factors identify a sexually active population.

The human papilloma virus, in particular, HPV types 16, 18, 31, and 35, has been implicated as a causative agent in cervical cancer (103). However, Tidy et al. (104) recently found HPV-16 in the cervical tissue biopsies of 80% of normal women, suggesting that HPV alone is not sufficient to be carcinogenic. The HPV virus may function as a cocarcinogen or may be only another marker of a sexually active population.

To date, more than 30 epidemiological studies have examined the association of cigarette smoking and cervical cancer (105). Smoking remains a significant risk factor in multiple regression analyses after controlling for other behavioral influences, such as the number of sexual partners and age at first intercourse. Cigarette smoking has been shown to result in immune suppression. Since immunosuppressed women have both an increased incidence and virulence of lower genital tract neoplasia, this association may be causal. In a recent study, passive cigarette smoke exposure

for 3 hr daily was associated with an elevated risk for the development of cervical cancer (106). Alcohol consumption has not been shown to increase the risk of cervical cancer.

There are reports that cervical cancer patients had more commonly used vaginal douches (107) and four times as frequently reported douching with Lysol, a coal tar substance.

## VULVAR AND VAGINAL CANCER

Because of their relative infrequence, few studies have addressed the epidemiological risk factors for vulvar and vaginal cancer. Patients with vulvar cancer often have a history of young age at first intercourse, multiple sex partners, and/or low socioeconomic status (108); syphilis and condyloma (109); or HSV-2 infections (110). A history of genital warts (RR = 15.2) was a major risk factor, particularly in patients who smoked (RR = 35) (108).

## TROPHOBLASTIC DISEASE

Gestational trophoblastic disease (GTD) encompasses a spectrum of diseases including partial and complete hydatiform molar pregnancies, placental site trophoblastic tumor, and choriocarcinoma. A dramatic variation in the worldwide incidence of GTD has been reported. In the U.S., the incidence of GTD in the black population is half that of the white population.

Advanced maternal age has been repeatedly associated with an increased risk of GTD. Although professional occupations may result in delayed childbearing, a recent case-control study matched for gestational age found professional occupation to be an independent risk factor (RR = 2.56) (111).

In a multicentered case-control study of gestational choriocarcinoma, features of subnormal estrogen level, including delayed menarche, light menstruation, and lower body mass index, were more often reported by cases than controls (112). Although smoking can reduce estrogen levels, it is not clearly related to GTD. In a study from China, the use of oral contraceptives for more than 4 yr in duration increased the risk of GTD (RR = 2.2) (113). Recently, however, the Gynecologic Oncology

Group found no association of trophoblastic disease with oral contraceptive use following molar evacuation (114). Dietary vitamin A has been reported to protect against the development of GTD (115).

## SUMMARY AND CONCLUSIONS

There is now substantial evidence that some cancers of the reproductive tract are associated with occupational and/or environmental exposures to chemicals, viruses, or radiations, and that some nonreproductive tract tumors may be caused by similar factors operating during the reproductive process.

This chapter has addressed three modes of exposure and initiation of carcinogenesis: (a) initiation of reproductive tract cancers in the conceptus after the transplacental transport of the offending agent from the pregnant woman to the fetus; (b) initiation of nonreproductive tract cancer in children as the result of parental exposure in the workplace, presumably acting in some manner intimately related to reproduction per se; and finally, (c) initiation in adults of reproductive tract cancer as the result of direct occupational or environmental exposure.

While the relationships of each individual cancer and its possible risk factors are of great interest, one must be impressed by the wide variety of reproductive tract tumors that may be of occupational or environmental origin. Protection of individuals from these carcinogens has the potential to reduce the incidence of at least some of these many and diverse forms of cancer.

## REFERENCES

1. Herbst AL, Ulfelder H. Poskanzer DC. Adenocarcinoma of the vagina: association of maternal stilbestrol therapy with tumor appearance in young women. N Engl J Med 1971;284:878–881.
2. Noller KL, Decker DG, Dockerty MG, Lanier AP, Smith RA, Symmonds RE. Mesonephric (clear-cell) carcinoma of the vagina and cervix: a retrospective analysis. Obstet Gynecol 1974;43:640–644.
3. Lanier AP, Noller KL, Decker DG, Elveback LR, Kurland LT. Cancer and stilbestrol: a follow-up of 1,719 persons exposed to estrogens in utero and born 1943–1959. Mayo Clin Proc 1973;48:793–799.
4. Rice JM. An overview of transplacental chemical carcinogenesis. Teratology 1973;8:113–126.
5. Herbst AL, Anderson S, Hubby MM, Haenszel WM, Kaufman RH, Noller KL. Risk factors for the development of diethylstilbestrol-associated clear cell adenocarcinoma: a case-control study. Am J Obstet Gynecol 1986;154:814–822.
6. O'Brien PC, Noller KL, Robboy SJ, et al. Vaginal epithelial changes in young women enrolled in a national cooperative diethylstilbestrol adenosis (DESAD) project. Obstet Gynecol 1979;53:300–308.
7. Herbst AL, Cole P, Colton T, Robboy SJ, Scully RE. Age incidence and risk of diethylstilbestrol-related clear cell adenocarcinoma of the vagina and cervix. Am J Obstet Gynecol 1977;128:43–50.
8. Fabia J, Thuy TD. Occupation of father at time of birth of children dying of malignant diseases. Br J Prev Soc Med 1974;28:98–100.
9. Sanders BM, White GC, Draper GC. Occupations of fathers of children dying from neoplasms. J Epidemiol Community Health 1981;35:245–250.
10. Hakulinen T, Salonen T, Teppo L. Cancer in the offspring of fathers in hydrocarbon-related occupations. Br J Prev Soc Med 1976;30:138–140.
11. Kwa SL, Fine LJ. The association between parental occupation and childhood malignancy. J Occup Med 1980;22:792–794.
12. Zack M, Cannon S, Loyd D, et al. Cancer in children of parents exposed to hydrocarbon-related industries and occupations. Am J Epidemiol 1980;111:329–336.
13. Hemminki K, Saloniemi I, Salonen T, et al. Childhood cancer and parental occupation in Finland. J Epidemiol Community Health 1981;35:11–15.
14. Gold EB, Diener MD, Szklo M. Parental occupations and cancer in children. J Occup Med 1982;24:578–584.
15. Dryja TP, Mukai S, Petersen R, Rapaport JM, Walton D, Yandell DW. Parental origin of mutations of the retinoblastoma gene. Nature 1989;339:556–558.
16. Butler M, Palmer C. Parental origin of chromosome 15 deletion in Prader-Willi syndrome. Lancet 1983;1:1285–1286.
17. Jadayel D, Fair P, Upadhyaya M, et al. Paternal origin of new mutations in Von Recklinghausen neurofibromatosis. Nature 1990;343:558–559.
18. Knishkowy B, Baker E. Transmission of occupational disease to family contacts. Am J Ind Med 1986;9: 543–550.
19. Vianna N, Kovasznay B, Polan A, Ju C. Infant leukemia and paternal exposure to motor vehicle exhaust fumes. J Occup Med 1984;26:679–682.
20. Van Steensel-Moll HA, Valkenburg HA, Van Zanen GE. Childhood leukemia and parental occupation. Am J Epidemiol 1985;121:216–334.
21. Lowengart R, Peters J, Cicioni C, et al. Childhood leukemia and parents' occupational and home exposures. J Natl Cancer Inst 1987;79:39–46.
22. Buckley JD, Robison L, Swotinsky R, et al. Occupational exposures of parents of children with acute nonlymphocytic leukemia: a report from the Children's Cancer Study Group. Cancer Res 1989;49:4030–4037.
23. McKinney PA, Cartwright RA, Saiu JMT, et al. The inter-regional epidmeiological study of childhood cancer (IRESCC): a case-control study of aetiological factors

in leukaemia and lymphoma. Arch Dis Child 1987; 62:279–287.

24. Blair A. Cancer risks associated with agriculture. In: Fleck RF, Hollaender A, eds. Genetic toxicology: an agricultural perspective. New York: Plenum Press, 1982.

25. Shu XO, Gao YT, Brinton LA, et al. A population-based case-control study of childhood leukemia in Shanghai. Cancer 1988;62:635–644.

26. Gardner M, Snee M, Hall A, Powell C, Downes S, Terrell J. Results of case-control study of leukaemia and lymphoma among young people near Sellafield nuclear plant in West Cumbria. Br Med J 1990;300:423–429.

27. Peters JM, Preston-Martin S, Yu MC. Brain tumors in children and occupational exposure of parents. Science 1981;213:235–237.

28. Olshan AF, Breslow NE, Daling JR, Weiss NS, Leviton A. Childhood brain tumors and paternal occupation in the aerospace industry. J Natl Cancer Inst 1986;77: 17–19.

29. Johnson CC, Annegers JF, Frankowski RF, Spitz MR, Buffler PA. Childhood nervous system tumors—an evaluation of the association with paternal occupational exposure to hydrocarbons. Am J Epidemiol 1987;126: 605–613.

30. Wilkins JR, Sinks T. Parental occupation and intracranial neoplasms of childhood: results of a case-control interview study. Am J Epidemiol 1990;132:275–292.

31. Wilkins JR, Koutras RA. Paternal occupation and brain cancer in offspring: a mortality-based case-control study. Am J Ind Med 1988;14:299–318.

32. Howe GR, Burch JD, Chiarelli AM, Risch HA, Choi BCK. An exploratory case-control study of brain tumors in children. Cancer Res 1989;49:4349–4352.

33. Nasca PC, Baptiste MS, MacCubbin PA, et al. An epidemiologic case-control study of central nervous system tumors in children and parental occupational exposures. Am J Epidemiol 1988;128:1256–1265.

34. Hicks N, Zack M, Caldwell CG, et al. Childhood cancer and occupational radiation exposure in parents. Cancer 1984;53:1637–43.

35. Kantor A, Curnan M, Meigs J. Occupations of fathers of patients with Wilms' tumour. J Epidemiol Community Health 1979;33:253–256.

36. Wilkins JR, Sinks TH Jr. Paternal occupation and Wilms' tumor in offspring. J Epidemiol Community Health 1984;38:7–11.

37. Bunin GR, Nass CC, Kramer S, Meadows AT. Parental occupation and Wilms' tumor: results of a case-control study. Cancer Res 1989;49:725–729.

38. Olshan A, Breslow N, Daling J, et al. Wilms' tumor and paternal occupation. Cancer Res 1990;50:3212–3217.

39. Spitz MR, Johnson CC. Neuroblastoma and paternal occupation: a case-control analysis. Am J Epidemiol 1985;121:924–929.

40. Wilkins JR, Hundley VD. Paternal occupational exposure to electromagnetic fields and neuroblastoma in offspring. Am J Epidemiol 1990;131:995–1008.

41. Bunin G, Ward E, Kramer S, Rhee C, Meadows A. Neuroblastoma and parental occupation. Am J Epidemiol 1990;131:776–780.

42. Bunin G, Petrakova A, Meadows A, et al. Occupations of parents of children with retinoblastoma. Cancer Res 1990;50:7129–7133.

43. Knudson AG Jr. Mutation and cancer: statistical study of retinoblastoma. Proc Natl Acad Sci USA 1971;68: 820–823.

44. Boring CC, Squires TS, Tong T. Cancer statistics. Cancer 1991;41: 19–37.

45. Hsing AW, Comstock G. Serum hormone and risk of subsequent prostate cancer. Am J Epidemiol 1989;130:829.

46. Honda GD, Bernstein L, Ross RK, et al. Vasectomy, cigarette smoking, and age at first sexual intercourse as risk factors for prostate cancer in middle-aged men. Br J Cancer 1988;57:326–331.

47. Sidney S. Vasectomy and the risk of prostatic cancer and benign prostatic hypertrophy. J Urol 1987;138:795–797.

48. Rosenberg L, Palmer JR, Zauber AG, et al. Vasectomy and the risk of prostate cancer. Am J Epidemiol 1990;132:1051–1055.

49. Mettlin C, Natarajan N, Huben R. Vasectomy and prostate cancer risk. Am J Epidemiol 1990;132:1056–1061.

50. Armstrong B, Doll R. Environmental factors and cancer incidence and mortality in different countries, with special reference to dietary practices. Int J Cancer 1975;15:617–631.

51. Hill P, Wynder E, Garbaczewski L, et al. Diet and urinary steroids in black and white North American men and black South African men. Cancer Res 1979;39:5101–5105.

52. Reichman ME, Hayes RB, Ziegler RG, et al. Serum vitamin A and subsequent development of prostate cancer in the First National Health and Nutrition Examination Survey epidemiologic follow-up study. Cancer Res 1990;50:2311–2315.

53. Williams RR, Stegens NL, Goldsmith JR. Associations of cancer site and type with occupation and industry from the Third National Cancer Survey interview. J Natl Cancer Inst 1977;59:1147–1185.

54. Brownson RC, Chang JC, Davis JR et al. Occupational risk of prostate cancer: a cancer registry-based study. J Occup Med 1988;30:523–526.

55. Ernster VL, Selvin S, Brown SM, et al. Occupation and prostate cancer. A review and retrospective analysis based on the death certificates in two California counties. J Occup Med 1979;21:175–183.

56. Kolonel L, Winkelstein W Jr. Cadmium and prostate carcinoma. Lancet 1977;2:566–567.

57. Haughey BP, Graham S, Brasure J, et al. The epidemiology of testicular cancer in upstate New York. Am J Epidemiol 1989;130:25–36.

58. Pottern LM, Brown LM, Hoover RN, et al. Testicular cancer risk among young men: role of cryptorchidism and inguinal hernia. J Natl Cancer Inst 1985;74:377–384.

59. Cale ARJ, Farouk M, Prescott RJ, et al. Does vasectomy accelerate testicular tumor? Importance of testicular examinations before and after vasectomy. Br Med J 1990;300:370.

60. Leary FJ, Resseguie LJ, Kurland LT, et al. Males exposed in utero to diethylstilbestrol. JAMA 1984; 252: 2984–2989.

61. Mustacchi P, Millmore D. Racial and occupational variations in cancer of the testis, San Francisco 1956–1965. J Natl Cancer Inst 1976;56:717–733.

62. Mills PK, Newell GR, Johnson DE. Testicular cancer associated with employment in agriculture and oil natural gas extraction. Lancet 1984;1:207–209.

63. Jensen OM, Olsen JH, Osterlind A. Testis cancer risk among farmers in Denmark. Lancet 1984;1:794.

64. Sewell CM, Castle SP, Hull HF. Testicular cancer and employment in agriculture and oil and natural gas extraction. Lancet 1986;1:553.

65. Centers for Disease Control. Testicular cancer in leather workers—Fulton County, New York. MMWR 1989;38:105–114.

66. Wong O, Brocker W, Davies HV, et al. Mortality of workers potentially exposed to organic and inorganic brominated chemicals, DBCP, TRIS, PBB and DDT. Br J Ind Med 1984;41:15–24.

67. Swerdlow AJ, Huttly SRA, Smith PG. Is the incidence of testis cancer related to trauma or temperature? Br J Urol 1988;61:518–521.

68. Brown LM, Pottern LM, Hoover RN. Testicular cancer in young men: the search for causes of the epidemic increase in the United States. J Epidemiol Community Health 1987;41:349–354.

69. Verreault R, Weiss N, Hollenbach KA, et al. Use of electric blankets and risk of testicular cancer. Am J Epidemiol 1990;131:759–762.

70. Barrasso R, Brux JD, Croissant O, et al. High prevalence of papillomavirus-associated penile intraepithelial neoplasia in sexual partners of women with cervical intraepithelial neoplasia. N Engl J Med 1987;317:916–923.

71. Hellberg D, Valentin J, Eklund T, et al. Penile cancer: is there an epidemiologic role for smoking and sexual behavior? Br Med J 1987;295:1306–1308.

72. Stern RS. Genital tumors among men with psoriasis exposed to psoralens and ultraviolet A radiation (puva) and ultraviolet B radiation. N Engl J Med 1990; 322: 1093–1097.

73. Roush GC, Kelly JA, Meigs JW. Scrotal carcinoma in Connecticut metal workers:sequel to a study of sinonasal cancer. Am J Epidemiol 1982;116:76–85.

74. Sorahan T, Cooke MA, Wilson S. Incidence of cancer of the scrotum 1971–1984. Br J Ind Med 1989;46:430–431.

75. McMahon B. Risk factors for endometrial cancer. Gynecol Oncol 1974;2:122–129.

76. Wynder EL, Escher GC and Mantel N. An epidemiologic investigation of cancer of the endometrium. Cancer 1966;19:489–520.

77. Mack TM, Pike MC, Henderson BE, et al. Estrogens and endometrial cancer in a retirement community. N Engl J Med 1976;294:1262–1267.

78. Phillips RL. Role of life-style and dietary habits in risk of cancer among Seventh-Day Adventists. Cancer Res 1976;35:3513–3522.

79. La Vecchia C, Decarli A, Fasoli M, et al. Nutrition and diet in the etiology of endometrial cancer. Cancer 1986;57:1248–1253.

80. Ory HW. Oral contraceptive use and the risk of endometrial cancer. JAMA 1983;249:1600–1604.

81. Lesko SM, Rosenberg L, Kaufman DW, et al. Cigarette smoking and the risk of endometrial cancer. N Engl J Med 1985;313:593–596.

82. Boice JD, Day NE, Anderson A, et al. Second cancers following radiation treatment of cervical cancer: an international collaboration among cancer registries. J Natl Cancer Inst 1985;74:995–975.

83. Ory HW, Layde PM, Rubin GL, et al. The reduction in risk of ovarian cancer associated with oral-contraceptive use. N Engl J Med 1987;316:650–655.

84. Parazzini F, La Vecchia C, Negri E, et al. Menstrual factors and the risk of epithelial ovarian cancer. J Clin Epidemiol 1989;42:443–448.

85. Walker AH, Ross RK, Haile RWC, et al. Hormonal factors and risk of ovarian germ cell cancer in young women. Br J Cancer 1988;57:418–422.

86. Cramer DW, Welch WR, Hutchison GB, et al. Dietary animal fat in relation to ovarian cancer risk. Obstet Gynecol 1984;63:833–838.

87. La Vecchia C, Decarli A, Negri E, et al. Dietary factors and the risk epithelial ovarian cancer. J Natl Cancer Inst 1987;79:663–669.

88. Farrow DC, Weiss NS, Lyon JL, et al. Association of obesity and ovarian cancer in a case-control study. Am J Epidemiol 1989; 129:1300–1304.

89. Stocks P. Cancer mortality in relation to national consumption of cigarettes, solid fuel, tea and coffee. Br J Cancer 1970;24:215–225.

90. Trichopoulos D, Papapostolou M, Polychronopoulou A. Coffee and ovarian cancer. Int J Cancer 1981;28: 691–693.

91. Kinlen LJ. Mortality in relation to abstinence from meat in certain orders of religious sisters in Britain. In: Cairns J, Lyon JL, Skolnick M., eds. Cancer incidence in defined populations. New York: Cold Spring Harbor Laboratory, 1980:135–143.

92. Slattery ML, Schuman KL, West DW, et al. Nutrient intake and ovarian cancer. Am J Epidemiol 1989;130:497–502.

93. Graham J, Graham R. Ovarian cancer and asbestos. Environ Res 1967;1:115–128.

94. Newhouse ML, Berry G, Wagner JC, et al. A study of the mortality of female asbestos workers. Br J Ind Med 1972;29:134–141.

95. Cramer DW, Welch WR, Skully RE, et al. Ovarian cancer and talc. A case control study. Cancer 1982;50:372–376.

96. Cramer DW, Welch WD, Cassells S, et al. Mumps, menarche, menopause, and ovarian cancer. Am J Obstet Gynecol 1983;147:1–6.

97. Hartge P, Schiffman MH, Hoover R, et al. A case-control study of epithelial ovarian cancer. Am J Obstet Gynecol 1989;161:10–16.

98. Shimizu Y, Kato H, Schull WJ. Studies of the mortality of A-bomb survivors. 9. Mortality, 1950–1985: part 2. Cancer mortality based on the recently revised doses (DS 86). Radiat Res 1990;121:120–141.

99. Peters RK, Thomas D, Hagan DG, et al. Risk factors for invasive cervical cancer among Latinas and non-Latinas in Los Angeles County. J Natl Cancer Inst 1986;77:1063–1077.

100. Noller KL, O'Brien PC, Melton LJ, et al. Coital risk factors for cervical cancer. Am J Clin Oncol 1987;10:222–226.

101. Catalano LW, Johnson LD. Herpesvirus antibody and carcinoma in situ of the cervix. JAMA 1971;217:447–450.

102. Nahmias AJ, Naib AM, Josey WE, et al. Prospective studies of the association of genital herpes simplex infection and cervical anaplasia. Cancer Res 1973;33:1491–1497.

103. Crum CP, Ikenberg H, Richart R, et al. Human papillomavirus type 16 and early cervical neoplasia. N Engl J Med 1984;310:880–883.

104. Tidy J, Parry GCN, Ward P, et al. High rate of human papillomavirus type 16 infection in cytologically normal cervices. Lancet 1989;1:434.

105. Winkelstein W. Smoking and cervical cancer-current status: a review. Am J Epidemiol 1990;131:945–957.

106. Slattery ML, Robison LM, Schuman KL, et al. Cigarette smoking and exposure to passive smoke are risk factors for cervical cancer. JAMA 1989;261:1593–1598.

107. Graham S, Schotz W. Epidemiology of cancer of the cervix in Buffalo, New York. J Natl Cancer Inst 1979;63:23–27.

108. Brinton LA, Nasca PC, Mallin K, et al. Case-control study of cancer of the vulva. Obstet Gynecol 1990;75:859–866.

109. Franklin EW, Rutledge F. Epidemiology of epidermoid carcinoma of the vulva. Am J Obstet Gynecol 1972;39:165–172.

110. Kaufman RH, Dreesman GR, Burek J, et al. Herpesvirus-induced antigens in squamous-cell carcinoma in situ of the vulva. N Engl J Med 1981;305:483–488.

111. Messerli L, Lilienfield AM, Parmley T, et al. Risk factors for gestational trophoblastic neoplasia. Am J Obstet Gynecol 1985;153:294–300.

112. Buckley JD, Henderson BE, Marrow CP, et al. Case-control study of gestational choriocarcinoma. Cancer Res 1988;48:1004–1010.

113. Brinton LA, Wu B, Wang W, et al. Gestational trophoblastic disease: a case-control study from the People's Republic of China. Am J Obstet Gynecol 1989;161:121–127.

114. Curry SL, Schlaerth JB, Kohorn EI, et al. Hormonal contraception and trophoblastic sequelae after hydatidiform mole. Am J Obstet Gynecol 1989;160:805–809.

115. Parazzini F, La Vecchia C, Mangili G, et al. Dietary factors and risk of trophoblastic disease. Am J Obstet Gynecol 1988;158:93–100.

**II**

································································

# Research Methods

# Reproductive and Developmental Toxicity Testing Methods in Animals

PETER K. WORKING, DONALD R. MATTISON

Regulatory agencies have developed systematic scientific and administrative approaches to assess risks associated with exposures to chemicals (1). The process begins with *hazard identification* followed by *dose-response assessment*, *exposure assessment*, and *risk characterization*. If good quantitative human data exist, they can be used for hazard identification and for determining an acceptable human exposure level. However, risk assessment is much more often based on findings from laboratory animal studies. Therefore, risk assessors and clinicians will confront difficult issues as they attempt to extrapolate from animal to human. In this chapter, we discuss some of these issues, emphasizing the evaluation of the study's quality and its relevance to humans, and describe some commonly used methods for assessing reproductive and developmental effects in animals.

## USE OF ANIMAL STUDIES TO DEFINE HUMAN RISK

When adequate human data are not available, animal studies must be used to protect human reproductive and developmental health. Unfortunately, the quality and quantity of animal data vary considerably among tested substances, and data are often nonexistent or in-

sufficient to evaluate potential reproductive or developmental toxicity. For example, it is estimated that only 34% of pesticides and inerts, 22% of cosmetics, 45% of drugs, and 20% of food additives have sufficient data for evaluation of reproductive or developmental toxicity (2). A recent survey of the Organization for Economic Cooperation and Development (OECD) member countries found that for high production volume chemicals, 367 of 948 organic chemicals and 148 of 390 inorganic chemicals had sufficient data for determining reproductive or developmental hazard (3). Therefore, even for chemicals with high production volumes and likely human exposure, there is apt to be little available data for assessing the potential risk to reproduction and development.

It is customary to conduct animal experiments at dosages exceeding estimated levels of human exposure, both to increase the likelihood that a weak toxicant will produce a detectable effect and to compensate for the relatively small numbers of animals used in the assay. Thus, it is necessary to extrapolate results from experimental dosage levels to the normally lower levels of human exposure.

An important step in characterizing the

dose-response relationship in these studies is to determine the "no-observed-effect level" (NOEL), i.e., the highest exposure level at which no morphological, physiological, or functional modification of any kind is detectable under the test conditions. Another widely used concept in toxicology is the "no-observed-adverse-effect level" (NOAEL), i.e., the highest dose level at which no biologically adverse effects occur. In many cases, both the NOEL and NOAEL refer to the same exposure level. If not, the NOAEL is typically used as the basis for establishing permissible levels for human exposure, since it is possible for a substance to have a nonadverse effect at a low-dose level and an adverse effect at a higher dose. However, it is essential to determine that the "effect" observed is not a precursor to, or more sensitive biomarker of, reproductive or developmental disease.

Depending upon the sensitivity of the endpoint monitored and the test species utilized, different NOAELs may be derived for the same chemical. Generally, if multiple endpoints suggest that the chemical is a reproductive or developmental toxicant, then the most sensitive one (i.e., the one that occurs at the lowest exposure level) should be used to establish the NOAEL. In defining the appropriate NOAEL, the study selected should use an exposure route relevant to the human exposure whenever possible. If data from several species/strains are available, the most sensitive species should be used in determining the NOAEL, unless data from that species are not relevant to the human. A determination of relevance is based on the effect measured and the existence of comparable anatomical, physiological, toxicological, toxicokinetic, metabolic, and toxicodynamic processes for the effect in the test animal and in humans.

If sufficient data do not exist to determine the NOAEL for an endpoint, then the "lowest-observed-adverse-effect level" (LOAEL) should be used. Regardless of whether the NOAEL or the LOAEL is used, uncertainty or safety factors are typically applied to estimate an exposure level for humans at or below which there should be no adverse reproductive or developmental effects. This exposure level is often referred to as the reference dose or $R_f D$

(4). The total uncertainty factor usually ranges from 10–1000. Uncertainty factors of 10 each are applied (a) when the LOAEL must be used because a NOAEL was not established, (b) to account for differences between species, and (c) to provide an intraspecies adjustment for variable sensitivity among individuals. Additional adjustments may be made for length of exposure, inadequacy of the NOAEL or LOAEL, deficiencies in study design, or to account for special "sensitivity" of the human. Alternative approaches to the use of safety factors are being explored for both reproductive (5–7) and developmental toxicity (8–11).

## ASSESSING REPRODUCTIVE TOXICITY IN ANIMALS

### Endpoints Used in Reproductive Toxicity Studies

Alterations in reproductive capacity measured in animals may be sufficient to classify an agent as a hazard to reproduction in humans. Less conclusive results may indicate potential hazard and suggest the need for further investigation.

Some chemicals cause reversible reproductive effects in the adult male and female or developing offspring. Exposures leading to effects in this category are likely to be of lower risk to human reproduction than those that cause permanent damage. However, exposure to even a reversible reproductive toxicant results in a shifting of couples to a smaller completed family size. In other words, a temporary effect on fertility may permanently alter family size if that transient effect occurs during attempted reproduction.

### Animal Breeding Studies

Endpoints that are commonly determined in animal breeding studies and that may be most useful in identifying a potential human reproductive hazard are summarized in Table 8.1. The first eight endpoints indicate the ability of animals to mate, to conceive, or to deliver live offspring and, as such, measure overall effects on male and female fertility. These endpoints should be considered collectively when evaluating study results. The survival indices, expressed in increments over the time period, measure pup survival from birth through postnatal day 21. The body weights and growth of offspring are likely to be insufficient to identify a hazard definitively because of the myriad factors that are independent of test substance exposure and that may affect these endpoints.

## Male Reproductive Toxicity Studies

Endpoints that can be used as biomarkers of fecundity in male animals are summarized in Table 8.2. Subjective endpoints, such as those evaluated by histopathological techniques, must be interpreted with caution before concluding that a substance is a reproductive hazard. Recent developments in quantitative evaluation of testis histopathology, however, promise to increase the utility of these methods (12, 13). Endpoints that are more easily quantified, such as testicular spermatid number or the sperm count in the ejaculate, provide more compelling evidence, if the effects are both statistically significant and dose-dependent. A significant increase in the proportion of sperm

**Table 8.1.**
**Reproductive Indices Commonly Used in Animal Breeding Studies[a]**

| | | |
|---|---|---|
| Male (female) mating index | = | $\dfrac{\text{Number of males (females) for which mating was confirmed} \times 100}{\text{Number of males (females) used for mating}}$ |
| Male fertility index | = | $\dfrac{\text{Number of males producing a pregnant female} \times 100}{\text{Number of males for which mating was confirmed}}$ |
| Female fertility index | = | $\dfrac{\text{Number of females confirmed pregnant} \times 100}{\text{Number of females for which mating was confirmed}}$ |
| Gestation index | = | $\dfrac{\text{Number of females delivering at least one live offspring} \times 100}{\text{Number of females confirmed pregnant}}$ |

Number of implantations per pregnant female
Number of pre- and post implantation losses
Litter size at birth

| | | |
|---|---|---|
| Live birth index | = | $\dfrac{\text{Mean number of live offspring per litter} \times 100}{\text{Mean number of offspring per litter}}$ |
| Survival indices | = | $\dfrac{\text{Number of live offspring on postnatal day 4} \times 100}{\text{Number of live offspring born}}$ |
| | = | $\dfrac{\text{Number of live offspring on postnatal day 7} \times 100}{\text{Number of live offspring on postnatal day 4}}$ |
| | = | $\dfrac{\text{Number of live offspring on postnatal day 14} \times 100}{\text{Number of live offspring on postnatal day 7}}$ |
| | = | $\dfrac{\text{Number of live offspring on postnatal day 21} \times 100}{\text{Number of live offspring on postnatal day 14}}$ |

Reproductive capacity of $F_1$ offspring of exposed males and/or females (as measured by indices listed above)

[a]Adapted from Mattison DR, Working PK, Hughes CL Jr, Killinger JM, Olive DL, Rao KS. Criteria for identifying and listing substances known to cause reproductive toxicity under California's Proposition 65. Repro Toxicol 1990;4:163–165.

**Table 8.2.**
**Indices of Male Fecundity in Laboratory Animals[a]**

Disruption of seminiferous epithelium
Alterations in gonadal function causing decreased testicular spermatid number or decreased sperm count in the epididymis, vas deferens, or ejaculate
Decrease in percentage of motile spermatozoa
Significant change in sperm morphology
Alterations in reproductive organ weight (e.g., testes, epididymides, seminal vesicles, or prostate)
Altered concentration or temporal patterns of testosterone, luteinizing hormone (LH), or follicle-stimulating hormone (FSH)

[a]Adapted from Mattison DR, Working PK, Hughes CL Jr, Killinger JM, Olive DL, Rao KS. Criteria for identifying and listing substances known to cause reproductive toxicity under California's Proposition 65. Reprod Toxicol 1990;4:163–165.

with morphological abnormalities is also good evidence that a substance is a male reproductive hazard. Endpoints such as changes in reproductive organ weights and hormone profiles, which either are highly variable in humans and laboratory animals or are inconsistent indicators of changes in reproductive potential, should be considered only suggestive of potential reproductive hazard.

## Female Reproductive Toxicity Studies

Biomarkers of female fecundity are listed in Table 8.3. Inhibition of ovulation, inhibition of implantation, delayed puberty, and early reproductive senescence (14, 15) are the most compelling endpoints in defining a potential female reproductive hazard. The other endpoints listed are more difficult to interpret in terms of human reproductive risk. Recently, quantitative morphometric approaches have been developed to characterize the individual ovarian compartments affected by toxicants and the dynamic processes of ovarian toxicity (16–18).

## Study Design and Statistical Issues

Several general principles guide the use of animal studies to assess potential human reproductive risk. In general, the relevance of animal studies to humans is based on (*a*) consistency among animal studies of patterns of exposure, abnormal outcomes, and causal associations; (*b*) concordance of reproductive biology; and (*c*) evidence indicating biological plausibility of mechanism of action. These factors must be consistent with human biological principles.

In the interpretation of data from animal reproductive toxicology studies, the quality, design, conduct, and statistical analyses of the study must be taken into consideration; deficiencies in these factors may lead to the application of additional safety factors. The data used should be derived from studies of acceptable quality in mammalian species that are predictive of human responses. Animals should be exposed to the test compound by a route of administration relevant to the human route of exposure. Other routes may be relied upon by taking into consideration physiological and toxicological information. Also, exposures should be at the proper time and for the proper duration so as to maximize detection of an effect. In all cases, endpoints evaluated in animal reproduction studies should be predictive of adverse reproductive outcomes (Tables 8.1–8.3).

For an agent to be identified as a reproductive hazard, adverse reproductive effects should occur at doses that do not cause systemic toxicity significant enough to interfere with mating ability or frequency. When reproductive and systemic effects occur concomitantly, scientific judgment is needed to determine the probability of reproductive toxicity at lower doses.

Another important consideration is the power of the study, or the probability that the study demonstrates a true effect. Power is dependent on sample size, as well as on the background incidence and variability of the endpoint(s) examined. The apparent lack of an effect may be due to a true absence of activity or to the inability to identify an effect because of small sample size. Conversely, some statistically significant effects may arise by chance, especially if a large number of endpoints are

**Table 8.3.**
**Indices of Female Fecundity in Laboratory Animals[a]**

Estrous cycle disruption resulting in anovulation
Significant reduction in the number of ovarian follicles or oocytes
Altered uterine histology
Altered ovarian histology characterized by reduced corpora lutea or increased number of ovarian cysts
Altered concentration or temporal patterns of testosterone, luteinizing hormone (LH), or follicle-stimulating hormone (FSH)
Alterations in ovarian or uterine weight
Delayed puberty
Premature reproductive senescence

[a]Adapted from Mattison DR, Working PK, Hughes CL Jr, Killinger JM, Olive DL, Rao KS. Criteria for identifying and listing substances known to cause reproductive toxicity under California's Proposition 65. Reprod Toxicol 1990;4:163–165.

analyzed. The use of appropriate historical control data and critical attention to toxicological and reproductive biological principles may prevent false assumptions in such cases.

The number of animals per dose group should be determined after consideration of a variety of factors. These include the general toxicity of the substance being tested, which will affect the number of animals that survive to provide data, and the expected variation of the reproductive and developmental endpoints being measured. The likely magnitude of the effect should also be considered, as well as the level of significance desired to establish a positive finding.

Reproductive and developmental toxicity studies often involve observations on animals from the same litter. Litter mates tend to respond more similarly to a test substance than animals from different litters (19, 20). This litter effect is taken into account by using the variation between litters, rather than the variation within litters, as the basis for statistical analysis (21).

Data from replicate studies and multiple independent study types should be consistent and reinforcing. When data are discordant, sufficient additional evidence should be available to reconcile the differences. Confidence in a study outcome may be increased by the demonstration of a dose-response relationship. However, competing endpoints may obscure dose-response relationships in some cases (22). Negative findings deserve special scrutiny regarding study design and conduct. In general, the highest dose used should produce systemic toxicity in the sexually mature animal. These studies must include sufficient numbers of animals to detect an adverse effect, appropriate dose levels and exposure routes, and appropriate statistical methods. Negative studies should also indicate the power to define an adverse effect or the confidence interval on the null hypothesis.

## ASSESSING DEVELOPMENTAL TOXICITY IN ANIMALS

### Endpoints Used in Developmental Toxicity Studies

Endpoints for developmental toxicity include growth retardation, death of the conceptus,

deleterious structural malformations (teratogenesis), and functional deficits. Table 8.4 presents examples of developmental endpoints often observed in laboratory animals.

A structural abnormality in animals is generally classified as a malformation or a variation. A malformation is defined as a permanent structural change that adversely affects survival, development, or function. A variation is a divergence beyond the usual range of structural constitution that does not usually affect survival or health. Altered growth frequently manifests as a decrease in offspring organ or body size and, in some instances, is reversible. Functional deficiency is a delay or deficit in functional competence of the organism or organ system and may also be reversible. In general, reversible effects that occur in the presence of maternal toxicity are of less concern in the determination of potential human risks.

The developmental toxicity endpoints encountered in experimental animals do not necessarily mimic either qualitatively or quantitatively those observed in humans exposed to the same toxicant (although in some cases there is remarkable concordance). Similarly, specific toxicant-induced developmental endpoints in humans are not always reproduced in experimental animals (23). The lack of absolute uniformity of response is not surprising, however,

**Table 8.4.**
**Examples of Developmental Alterations Observed in Laboratory Animals[a]**

| Major Effects | Variations |
| --- | --- |
| Cleft palate | Delayed ossification of |
| Aphakia | bones |
| Anophthalmia | Lumbar ribs |
| Renal agenesis | Wavy ribs |
| Malformed heart- | Unfused centers of |
| valves, vessels | ossification |
| Gastroscisis | Extra center of sternebral |
| Missing ribs, vertebrae | ossification |
| Exencephaly | Increased renal pelvic |
| Spinal bifida | cavitation |
| Missing limbs | Hemorrhages at some |
| Fetal death | sites |
| Increased number of | Some displaced testes |
| resorptions | Some types of |
| | hydroureter |

[a]Adapted from Wang GM, Schwetz BA. An evaluation system for ranking chemicals with teratogenic potential. Teratogenesis Carcinog Mutag 1987;7:133–139.

given the critical differences that exist between the conditions of human and animal model exposure. For example, differences in dosage, placentation, metabolism, toxicokinetics, critical periods of development, and durations of gestation can be expected to affect the expression of developmental toxicity.

From a given data set, a "consistent pattern of outcome" might include findings of adverse developmental effects in multiple species tested or adverse effects in multiple strains or multiple studies of the same strain of a single species. The types of developmental effects seen in different species/strains need not be the same to satisfy this requirement. In judging consistency, many well-conducted studies showing an absence of adverse effects on development, even in the presence of studies with positive findings, warrant careful evaluation of the biological plausibility and human relevancy of the observation of adverse effects. In all of these determinations, differences in dosing and/or exposure regimen need to be factored into a finding of "consistent" results.

Measures of functional and behavioral toxicity are sometimes compromised by deficiencies in study protocols, data collection methods, and identification of appropriate endpoints, and these data must be utilized with caution in classifying a chemical as a developmental toxicant. However, the relevance of findings of behavioral and functional deficits is strengthened when corroborated by data from neurological, neurophysiological, neuropathological, and/or neurochemical studies (24, 25).

## Study Design and Statistical Issues

Many of the general principles that guide the design and interpretation of animal reproductive toxicity studies also apply to developmental toxicity investigations. In general, the minimum data set should include results from developmental toxicity studies in two species, preferably rodent and nonrodent. Treatment should be via the likely route of human exposure. The highest dose should be the one that causes measurable maternal toxicity. Results should permit identification of the NOAEL and LOAEL for maternal and/or developmental toxicity. Statistical factors should be given special consideration, and studies should have reasonable power to detect true adverse effects. When these criteria are satisfied, animal data are relatively good predictors of human developmental hazards (26–28).

One criterion for identifying a developmental toxicant is determination of the relative toxicity of the substance to the adult mother and the developing conceptus. In humans, there are both substances that are toxic to conceptuses in the absence of apparent maternal toxicity (e.g., thalidomide, diethylstilbestrol, chloroquine, phenytoin, iodine, lithium carbonate, doxycycline, retinoic acid, tetracycline, carbamazepine, valproic acid) and substances that are toxic to the conceptus at doses that result in maternal toxicity (e.g., aminopterin, 6-azauridine, busulfan, chlorambucil, cyclophosphamide, cytarabine, ethanol, 5-fluorouracil, methotrexate, methylmercury).

To address this issue, developmental toxicity tests should be conducted at a range of doses, including one toxic to the mother. Common markers of maternal toxicity are provided in Table 8.5. Adverse effects on development that occur only with maternal toxicity may not indicate a specific hazard to the conceptus (29). In contrast, developmental toxicity in the absence of maternal toxicity implies unique susceptibility of the conceptus. Most risk assessors assign

**Table 8.5.**
**Indices of Maternal Toxicity**[a]

Effects on food and water consumption
Loss of body weight or decreased body weight gain
Changes in respiration, motor activity, posture, alertness, behavior, hair or coat appearance, frequency of urination or color of urine
Excess salivation, tremor, nasal discharge, diarrhea, convulsions, and coma
Death and necropsy findings

[a]Adapted from Khera KS. Maternal toxicity in humans and animals: effects on fetal development and criteria for detection. Teratogenesis Carcinog Mutagen 1987;7:287–295.

a low level of concern to developmental effects that occur only at doses toxic to the mother, unless human exposure occurs at these doses.

Calculation of the ratio of the largest dose that produces no adverse effect in the mother to the largest dose that produces no adverse effect in the conceptus is important in assessing the extent of differential susceptibility (the adult toxicity:developmental toxicity ratio or A/D ratio). A large ratio (greater than 2) means that developmental toxicity occurs at doses far lower than those producing toxicity to the mother. A small ratio (approximately 1) implies that the dose that exerts toxicity in the conceptus may be close to the dose that produces toxicity in the adult (30). Different methods for evaluating the relationship between maternal and developmental toxicity have been suggested; thus, different ratios can be derived. The range of these methods should be considered when evaluating the developmental hazard of a substance.

An approach to applying this criterion is to examine all data available from animal studies, to determine the NOAELs for maternal and developmental toxicity, and to consider the human exposure potential for that substance and its relationship to the NOAELs. Substances with high maternal-to-conceptus toxicity ratios are more likely to be developmental toxicants in humans exposed to levels of the substance well below the maternal toxic dose. If humans are exposed to a substance with a low ratio at levels that approximate the maternal toxic dose, (e.g., many drugs produce therapeutic effects and developmental toxicity at the same concentration or dose), the requirement of a high toxicity ratio would be ignored. Despite the usual warnings found in the package insert and *Physicians Desk Reference*, many drugs appear safe for use during pregnancy (27, 28). When addressing the issue of drug use during pregnancy, it is important to conduct a careful, quantitative risk assessment (31).

## CONCLUSIONS

When attempting to characterize the potential hazard of a drug or chemical exposure on reproduction or development, it is necessary to evaluate a hierarchy of information. In a very few cases, sufficient human data are available

to accomplish this task. It may then be a relatively simple exercise to counsel the patient appropriately (5, 31) or to define an exposure level that protects public health.

More often, it is necessary to rely on animal data. In general, animal studies correctly identify most human reproductive or developmental toxicants (26, 27). However, animal studies also identify many more chemicals as reproductive or developmental toxicants than have been confirmed in humans (27, 32, 33). This may not be a problem from a public health perspective, as it is probably better to overestimate risk to humans than underestimate it.

After the chemical has been identified as a potential hazard, it is necessary to characterize the dose-response relationship, as well as the site and mechanism of action. These steps are necessary to extrapolate the animal data to humans appropriately to estimate qualitatively or quantitatively the risk to reproduction or development. After hazard identification and hazard characterization have been completed, the next step is characterization of exposure. What was the concentration, duration, and relationship of the exposure to the critical milestones of reproduction or development? Most chemicals that are reproductive or developmental toxicants have biological windows during which they produce their adverse effects. Exposure outside of these windows is associated with substantially smaller risks or no risk to the reproductive or developmental process.

Unfortunately, there are often insufficient data even to characterize a chemical as a reproductive or developmental toxicant. In these cases, proper guidance is difficult indeed. It has been suggested that protection against cancer also prevents reproductive and developmental toxicity; unfortunately, this assertion does not seem to be correct (9). In some cases, careful comparison of the structure of the chemical to that of known reproductive or developmental toxicants may be useful in estimating the potential for harm. Other factors that may be of value in determining whether the exposure or treatment carries risk include timing and duration of exposure and the presence or absence of systemic toxicity.

In the face of inadequate data, two different approaches may be useful in protecting public health. One approach assumes that the chemical is a potent reproductive and developmental toxicant until proven otherwise and allows *no* human exposure. Another approach, employed in California's Safe Drinking Water and Toxics Enforcement Act of 1986 (Proposition 65), assumes that a stringent safety factor (at least 1000-fold) applied to the NOEL will protect human reproductive and developmental health. However, this method may be insufficient for some chemicals or for sensitive subpopulations. For those chemicals to which large numbers of humans are exposed, or where human exposure is to high concentrations, even more stringent safety factors may be necessary until adequate testing is available.

Consideration should be given to the redesign of many of the existing toxicological testing protocols with reproductive and developmental endpoints specifically in mind. However, it will still be many years before the large number of untested chemicals receives any evaluation in a bioassay. Rapid and inexpensive alternative approaches are needed to screen chemicals for reproductive and developmental toxicity and to prioritize chemicals for the more expensive and time-consuming bioassays.

## REFERENCES

1. National Research Council. Risk assessment in the federal government: managing the process. Washington, DC: National Academy Press, 1983.
2. National Research Council. Toxicity testing: strategies to determine needs and priorities. Washington, DC: National Academy Press, 1984.
3. Brydon JE, Morgenroth VH, Smith A, Visser R. OECD's work on investigation of high production volume chemicals. Report prepared for the Organization for Economic Cooperation and Development (OECD), May 2, 1990.
4. Barnes DG, Dourson M. Reference dose ($R_fD$): description and use in health risk assessments. Regul Toxicol Pharmacol 1988; 8:471–486.
5. Mattison DR. An overview on biological markers in reproductive and developmental toxicology: concepts, definitions and use in risk assessment. Biomed Environ Sci 1991;4:8–34.
6. Meistrich ML. Calculations of the incidence of infertility in human populations from sperm measures using the two distribution model. In: Burger EJ, Tardiff RG, Scialli AR, Zenick H, eds. Sperm measures and reproductive success: Institute for Health Policy Analysis forum on science, health and environmental risk analysis. New York: Alan R. Liss, 1989:275–290.
7. Pease W, Vandenberg J, Hooper K. Comparing alternative approaches to establishing regulatory levels for reproductive toxicants: DBCP as a case study. Environ Health Perspect 1991;91:141–155.
8. Faustman EM, Wellington DG, Smith WP, Kimmel CA. Characterization of a developmental toxicity dose-response model. Environ Health Perspect 1989;79: 229–241.
9. Gaylor DW. Quantitative risk analysis for quantal reproductive and developmental effects. Environ Health Perspect 1989;79:243–246.
10. Rai K, Van Ryzin J. A dose-response model for teratological experiments involving quantal responses. Biometrics 1985;41:1–9.
11. Van Ryzin J. Risk assessment for fetal toxicity. Toxicol Ind Health 1985;1:299–310.
12. Sinha Hakim AP, Amador AG, Klemcke HG, Bartke A, Russell LD. Correlative morphology and endocrinology of sertoli cells in hamster testes in active and inactive states of spermatogenesis. Endocrinology 1989;125: 1829–1843.
13. Russell LD, Ettlin RA, Sinha Hakim AP, Clegg ED. Histopathologic evaluation of the testis in toxicologic testing and risk assessment. In: Histological and histopathological evaluation of the testis. Clearwater: Cache River Press, 1990:267–276.
14. Greep RO, ed. Recent progress in hormone research. Proceedings of the 1985 Laurentian hormone conference, vol. 42. Orlando: Academic Press, 1986: Chaps. 8–9.
15. Mastroianni L Jr, Paulsen CA, eds. Aging, reproduction, and the climacteric. New York: Plenum Press, 1986: Chap. 11.
16. Plowchalk DR, Mattison DR. Ovarian morphometric changes following cyclophosphamide treatment. In: Hirshfield AN, ed. Growth factors and the ovary. New York: Plenum Press, 1989:427–432.
17. Plowchalk DR, Mattison DR. Phosphoramide mustard is responsible for the ovarian toxicity of cyclophosphamide. Toxicol Appl Pharmacol 1991;107:472–481.
18. Weitzman GA, Miller MM, London SN, Mattison DR. Morphometric assessment of the murine ovarian toxicity of 7,12-dimethylbenz(a)anthracene. Reprod Toxicol 1992; 6:137–141.
19. Mantel N. Some statistical viewpoints in the study of carcinogenesis. In: Progress in experimental tumor research, vol. 11. New York: S. Karger, 1969:431–443.
20. Weil CS. Selection of a valid number of sampling units and a consideration of their combination in toxicological studies involving reproduction, teratogenesis or carcinogenesis. Food Cosmet Toxicol 1970;8:177–182.
21. Gad SC, Weil CS. Statistics for toxicologists. In: Hayes AW, ed. Principles and methods of toxicology. 2nd ed. New York: Raven Press, 1989:435–483.
22. Selevan SG, Lemasters GK. The dose-response fallacy in human reproductive studies of toxic exposures. J Occup Med 1987;29:451–454.
23. Jelovsek FR, Mattison DR, Young JF. Eliciting principles of hazard identification from experts. Teratology 1990;42:521–533.
24. Federation of American Societies for Experimental Biology (FASEB). Predicting neurotoxicity and behavioral dysfunction from preclinical toxicologic data. Bethesda: Life Sciences Research Office, 1986.

25. Kimmel CA, Rees DC, Francis EZ (eds). Qualitative and quantitative comparability of human and animal developmental neurotoxicology. Neurotoxicol Teratol 1990;12:285–292.

26. Frankos VH. FDA perspectives on the use of teratology data for risk assessment. Fundam Appl Toxicol 1985;5:615–25.

27. Jelovsek FR, Mattison DR, Chen JJ. Prediction of risk for human developmental toxicity: how important are animal studies for hazard identification? Obstet Gynecol 1989;74:624–636.

28. Friedman JM, Little BB, Brent RL, Cordero JF, Hanson JW, Shepard TH. Potential human teratogenicity of frequently prescribed drugs. Obstet Gynecol 1990;75:594–599.

29. Khera KS. Maternal toxicity: a possible etiological factor in embryo fetal deaths and fetal malformations of rodent rabbit species. Teratology 1985;31:129–153.

30. Fabro S, Schull G, Brown NA. The relative teratogenic index and teratogenic potency: proposed components of developmental toxicity risk assessment. Teratogenesis Carcinog Mutagen 1982;2:61–76.

31. Mattison DR. Drug effects on the fetus. In: Rayburn WF, Zuspan FP, eds. Drug therapy in obstetrics and gynecology. 3rd ed. St. Louis: Mosby-Year Book, Inc. 1992:13–31.

32. Shepard TH. Catalog of teratogenic agents. 5th ed. Baltimore: Johns Hopkins University Press, 1989.

33. Schardein JL. Chemically induced birth defects. New York: Marcel Dekker, 1985.

# 9

# Epidemiology[a]

## SHERRY G. SELEVAN

With the discovery of the human teratogenic effects of thalidomide in the 1950s, drugs became a primary focus of study for reproductive/developmental toxicologists and epidemiologists. In recent years, these fields have grown to encompass the study of a much wider range of environmental and occupational toxicants. In addition, a much broader spectrum of developmental effects is now considered. As explained in Chapter 4, developmental toxicity may result from preconceptional, prenatal, or postnatal exposures; major manifestations of developmental toxicity include death of the developing organism, structural abnormality, altered growth, and functional deficiency (1). Toxicant-induced reproductive effects are also broad in range and include, for example, reduced fertility, semen changes in males, and oocyte toxicity in females.

Unlike the controlled conditions found in laboratory animal experiments, multiple human exposures typically occur together, and they may occur sporadically or continuously over a wide dose range. The complexities inherent in the study of human populations require that epidemiological studies be carefully examined to assess the relationship between exposure and health effects. This chapter provides information for clinicians to evaluate available human data on reproductive and developmental toxicants.

[a]The views expressed in this chapter are those of the author and do not necessarily reflect the views or policies of the U.S. Environmental Protection Agency.

## PURPOSE OF EPIDEMIOLOGY: ASSOCIATION VS. CAUSATION

Consider this familiar scenario. A study is published assessing the relationship between contamination of community drinking water and fetal loss. Ingestion of contaminated water is associated with a two-fold increase in risk for spontaneous abortion in this study. The following day, local newspapers carry headlines that create considerable turmoil in the community: "Polluted drinking water causes miscarriages."

This case illustrates a common misconception about epidemiological studies, i.e., that any one study proves causation. In fact, the purpose of an epidemiological study is to evaluate the association among various factors and one or more outcomes. Determining whether or not these associations are causal is a much more complex process. The following precepts for causality have been proposed (2):

(a) *Strength of the association*. The greater the magnitude of effect observed with the exposure, the more likely it is to be causal.
(b) *Consistency*. The association has been observed in a variety of populations under a variety of circumstances.
(c) *Specificity*. The agent causes a specific effect. (While true for most infectious agents, experience demonstrates that specificity does not apply to many toxicants.)
(d) *Temporality*. The cause precedes the effect.
(e) *Biological Gradient*. There is evidence of an increasing dose-response relationship.

(Exceptions in the area of developmental toxicity will be discussed.)

(e) *Coherence.* The findings are plausible given existing knowledge about biology, mechanisms, etc. of the agent and the outcome.

(f) *Experimental evidence.* Laboratory data support the human findings.

(g) *Analogy.* Similar agents are associated with similar effects.

While temporality is an unquestionable criteria for causality, the other precepts may have exceptions. In general, evaluation of data for causality is based on the body of evidence. Evaluation is more meaningful when the body of evidence consists of a number of well-designed epidemiological and laboratory studies. Usually, it takes many years of study to establish causality (e.g., smoking and lung cancer). Occasionally, when an outcome occurs rarely in an unexposed population, causality is more easily established (e.g., diethylstilbestrol and adenocarcinoma of the vagina).

## EPIDEMIOLOGICAL STUDY DESIGNS

Typical epidemiological study designs include cross-sectional, case-control, cohort, and ecological studies. The basic differences among the first three types of studies are illustrated in Figure 9.1.

### Cross-sectional Studies

Cross-sectional studies measure both the exposure and the outcome at the same time. For example, Needleman et al. (3) used a cross-sectional design to study the relationship between prenatal lead exposure and congenital anomalies. At the time of birth, lead was measured in umbilical cord blood samples, and congenital malformation data were abstracted from newborn hospital records. After application of statistical methods to control for potential confounders, lead exposure was found to be associated with an increased risk for minor anomalies.

Cross-sectional studies increase the ease of obtaining quality exposure data through inter-

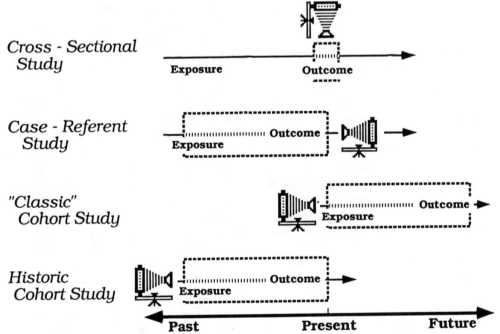

**Figure 9.1.** Common epidemiological study designs. The *cross-sectional study* takes a snapshot of both exposure and outcome at a particular point in time. In the *case-referent study*, the investigator identifies the outcome and looks back at the exposure. The *cohort study* can be done from two perspectives. Both approaches identify exposure groups and follow them to observe outcomes; however, one is done historically on past events, and the other identifies current exposures and follows the study members forward.

view, industrial or environmental monitoring, or biological measurements. These studies assume relatively consistent exposure levels, because the exposure is typically measured after the critical period for the outcome.

## Case-Referent Studies

Case-referent (case-control) studies assign individuals to one of two groups based upon the presence (case) or absence (referent) of the health outcome of interest. Exposure histories are compared in the two groups. This study design, for instance, was used to investigate the relationship between occupational exposure to chemotherapeutic agents and fetal loss in nurses employed in Finnish hospitals (4). *Cases* were nurses who experienced fetal loss while working on hospital wards that used antineoplastics; *referents* were age-matched nurses from the same hospital who gave birth. Data on exposure were obtained by self-administered, mailed questionnaires. In this study, the odds ratio for first trimester exposure to antineoplastic drugs was 2.3, i.e., nurses who aborted were more than twice as likely to have reported first trimester exposure to antineoplastics as were controls.

Case-referent studies more efficiently examine an exposure-outcome relationship for rarer events (e.g., birth defects). Because these studies are limited to the specific outcome for which cases are selected, they may miss effects of exposure that a cohort study, which can examine multiple outcomes, might identify. In case-referent studies, the exposures of interest are typically measured at some time after the critical period for the outcome. This estimate is useful if the exposure is close to steady-state, but determinations of variable exposures may be far less accurate. Case-referent studies that base exposure definition on biological or ambient data collected during the critical period are the most informative.

## Cohort Studies

Cohort studies define groups by exposure status and follow the members over time to determine the occurrence of certain outcomes.

If these studies are prospective, i.e., the groups are defined in the present and followed into the future, the investigators have an opportunity to obtain contemporary, quality exposure data. Unfortunately, prospective cohort studies require considerable time and money, and subjects may be lost to follow-up. In addition, occupational cohorts are typically limited in size. Due to these factors, researchers may assess exposure historically and follow the population to the present. In these situations, exposure data are limited in ways similar to case-control studies. Few environmental agents have been evaluated in cohort studies. Lead is a notable exception, with a number of prospective cohort studies assessing the effects of lead on child development (5–7). A major advantage to this study design is the ability to examine more than one outcome in the same population; however, large sample sizes are required to study rare events.

## Ecological Studies

Ecological studies assign exposure to groups by residential history or some other shared characteristic, while rates of the outcome in each group are compared within broad exposure designations. For example, Hanify et al. (8) used an ecological study design to investigate the relationship between community exposure to phenoxyherbicides and rates of human malformations. Hospital records were used to identify the incidence of malformations in specific areas of New Zealand subject to aerial spraying of 2,4,5-trichlorophenoxyacetic acid (2,4,5-T). Malformation rates were compared for the years before and after spraying; area-specific malformation rates were compared with the density of spray applications in the areas, as determined by company records.

Data from ecological studies are limited by misclassification of individual exposures and other characteristics (e.g., basic demographic data) that are typically not determined (9). While these studies can generate important hypotheses, they are of limited use for suggesting causality. Environmental studies are more likely than occupational studies to use an ecological design.

## GENERAL DESIGN CONSIDERATIONS

### Occupational vs. Environmental Studies

Occupational and environmental studies are similar in that they both examine the same types of exposures. However, major characteristics that may vary in the two types of settings include sizes of the study groups (and, consequently, the power of the study to detect various outcomes) and the magnitude and frequency of exposure. These factors affect the research designs typically used in each setting.

### Sizes of the Study Groups

Occupational populations are usually smaller than groups of people exposed to environmental toxicants. When the study group is small, the ability to examine rare events is severely affected. This factor affects the type of study design that is possible; in most cases, cohort studies are confined to events that occur frequently (e.g., early fetal loss), while case-referent studies are useful in evaluation of rarer outcomes (e.g., birth defects).

### Statistical Considerations: Significance and Power

Statistical tests of significance are used to determine whether the findings of an epidemiological study are likely to have occurred by chance. This testing consists of evaluation of the null hypothesis, i.e., that there is no relationship between exposure and the health outcome under study. A $p$ value (or probability) of 0.05 ($\alpha$) has been traditionally used to reject the null hypothesis. This cutoff suggests that a statistically significant association will be found by chance 5% of the time, and the null hypothesis will be erroneously rejected (Type I error). It is important to note that this convention is an arbitrary cutoff point that does not carry any biological significance. Type II error ($\beta$) is the probability that the null hypothesis is accepted when it should not be. The $\beta$ is also arbitrarily set, frequently at 0.1 or 0.2. A better alternative is the determination of confidence intervals (CI) around the estimate of risk. Confidence intervals provide information on statistical significance (if the CI includes 1.0, $p > 0.05$), the potential extremes of risk consistent with the findings, and the variability of the data (the narrower the CI, the less variability). An in-depth discussion of these issues can be found elsewhere (2).

The power, or ability of a study to detect a true effect, is the complement of $\beta$ (i.e., power = 1-$\beta$). It is dependent on the size of the study group, the frequency of the outcome in the general population, and the level of excess risk to be identified. For different study designs, curves can be calculated to estimate sample sizes required to detect certain levels of effect. Examples of curves for cohort studies assessing various developmental outcomes are provided in Figure 9.2. As the figure illustrates, common outcomes, such as recognized fetal loss, require hundreds of pregnancies to have a high probability of detecting a modest increase in risk; while less common outcomes, such as major malformations recognized at birth, require thousands of pregnancies to have the same probability (10–12). In case-referent investigations, study sizes are dependent upon the frequency of exposure within the source population. Confidence in the results of a study with negative findings is directly related to the power of the study to detect meaningful differences in the health effects under investigation.

Power can be enhanced by combining populations from several studies using a meta-analysis (13). The combined analysis increases confidence in the absence of risk for agents with nonpositive findings. However, care must be exercised to avoid combination of potentially dissimilar study groups.

A posteriori determination of a study's power can be helpful in evaluating findings that do not reject the null hypothesis. Nonpositive findings in a study of low power would be given less weight than either a positive study or a nonpositive study with high power. Positive findings from very small studies are open to question due to the instability of the risk estimates and the potentially highly selected nature of the population.

### Magnitude and Frequency of Exposure

The potential routes of exposure to toxicants include inhalation, ingestion, and dermal ab-

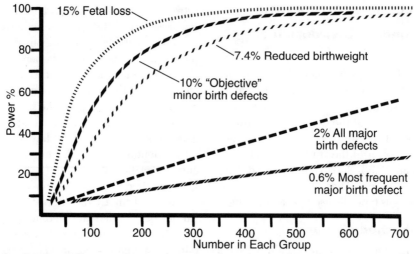

**Figure 9.2.** This figure illustrates the population size for cohort studies assessing various developmental outcomes. Studies of outcomes that occur rarely in the general population (e.g., major malformations) require larger numbers of subjects in the exposed and unexposed groups to detect an effect than studies of outcomes that occur more frequently (e.g., fetal loss). The figure assumes a two-sided $\alpha = 0.05$ and a doubling of risk. Reproduced from Selevan SG. Design of pregnancy outcome studies of industrial exposure. In: Hemminki K, Sorsa M, Vainio H, eds. Occupational hazards and reproduction. Washington, DC: Hemisphere Publishing Co, 1985: 221, with permission. Calculated using formulas from Schlesselman (37) and the following rates: fetal loss (38), reduced birthweight (39), and rates for all birth defects (40).

sorption. In general, occupational exposures tend to be higher than those found in the general environment. Of course, exceptions exist; for example, massive environmental exposure followed the industrial accident in Bhopal, India (14, 15).

While environmental levels tend to be lower, the time exposed is potentially greater, and exposure is not limited to relatively healthy employed populations. All segments of the population may be exposed, including more sensitive subgroups, such as the very young and very old. In addition, studies of industrial populations may have one clearly dominant exposure (e.g., lead in a lead battery plant), while multiple exposures are very common in environmental studies.

Identification of exposure levels in epidemiological studies may vary from broad and indirect descriptors, to ambient/area measures, to environmental measurements related to specific individuals, and finally, to individual biological measurements. Examples of these exposure indices are listed in Table 9.1. As one moves down the list, the measurement becomes more representative of the individual's actual exposure. More representative data in-

**Table 9.1.**
**Comparison of Exposures for Industrial and Environmental Studies.**

| Exposure Measures | Environmental Studies | Industrial Studies |
|---|---|---|
| Indirect descriptors | Gallons of gasoline used Distance from point source (e.g., factories) | Production figures Process information |
| Ambient measurement | Air or water levels | Area industrial hygiene samples |
| Measurements related to individual | Home tap water House dust Food | Personal industrial hygiene samples |
| Biological measurements | Blood Urine Hair Breast milk | Blood Urine Hair Breast milk |

crease confidence in the findings on the exposure-outcome relationship.

The ability to develop good measures of exposure varies widely in occupational and environmental settings, due to differences in existing data and in opportunities to generate high-quality exposure information. In workplace studies, occupational histories may be used along with some knowledge of the functioning of different departments to group areas into high, medium, and low exposure categories. The combination of individual work histories plus historical industrial hygiene data may establish these groups more accurately. Finally, the use of biological monitoring data on individual workers gives a much more direct measurement of internal dose, and, if taken on a relatively frequent schedule, produce the best information. In environmental settings, exposure to toxicants can be estimated by usage patterns (e.g., gallons of leaded gasoline purchased in a certain area), by measurements of environmental levels (e.g., levels of lead in drinking water), by environmental measurements pertinent to individuals (e.g., lead in house dust), and finally, through individual biological indices (e.g., blood lead values). These examples range from the least to the most biologically relevant.

## Potential Bias in Data Collection

Important sources of bias in epidemiological studies include selection bias and information bias (2).

## SELECTION BIAS

Selection bias can occur when an individual's willingness to participate varies with certain characteristics relating to his or her exposure or health status. In addition, selection bias can operate in the identification of subjects for study. For example, in spontaneous abortion studies, use of hospital records to identify embryonic or early fetal loss will underascertain events, because women are not always hospitalized for these outcomes. A more complete ascertainment of pregnancies can be obtained by collecting biological data on pregnancy status through human chorionic gonadotropin (HCG) measurements. These studies, however, may also be affected by selection factors related to the willingness of different groups of women to continue participation over the total length of the study. Interview data result in more complete ascertainment; however, this

strategy carries with it the potential for recall bias, as discussed below.

Studies of working women present the potential for additional bias, since some factors that influence employment status may also be associated with reproductive endpoints. For example, due to child care responsibilities, women may terminate employment, as might women with a history of reproductive problems who wish to have children and are concerned about workplace exposures (16).

## INFORMATION BIAS

Information bias results from misclassification of characteristics of individuals or events identified for study. Recall bias, one type of information bias, may occur when respondents with specific exposures or outcomes recall information differently than those without the exposures or outcomes. For example, women with malformed children may closely examine their histories for possible causes and, thus, more completely report exposures than women with healthy children. Interview bias may result when the interviewer knows a priori the category of exposure (for cohort studies) or outcome (for case-referent studies) in which the respondent belongs. Use of highly structured questionnaires or "blinding" of the interviewer reduces the likelihood of interview bias.

When data are collected by interview or questionnaire, choosing the appropriate respondent is important. For example, a comparison of husband-wife interviews on reproduction found the wives' responses to questions on pregnancy-related events to be considerably more complete and valid than those of the husbands (17). Studies based on data from the appropriate respondent(s) carry more weight than those from proxy respondents.

Data from any source may be prone to errors or bias. All types of bias are difficult to assess; however, validation with an independent data source (e.g., vital or hospital records) or use of biomarkers of exposure or outcome may indicate the degree of bias present. Studies with a low probability of biased data increase confidence in the findings (18, 19).

Some misclassification of data is not uncommon; for example, some subjects may not report an exposure that did, in fact, occur or vice versa. Misclassification may be nondifferential (random) or differential (certain subgroups are more likely than others to have misclassified data). Differential misclassification may either raise or lower the estimate of risk. Nondifferential misclassification lowers the estimate of risk, biasing the results toward a finding of "no effect" (2).

## Effect Modifiers and Confounders

Risk factors for reproductive and developmental toxicity include such characteristics as age, smoking, alcohol consumption, drug use, and past reproductive history, as well as occupational and environmental exposures. Known and potential risk factors should be examined to identify those that may be confounders or effect modifiers. An *effect modifier* is a factor that produces different exposure-response relationships at different levels of that factor. For example, in a study assessing the relationship of lead exposure to hypertension in pregnant women, maternal age could be an effect modifier, inasmuch as the risk of hypertension increases with age. A *confounder* is a variable that is a risk factor for the disease under study and is associated with the exposure under study, but is not a consequence of the exposure. For example, smoking might be a confounder in a study of the association of socioeconomic status and fertility, because smoking is associated with both. A confounder may distort both the magnitude and direction of the association between the exposure of interest and the outcome.

Both effect modifiers and confounders must be controlled in the study design or analysis to improve the estimate of the effects of exposure (2, 19, 20). The statistical techniques used to control for these factors require careful consideration in their application and interpretation (2, 20). Studies that fail to account for these important factors should be given less weight in an assessment of the data.

## REPRODUCTIVE EPIDEMIOLOGY: SPECIAL CONSIDERATIONS

### Identification of Exposure

Unlike studies of other health effects (e.g., chronic respiratory disease, cancer), where lifetime exposures are considered important, dif-

ferences in timing and intensity of exposure can have a substantial effect on the presence and types of reproductive or developmental outcomes observed. For example, birth defects may be caused by insults to the conceptus during critical periods of differentiation and development of the organ systems. The different organ systems are on different "schedules"; a brief exposure early in pregnancy may cause specific effects in certain organ systems, while exposures later in gestation may produce a very different group of effects (21).

Similarly, reproductive effects may result from exposures during certain key stages. For example, exposures to different stages in the maturation of sperm can produce different effects depending on survival and repair capacity at that stage. For other reproductive outcomes, effects may result from cumulative exposure. For example, the effects of an agent that causes oocyte death at any time would be both irreversible and cumulative.

Consideration of the effects of any reproductive or developmental toxicant also requires knowledge of the fate and disposition of the agent in the body. For example, an agent with a long half-life, such as lead, will accumulate in the body. Thus, the actual exposure to the toxicant during the time of interest for an outcome may be more than that measured externally.

In summary, the appropriate exposure classification in reproductive/developmental epidemiological studies depends on the outcome(s) of interest, the biological mechanism affected by exposure, and the biological half-life of the agent. The biological half-life, in combination with the patterns of exposure, affect the individual's body burden and, consequently, the actual dose during the critical period. Misclassification of exposure status may affect the ability to recognize a true effect in a study (22).

### Selection of Outcomes for Study

A number of endpoints can be considered in the evaluation of adverse reproductive or developmental effects. However, some outcomes are not easily observed in humans, such as early embryonic loss and reproductive capacity of offspring. Others require invasive techniques to obtain samples (e.g., testicular histopathology) or have high intra- and/or interindividual variability (e.g., serum hormone levels, sperm count).

Additional factors that limit the reproductive outcomes available for epidemiological examination include the relative magnitude of the exposure and the size and demographic characteristics of the population. Demographic factors such as marital status, age distribution, education, socioeconomic status, and prior reproductive history, influence whether couples will attempt to have children. Differences in contraceptive use also affect the number of outcomes available for study. In addition, women with livebirths are more likely to terminate employment than are those with other outcomes, such as infertility or early fetal loss. Retrospective studies of female exposures that do not include women who terminated employment may be of limited value, because the level of risk for these latter outcomes is likely to be overestimated (23).

A reproductive endpoint can be envisioned as an effect recognized at a specific point in a continuum of events that start preconceptionally and continue through death of the offspring. In utero exposures may cause a variety of effects that are part of the same causal chain. If malformations are very severe, for instance, fetal death can result. The definition of the study population affects which events are ascertained. Thus, a malformed stillbirth would not be included in a study of defects observed at live birth, even if the etiology were identical (10).

Below are descriptions of some male, female, and couple-dependent biological endpoints commonly measured in reproductive epidemiological studies. Methods of ascertainment range from biological indices to indirect measures of fertility and pregnancy outcome typically used in reproductive history studies.

## MALE REPRODUCTIVE ENDPOINTS: SEMEN EVALUATIONS

Most epidemiological studies of semen characteristics have been conducted in occupational groups or in patients receiving drug therapy. In the workforce, it is difficult to attain a high level of participation in studies requiring semen specimens. Response rates are typically less than 70% in these studies, and may be even lower in the comparison group. Some low response rates may be due to inclusion of vasectomized men in the total population, although this varies widely by population (24). Men who are planning to have children or who are concerned about pre-existing reproductive problems or possible deleterious exposures may be more likely to participate. Unless controlled, this biased participation can yield unrepresentative estimates of risk associated with exposure. Response rates can be substantially improved with proper education and payment of subjects (25).

Semen parameters are influenced by several factors including the period of abstinence preceding collection of the sample, health status, and social habits (e.g., alcohol, drugs, smoking). Data on these factors may be collected by interview.

## FEMALE REPRODUCTIVE ENDPOINTS

Reproductive effects may result from exposure to developmental toxicants. For example, prenatal exposures that result in a significant loss of primordial oocytes irreversibly affect female fertility. Although oocyte depletion is difficult to examine directly in women due to the invasiveness of the tests required, it can be studied indirectly through evaluation of the age at menopause (26).

Menstrual history data were used to examine adverse reproductive effects in women occupationally exposed to styrene (27). Studies that collect data prospectively are most useful, but they are difficult to perform (28).

## COUPLE-DEPENDENT ENDPOINTS

### Measures of Fertility

Infertility or subfertility may be thought of as a "nonevent," i.e., a couple is unable to have children within a specific period. Therefore, the epidemiological measurement of reduced fertility is typically indirect and is accomplished by comparing birth rates or time intervals between births or pregnancies. These evaluations estimate the couple's joint ability to procreate.

One method, the Standardized Birth Ratio (SBR), compares the number of births observed to those expected based on the person-years of observation and stratified by factors such as time period, age, race, marital status, parity, and contraceptive use (29, 30). Analysis of the time between recognized pregnancies or live births is another indirect measure of fertility (31, 32). Because the interval between births increases with increasing parity, comparisons within birth order (parity) are more appropriate.

## Pregnancy Outcomes

Pregnancy outcomes commonly examined in human studies of parental exposures include embryofetal loss, congenital malformations, birth weight effects, sex ratio at birth, and postnatal effects (e.g., physical growth and development, organ or system function, and behavioral effects). Hospital and vital records provide good information for some of these outcomes (e.g., birth weight, sex ratio), but not others (e.g., embryofetal loss). Early pregnancy loss can be evaluated by the presence of HCG in the blood or urine. Recently, Wilcox et al. (33) showed the utility of daily urine monitoring in the identification of very early loss (as soon as day 9 postconception). Several ongoing studies are using HCG assays as a measure of the health outcome of the study.

Epidemiological studies that focus on only one type of pregnancy outcome may miss a true effect of exposure. Studies that examine multiple endpoints yield more information, but results may be difficult to interpret. Evidence of a dose-response relationship is usually an important criterion in the assessment of exposure to a potentially toxic agent. However, traditional dose-response relationships may not always be observed for some developmental endpoints (34). For example, with increasing dose, a pregnancy may end in an embryofetal loss, rather than a livebirth with malformations. A shift in the patterns of outcomes can result from differences in magnitude or timing of exposure. An assessment should, when possible, attempt to look at the interrelationship of different reproductive endpoints and patterns of exposure.

## Statistical Factors

Pregnancies experienced by the same woman are not independent events (11, 35). Women who have had embryofetal loss are more likely to have subsequent losses (12). In laboratory animal studies, the litter is generally used as the unit of measure to deal with nonindependence of events. Human pregnancies, however, are sequential, and the risk factors change for different pregnancies, making analyses considering nonindependence of events very difficult (35). Including more than one pregnancy per woman is often necessary due to small study groups. This use of nonindependent observations overestimates the true size of the groups being compared, thus artificially increasing the probability of attaining statistical significance (36). Biased estimates of risk can also result, if family size confounds the relationship between exposure and outcome. Approaches to address these issues have been suggested (11, 35, 36). At this point in time, however, a generally accepted solution to this problem has not been developed.

## SUMMARY

This chapter introduces clinicians to the basic concepts of epidemiology, especially as they pertain to the study of effects of toxicants on reproduction and development. This information should aid in the evaluation of epidemiological studies and allow both health care providers and patients to understand better the possible risks associated with these exposures.

When interpreting epidemiological data, it is important to note whether there are several studies with consistent results and, in particular, what the "stronger" studies say. Questions that are useful in evaluating the strength of a study include the following:

(a) Is it a cohort or case-referent study? (These are generally more useful than ecological or cross-sectional studies.)

(b) How well has the exposure been characterized? (Exposure measures determined by direct information on the individual are preferable to surrogate measures.)

(c) Are there sufficient data on various outcomes to identify critical periods of concern?

(d) Have effect modifiers, confounders, and other risk factors been adequately addressed?

(e) Are the data biased, and, if so, how might the bias affect the findings?

(f) How big is the risk (if any), and how tight are the confidence intervals around the risk estimate?

The epidemiological examination of reproductive and developmental effects of occupational and environmental toxicants has a relatively short history. Given the increased concern and research in this area, improved methods to assess human risks will be available in the future. For the present, an examination of both laboratory and human data provides a starting place for the understanding of possible risks of environmental and occupational exposures to human reproduction and development.

## REFERENCES

1. Environmental Protection Agency. Guidelines for developmental toxicity risk assessment. 56 Fed Reg 63798–63826, 1991.
2. Rothman KJ. Modern epidemiology. Boston: Little, Brown, and Co., 1986:83–94.
3. Needleman HL, Rabinowitz M, Leviton A, Linn S, Schoenbaum S. The relationship between prenatal exposure to lead and congenital anomalies. JAMA 1984; 251: 2956–2959.
4. Selevan SG, Lindbohm M-L, Hornung RW, Hemminki K. A study of occupational exposure to antineoplastic drugs and fetal loss in nurses. N Engl J Med 1985; 313: 1173–1178.
5. Wigg N, Vimpani G, McMichael AJ, et al. Port Pirie cohort study: childhood blood lead and neuropsychological development at age two years. Epidemiol Community Health 1988;42:213–219.
6. Dietrich KN, Succop P, Bornschein RL, et al. Lead exposure and neurobehavioral development in later infancy. Environ Health Perspect 1990;89:13–19.
7. Bellinger D, Sloman J, Leviton A, Rabinowitz M, Needleman HL, Waternaux C. Low-level lead exposure and children's cognitive function in the preschool years. Pediatrics 1991;87:219–227.
8. Hanify JA, Metcalf P, Nobbs CL, Worsley RJ. Aerial spraying of 2,4,5-T and human birth malformations: an epidemiological investigation. Science 1981;212: 349–351.
9. Walter SD. The ecologic method in the study of environmental health. II. Methodologic issues and feasibility. Environ Health Perspect 1991;94:67–73.
10. Bloom AD. Guidelines for reproductive studies in exposed human populations. Guideline for studies of populations exposed to mutagenic and reproductive hazards. Report of Panel II. White Plains, NY: March of Dimes Birth Defects Foundation, 1981:37–110.
11. Selevan SG. Design of pregnancy outcome studies of industrial exposure. In: Hemminki K, Sorsa M, Vainio H, eds. Occupational hazards and reproduction. Washington, DC: Hemisphere Publishing Co., 1985;219–229.
12. Stein Z, Kline J, Shrout P. Power in surveillance. In: Hemminki K, Sorsa M, Vainio H, eds. Occupational hazards and reproduction. Washington, DC: Hemisphere Publishing Co., 1985:203–208.
13. Greenland S. Quantitative methods in the review of epidemiologic literature. Epidemiol Rev 1987;9:1–30.
14. Daniel CS, Singh AK, Siddiqui P, Mathur BBL, Das SK, Agarwal SS. Preliminary report on the spermatogenic function of male subjects exposed to gas at Bhopal. Indian J Med Res 1987;86(Suppl):83–86.
15. Varma DR. Epidemiological and experimental studies on the effects of methyl isocyanate on the course of pregnancy. Environ Health Perspect 1987;72:153–157.
16. Joffe M. Biases in research on reproduction and women's work. Int J Epidemiol 1985;14:118–123.
17. Selevan SG. Evaluation of data sources for occupational pregnancy outcome studies [Dissertation]. Cincinnati, OH: University of Cincinnati, 1980.
18. Axelson O. Epidemiologic methods in the study of spontaneous abortions: sources of data, methods, and sources of error. In: Hemminki K, Sorsa M, Vainio H, eds. Occupational hazards and reproduction. Washington, DC: Hemisphere Publishing Co., 1986:231–236.
19. Stein A, Hatch M. Biological markers in reproductive epidemiology: prospects and precautions. Environ Health Perspect 1987;74:67–75.
20. Kleinbaum DG, Kupper LL, Morgenstern H. Epidemiologic research: principles and quantitative methods. London, England: Lifetime Learning Publications, 1982.
21. Wilson JG. Environment and birth defects. New York: Academic Press, 1973:30–32.
22. Lemasters GK, Selevan SG. Use of exposure data in occupational reproductive studies. Scand J Work Environ Health 1984;10:1–6.
23. Lemasters GK, Pinney SM. Employment status as a confounder when assessing occupational exposures and spontaneous abortion. J Clin Epidemiol 1989;42:975–981.
24. Milby TH, Whorton D. Epidemiological assessment of occupationally related, chemically induced sperm count suppression. J Occup Med 1980;22:77–82.
25. Ratcliffe JM, Schrader SM, Steenland K, Clapp DE, Turner T, Hornung RW. Semen study of papaya workers exposed to ethylene dibromide. Br J Ind Med 1987;44:317–326.
26. Everson RB, Sandler DP, Wilcox AJ, et al. Effect of passive exposure to smoking on age at natural menopause. Br Med J 1986;293:792.
27. Lemasters GK, Hagen A, Samuels S. Reproductive outcomes in women exposed to solvents in 36 reinforced plastics companies. I. Menstrual dysfunction. J Occup Med 1985;27:490–494.
28. Burch TK, Macisco JJ, Parker MP. Some methodologic problems in the analysis of menstrual data. Int J Fertil 1967;12:67–76.
29. Levine RJ. Methods for detecting occupational causes of male infertility: reproductive history versus semen analysis. Scand J Work Environ Health 1983;9:371–376.

30. Starr TB, Dalcorso RD, Levine RJ. Fertility of workers: a comparison of logistic regression and indirect standardization. Am J Epidemiol 1986;123:490–498.

31. Baird DD, Wilcox AJ, Weinberg CR. Using time to pregnancy to study environmental exposures. Am J Epidemiol 1986;124:470–480.

32. Weinberg CR, Gladen BC. The β-geometric distribution applied to comparative fecundability studies. Biometrics 1986;42:547–60.

33. Wilcox AJ, Weinberg CR, Wehmann RE, Armstrong EG, Canfield RE, Nisula BC. Measuring early pregnancy loss: laboratory and field methods. Fertil Steril 1985;44:366–374.

34. Selevan SG, Lemasters GK. The dose-response fallacy in human reproductive studies of toxic exposures. J Occup Med 1987;29:451–454.

35. Kissling G. A generalized model for analysis of nonindependent observations [Dissertation]. Chapel Hill, NC: University of North Carolina, 1981.

36. Stiratelli R, Laird N, Ware JH. Random-effects models for serial observations with binary responses. Biometrics 1984;40:961–971.

37. Schlesselman JJ. Sample size requirements in cohort and case-control studies of disease. Am J Epidemiol 1974;99:381–384.

38. Buffler PA. Some problems involved in recognizing teratogens used in industry. Contrib Epidemiol Biostat 1979;1:118–137.

39. U.S. Department of Health Education and Welfare (DHEW), National Center for Health Statistics. Vital statistics of the United States, 1974, vol. 1, natality. PHS 78–1100. Hyattsville, MD: U.S. DHEW (PHS), 1978.

40. Hook EB. Some general considerations concerning monitoring. Applications to utility of minor birth defects as markers. In: Hook EB, Janerick DT, Porter IH, eds. Monitoring, birth defects, and environment: the problem of surveillance. New York: Academic Press, 1971: 177–192.

# III

# Clinical Assessment and Management

# 10

.................................................

# Clinical Evaluation and Management

## MAUREEN PAUL

Patients are turning increasingly to the health care system for information regarding occupational and environmental reproductive hazards. Counseling and appropriate intervention can provide patient reassurance and can result in changes beneficial to both individual and public health.

In many ways, the clinical approach to concerns about workplace and community exposures is similar to the evaluation of prescription drug use by patients. Common to each situation is the need to identify the chemical ingredients of products, determine how and where they exert their effects in the body, and to assess timing and doses of exposure. Decision-making requires careful weighing of risks and benefits, with modification or elimination of exposure if deleterious effects outweigh the advantages.

However, there are also important differences. While drug dosage is uniform and easy to quantify, environmental exposures are often diverse, occur via multiple routes, and are difficult to precisely measure. In contrast to vigorous premarket testing requirements for prescription medications, toxicity data on industrial chemicals are frequently inadequate. Finally, the involuntary nature of exposure to workplace or community contamination complicates the risk-benefit equation.

While details vary according to the clinical problem at hand, this chapter provides an overall framework for patient evaluation and management. Specific clinical problems are presented in Chapter 11.

## CLINICAL RISK ASSESSMENT

Clinical risk assessment involves three steps: (a) detecting and characterizing potential hazards; (b) evaluating the degree and timing of patient exposure; and (c) using the accumulated information to estimate the risk to the patient. As depicted in Figure 10.1, this process often requires a multidisciplinary effort involving occupational health specialists, toxicologists, government agencies, and others. The primary practitioner's role in the work-up will vary according to time, interest, and complexity of the problem, but invariably includes the initial screening and coordination of patient care. Identifying referral resources in the local community facilitates an effective and timely response to patient concerns.

### Step 1: Detecting and Characterizing Potential Hazards

The initial step in patient evaluation is to identify agents that have the potential to cause harmful reproductive or developmental effects. Through a process of information gathering, the clinician attempts to answer some fun-

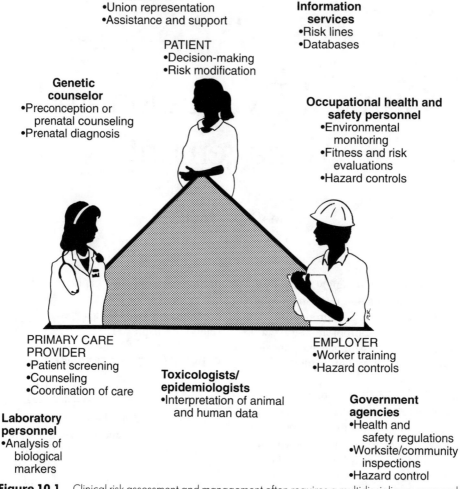

**Figure 10.1.** Clinical risk assessment and management often requires a multidisciplinary approach.

damental questions: What is the name of the agent(s) to which the patient is potentially exposed? Is there any evidence that this substance(s) causes adverse reproductive or developmental effects in experimental animals or humans? If so, what kinds of effects are observed and at what doses and stages of development? If not, are there any properties of the agent (e.g., chemical similarity to a known reproductive toxicant) that raise concerns? Answers to these questions are relatively straightforward when human toxicity data are adequate. However, if experimental animal studies are the primary sources of information, consultation with toxicologists or other experts may be necessary to determine their relevance for humans.

Clinical evaluation includes independent assessment of the male and female, as well as consideration of couple-dependent factors (1). Reproductive and developmental harm can result from paternal exposure (Chapters 1 and 5), and coexposure to both members of a couple may increase the risk of adverse pregnancy outcomes (2).

Following are some resources available to the clinician to assist in hazard detection and characterization.

## HISTORY

Table 10.1 delineates the essentials of the occupational and environmental history that help characterize patients' job tasks and potential exposures in the home or community (3, 4).

**Table 10.1.**
**Occupational/Environmental History[a]**

I.   Current job
   A.  Job title
   B.  Employer
   C.  Duration of employment
   D.  Description of job tasks
   E.  Occupational exposures
      1.  Chemical, e.g., vapors, fumes
      2.  Physical, e.g., noise, radiation, heat, heavy lifting
      3.  Biological, e.g., viruses
      4.  Psychological, e.g., stress
   F.  Protective measures used to minimize exposures, e.g., personal protective equipment (gloves, respirators), engineering controls (e.g., ventilation, lifting devices)
   G.  Temporal relationship of symptoms to work exposures
II.  Prior work experience
   Details as in I (above) may be relevant if employment at current job brief or for chemicals that bioaccumulate or have prolonged half-lives (e.g., lead, polychlorinated biphenyls)
III. Community/home exposures
   A.  Proximity to toxic waste site or incinerator
   B.  Pesticide application
   C.  Air pollution
   D.  Excessive noise (e.g., proximity to airports)
   E.  Known water contamination
   F.  Household products (e.g., cleaning solvents, paints, and varnishes)
   G.  Hobbies (e.g., ceramics, photography) and home renovations
   H.  Exposure to hazardous substances from household members (e.g., environmental tobacco smoke, lead, or other toxic dusts brought home on workclothes)

[a]Adapted from Paul M, Himmelstein J. Reproductive hazards in the workplace: what the practitioner needs to know about chemical exposures. Obstet Gynecol 1988;71:921–938.

Taking an adequate work history may feel a bit intimidating to the clinician inexperienced in occupational medicine. Few primary practitioners know what is entailed in industrial processes such as brazing, photolithography, or tool and die operations. Here, requesting details about job tasks in an interested manner provides the opportunity for patients to share their experiences and expertise. Ask the patient to list products used on the job and describe how they are handled. If the patient complains of musculoskeletal pain, role-playing certain job tasks can provide insight into problematic positions and postures. These efforts often result in identification of hazards unanticipated from the simple job title. The title "solderer," for instance, readily evokes suspicions of metal exposure. Frequently, however, other chemicals are used to clean metals before soldering.

A careful review of systems provides important clues to the identification of work-related hazards. Systemic symptoms that recede on weekends or vacations and are exacerbated upon return to work are likely to have occupational etiologies. Since significant exposures to reproductive or developmental toxicants may also affect other organ systems, attention to these temporal relationships is important. For example, workers exposed to organic solvents frequently complain of mucous membrane irritation or headaches that improve when away from the worksite.

In addition, patients may be aware of coworkers experiencing similar symptoms to their own. Personal sharing of infertility problems among workers at a California pesticide formulation plant led to the discovery of 1,2-dibromo-3-chloropropane (DBCP) as a spermatotoxin (5). While such "clusters" are not proof of a cause-and-effect relationship, they can generate important suspicions about potential occupational hazards.

Identification of hazards in the home or community is often more challenging. Frequent use of household products such as cleaning solvents or insecticides, engagement in hobbies involving chemical exposures, and even dust brought home on workclothes (6) can result in significant exposures to toxicants. While environmental poisoning epidemics are rare, patients may be concerned about chronic, low-level contamination from neighborhood factory discharges, toxic waste sites, or incinerators. These home and community exposures are covered in Chapters 26 and 27.

The history should also include medical, genetic, demographic, and lifestyle factors that influence reproductive or developmental outcomes. Maternal age, for example, affects the risk of fetal chromosomal anomalies (7). The incidence of congenital malformations is significantly increased in offspring born to women with poorly controlled diabetes mellitus (8). Cigarette smoking has been associated with subfertility, decreased age at menopause, spontaneous abortion, and placental abruption (9,

10). Low socioeconomic status has significant health consequences (11) and may limit a concerned worker's options to transfer or to discontinue employment. Careful consideration of these types of factors is essential to a balanced and comprehensive assessment of reproductive risk.

## MATERIAL SAFETY DATA SHEETS

Even after taking a thorough occupational and environmental history, questions frequently remain about the exact identity of chemical products handled on the job. Material Safety Data Sheets (MSDSs) are important sources of information concerning industrial chemicals.

MSDSs are prepared by chemical manufacturers and importers to describe the hazardous ingredients, properties, and acute and chronic health effects associated with their products. Under the Occupational Safety and Health Administration (OSHA) Hazard Communication Standard (12) and state right-to-know laws, the employer must keep on file updated MSDSs for all hazardous chemicals used at the worksite. Copies must be made readily available to employees upon request (13). Title III of the Superfund Amendments and Reauthorization Act (14) gives citizens concerned about community contamination the right to access MSDSs and chemical and toxic release inventories from local facilities. When patients call for appointments, ask them to obtain relevant MSDSs from employers and bring them to the office visit.

Appendix A describes the type of information provided on MSDSs. The important section entitled "Product Identification" specifies the company that prepared the MSDS, a phone number for additional information, and hazardous chemical constituents of the product. However, specific ingredients of products approved as "proprietary formulations" or "trade secrets" are not listed on the supposition that supplying these data places the company at a commercial disadvantage relative to its competitors. Physicians can access information about trade secrets through a formal mechanism involving written justification for the request and signing of a confidentiality statement. In medical emergencies, the product supplier must immediately provide essential information to the treating physician or nurse by telephone.

Because MSDSs are prepared by individual suppliers, the quality of information they provide varies tremendously. While most MSDSs identify hazardous product constituents, they provide inadequate data to assess toxicity. Even the best of MSDSs contain only broad generalities about health effects and lack dose-response information. In particular, they cannot be trusted to identify reproductive or developmental toxicants. In our recent study of nearly 1000 MSDSs for lead and the ethylene glycol ethers, 57% failed to make any mention whatsoever of effects on the adult reproductive system or fetus. When reproductive hazards were addressed, prenatal effects were significantly more likely to be reported than were male reproductive disorders. Obviously, clinicians need to access other information sources for comprehensive data on health effects.

Identifying potentially hazardous constituents of household products is more problematic, as many products are inadequately labeled. Clinicians may obtain MSDSs and other useful information by calling the manufacturer listed on the product label. Other helpful resources include poison control centers, the Consumer Product Safety Hotline (Appendix B), and texts such as *The Handbook of Poisoning* (15) or *The Clinical Toxicology of Commercial Products* (16).

## HEALTH EFFECTS DATA

At this point in the work-up, the clinician has utilized the history, MSDSs, and other resources to generate a list of agents to which the patient may be exposed. The next step is to determine if, and under what conditions, the agents pose risks to human reproduction or development. Two approaches are helpful here. The first is to assess the patient to determine if untoward effects have occurred. The second includes use of available information resources to research toxicant-induced health effects. This information can then be applied to the patient's specific clinical concerns and findings.

### Physical Findings and Laboratory Data

A complete physical examination should be performed. Its purpose is to assess general health status, verify complaints, look for signs of overexposure, and to rule out other medical or reproductive conditions that may contribute to the etiology of the problem. While no physical findings are pathognomonic for environmentally induced disease, this etiology is suggested if certain findings are combined with evidence of exposure. For example, the dermatological condition, chloracne, raises concerns about exposure to polyhalogenated aromatic compounds (17). Gynecomastia may prompt a search for environmental or occupational exposure to sex steroid hormones (18).

A variety of laboratory tests is available to document alterations in adult reproductive function or fetal development (19). For instance, anovulation can be diagnosed by basal body temperature measurements, gonadotropic and sex steroid hormone assays, and endometrial biopsy. Semen analysis measures a number of sperm parameters that can be affected by exposure to xenobiotics. Serological antibody testing can document susceptibility or recent infection in patients exposed to viral teratogens. The early pregnancy marker, human chorionic gonadotropin (HCG), is useful in the diagnosis of aberrant implantation or early embryonic loss. Advances in sonographic imaging techniques allow for increasingly sophisticated observations of fetal growth, morphology, and function. α-fetoprotein in maternal serum and amniotic fluid is well validated as a screen for fetal neural tube defects. Choosing which of the many available tests to perform depends on the specifics of the clinical problem.

## Researching Toxicants

Data regarding the reproductive and developmental health effects of specific toxicants are available from many sources including computerized databases, toxicology "hotlines," published texts, and government agencies. A selected list of helpful resources is presented in Appendix B. Practitioners who frequently care for patients concerned about reproductive risks may wish to subscribe to on-line databases with ready access via an office computer system. Some databases, such as REPROTOX and the Teratogen Information System (TERIS), provide summary data for clinicians on toxicant-induced developmental (both databases) and reproductive (REPROTOX) effects. Bibliographic information is available through the National Library of Medicine's Toxicology Information Program, which includes databases such as the Environmental Teratology Information Backfile (ETICBACK) and Developmental and Reproductive Toxicology (DART). At present, most databases focus on maternal exposures and developmental outcomes. Obtaining information on male-mediated effects may require more complex searches.

A significant amount of human data is available for a few chemicals such as lead, ethanol, and methyl mercury. In these cases, the following should be noted: the types of effects induced by the toxicant; the doses at which specific effects (or their absence) are observed and whether developmental toxicity occurs at or below levels causing maternal toxicity; routes of exposure; critical time periods of exposure; and important pharmacokinetic data, e.g., whether the toxic parent compound or metabolite is known to cross the placenta. It is also important to remember that many developmental endpoints are interrelated and dose-dependent (20). For example, low-dose exposure to a teratogen may produce subtle growth deficits. As dose increases, the frequency and severity of malformations may rise. However, most severely anomalous fetuses spontaneously abort. Therefore, developmental toxicity encompasses a range of outcomes that may be relevant in the clinical setting.

For the majority of industrial chemicals, the practitioner is likely to find that data are lacking or confined to studies on laboratory animals. Of the more than 90,000 chemicals in widespread commercial use in the U.S., published results of animal developmental toxicity testing are available for approximately 3000 (21, 22). Analyzing experimental animal data to predict potential human reproductive or developmental impairment is exceedingly complex. Attention must be paid to a number of factors including the adequacy of study design, species and strain characteristics, toxicokinetics, timing and dose considerations, and outcome patterns (Chapter 8). Interpretation of developmental toxicity studies is particularly difficult, because dose-response relationships may differ for the pregnant adult and fetus, for specific end-

**Table 10.2.**
**Proposed Risk Classification System**

| Human Risk Potential | Criteria | Examples and Some Reported Effects |
| --- | --- | --- |
| Positive | Adequate, well-controlled human studies show reproducible patterns of adverse effects | Lead (spermatotoxicity, developmental toxicity)<br>Methyl mercury (developmental toxicity)<br>Dibromochloropropane (spermatotoxicity) |
| Suspicious | Human studies are lacking or inadequate, but well-designed animal studies show consistent, biologically plausible adverse effects in at least two species; suspicion is increased when:<br>  There are some supporting human data<br>  A dose-response relationship is demonstrated<br>  Developmental effects occur at doses below those causing maternal toxicity<br>  Results are positive in subhuman primates or in a species known to handle the toxicant in a manner similar to humans<br>  Effects are demonstrated at doses and via routes of administration likely to be encountered by humans | Ethylene glycol ethers (spermatotoxicity, teratogenesis)<br>Carbon disulfide (spermatotoxicity, embryo lethality)<br>Cadmium (spermatotoxicity, developmental toxicity)<br>Waste anesthetic gases (fetal loss)<br>Toluene (developmental toxicity) |
| Uncertain | Human and animal data are lacking or inadequate, or human data show conflicting results | Styrene (menstrual abnormalities)<br>Ethylene oxide (spermatotoxicity, developmental toxicity) |
| Probable negative | Well-designed animal studies are negative at doses encountered in human environments, but human studies are lacking or inadequate<br>or<br>Well-designed human investigations consistently fail to demonstrate risk | Organic acids |

points, and for different developmental periods. Given these complexities, interpretation of animal data requires input from experts adequately trained in toxicology and risk assessment methodology.

When explicit health effects data are unavailable, the chemical structure or mechanism of action of an agent may raise suspicion about reproductive toxicity. Chemicals that have structures or activities similar to reproductive hormones may exert adverse effects. For example, stilbenes or the pesticides dichlorodiphenyltrichloroethane (DDT) and chlordecone bind to endogenous estrogen receptors and may interfere with hormonal regulation of the hypothalamic-pituitary-gonadal axis (23, 24). Identification of a chemical as an alkylating agent implies genotoxicity and heightens suspicion about potential developmental or carcino-

genic effects. On the other hand, organic acids are well known for their acute irritant effects, but rarely cause chronic toxic effects other than sensitization (25).

Based on the information collected, clinicians may find it helpful to categorize agents broadly according to their potential human reproductive or developmental toxicity. Practitioners are familiar with the U.S. Food and Drug Administration's (FDA) Usage-in-Pregnancy Ratings delineated in the *Physicians' Desk Reference* (26) to estimate risks of medication use during gestation. No analogous, standardized classification scheme is yet available for industrial chemicals. Table 10.2 proposes one ranking system for consideration.

For the initiate, researching chemicals is quite burdensome at first. Patients often work with multiple diverse chemicals that require investigation. To ease the task, a few points should be kept in mind. First, most clinicians practice within limited localities where one or a few types of industry predominate. It does not take long to develop familiarity with work processes and exposures common to patients from local communities. Second, maintaining a file of health effects data for specific toxicants avoids repetitive searches (although information must be periodically updated). With time, the number of unfamiliar substances requiring extensive research decreases. Finally, use of information services such as pregnancy risk lines (hotlines), clinically oriented computer databases, and government agencies is time-saving.

## Step 2: Evaluate the Extent of Exposure

The mere presence of a toxicant in the workplace or community is not necessarily equated with significant exposure. A common error made by clinicians is to infer risk without adequate attention to the levels of exposure actually experienced by patients. In the industrial setting, absorption of xenobiotics can be reduced by measures such as enclosure of work processes, effective ventilation, and the use of personal protective equipment. Therefore, the next step in clinical assessment involves gathering data to characterize the patient's extent of exposure better.

Toxicants enter the body by three main routes. Inhalation represents the most common route of industrial exposure, but skin absorption should also be assessed, especially for organic solvents and pesticides. Ingestion of toxicants occurs rarely in industry and is most often secondary to inadequate hygiene practices or to inappropriate eating or smoking in contaminated areas.

Work processes may change the properties of an agent and thereby modify routes of exposure. For instance, volatilization of molten lead produces toxic fumes during welding or other processes involving high temperatures. Hand soldering operations involving lead often occur at low enough temperatures to prevent volatilization. However, contamination of work surfaces or clothing by lead particles can result in exposure through ingestion.

## GATHERING EXPOSURE DATA

Two major characteristics of exposure are important to consider in the clinical setting—timing and dose.

### Timing

Information about timing of exposure derives primarily from the history. Exposures may be brief, occurring once or on an episodic basis. Others will be chronic, and their duration should be documented.

Most teratogens exert their effects during specific critical periods of fetal organogenesis. For example, the thalidomide embryopathy occurred only in offspring exposed in utero from days 38–50 of gestation. Therefore, every effort must be made to establish gestational age at the time of exposure precisely. Decreased sperm count should prompt a search for gametotoxic exposures in the several months before the onset of the problem. In the human, spermatogenesis requires about 74 days (27). Depending on the germ cell types affected, the clinical expression of toxicant-induced injury becomes apparent within days to many weeks postexposure; serial semen analyses are often necessary to document the full extent of injury.

Occasionally, exposures in the more distant past can affect reproductive or developmental outcome. For example, in utero exposure to the transplacental carcinogen, diethylstilbestrol (DES), resulted in vaginal adenocarcinoma many years later. Some persistent lipid-soluble chemicals, such as the polychlorinated biphenyls, accumulate in adipose tissue. Later, lactation may result in release of these compounds from fat stores and excretion into breast milk (28). Similarly, more than 90% of absorbed lead is stored in bone. Conditions associated with heightened bone loss, such as menopause, may increase blood lead levels (29). Whenever possible, the history should include information about exposures to chemicals that bioaccumulate or have long half-lives. Unfortunately, however, disease that occurs long after exposure is difficult to relate to a toxicant unless the abnormal findings are pathognomonic or occur rarely in unexposed individuals.

## Dose

With the exception of mutagens and carcinogens, most toxicants must reach critical threshold concentrations at target tissues to induce ill effects. The type of effect seen may be highly dose-dependent. Clinical assessment includes efforts to estimate the dose of a toxicant to which the patient is exposed.

In some instances, merely taking a comprehensive history from a well-informed patient provides sufficient information about dose. Consider, for example, a hospital pharmacy worker who inquires about the risks of preparing chemotherapeutic agents during pregnancy. Careful questioning reveals that the preparation occurs under well-working fume hoods and that the guidelines regarding work practices recommended by OSHA are carefully followed (30). In this instance, the clinician can be reasonably sure that exposures are negligible without much further investigation.

More detailed dose information can be gained through arrangement of a worksite walk through by an industrial hygienist or occupational health specialist. These plant tours provide opportunities to assess first hand the patient's job tasks and potential routes and sources of exposure. Attention is paid to routine exposures, as well as to peak exposures that occur during cleaning and maintenance operations, accidents, or spills. Exposure control measures at the worksite are noted. In addition, the walk through provides an opportunity to gather information directly from management and workers.

Two general methods are available to quantify dose in the occupational setting more precisely. *Environmental monitoring* measures the concentration of contaminants in the air or on work surfaces. Techniques are also available to measure pollutant levels in air, soil, or water in the community or home environment. *Biological monitoring* of exposure, which is analogous to drug level testing, measures the individual absorbed dose of a toxicant (Fig. 10.2).

Environmental monitoring is usually performed by industrial hygienists who are trained in the identification, measurement, and control of hazards. If the patient is employed by a large company, periodic evaluations of the worksite may be performed by corporate health and safety personnel. These services are also available through many labor unions or academic or community-based occupational health programs. At the request of a concerned employee, OSHA will inspect the worksite, perform appropriate environmental monitoring, and cite employers for violations of OSHA regulations. These OSHA requests can be made confidentially and provide the worker with legal protection against employer retaliation for raising a health and safety complaint. In addition, OSHA contracts with certain state agencies (e.g., the Department of Labor in Massachusetts) to provide consultations for small businesses that may include environmental monitoring, employer education, and recommendations for voluntary abatement of concerning exposures. According to OSHA regulations (31), results of worksite testing must be made available to employees and health care providers upon request. Community or home monitoring is performed by government environmental agencies delineated in Appendix B or by private consulting firms.

Industrial hygienists utilize a variety of methods to assess exposure. The techniques used depend on the nature of the hazards and their potential routes of exposure (32). Air sampling measures the concentration of toxic particulates, vapors, or gases in the work area. Direct reading instruments are used to detect instantaneous concentrations of air contaminants, while sample collectors filter substances from the air for later analysis in the laboratory. Industrial hygienists usually sample at fixed locations throughout the workspace; in addition, employees may be asked to wear small sampling pumps or badges during performance of work tasks. Wipe sampling can be used to measure the concentration of toxicants on work surfaces (32).

Industrial hygienists also evaluate available hazard control methods at the worksite. They may test ventilation systems and assess the design and use of personal protective equipment or clothing. If monitoring suggests exposures that may cause concern, industrial hygienists can provide advice to employers, patients, and clinicians about appropriate controls and work practices necessary to decrease risk.

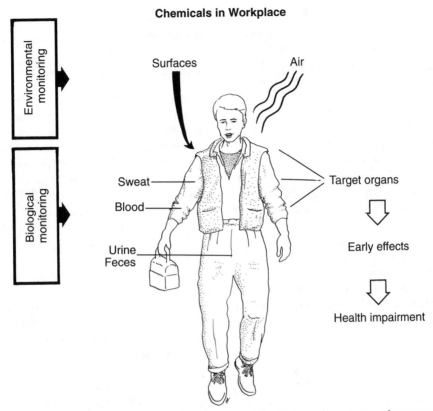

**Figure 10.2.** Environmental monitoring measures external dose. Biological monitoring of exposure assesses internal dose or toxicant-induced early effects.

The multiplicity of exposures in the community setting makes environmental monitoring both difficult and time-consuming. Toxic waste sites, for example, contain multiple diverse chemicals, and evaluation involves measurements of both surface contamination and of toxicant concentrations that have leached through the soil to pollute groundwater. Dispersion of chemicals into air is influenced by a number of factors including weather conditions and wind velocities. Environmental agencies often use complicated models to estimate the concentrations of toxicants reaching communities through air or drinking water. Therefore, the clinician rarely has access to environmental exposure data that are precise, interpretable, and timely.

While environmental monitoring is useful in the assessment of external toxic exposures, it does not take into consideration the many factors that influence individual absorption and metabolism of xenobiotics. In contrast, biological monitoring provides an individual estimate of the internal dose of a chemical (19). Biological indices measure absorption by all routes and from all sources and are particularly useful when the potential for ingestion or dermal exposure exists.

The best biological indicators of exposure derive from sampling at the site of action in the reproductive organs. Because these tissues are usually inaccessible, however, biological exposure monitoring most commonly involves testing of blood or urine from individuals to estimate body uptake of a toxicant. In some cases, early biochemical or cellular changes are used as markers of exposure. For example, the concentration of free erythrocyte protoporphyrin (FEP) in blood is commonly used as an indicator of lead absorption; the FEP level, however, actually reflects lead-induced heme enzyme inhibition.

Biological monitoring allows estimation of dose only when sufficient data are available regarding the pharmacokinetics, mechanisms of action, and rates of variation for a specific toxicant. Analysis of biological samples should be performed by qualified personnel at hospital or commercial toxicology laboratories. Interpretable results depend on many factors including methods of collection, storage, and transport; interindividual variability; and background levels from nonoccupational sources. In general, timing is not a critical consideration for agents with long biological half-lives. For exposures to toxicants with short half-lives and rapid elimination, however, sampling is best performed shortly after exposure. Serial sampling is sometimes necessary when high background levels or interindividual variations makes interpretation of a single measurement difficult. Problems can be avoided by contacting the laboratory before testing to obtain details about appropriate sampling procedures (33).

## INTERPRETING EXPOSURE DATA

The clinician who has obtained environmental or biological exposure data is next faced with the task of interpreting the information. Is a blood lead level of 30 μg/dl in a pregnant patient worrisome? Is an average air concentration of 100 parts per million (ppm) methyl ethyl ketone in an employee's work area excessive? The certainty with which these questions can be answered depends largely on whether adequate human data and valid biological indices are available for a specific toxicant. In the first example, human studies confirm that lead levels in fetal blood approximate those in the pregnant woman, and that concentrations well below 30 μg/dl can result in neurodevelopmental deficits in offspring. In the much more common second example, experimental animal studies are the primary sources of information regarding the chemical, and extrapolation to the human situation is more uncertain.

Reference values set by government agencies are the primary resources available to guide clinicians in the determination of acceptable patient exposure limits. When regulatory limits are lacking or inapplicable, it may be possible to apply quantitative risk assessment methods in the clinical setting, provided experienced toxicologists are available to analyze animal research findings.

## Regulatory or Recommended Limits

A number of regulatory agencies in the U.S. are responsible for setting acceptable exposure limits for workers and for the general public. Most workplace exposure limits are established and enforced by OSHA; the National Institute for Occupational Safety and Health (NIOSH) advises OSHA in this capacity. The Environmental Protection Agency (EPA) sets standards for community exposures, while the FDA regulates medications, medical devices, and food additives. Some exceptions exist. For example, the Nuclear Regulatory Commission is responsible for the protection of most federal nuclear radiation workers (Chapter 13). While OSHA regulates exposures to pesticide production workers, field workers and applicators fall under the auspices of the EPA. In general, regulatory limits pertain to toxicant concentrations in environmental media (e.g., air or water) and not in biological tissues.

The main advantage of this approach is that regulatory limits are backed by the force of law. Measured patient exposures that exceed established limits are clearly excessive and warrant intervention. However, clinical use of these standards is also problematic. There are very few substances that are specifically regulated to protect against harm to the reproductive system. The U.S. General Accounting Office recently published an evaluation of regulatory actions in relation to 30 chemicals widely acknowledged to be reproductive hazards (34). Government agencies reported examining reproductive or developmental toxicity data only 44% of the time when they made major regulatory decisions concerning these chemicals. To date, in fact, only four OSHA standards are based in part on consideration of adverse reproductive or developmental effects (lead, ethylene oxide, DBCP, and ionizing radiation) (35), and even some of these require modification based on newly accumulated data. Moreover, the process of standard setting in the U.S. is not free from political influence. Enforceable exposure limits are generally not based solely on consideration of scientific data.

Rather, they represent values compromised by competing interests and consideration of costs to industry (36). Against this background, limits espoused by regulatory experts may diverge from those considered acceptable by clinicians and patients.

The Appendix (at the end of the book) presents a select list of known or suspected reproductive and developmental toxicants, along with the most recent exposure limits mandated or recommended by government agencies. Exposure limits for specific substances are also designated on MSDSs, and comprehensive tables are available free of charge from regulatory agencies.

The OSHA Permissible Exposure Limits (PELs) delineated in the Appendix are legally enforceable (37). In its advisory capacity to OSHA, NIOSH has developed Recommended Exposure Limits (RELs) for some of these substances (38). The REL is based solely on scientific information relevant to the potential hazard, including available data on reproductive and developmental effects. The NIOSH RELs are included in the Appendix for comparison with the OSHA limits. Where a significant discrepancy exists, the RELs are assumed to be more health protective, although they are, unfortunately, not legally mandated.

Because EPA exposure limits for the general public are based on heterogeneous populations, some of whose members are considered more sensitive to toxicant-induced health effects than the average worker, EPA limits are often below those set by OSHA. For example, annual whole body ionizing radiation limits for members of the general public are currently set by the EPA at 0.1 of the allowable occupational limit. The EPA has also established enforceable Maximum Contaminant Levels (MCLs) for many chemicals found in drinking water. For some nonregulated contaminants, the EPA has published "health advisories" that summarize available information on toxicokinetics, health effects (including those pertaining to reproduction and development), and mitigation technologies, and provide recommended contaminant limits. Clinicians can obtain health advisories for specific contaminants by calling the EPA's Safe Drinking Water Hotline (Appendix B).

For workplace toxicants amenable to biological monitoring, Biological Exposure Indices (BEIs) recommended by the American Conference of Governmental Industrial Hygienists (ACGIH) are provided in the Appendix (39). While not a regulatory body, ACGIH has considerable influence on OSHA standard setting activities (36). An excessive biological value in a patient whose inhalation exposure is at or below the ACGIH air limit usually indicates additional absorption by some other route (most commonly, the skin). This situation should prompt careful investigation of control measures at the worksite, as well as potential nonoccupational sources of exposure to the toxicant.

## Risk Assessment Methods in the Clinical Setting

When adequate human studies are lacking but a chemical has been tested for reproductive or developmental toxicity at various doses in laboratory animal species, it may be possible to estimate whether or not a patient's exposure level is concerning. This approach is useful for endpoints that are assumed to have a threshold below which toxicity does not occur. It involves calculation of the patient's absorbed dose in units comparable to the test species, then comparison of the patient dose to the animal dose that caused no observed adverse effects. Again, a prerequisite for application of this method is an analysis of the animal literature on the agent by a toxicologist or qualified expert. While this approach is controversial, some attempt at quantitative assessment is perhaps better than conclusions based solely on gross qualitative assumptions.

Let's consider a hypothetical example. Suppose a patient is exposed to an air-borne contaminant at a constant dose of 400 $\mu g/m^3$ (0.4 $mg/m^3$) for an 8-hr workday. The patient is 10 weeks pregnant and wants to know if this level of exposure is worrisome. No human data are available, but your research reveals the chemical to be a developmental hazard in experimental rodent studies. Your first step is to establish the "no-observed-adverse-effect level" (NOAEL) for the most sensitive endpoint in the most sensitive species tested. The NOAEL refers to the highest dose of chemical at which there is no increase in frequency or severity of adverse effects between the exposed and control groups (40). In this case, let's assume that the most sensitive endpoint is embryolethality, and that this outcome occurs at the lowest dose in pregnant rats (i.e., the most sensitive species) in the absence of maternal toxicity. The highest oral dose at which embryolethality does not occur in rats is 20 mg/kg/day (i.e., the NOAEL). Other adverse systemic or developmental outcomes are observed in a variety of species, but only at higher doses.

You now must carry out some calculations to convert the patient's occupational respiratory dose to an absorbed dose for comparison with the rat's oral dose. The patient's daily absorbed dose of the toxicant is determined primarily by its concentration in air and the amount of air that the worker breathes in during the workday. In the absence of data to the contrary, assume that the total inhaled dose is absorbed. The following formula is used:

$$Dose = C \times t \times MV \times CF \times A \times bw^{-1}$$

where: $Dose$ = patient's estimated absorbed dose in mg/kg/day; $C$ = 8-hr average air concentration of the toxicant in mg/m$^3$; $t$ = exposure time in minutes (480 min for an 8-hr workday); $MV$ = minute ventilation in liters/min (assume 11 liters/min for a pregnant woman performing light activities; increases with higher intensities of work); $CF$ = conversion factor (0.00l m$^3$/liter); $A$ = percent absorbed via respiratory route; $bw$ = patient's body weight in kg (assume 58 kg in this case).

Substituting the appropriate values, we have the following:

$$Dose = (0.4 \text{ mg/m}^3 \times 480 \text{ min/day} \times 11 \text{ liters/min} \times 0.001 \text{ m}^3/\text{liter} \times 1.00) / 58 \text{ kg} = 0.036 \text{ mg/kg/day}$$

The patient's daily absorbed dose from occupational exposure to the chemical (0.036 mg/kg/day) is approximately 1/500th of the dose that caused no adverse developmental effects in the the most sensitive animal species tested (20 mg/kg/day). In the absence of an established occupational limit based on consideration of developmental effects, this estimate provides some reassurance. Risk assessors gen-

erally hold that a 100-fold safety margin provides adequate protection if the NOAEL is established through well-designed chronic dosing studies in appropriate animal species (41). However, because some regulatory agencies employ a more conservative safety margin of 1/1000 for irreversible developmental effects (41, 42), it is reasonable to recommend follow-up (e.g., ultrasound to detect developmental aberrations) and to explore control measures that can lower the exposure (e.g., better ventilation, personal protective equipment).

In the case of drinking water contamination, the route of exposure to the toxicant (ingestion) is usually similar for patient and test species. It is simple to convert the units commonly used to measure water contamination (mg/liter) into those employed in animal testing (mg/kg/day) for comparison purposes. Let's assume that the same chemical as above is found in contaminated drinking water at a level of 0.6 mg/liter. The following formula is employed:

$$\textit{Patient's daily dose} \text{ (mg/kg/day)} = C \times V \times bw^{-1}$$

where: $C$ = concentration of contaminant in water in mg/liter; $V$ = volume of water consumed daily by patient (assume 2 liters/day); $bw$ = patient's body weight in kg (58 kg).

Substituting, we have:

$$Dose = 0.6 \text{ mg/liter} \times 2 \text{ liters/day} /58 \text{ kg} = 0.02 \text{ mg/kg/day}$$

which is 1/1000th of the animal NOAEL.

The primary advantage of this method is that it provides some quantitative basis for comparison of animal and patient data. The method can easily be adapted to accommodate a range of doses (more common in the occupational setting) or incomplete absorption. The fact that animals are often administered doses via the oral route while inhalation is the most common exposure route for workers does not negate the usefulness of the method, because the portion of chemical that fails to reach the lower airways is either expelled or swallowed.

There are also a number of problems with this approach. First, considerable research is required, and the clinician must have an expert consultant available to assist in interpretation of animal data. Second, there is no firm guarantee that patient doses below those causing adverse effects in laboratory animals are "safe." The NOAEL is a statistical construct based on study of a limited number of biological endpoints; experiments with larger numbers of animals, more diverse species, or with other endpoints might reveal a lower NOAEL (43). Moreover, the appropriate "safety factor" to apply to the NOAEL depends on interspecies and intraspecies variations in sensitivity to a toxicant, the quality of the experimental data, and other variables (40). Based on these factors, the dose considered safe for humans generally ranges from 1/10th to 1/1000th of the no-effect animal dose, but may occasionally be less. Finally, many criticize this method in favor of more sophisticated techniques that consider mechanisms of action, detailed dose-response relationships, and other toxicokinetic factors of importance (41, 42). More complex models are, however, not applicable to most chemicals due to insufficient data regarding these parameters and are certainly well beyond the reach of clinicians.

## Step 3: Estimate the Risk

The final step in clinical risk evaluation involves assimilating exposure and health effects data to estimate the degree of risk to the patient. Scarcity of scientific data is a serious hindrance to accurate risk assessment. While quantitative risk estimates based on human studies are available for ionizing radiation and some viral teratogens, this is not the case for most industrial chemicals. When reliable animal data are available, clinical consultation with toxicologists may result in reasonable estimations of risk. In may cases, however, the risk will simply be unknown.

In addition to the characteristics of the toxicant and exposure conditions, individual biological responses are modified by factors such as age, nutritional status, genetic constitution, and pre-existing medical or reproductive problems (44). Figure 10.3 summarizes important factors that influence the risk posed by exposure to a xenobiotic. For example, exposures potentially associated with preterm labor, such as physically strenuous work, are of particular concern for women with a history of early delivery (45). Deficiencies of iron, zinc, and calcium are associated with increased gastrointestinal lead absorption (46). The solvent, methylene chloride, is rapidly metabolized to carbon monoxide in vivo, so that cigarette smoking can exacerbate the toxic effects of this

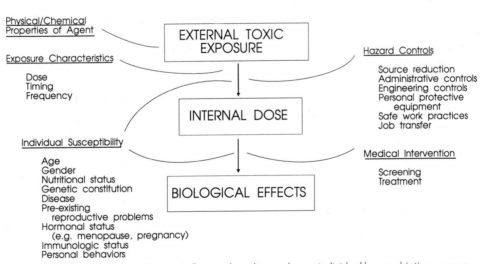

**Figure 10.3.** A number of factors influence the risk posed to an individual by xenobiotic exposure.

agent (47). The principle of genetic variability in response to xenobiotic exposure is well established, and evidence is accumulating to suggest genetic influences on teratological outcomes. For example, the anticonvulsant medication, phenytoin, is metabolized to reactive epoxide intermediates. Genetic differences have been identified in the activity of epoxide hydrolase, the enzyme that detoxifies these reactive metabolites, and may influence fetal susceptibility to the teratogenic effects of this agent (48). Consideration of interactions between extrinsic and intrinsic factors is important to a comprehensive determination of risk.

For purposes of general health protection, intervention is clearly warranted when exposure to any chemical or physical agent exceeds regulatory exposure limits. Because few legally mandated limits are based on adequate consideration of reproductive system effects, even lesser exposures to known or suspected human reproductive or developmental toxicants may deserve attention. Conversely, negligible exposures warrant no action.

When uncertainty exists because of insufficient toxicity or exposure data, decisions regarding reproductive and employment options belong to the well-counseled patient. Because workers' compensation or disability benefits are difficult to obtain in this setting (Chapter 12), some patients may feel that loss of income and benefits due to job removal far outweigh uncertain health risks in the workplace. With the help of the physician, workers may be able to negotiate reasonable accommodations with their employers that allow for continued employment. Some patients may choose to leave their jobs if no other options are available to minimize risk. In the face of uncertainty, the patient is in the best position to weigh the implications of each decision alternative in the context of his or her own life circumstances and resources. Counseling and support by the health care provider can assist patients in making these difficult decisions.

## CLINICAL RISK MANAGEMENT

The primary objectives of risk management in the clinical setting are to educate the patient and to decrease risk. These objectives can be achieved through effective patient counseling and, when appropriate, through intervention strategies in the workplace or community aimed at reducing concerning exposures.

## Patient Counseling

Patients experiencing pregnancy or reproductive disorders who seek medical advice about environmental exposures are likely to harbor considerable anxiety. Reproductive events may catalyze fears that have remained otherwise quiescent. In addition, patients' perceptions of risk are influenced by a variety of economic, social, ethical, and cultural factors. Situations involving involuntary exposure, lack of personal control over the risk, and the potential for damage to future generations may result in amplification of risk (49).

Effective counseling can significantly influence patients' perceptions of risk. One study (50) of 80 women attending an antenatal consultation service revealed that women exposed to nonteratogenic agents during pregnancy assigned a mean risk for major malformations of 24% before counseling and 14% after. The tendency to terminate the pregnancy due to exposure-related concerns decreased significantly after consultation. On the other hand, counseling had no effect on the risk women assigned to drugs known to be teratogenic. In this latter circumstance, the counselor can still provide vital information to the patient regarding risks, prognosis, and follow-up; can assist in patient decision-making; and can offer emotional support.

Guidelines for effective counseling include consideration of setting, style, content, and follow-up (51). A basic prerequisite is a quiet, private space free from distractions. Ample time is necessary to discuss patient questions and concerns in a relaxed, unhurried manner; an hour or more may be necessary for the clinical assessment and counseling of a new patient. If it is necessary to gather additional toxicological or exposure data before counseling can take place, the patient can be scheduled for a follow-up appointment in a reasonable amount of time. In complex cases, collaboration with a genetic counselor eases time restraints on the busy provider.

Counseling is a form of communication that is educative and supportive, but not judgmental or coercive. Patients' concerns, needs, and expectations can only be identified by an attentive listener. Health care providers may harbor personal prejudices that can interfere with the patient-counselor interaction. For example, clinicians may feel that patients who are concerned about their working conditions but continue to smoke cigarettes are less deserving of interventions to reduce exposures on the job. Providers may disagree with a patient's decision to terminate a pregnancy or to continue to work in the face of uncertain, but potential, risk. While counselors can assure that patient decisions are as well-informed as possible and can encourage health-protective behaviors, respecting the patient's right to autonomous decision-making is crucial.

Effective patient education requires that information be provided in a manner that is both understandable and likely to be remembered. Patient anxiety may interfere with recall or comprehension. The language used by counselors should be sensitive to the patient's educational status and cultural background. For couple exposures, counseling both partners is essential to effective management. If only one patient is involved, the presence of a close friend or relative can aid recall and provide support. Important main points of the discussion are reviewed at the end of the counseling session. In addition, a follow-up letter summarizing the discussion reinforces important information and helps avoid miscommunications. Copies of written communications are useful for patient follow-up and essential for liability purposes.

The counselor should provide an honest appraisal of risk based on available data regarding the toxicant(s), its potential effects, and the dose and timing of the patient's exposure. Uncertainties inherent in the extrapolation of animal findings to humans must be explained, as well as the limitations of available epidemiological studies. Interpreting specific relative risks is important. For example, a two-fold increased risk for spontaneous abortion that increases the rate of miscarriage from 15% to 30% is quite dramatic. On the other hand, a two-fold increased risk for a malformation that occurs with a baseline frequency of 1 in 1000 live-births would result in one additional affected infant in this population.

Once all pertinent information has been conveyed, the health care provider makes medical recommendations to the patient and devises a follow-up plan. A variety of health-protective behaviors can be suggested, ranging from changes in work practices to cessation of cigarette smoking or curtailment of potentially deleterious hobbies. Appropriate diagnostic tests are offered. For instance, Level II ultrasounds are advisable when pregnant patients are significantly exposed to agents that may increase the risk of congenital anomalies, such as organic solvents or high-dose radiation.

When intervention in the workplace is contemplated, the clinician should inquire about patient needs for confidentiality and discuss the likelihood of employer cooperation or reprisal. In addition, economic restraints may limit the options available to patients. Except in the rare instance of a significant threat to patient and public health, interventions are carried out only with the full permission and cooperation of the patient. Appropriate referrals are sometimes warranted to assist patients with legal or financial problems.

Even in the absence of concerning exposures, a healthy reproductive or pregnancy outcome can never be guaranteed due to the background rates of adverse outcomes. The patient is informed that 1 of 12 couples of reproductive age in the U.S. is diagnosed as infertile (52), that 12–15% of clinically recognized pregnancies end in spontaneous abortion (53), and that 2–3% of newborns are diagnosed with major anomalies (54). Through this explanation, patients can better accept clinicians as educators and advocates without harboring unrealistic expectations about outcomes.

## Hazard Control

When exposures are of concern, clinicians may be able to work with employers and other consultants to reduce or eliminate potential hazards. Occupational and environmental health specialists, industrial hygienists, and government regulatory agencies can be helpful in the assessment and implementation of exposure control strategies.

There are three general methods available to control exposures (55). As illustrated in Figure 10.4, these methods include removing the source of the hazard, interrupting the pathway from the source to the individual, and personal protection of the worker. From a health perspective, source reduction is the preferred option. Conversely, measures that depend on individual compliance are most subject to failure. Often, a combination of methods is used.

Removing the source of the hazard involves substituting the chemical of concern for a less toxic one or redesigning work processes to eliminate use of hazardous substances. For example, new oxidation techniques are available to bleach paper products that eliminate the use of chlorine. Many manufacturers have reformulated products to eliminate the ethylene glycol ethers, suspected reproductive and developmental toxicants. While source reduction focuses on primary prevention, its limitations include the time required to institute changes and the possibility that alternative agents or processes will introduce new, unforeseen hazards.

Interrupting the flow of contaminants from the source to the individual most commonly involves enclosure of work processes or effective ventilation. Local exhaust ventilation captures and removes contaminants before they are released into the worker's breathing zone. The use of fume hoods in research laboratories is an excellent example of local exhaust ventilation familiar to medical personnel. Slotted vents around chemical sinks are also common. Ventilation systems must be periodically tested and maintained to assure continued efficiency. Patients may know the most recent date and the results of ventilation testing. This information is also available from employers.

Control methods that focus on the individual worker include administrative controls and the use of personal protective equipment. Rotating workers to limit time spent by any one individual in contaminated areas is one common administrative method. Unfortunately, administrative controls do not prevent acute exposures that can result in reproductive or developmental harm.

Generally, personal protective equipment should be used as a "last resort" when other methods fail to control exposures adequately. Bulky protective clothing and respirators may be uncomfortable for workers, especially during the latter part of pregnancy. In some situations, however, short-term use of personal protective equipment, combined with other more effective controls, provides a satisfactory alternative to removing patients from their jobs.

Personal protective equipment includes clothing and respirators that decrease worker contact with contaminants and lifting devices to avoid musculoskeletal injury. Personal protective equipment must be carefully selected to

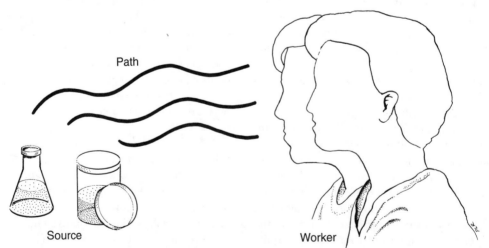

Path

Source

Worker

**Figure 10.4.** Hazard control methods include reduction of the source of the hazard, interrupting the flow of contaminants from source to worker, and personal protection of the worker.

match the hazards of the job. The permeability of chemicals through gloves, for instance, depends on the glove material. Even when the glove is compatible for the chemical of interest, permeation eventually occurs, and gloves may need to be changed frequently to protect against contamination.

There are two main types of respirators. *Air-supplied* respirators deliver uncontaminated air from an external source to the breathing zone of the worker. With *air-purifying* respirators, inhaled air passes through a filter or cartridge to remove toxic aerosols, vapors, or gases; the filtering material must be specifically selective against the chemical(s) of concern. Air-purifying respirators are less cumbersome, less expensive, and easier to use, but have limited utility in industrial settings where occupational limits are approached or exceeded. In these situations, engineering controls and, if necessary, air-supplied respirators are better alternatives. The Mine Safety and Health Administration and NIOSH test and certify respirators for specific uses. Only approved respirators should be used in toxic environments; in addition, OSHA guidelines for proper respirator fit, training, use, and maintenance should be carefully followed (56).

If these control measures are infeasible or fail to curtail exposure satisfactorily, the clinician can recommend temporary job transfer or leave. Because economic and job security are integral to workers' general and reproductive health (11), practitioners must remain sensitive to the degree of job protection and compensation available to patients in these circumstances. As discussed in Chapter 12, current disability and workers' compensation programs often inadequately address the problem of reproductive hazards. However, letters and calls by health care providers to employers, insurance carriers, and union representatives may help the patient obtain alternative work assignments or disability or unemployment benefits. In some circumstances, legal consultation will be necessary to assure the protection of employee rights.

One common error made by clinicians writing pregnancy disability letters is to emphasize concerns about potential fetal damage from workplace exposures while ignoring symptoms referrable to the pregnant woman herself. This oversight may result in denial of disability benefits, because the woman, but not the fetus, is considered the insured worker. A letter detailing maternal toxicant-induced symptoms is more likely to be accommodated by insurance carriers than one focused solely on conjectural fetal effects.

Control of community exposures is usually limited to removal or containment of environmental contaminants. Effective control is difficult to attain. Clean-up of toxic waste sites, for example, is both expensive and time-consuming. Moreover, considerable controversy has arisen between regulatory agencies and concerned citizens over the extent of clean-up necessary to protect health. In rare instances, widespread contamination has resulted in removal of citizens from their homes, as at Love Canal, New York. Such actions result in serious economic losses for patients, in addition to disruption of friendships and community. Scientific uncertainties, combined with these other factors, make clinical management of the environmentally exposed patient particularly difficult. While the clinician can play an important supportive role, the degree of risk is seldom clear and protection from exposure is difficult to attain in a timely fashion.

## SUMMARY

Evaluation of patients exposed to potential reproductive or developmental toxicants is a complex process that usually requires a team effort. The primary clinician can play a vital role in identifying risk factors, making appropriate referrals, providing support and counseling, and coordinating overall patient care. This chapter provided a general framework for addressing these problems; in the following chapter, some occupational case histories are presented to illustrate important aspects of the work-up.

## ACKNOWLEDGMENTS

My appreciation to Drs. Jay Himmelstein, Robert Vanderslice, and Anthony Scialli for their insightful commentary on this chapter.

## REFERENCES

1. Mattison DR. An overview of biological markers in reproductive and developmental toxicology: concepts, definitions and use in risk assessment. Biomed Environ Sci 1991;4:8–34.

2. Hemminki K, Kyyronen P, Marja-Liisa N, Koskinen K, Sallmen M, Vainio H. Spontaneous abortions in an industrialized community in Finland. Am J Public Health 1983;73:32–37.

3. Paul M, Himmelstein J. Reproductive hazards in the workplace: what the practitioner needs to know about chemical exposures. Obstet Gynecol 1988;71:921–938.

4. Goldman RH, Peters JM. The occupational and environmental health history. JAMA 1981;246:2831–2836.

5. Whorton D, Krauss RM, Marshall S, Milby T. Infertility in male pesticide workers. Lancet 1977;2:1259–1261.

6. Baker EL Jr, Folland DS, Taylor TA, et al. Lead poisoning in lead workers and their children: home contamination with industrial dust. N Engl J Med 1977;296:260–261.

7. Hook EB. Rates of chromosome abnormalities at different maternal ages. Obstet Gynecol 1981;58:282–285.

8. Mills JL, Knopp RH, Simpson JL, et al. Lack of relation of increased malformation rates in infants of diabetic mothers to glycemic control during organogenesis. N Engl J Med 1988;318:671–676.

9. Mattison DR. The effects of smoking on fertility from gametogenesis to implantation. Environ Res 1982;28:410–433.

10. Werler MM, Pober BR, Holmes LB. Smoking and pregnancy. In: Sever JL, Brent RL, eds. Teratogen update: environmentally induced birth defect risks. New York: Alan R. Liss Inc, 1986:131–139.

11. Catalano R. The health effects of economic insecurity. Am J Public Health 1991;81:1148–1152.

12. Occupational Safety and Health Administration. 29 CFR: Sec 1910.1200. Washington, DC: Office of the Federal Register, 1988.

13. Himmelstein JS, Frumkin H. The right to know about toxic exposures: implications for physicians. N Engl J Med 1985;312:687–690.

14. U.S. Congress: Superfund Amendments and Authorization Act, title III, public law 99–499, October 17, 1986.

15. Dreisbach R, Robertson W. Handbook of poisoning: prevention, diagnosis and treatment. 12th ed. Norwalk, CT: Appleton & Lange, 1987.

16. Gosselin RE, Smith RP, Hodge HC. Clinical toxicology of commercial products. 5th ed. Baltimore: Williams & Wilkins, 1984.

17. Suskind RR. Chloracne, "the hallmark of dioxin intoxication." Scand J Work Environ Health 1985;11:165–171.

18. Harrington JM, Stein GF, Rivera RO, deMorales AV. The occupational hazards of formulating oral contraceptives: a survey of plant employees. Arch Environ Health 1978;33:12–15.

19. National Research Council. Biologic markers in reproductive toxicology. Washington, DC: National Academy Press, 1989.

20. Selevan SG, Lemasters GK. The dose-response fallacy in human reproductive studies of toxic exposures. J Occup Med 1987;29:451–454.

21. Schardein JL. Chemically induced birth defects. New York: Marcel Dekker, 1985.

22. Shepard TH. Catalog of teratologic agents. 6th ed. Baltimore: Johns Hopkins University Press, 1989.

23. Mattison DR. The mechanisms of action of reproductive toxins. Am J Ind Med 1983;4:65–79.

24. Kupfer D. Critical evaluation of methods for detection and assessment of estrogenic compounds in mammals: strengths and limitations for application to risk assessment. Reprod Toxicol 1988;1:147–153.

25. Leung H-W, Paustenbach DJ. Organic acids and bases: review of toxicological studies. Am J Ind Med 1990;18:717–735.

26. Huff B, ed. Physicians' desk reference. 44th ed. Oradell, NJ: Medical Economics Company, Inc., 1990.

27. Heller CG, Clermont Y. Kinetics of the germinal epithelium in man. Recent Prog Horm Res 1964;20:545–575.

28. Rogan WJ, Gladen BC, McKinney JD, et al. Polychlorinated biphenyls (PCBs) and dichlorodiphenyl dichloroethene (DDE) in human milk: effects of maternal factors and previous lactation. Am J Public Health 1986;76:172–177.

29. Silbergeld EK, Schwartz J, Mahaffey K. Lead and osteoporosis: mobilization of lead from bone in postmenopausal women. Environ Res 1988;47:79–94.

30. Occupational Safety and Health Administration. Guidelines for cytotoxic (antineoplastic) drugs: OSHA instruction Pub. 8–1.1. Washington, DC: Occupational Safety and Health Administration, 1986.

31. Occupational Safety and Health Administration, 29 CFR:Sec 1910.20. Washington, DC: Office of the Federal Register, 1986.

32. Smith TJ. Industrial hygiene. In Levy BS, Wegman DH, eds. Occupational health: recognizing and preventing work-related disease. 2nd ed. Boston: Little, Brown, & Co, 1988:87–103.

33. Kneip TJ, Crable JV, eds. Methods for biological monitoring: a manual for assessing human exposure to hazardous substances. Washington, DC: American Public Health Association, 1988.

34. U.S. General Accounting Office, Program Evaluation and Methodology Division. Reproductive and developmental toxicants: regulatory actions provide uncertain protection. Washington, DC: U.S. General Accounting Office, 1991.

35. U.S. Congress, Office of Technology Assessment. Reproductive health hazards in the workplace. Washington, DC: Office of Technology Assessment, OTA-BA-266, 1985:199.

36. Castleman BI, Ziem GE. Corporate influence on threshold limit values. Am J Ind Med 1988;13:531–559.

37. Occupational Safety and Health Administration. 29 CFR: Sec 1910.1000. Washington, DC: Office of the Federal Register, 1989.

38. Centers for Disease Control. NIOSH recommendations for occupational safety and health standards. MMWR 1988;37(suppl S-7):1–29.

39. American Conferences of Governmental Industrial Hygienists. 1991–1992 threshold limit values for chemical substances and physical agents and biological exposure

indices. Cincinnati: American Conference of Governmental Industrial Hygienists, 1991.

40. Hallenbeck WH, Cunningham KM. Quantitative risk assessment for environmental and occupational health. Chelsea, MI: Lewis Publishers Inc., 1988.

41. Pease W, Vandenberg J, Hooper K. Comparing alternative approaches to establishing regulatory levels for reproductive toxicants: DBCP as a case study. Environ Health Perspect 1991;91:141–155.

42. Frankos VH. FDA perspectives on the use of teratology data for human risk assessment. Fund Appl Toxicol 1985;5:615–625.

43. Kimmel CA, Gaylor DW. Issues in qualitative and quantitative risk analysis for developmental toxicity. Risk Analysis 1988;8:15–20.

44. Omenn GS. Susceptibility to occupational and environmental exposure to chemicals. Prog Clin Biol Res 1986;214:527–545.

45. Mamelle N, Laumon B, Lazar P. Prematurity and occupational activity during pregnancy. Am J Epidemiol 1984;119:309–322.

46. Mahaffey KR. Nutritional factors in lead poisoning. Nutr Rev 1981;39:353–362.

47. Ott MG, Skory LK, Holder BB, Bronson JM, Williams PR. Health evaluation of employees occupationally exposed to methylene chloride: metabolism data and oxygen half-saturation pressures. Scand J Work Environ Health 1983; 9(Suppl 1):31–38.

48. Buehler BA, Delimont D, won Waes M, Finnell RH. Prenatal prediction of risk of the fetal hydantoin syndrome. N Engl J Med 1990;322:1567–1572.

49. Slovik P. Perception of risk. Science 1987;236:280–285.

50. Koren G, Bologa M, Long D, Feldman Y, Shear NH. Perception of teratogenic risk by pregnant women exposed to drugs and chemicals during the first trimester. Am J Obstet Gynecol 1989;160:1190–1194.

51. Shepard TH. Counseling pregnant women exposed to potentially harmful agents during pregnancy. Clin Obstet Gynecol 1983;26:478–483.

52. Mosher WD, Pratt WF. Fecundity, infertility and reproductive health in the United States, 1982. Washington, DC: National Center for Health Statistics, 1987.

53. Kline J, Stein Z, Susser M. Conception to birth: epidemiology of prenatal development. New York: Oxford University Press, 1989:43–68.

54. Holmes LB. Congenital anomalies. In Oski FA, ed. Principles and practice of pediatrics. Philadelphia: JB Lippincott, 1990:258–261.

55. U.S. Congress, Office of Technology Assessment. Preventing illness and injury in the workplace. Washington, DC: Office of Technology Assessment, OTA-H-256, 1985:77–85.

56. Occupational Safety and Health Administration. 29 CFR: Sec 1910.134. Washington, DC: Office of the Federal Register, 1988.

···········································

# Material Safety Data Sheet

## SECTION I.  PRODUCT IDENTIFICATION

The name, address, and telephone number of the manufacturer is provided in this section, along with the date that the MSDS was prepared or revised and an emergency phone number. Chemical products are identified by formal chemical name, trade name, chemical family, and chemical formula.

## SECTION II.  HAZARDOUS INGREDIENTS

Each hazardous ingredient of a product is listed by generic chemical name, Chemical Abstract Service (CAS) number, and percent make-up. The CAS number is unique to each chemical and can be used when researching a substance. When "trade secret" or "proprietary formulation" is noted, the ingredients are omitted. However, physicians can obtain this information through a phone call or written request to the manufacturer.

Recommended air-borne exposure limits are provided if available. Threshold Limit Values (TLVs) are recommended by the American Conference of Governmental Industrial Hygienists and are not legally enforceable. Permissible Exposure Limits (PELs) are enforceable OSHA limits. Values refer to time-weighted average air-borne concentrations for a normal 8-hr workday and a 40-hr work week to which nearly all workers may be repeatedly exposed without adverse effects. However, reproductive and developmental effects may not have been adequately assessed when setting these limits.

## SECTION III.  PHYSICAL DATA

Information about the physical properties of the product is useful in determining potential routes of exposure. In general, a substance with a low *boiling point* or high *vapor pressure* tends to evaporate and present an inhalation hazard.

*Evaporation rate* indicates how fast a substance evaporates as compared to butyl acetate (slow) or ether (rapid). Agents that do not readily evaporate may still be absorbed through dermal contact. *Appearance and Odor* describe characteristic qualities that may allow for sensory identification of a chemical. However, some hazardous substances, such as carbon monoxide, are odorless. Tolerance to odors or olfactory fatigue may occur, allowing hazardous concentrations of some chemicals to go unnoticed.

## SECTION IV.  FIRE AND EXPLOSION HAZARD DATA

This section provides information on how to avoid and how to contain fires involving the product.

## SECTION V.  HEALTH HAZARD DATA

This section provides information on acute and chronic health effects, along with emergency and first aid procedures. Unfortunately, reproductive and developmental health risks are seldom adequately addressed.

## SECTION VI.  REACTIVITY DATA

This section indicates the tendency of the product to react with other substances. Conditions to avoid are noted along with a list of *Incompatible Substances*. *Hazardous Decomposition Products* describe reaction byproducts. *Hazardous Polymerization* describes reactions that result in release of excess heat or toxic gases. If the "may occur" box is checked, special storage procedures are required.

## SECTION VII.  SPILL OR LEAK PROCEDURES

This section describes important waste disposal methods and steps to be taken if material is accidentally released or spilled.

## SECTION VIII. SPECIAL PROTECTIVE INFORMATION

This important section describes the type of ventilation and personal protective equipment (e.g., gloves, respirators, eyewear) that should be utilized to reduce exposure to hazardous constituents.

## SECTION IX. SPECIAL PRECAUTIONS

Relevant information not discussed in the previous sections is presented here.

· · · · · · · · · · · · · · · · · · · · · · · · · · · · · · · · · · · · · · · · · · · · · · · · · · · · · · · · · · · ·

# Resources

## COMPUTER DATABASES

MEDLINE, National Library of Medicine, Bethesda, MD (800) 638–8480

> Contains references from over 3000 biomedical journals

REPROTOX, Reproductive Toxicology Center, Washington, DC (202) 293–5946

> Contains referenced summaries of reproductive and developmental data for over 3000 physical and chemical agents

TERIS (Teratogen Information System), Seattle, WA

> Provides summaries and risk ratings for drugs and some industrial chemicals; includes Shepards's on-line *Catalog of Teratogenic Agents*

Toxicology Information Program, National Library of Medicine, Bethesda, MD (301) 496–1131. Maintains the following relevant databases:

> ETICBACK (Environmental Teratology Information Backfile): Bibliographic database containing over 46,000 citations to publications concerning teratology and developmental toxicology (pre-1950 through 1988)
>
> DART (Developmental and Reproductive Toxicology): Bibliographic database on agents that may cause birth defects (1989 on): continuation of ETICBACK
>
> HSDB (Hazardous Substances Data Bank): Factual, nonbibliographic data bank including toxicologic and biomedical information on over 4000 chemicals
>
> RTECS (Registry of Toxic Effects of Chemical Substances): On-line version of the NIOSH compilation of potentially toxic substances; contains acute and chronic health effects data on more than 100,000 chemicals
>
> TOXLINE (Toxicology Information On-line): Extensive collection of bibliographic information covering the pharmacological, biochemical, physiological, and toxicological effects of chemicals and drugs
>
> IRIS (Integrated Risk Information System): Database containing EPA health risk and regulatory information on approximately 400 chemicals; includes EPA Drinking Water Health Advisories; integrated into TOXNET system

## RISKLINES

### Nationwide

National Pesticides Telecommunications Network; Lubbock, TX

> (800) 858–7378

NIOSH Information Hotline, Cincinnati, OH

> (800) 356–4674

U.S. Consumer Product Safety Commission Hotline, Washington, DC

> (800) 638–2772

U.S. EPA Air RISC Hotline, Durham, NC

> (919) 541–0888

U.S. EPA Safe Drinking Water Hotline, Washington, DC

> (800) 426–4791

### Eastern United States

Teratogen Counseling Service, Arkansas Genetics Program, University of Arkansas for Medical Sciences, Little Rock, AR

> Serves primarily Arkansas: (501) 686–5994

Connecticut Pregnancy Exposure Information Service, University of Connecticut Health Center, Farmington, CT

> Serves Connecticut only: (203) 679–1502, (800) 325–5391

Teratogen Information Services, University of Florida, Gainesville, FL

Serves primarily Florida: (904) 392–4104

Massachusetts Teratogen Information Service, Franciscan Children's Hospital, Boston, MA

Serves primarily Massachusetts, but will accept calls from practitioners nationwide: (617) 787–4957, (800) 322–5014 (MA only)

Occupational and Environmental Reproductive Hazards Center, University of Massachusetts Medical Center, Worcester, MA

Provides clinical consultations and health provider educational sessions regarding reproductive hazards: (508) 856–6162

New Jersey Pregnancy Risk Information Service, University of Medicine and Dentistry of New Jersey, Camden, NJ

Serves New Jersey only: (609) 757–7812, (800) 441–0025

Western New York Teratogen Information Service, Amherst, NY

Serves western New York only: (716) 833–9359, (800) 869–9606

Pregnancy Safety Hotline, West Penn Hospital, Pittsburgh, PA

Serves Western Pennsylvania, Eastern Ohio, and West Virginia: (412) 687–SAFE

Vermont Pregnancy Risk Information Service, University of Vermont, Burlington, VT

Serves Vermont only: (802) 658–4310, (800) 531–9800

## Central United States

Illinois Teratogen Information Service, Northwestern University, Chicago, IL

Serves Illinois only: (312) 908–7441, (800) 252–4847

Genetics and Environmental Information Service, Washington University School of Medicine, St. Louis, MO

Serves central United States: (314) 454–8172

Nebraska Teratogen Project, University of Nebraska Medical Center, Omaha, NE

Serves primarily Nebraska, but will accept calls from practitioners in surrounding states: (402) 559–5071

South Dakota Teratogen and Birth Defects Information Project, University of South Dakota School of Medicine, Vermillion, SD

Serves primarily South Dakota: (605) 677–5623, (800) 962–1642 (SD only)

Wisconsin Teratogen Project, University of Wisconsin, Madison, WI

Serves primarily Wisconsin: (608) 262–4719, (800) 362–3020 (WI only, ask for Pregnancy Exposure Support Line)

## Western United States

Arizona Teratogen Information Service, University of Arizona Health Sciences Center, Tucson, AZ

Serves Arizona only, (602) 795–5675, (800) 362–0101

Teratogen Information and Education Service, Rocky Mountain Poison Center and the University of Colorado Genetics Division, Denver, CO

Serves Colorado, Montana, Wyoming, and Nevada: (303) 629–1123, (800) 332–2082 (CO only), (800) 525–5042 (MT only), (800) 442–2701 (WY only), (800) 446–6179 (NV only)

Hazard Evaluation System and Information Service, California Department of Health Services, Berkeley, CA

Serves California only: (415) 540–3014 (collect calls accepted from California physicians)

Pregnancy Riskline, Utah Department of Health and University of Utah, Salt Lake City, UT

Serves Utah, Nevada, and Montana: (801) 583–2229, (800) 822–2229 (UT only), (800) 521–2229 (MT and NV only)

Washington State Poison Control Network, Children's Hospital and Medical Center, Seattle, WA

(206) 526–2121, (800) 732–6985 (WA only)

## GOVERNMENT AGENCIES

Agency for Toxic Substances and Disease Registry (ATSDR), Atlanta, GA, (404) 639–0700

Provides consultation services and assessments of potential health threats at Superfund and Resource Conservation and Recovery toxic waste sites; develops and disseminates materials on health effects of toxic substances to health care providers

Environmental Protection Agency (EPA),

Washington DC, national and regional offices; (202) 382–2080

> Responsible for evaluation and control of environmental hazards including air and water pollution, waste management, pesticides, radiation, noise

National Institute for Occupational Safety and Health (NIOSH), Cincinnati, OH, national and regional offices; (404) 331–2396

> Develops scientific documents and recommended exposure limits for consideration in OSHA regulatory activities; performs health hazard evaluations in workplaces; provides for training of occupational health and safety personnel

Occupational Safety and Health Administration (OSHA), Washington DC, national and regional offices; (202) 523–8151

> Responsible for promulgation and enforcement of occupational health standards and permissible exposure limits; performs workplace inspections at request of employee, union, or health care provider; under section 7C1 of the Occupational Safety and Health Act, provides for state-based consultative services for employers to assess and control hazards voluntarily

## OTHER ORGANIZATIONS

American Association of Occupational Health Nurses, Atlanta, GA (800) 241–8014

> Professional organization of occupational health nurses; involved in educational activities and sets standards for practice

American College of Obstetricians and Gynecologists, Washington DC (800) 673–8444 or (202) 863–2518

> Professional organization of obstetricians and gynecologists; involved in continuing medical education activities; will accept calls from obstetricians regarding toxic exposures

American College of Occupational and Environmental Medicine, Arlington Heights, IL (708) 228–6850

> Professional organization of occupational medicine physicians; involved in continuing medical education activities related to occupational and environmental health

Association of Occupational and Environmental Clinics, Washington DC (202) 682–1807

> National organization of occupational and environmental clinics; makes referrals to qualified clinics in caller's region (all clinics have access to industrial hygiene services); involved in educational activities

Center for Occupational Hazards, New York, NY (212) 227–6220

> National clearinghouse for research and information on health hazards in the arts

Coalitions for Occupational Safety and Health (COSH), state offices

> Worker advocacy organizations involved in education, referral services, and political activities related to workplace health and safety

Citizens Clearinghouse for Hazardous Wastes, Arlington, VA (703) 276–7070

> National grassroots citizen advocacy organization; provides consultation and support for citizens concerned about community contamination

Nurses Association of the American College of Obstetricians and Gynecologists, Washington DC (800) 241–8014

> Professional obstetrical nursing association; involved in continuing medical educational activities

Pesticide Education Center, San Francisco, CA (415) 391–8511

> A nonprofit corporation that educates the public about use and health effects of pesticides

# 11

.....................................................

# Common Clinical Encounters

## MAUREEN PAUL

For obstetricians-gynecologists and other primary providers, the three most common clinical situations requiring knowledge of reproductive or developmental hazards include assessment of the infertile couple, preconception counseling, and evaluation of the pregnant woman. This chapter addresses each of these scenarios through some occupational case examples.

### INFERTILE COUPLE

Fertility is a measure of successful reproduction in a couple or population. Fecundity is the physiological capacity of an individual to produce a livebirth, and thus, is a measure of the biological competence of the male or female reproductive system (1).

An estimated one in 12 couples of reproductive age in the United States is infertile, i.e., they are unable to produce a viable pregnancy within 1 yr of unprotected intercourse (2). However, derivation of infertility rates is complicated by a number of factors including regional population differences, seasonal variations in conception rates, and by the influence of age on fertility. The risk of impaired fertility gradually increases with age, approximately doubling after women reach age 35 yr (3, 4).

Successful reproduction requires integration of a number of complex processes ranging from gametogenesis to release, transport, and union of the gametes to implantation and development of the conceptus. In the infertility work-up, the male and female are evaluated independently and as a couple. Using currently available technologies, the etiology of the fertility problem can be ascertained in 85–90% of couples. Approximately 30–40% of infertility is due to abnormal semen production, 10–15% is due to ovulatory disorders, 30–40% is caused by tubal disease or dysfunction, 10–15% is caused by cervical factors interfering with sperm transport, and 5% is due to uncommon or unknown causes (5).

Because of the multifactorial etiology of infertility, identification of potential reproductive toxicants must not curtail a detailed investigation of all possible sources of the problem. The comprehensive infertility work-up is detailed in a number of publications (5, 6), and a simplified outline is presented in Figure 11.1. In complex cases, referrals to reproductive endocrinologists or urologists is necessary for adequate evaluation and treatment of the couple. Primary clinicians involved in reproductive hazard evaluations should know the basic components of the infertility work-up and how to take a good history. Familiarity with interpretation of semen analysis and common tests of ovulatory dysfunction is also important.

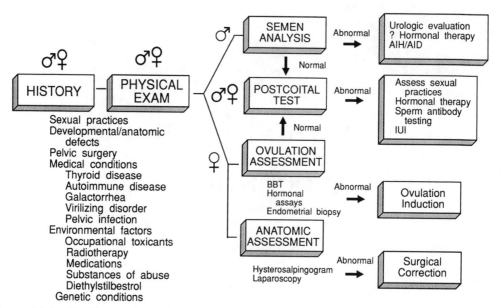

**Figure 11.1.** The basic work-up of the infertile couple. *BBT* = basal body temperatures; *AIH* = artificial insemination husband; *AID* = artificial insemination donor; *IUI* = intrauterine insemination.

## History

When assessing an infertility complaint, it is particularly important to ask about sexual practices and problems. Decreased libido, impotence, coital timing and frequency, and use of certain vaginal lubricants can influence the likelihood of conception. The reproductive history includes questions about sexual development, contraceptive practices, menstrual patterns, and reproductive and obstetrical outcomes. Prior trauma or surgery to the genital organs is noted. Particular attention must be paid to a history of sexually transmitted diseases and other medical conditions such as endometriosis (in the female) or mumps orchitis (in the male) that can affect gonadal function. Finally, certain chronic diseases (e.g., thyroid disorders, autoimmune disease) or genetic conditions may contribute to the fertility problem.

The occupational and environmental history seeks to identify toxicants that affect libido or gonadal or hormonal function and to characterize the timing and dose of exposure. Sperm production can be impaired by exposure to excessive heat, ionizing radiation, therapeutic medications, alcohol, smoking, illicit drugs, and a number of industrial chemicals such as lead,

ethylene dibromide, and the ethylene glycol ethers (7, 8). Oocyte toxicity resulting in earlier menopause has been demonstrated following exposure to high-dose ionizing radiation, alkylating agents, and cigarette smoke (9). Significant psychological or physical stress can interfere with hormonal regulation and can produce anovulation (10, 11), as can occupational exposure to sex steroid hormones, organohalide pesticides, and other agents (9, 12, 13). In addition, agents that interfere with tubal transport of the conceptus or that cause peri-implantation pregnancy loss result in clinical infertility. While these mechanisms have been well demonstrated in animal studies, little is known about toxicant-induced early pregnancy loss in humans.

## Physical Examination

Examination of the male and female may reveal physiological or anatomic abnormalities associated with impaired fecundity. Secondary sex characteristics are assessed, and aberrations such as gynecomastia are noted. In the male, the genitals are carefully inspected for size, consistency, and anatomic defects such as varicocele, hernia, undescended testes, and hypospadias. The pelvic examination may detect infection, tumors, or congenital anomalies of the reproductive tract. Neurological function is assessed, and signs associated with endocrine disorders such as thyroid disease, hyper-prolactinemia, or Cushing's syndrome are carefully noted.

## Laboratory Tests

A number of laboratory tests are available to evaluate gonadal function and couple-dependent factors (14). Only the most common tests are discussed here; more complex assessments, such as sperm penetration and immunological assays, may be indicated in some cases.

Basic laboratory investigations pertinent to the male patient include semen analysis and cultures to screen for infection. If the semen analysis is abnormal, gonadotropic and sex steroid hormonal assays may be helpful in identifying the source of the problem. Methods of collection and interpretation of these tests are addressed in Chapter l. Serial semen analyses are particularly important when assessing toxicant-induced injury, since a variable lag period exists between exposure and effect, depending on the germ cell types affected. Likewise, recovery from spermatotoxic insult may require appreciable time. In some cases, follow-up for months or years is required for full documentation of recovery.

In the female, the clinician seeks to identify abnormalities in structure or function of the three anatomic compartments of the reproductive tract: the uterus, fallopian tubes, and ovaries. Because of the relative inaccessibility of the female reproductive organs, many tests are designed to assess the function of the various compartments indirectly. Women who have regular periods (every 21–35 days) marked by premenstrual symptoms are usually ovulatory. Disturbances in ovulation may manifest as amenorrhea, oligomenorrhea, or as menstrual irregularity. Measurement of basal body temperature (BBT) is a somewhat imprecise indicator of ovulation but is considerably less expensive than other methods. In normal women, the BBT rises approximately 2 days after the midcycle luteinizing hormone (LH) surge; this is due to the thermogenic properties of progesterone. Ovulation probably occurs the day before the temperature elevation. The

temperature should remain elevated for 11–16 days; shorter elevations suggest an inadequate luteal phase due to deficient progesterone secretion by the corpus luteum (6). A number of more reliable tests are now available for ovulation prediction purposes. The most common are designed to detect the preovulatory LH surge through urine sampling (15). Progesterone concentrations in serum that are greater than 10 ng/ml measured in the midluteal phase also provide supportive evidence of ovulation. Because of the pulsatile release of progesterone during the luteal phase, however, this test alone is not sufficient to document ovulatory dysfunction. Recently, salivary progesterone tests have been developed as practical, noninvasive sampling alternatives (16).

Endometrial biopsy, performed 2–3 days before the expected menses, is a reliable method to assess ovulation and the adequacy of the luteal phase. Histological analysis reveals secretory endometrium in the ovulatory cycle. A discrepancy of more than 2 days between endometrial maturation and chronological data as determined by the onset of menses indicates an inadequate luteal phase. Inasmuch as deficient luteal phases occur occasionally in normal women, abnormal biopsies should be repeated during a second cycle for confirmation (17).

The amount and consistency of the cervical mucus vary with hormonal fluctuations of the menstrual cycle. With maximal estrogen levels, normal mucus is clear, watery, and has a spinnbarkeit (stretchability) of at least 6 cm just before ovulation. Microscopic examination of the mucus reveals a characteristic fern pattern.

Penetration of the cervical mucus by sperm is highly dependent on the changes that occur in conjunction with ovulation. The postcoital test assesses both the suitability of cervical mucus and the ability of sperm to penetrate and to survive within the mucus (6). At the time of optimal mucus production and 2–3 hr after intercourse, cervical mucus is aspirated and evaluated microscopically for the presence of motile sperm.

X-ray imaging of the uterus and fallopian tubes is possible with hysterosalpingography. This technique is useful in documenting tubal blockage and structural abnormalities of the uterus. The reproductive organs can also be directly evaluated through hysteroscopy and laparoscopy. In infertility patients undergoing ovulation induction, follicular development is often monitored with ultrasound.

## Management

Confronting a fertility problem is an emotionally trying experience for most couples. Feelings of vulnerability, embarrassment, and inadequacy are common; and the demands of the work-up may exacerbate sexual problems or strains in the relationship. Patients who believe that their fertility problem is related to workplace or environmental exposures may feel particularly anxious.

Counseling the infertile couple involves both objective sharing of information and support. The multifactorial etiology of infertility is explained, emphasizing the importance of age and male, female, and couple-dependent factors. The clinician reviews the overall work-up with the couple, placing the reproductive hazard assessment in the context of a more comprehensive exploration for all sources of the problem. Patients should understand that most occupational and environmental agents are inadequately tested for reproductive toxicity.

In the face of an unexplained abnormal semen analysis or ovulatory dysfunction, it is reasonable to reduce exposures to known or suspected gametotoxins in the workplace. In the absence of human data, experimental studies showing fertility deficits after exposure of male animals to a toxicant are worrisome. In most test species, several-fold declines in sperm count are required before infertility is observed; in contrast, human sperm concentrations are typically only two- to four-fold higher than the threshold at which fertility is significantly reduced (18).

Infertility is generally not considered a disabling condition by employers because it does not impair the worker's ability to carry out essential job tasks. Under most Workers Compensation statutes and employer disability insurance plans, the infertile worker is not entitled to compensated job leave or medical cost reimbursement. Even in states that do allow compensation for loss of function, the complex nature of infertility often makes it difficult to prove that exposures encountered in the workplace contributed to the problem.

## CASE 1

A.T. is a 26-yr-old white male who presented with the complaint that he and his spouse had not achieved pregnancy after 13 months of unprotected intercourse. A recent semen analysis obtained by his urologist revealed a sperm count of 12 million sperm/ml of ejaculate, with 30% motility and 40% abnormal forms. Repeat analysis confirmed the low sperm concentration and motility. His 24-yr-old partner is nulligravid, and her infertility work-up revealed no abnormalities. A.T. has never fathered children in the past.

A.T. works as a carpenter and house painter for a small construction company involved in home and commercial renovations. Over the past several months, he and two co-workers renovated and repainted a large wooden apartment complex slated for conversion into condominiums. When working in closets and other enclosed spaces, he wore a "dust mask" that he bought at a hardware store; he did not otherwise use personal protective equipment. A.T. ate lunch at the worksite and smoked cigarettes during breaks. He brought his work overalls home each day for his spouse to launder.

A.T.'s partner is a salesperson at a department store. The medical history for each member of the couple is negative, and neither takes medications. A.T. smokes one pack of cigarettes daily; both drink alcohol occasionally and in moderation. No other concerning exposures in the home or community were identified. During review of systems, A.T. complained of fatigue and intermittent abdominal discomfort, which he attributed to "indigestion."

A.T.'s physical examination was significant for facial pallor and mild abdominal tenderness without organomegaly; neurological and genital examinations were negative. A complete blood count (CBC) revealed a hemoglobin level of 9 g/100 ml; renal function tests were normal. A.T.'s blood lead level was 85 μg/dl with a free erythrocyte protoporphyrin (FEP) concentration of 230 μg/dl. His spouse had a slightly elevated blood lead level of 16 μg/dl with a FEP of 28 μg/dl.

Research reveals that excessive lead absorption is associated with anemia, gastrointestinal disturbances, nephrotoxicity, and neurological problems (19). Lead's spermatotoxicity is evident in both laboratory animal and human studies; occupational epidemiological investigations reveal oligospermia, decreased motility, and abnormal morphology at blood lead levels exceeding 35 μg/dl (20). Blood lead levels as low as 10–15 μg/dl have been associated with increases in blood pressure in adult males (21) and with developmental deficits in children exposed prenatally (22). One epidemiological study found an increased risk for spontaneous abortion in the wives of male workers with blood lead levels exceeding 30 μg/dl (23).

A.T. was informed that his clinical and laboratory findings were consistent with lead poisoning. His employer was contacted. Paint chips from the interior and exterior of the building tested positive for lead. A.T.'s co-worker was evaluated and found to also have excessive blood lead indices. With the help of the state Department of Labor, the employer was provided with information on lead toxicity and ways to minimize exposure including environmental and medical monitoring, provision of respirators and employer-laundered workclothes, housekeeping procedures, and prohibition of eating and smoking in contaminated areas. Fortunately, with the cold weather setting in, no painting projects were planned for the immediate future.

The couple was advised to use contraception until laboratory indices normalized. After a positive EDTA challenge test, A.T. underwent chelation therapy to decrease his lead body burden. A.T.'s blood lead indices gradually decreased, his abdominal pain subsided, and serial semen analyses showed eventual recovery. His wife's lead level also spontaneously decreased to 9 μg/dl.

This case involves excessive exposure to lead, a ubiquitous environmental contaminant also commonly used in a variety of industries. Although the use of lead in paint was restricted in the mid-1970s, scraping of lead paint from older building structures remains a significant source of exposure. This point is particularly relevant to patients who are undertaking home renovation projects in anticipation of pregnancy or childbirth. Before renovation, paint chips should be tested for lead. Lead paint removal should be performed only by qualified specialists using proper control measures.

A.T.'s excessive exposure was due to lack of adequate controls and improper work practices. Dust masks afford insufficient protection, and eating and smoking in contaminated work areas can result in ingestion of lead particles. Home laundering of lead dust-laden workclothes can result in exposure to family members. Chelation is indicated when systemic symptoms are severe or when a chelation challenge test results in ex-

cessive urinary excretion of lead. Without chelation, normalization of blood lead indices may require several months after removal from the source of exposure. To prevent deleterious effects on offspring, blood lead indices of both parents should be normalized before conception.

As a construction company, this employer was not subject to the provisions of the Occupational Safety and Health Administration's (OSHA's) general industry Lead Standard, which mandates monitoring, stringent control measures, and compensated medical removal of overexposed workers. In this case, a nonregulatory state agency was helpful in intervening and educating the employer. The current OSHA Lead Standard, promulgated in 1978, specifically recommends that blood lead levels of male and female prospective parents be maintained below 30 μg/dl. Given recent data about low-level health effects, however, the standard is in need of revision.

### CASE 2

B.C. is a 25-yr-old nulligravid white female with menarche at age 13 and a history of regular periods who presents with a 6-month history of amenorrhea. Eight months before her clinic visit, she started the first year of her residency in general surgery. She jogs approximately 20 miles per week and has maintained this activity despite the demands of her new position. She is 64 inches tall, and her weight has decreased from 120 lb to 113 lb since starting her residency. Her history is otherwise unremarkable. While B.C. is not now sexually active, she is concerned about the cessation of her periods. Physical examination is normal. Serum thyroid-stimulating hormone (TSH) and prolactin are within normal limits, but gonadotropin and estradiol levels are markedly low.

B.C. was given Provera 10 mg for 5 days with no withdrawal bleeding. Combined estrogen-progestin treatment resulted in withdrawal bleeding. The patient was counseled about the importance of maintaining her weight and referred to a stress reduction program. When conservative measures failed, she was offered calcium and hormonal replacement therapy, which she continued for 1 yr. At that time, her work schedule improved. She discontinued the medications and spontaneous menses resumed.

Ovulatory disorders can be of significant concern to patients, even in the absence of plans for pregnancy. In this case, the onset of the problem coincided with a dramatic increase in physical and psychological stress associated with medical training. Evaluation was consistent with hypothalamic amenorrhea secondary to stress. Because these patients are at risk for osteopenia secondary to chronic low estrogen levels (24), hormone replacement therapy is offered until the source of the problem is ameliorated. If the patient desires conception, ovulation induction is indicated.

## PRECONCEPTION COUNSELING

The goal of preconception counseling is to optimize the course and outcome of pregnancy through patient education and preventive medical intervention. Diseases such as diabetes mellitus or hypertension are identified so that adequate control can be achieved before conception. A comprehensive reproductive history may elucidate conditions, such as recurrent spontaneous abortion, that deserve further evaluation. The family history may suggest genetic conditions that warrant special counseling or diagnosis. Evaluation includes the work histories of both the male and female, along with potential adverse exposures in the community or home. All medications taken by patients are identified, as well as substances of abuse. The counselor reviews identified risk factors and encourages modification of harmful behaviors.

Laboratory tests are tailored to the specific needs of each patient. Women without prior documentation of rubella immunity are serologically tested, and, if sensitive, offered vaccination. In certain high-risk subgroups, tests are available to detect heterozygous carriers of serious genetic disorders such as sickle cell hemoglobinopathy or Tay-Sachs disease. Laboratory testing may be indicated in patients whose history indicates potential exposure to xenobiotics. For example, workers with potential exposure to blood and body fluids should be tested for hepatitis B surface antigen and, if susceptible, offered vaccination. Patients at high risk for lead exposure should be tested for blood lead and FEP concentrations. If excessive, the source of exposure is explored and eliminated to the extent feasible; the patient is counseled to delay conception until biological indices normalize.

The preconception period is an optimal time to evaluate workplace conditions and decrease hazardous exposures. However, success in this regard depends on a number of factors including employer responsibilities under federal regulations, economic restraints on the company, and the worker's financial situation and degree of job protection. Workplace exposure control measures are the best option, as compensated job leaves or transfers before pregnancy can be difficult to arrange. The variable responses of employers to preconception concerns are illustrated in Cases 3 and 4 below.

### CASE 3

S.B. is a 33-yr-old G1P0010 Asian immigrant employed for 4 yr in the central supply area of a medium-sized community hospital. She presents with concerns about her recent history of a first-trimester spontaneous abortion and desires evaluation and counseling before another conception.

S.B.'s job requires her to sterilize medical instruments in an ethylene oxide (EtO) sterilizer. She loads, operates, and unloads the sterilizer; transfers the instruments to an EtO aerator; unloads the aerator; then places the items in a sterile storage area. She wears no personal protective equipment and is sometimes expected to sterilize instruments on an emergency basis. She has not noted any chemical odors, but a sign in the sterilizer room warning of reproductive risks from EtO prompts her visit. S.B.'s husband works in the hospital laundry. Infection control measures are well established in the laundry, and there are no chemical exposures. However, he does complain of a hot work environment.

Paternal heat stress has been associated with decreased sperm count (Chapter 16); however, since the couple did not have problems conceiving, semen analysis was not performed. EtO is an alkylating agent and is mutagenic in a number of test systems. Limited developmental studies in rats reveal fetal resorptions and growth deficits at more than 100 ppm EtO via inhalation with an apparent no-observed-adverse-effect-level (NOAEL) of 33 ppm (25). One epidemiological study found a higher rate of spontaneous abortion among hospital workers involved in EtO sterilization procedures compared with controls (26), but individual exposure data were not collected. EtO is regulated as a potential human carcinogen (25). Some provisions of the OSHA Standard for EtO address reproductive concerns. The OSHA 8-hr Permissible Exposure Limit (PEL) for EtO is 1 ppm with a Short

Term Exposure Limit (STEL) of 5 ppm. NIOSH recommends an 8-hr TWA limit of less than 0.1 ppm.

With the patient's permission, a call was made to the hospital's Safety Office. Personal monitoring of S.B. revealed an 8-hr TWA exposure of 0.6 ppm with peak levels of 101 ppm when she opened the sterilizer door. When observing S.B.'s work practices, the safety officer noted that S.B. opened the door widely and did not subsequently vacate the room. A leaky seal on the sterilizer was also detected and replaced. S.B. was provided with intensive training regarding safe work practices, including cracking the sterilizer door and leaving the room during the evacuation phase of the cycle to allow exhaust ventilation to clear EtO-laden air from the area. A respirator was provided for those rare instances requiring emergency sterilization of surgical instruments. Subsequent personal and environmental monitoring revealed negligible EtO exposure. S.B. conceived and was delivered of an apparently normal infant at term.

In this case, the patient was protected by an enforceable OSHA standard that partially addresses reproductive concerns. Under the standard, the employer must institute a medical surveillance program for employees who work in areas where EtO concentrations exceed an "action level" of 0.5 ppm 8-hr TWA for more than 30 days per year. Medical consultation must be made available as soon as possible to an employee who desires advice concerning the effects of EtO on the ability to produce a healthy child. The intent of the OSHA PEL and STEL is to decrease the risk of nonthreshold biological effects (mutagenesis, carcinogenesis) to "acceptably" low levels, and the standard mandates workplace controls to accomplish this goal. However, based on review of the toxicity data, NIOSH recommends an exposure limit well below that of OSHA. Medium- to large-sized facilities often have health and safety personnel who can institute monitoring and appropriate controls in an expeditious fashion.

In this case, S.B.'s 8-hr average exposure exceeded the OSHA "action level," and her peak exposures were clearly concerning. While spontaneous abortion is a common occurrence that could not be definitely linked to EtO in this case, S.B.'s reproductive concerns became the catalyst for discovery of poorly controlled working conditions. The employer went be-

yond the responsibilities mandated by OSHA to lower limits to those consistent with the more protective NIOSH recommendations. Practitioners will not always encounter such cooperation, as illustrated in the following case.

## CASE 4

C.P. is a 25-yr-old G3P0120 white assembler at a small electronics plant. She has had two 10- to 14-week spontaneous abortions and a 36-week stillborn infant since starting employment at the firm. Desiring another pregnancy, she presented with concerns about the potential association between her workplace exposures and her poor obstetrical history.

The patient's medical history is unremarkable. Neither she nor her spouse take medications or engage in substance abuse. Physical examinations are within normal limits. A recurrent abortion work-up by C.P.'s referring physician, including a glucose screen, autoimmune indices, thyroid function tests, cervical cultures, hysterosalpingogram, and parental karyotypes, is negative.

C.P.'s spouse works as a cashier at a restaurant. C.P.'s job involves cleaning and assembling electronic parts while sitting at a bench with other assemblers. She handles several chemicals that are in open jars at the workbench and uses a brush to apply the solutions to the electronic constituents. A few times a day she also lowers a rackful of electronic components into a degreasing tank and retrieves the parts 30 min later. In the same room, other workers are engaged in chemically intensive job tasks. From the container labels, C.P. thinks that she is exposed to 1,1,1-trichloroethane, methylene chloride, toluene, and freons, but suspects other chemical exposures as well. No personal protective equipment is available. The room ventilation is poor; there are two small fans on the assembly bench, but she claims, "they just blow the chemicals right at me." She particularly complains about strong chemical odors when she removes the lid from the degreasing tank. She sometimes experiences headaches and feelings of "being high" that subside when away from the worksite.

In this small, nonunionized setting, C.P. was reluctant to ask for Material Safety Data Sheets (MSDSs) or to request an OSHA inspection for fear of retaliation by the employer. She could not afford to lose her job and health insurance benefits. She has never observed anyone performing environmental monitoring in her work area.

In a few epidemiological studies, laboratory work with mixed organic solvents during pregnancy has been associated with a modest increased risk for major congenital malformations including facial clefts, gastrointestinal atresia, and central nervous system (CNS) defects; however, quantitative exposure data are limited (Chapter 19). In the largest case-control study to date (27), an elevated risk of borderline significance was found for all malformations pooled, but not for specific defects, among women with "significant" solvent exposure (more than two-thirds of the Threshold Limit Values) during the first trimester. Studies assessing spontaneous abortion risks among laboratory workers have shown conflicting results; two recent, methodologically limited studies found increased rates of fetal loss among female electronics production workers (28, 29). Again, precise identification and quantification of exposures are lacking. Teratogenic effects have been reported in the offspring of women who recreationally abuse toluene during pregnancy; in a few studies of solvent-exposed workers, a specific association between toluene exposure and birth defects has been noted (Chapter 19). In rodents, toluene does not appear to be teratogenic even at maternally toxic doses; however, reduced fetal weight and retarded skeletal development are observed at lower exposures, with a NOAEL in rats of 112.5 mg/kg/day. Based on these animal data, risk assessors at the California Department of Health Services recently determined that the estimated daily absorbed dose for a 55-kg human female exposed at the OSHA PEL of 100 ppm is within an order of magnitude of the exposure level that caused adverse effects in mice and rats (30). Limited experimental animal studies provide no evidence for teratogenicity of 1,1,1-trichloroethane (31). Methylene chloride is mutagenic in some test systems and is an animal carcinogen; it is also metabolized to carbon monoxide in vivo (32). Developmental data on freons are extremely limited.

In view of the potential developmental effects of organic solvents, the patient's description of her working conditions, lack of environmental exposure data, and her unexplained poor reproductive history, a letter was sent to C.P.'s employer requesting transfer to a nonchemical position or paid leave while she attempted conception. The request was denied on the assertion that no alternative work was available and that a mere history of fetal losses did not constitute grounds for disability. The patient did conceive and, at 4 weeks' gestation, another request for leave was submitted. The request was denied by the company's disability insurance carrier, because *potential* harm to the pregnancy was not compensable. At 6 weeks' gestation, the patient developed moderate vaginal bleeding. Ultrasound demonstrated a viable conceptus. Disability leave at partial pay was granted for the duration of the pregnancy.

C.P. was placed on bedrest, and the bleeding resolved over a 2-week period. The patient was hospitalized at 26 weeks' gestation with a urinary tract infection and premature contractions, which resolved with hydration and antibiotic treatment. She was delivered vaginally at term of a healthy male infant.

Due to inadequate scientific and exposure data, no clear association can be drawn between this patient's occupational exposures and her prior history of fetal wastage. However, an attempt to effect transfer to a safer position or compensated leave for this high-risk patient is certainly reasonable. This case illustrates the limitations imposed on practitioners and patients faced with an uncooperative management. The fear of employer retaliation exhibited by this worker is not uncommon in small, nonunionized companies where job protections and transfer options are minimal. In addition, this case depicts poignantly the limited options available to workers concerned about reproductive or developmental hazards. Disability is usually narrowly defined by insurance carriers to cover identifiable medical conditions that interfere with ability to work; it does not cover situations involving *potential* harm to the pregnancy. Even when disability leave is granted, compensation is often inadequate to assure economic security, especially for the already low-paid worker. Given the difficulty in proving causation in this case, remediation under workers compensation is also unlikely. In retrospect, placing more emphasis on the patient's neurological symptoms (headache, feeling high), which are common complaints among solvent-exposed workers, may have been a more successful strategy than emphasizing potential risks to an anticipated pregnancy.

## CASE 5

D.V. is a 28-yr-old G1P0010 black female nurse employed at a large tertiary care hospital. Her partner is an internist in the same facility. D.V. has a remote history of a first trimester induced abortion, and the couple is now interested in having a child. It is winter, and an epidemic of respiratory syncytial virus (RSV) is occurring among children in the community. D.V. works in the pediatric ICU where she administers the antiviral agent, ribavirin aerosol, primarily via mist tent to patients with RSV. Ribavirin is administered for 12–18 hr/day, and she estimates that she typically spends 8 hr of her 12-hr shift in the room or at the bedside of a critically ill child receiving the drug. She usually wears gloves but no respiratory protection. She has noticed that the aerosol readily leaks from the mist tents during patient care, and that the package insert for ribavirin warns against its therapeutic use in pregnant women. She seeks advice about the safety of ribavirin and whether she should attempt to transfer to another area of the hospital before conception. The couple's history is otherwise unremarkable, and physical examinations are negative.

No systematic human data are available on the reproductive or developmental effects of ribavirin, and there is no established occupational safety limit. Available pharmacokinetic data indicate that 70% of the inhaled dose is deposited in the respiratory tract of patients, with the excess either swallowed or expelled. The medication is systemically absorbed and concentrates in erythrocytes, with an apparent half-life of 40 days (33). Ribavirin is fetotoxic and teratogenic in several animal species. The rabbit appears to be most sensitive to the developmental effects of ribavirin, with a NOAEL for embryo lethality of 0.3 mg/kg/day administered orally (34). In some studies, testicular lesions are induced in adult rats at chronic daily doses $\geq$ 16 mg/kg (35). Using the NOAEL for developmental toxicity in rabbits, the California Department of Health Services recommends an occupational air-borne exposure limit of 2.7 $\mu$g/m$^3$ (36). In an occupational study of 12 nurses and respiratory therapists administering ribavirin, this same agency found detectable levels of the drug in the red blood cells of one nurse whose average air-borne exposure level exceeded 300 $\mu$g/m$^3$ (37).

With the help of the hospital's industrial hygienist, D.V. was personally monitored during a typical workshift involving ribavirin administration. Her 8-hr time-weighted average (TWA) exposure to the drug was 200 $\mu$g/m$^3$. D.V. was advised either to delay conception or to consider transfer options while the safety officer explored better means of controlling occupational exposure to ribavirin.

This case illustrates the problems that arise in the absence of occupational exposure limits for potential developmental toxicants. Although the U.S. Food and Drug Administration licensed ribavirin for treatment of severe RSV in 1986, no considerations were given to the potential occupational hazards of aerosol administration. From both medical and legal perspectives, it is disconcerting to learn of the potential risk after thousands of caregivers, and many more visitors, have been exposed to aerosolized ribavirin. At the same time, ribavirin is by no means an established human teratogen, and exaggerating its toxicity may lead to unwarranted decisions regarding pregnancy or employment options or withdrawal of the drug from critically ill patients.

For the sake of learning, let's apply the risk assessment method used by the California Department of Health Services to the patient in this case. The following calculations are based on the formula presented in Chapter 10.

$$\text{Animal NOAEL for ribavirin}$$
$$= 0.3 \text{ mg/kg/day } (300 \text{ } \mu\text{g/kg/day})$$

$$\text{Patient's average air-borne exposure}$$
$$= 200 \text{ } \mu\text{g/m}^3$$

$$\text{Patient's absorbed dose} = C \times t \times MV$$
$$\times CF \times A \times bw^{-1}$$

where: $C$ = 8-hr TWA air concentration in $\mu$g/m$^3$; $t$ = exposure duration in minutes (480 min for 8-hr exposure); $MV$ = minute ventilation in liters/min (according to NIOSH, 19 liters/min for moderate work) (38); $CF$ = conversion factor (0.001 m$^3$/liter); $A$ = percent absorbed via respiratory route (70%); $bw$ = patient's body weight (56 kg in this case).

Substituting these values yields the following:

$$\text{Dose} = 200 \text{ } \mu\text{g/m}^3 \times 480 \text{ min} \times 19 \text{ liters/min}$$
$$\times 0.001 \text{ m}^3\text{/liter} \times 0.70 / 56 \text{ kg}$$
$$= 22.8 \text{ } \mu\text{g/kg/day}$$

According to these calculations, the patient's daily absorbed dose of ribavirin significantly exceeds 1/100th of the no-effect animal dose (300 $\mu$g/kg) and, thus, warrants caution. The values used here (e.g., percent absorption) have been criticized as high (39), but in the absence of adequate pharmacokinetic data, the use of conservative values in the clinical setting is not unreasonable.

Methods to control occupational exposure to ribavirin are being developed and tested

(40). At the same time, marketing of other therapeutic aerosolized medications is burgeoning. Whether or not the safety of ribavirin is ultimately confirmed in humans, these better control methods will have important broader applications in protecting workers who administer these types of agents.

## PREGNANCY

Perhaps the most difficult situation confronting the clinician involves risk evaluation and management of the pregnant patient. Because many women do not seek prenatal care until well past the first trimester, patients may be fearful that exposure-related harm to the pregnancy has already occurred. Decisions to terminate or to continue the pregnancy are significantly influenced by opinions and risk estimates provided by health care professionals. Given the litigious climate in which medical care is practiced, fear of a deleterious outcome also creates considerable anxiety for providers.

This complex situation warrants as efficient and accurate an evaluation as possible. The clinician should thoroughly explore all potentially harmful exposures in and out of the workplace and gather information about medical, obstetric, and demographic factors that can affect pregnancy outcome. Efforts should be made to quantify patient exposures; gestational age should be precisely established because timing of exposure may be critical in this setting. Expert consultation may be necessary for exposure assessment and interpretation of developmental toxicity data.

Patient counseling includes a critical summary of current data regarding known or suspected hazards in light of patient exposure levels. In all cases, the patient should be informed about the background frequency of adverse developmental outcomes. Because of considerable data gaps, precise risk estimates for exposure to most industrial chemicals are not possible. As in other cases of uncertain risk, responsibility for choices regarding pregnancy and employment options belong to the well-informed patient.

## CASE 6

C.T. is a 30-yr-old G2P1001 white female at 9 weeks' gestation employed for the past 8 months as a childcare worker in an after-school program. The program services children from a number of surrounding elementary schools. She is concerned about an epidemic of fifth disease affecting three of the schools that utilize her program. Two children from the after-school program are currently ill with the disease. C.T.'s job involves close contact with the children for 4 hr/day. Her 8-yr-old child, the product of a full-term uncomplicated vaginal delivery, attends one of the schools where the disease is prevalent. C.T. is asymptomatic but is concerned about her risk of infection and potential effects on her pregnancy. Her partner is a media and computer consultant. He smokes approximately one pack of cigarettes daily. The history is otherwise unremarkable. Physical examination is negative.

A blood sample was collected from CT and sent to the Centers for Disease Control (CDC) for human parvovirus B19 IgM and IgG antibody analysis. Results were expected in 6–8 weeks. The couple was extensively counseled about human parvovirus B19, the etiological agent in fifth disease. Current data suggest the following important points (41): (a) 30–60% of adults in the U.S. are susceptible to infection; (b) the virus is transmitted effectively after close-contact exposures; in schools with widespread student infection, secondary attack rates among susceptible staff are approximately 20–30% compared to approximately 50% among susceptible household contacts; (c) the greatest risk of transmission occurs before the development of clinical symptoms; (d) less than one-third of maternal infections result in fetal infection; (e) fetal infection is a risk factor for nonimmune hydrops and fetal loss. Studies to date suggest that the risk of B19-associated fetal death after documented maternal infection is less than 10%. In cases where the antibody status of the pregnant woman is unknown, the upper estimate of the risk of fetal death is less than 2.5% after exposure to infected household members (less than 0.1 risk of fetal death × 0.5 rate of susceptibility × 0.5 rate of infection × 100) and less than 1.5% after prolonged exposure at schools with widespread student infection (less than 0.1 risk of fetal death × 0.5 rate of susceptibility × 0.3 rate of infection × 100). The couple was also counseled about health risks from active and passive tobacco smoke exposure. In some studies, passive smoke exposure has been associated with decreased birthweight and a possible increased risk for childhood cancer (Chapter 25). C.P.'s partner was advised to discontinue smoking or, at least, to not smoke in the presence of C.P.

A letter was sent to the after-school program

administrator requesting that C.P. be transferred to a position without close contact with the children until her serological results were available. If susceptible, she would be maintained in this position until the epidemic subsided. The request was denied. After much deliberation, C.T. decided to quit her job. A few weeks later, her serological studies returned negative for both B19 IgM and IgG, indicating susceptibility but no recent infection. Her pregnancy remained uneventful until 34 weeks' gestation at which time she delivered a preterm but healthy infant.

According to the CDC (41), the decision to try to decrease the risk of B19 infection by avoidance of high-risk occupational settings should be made by the patient after consultation with family members, health specialists, and others. The agency does not support policies that routinely exclude members of high-risk groups from work environments where human parvovirus B19 infection is prevalent. In fact, the risk of transmission is more likely from household contact with infected individuals than from exposure in the work environment. In the clinical setting, the 6- to 8-week waiting period required for analysis of maternal serological studies presents difficult choices for the patient. In this case, the patient chose to minimize her occupational risk even though it presented some financial hardship and could not prevent infection from household contact, should her daughter become ill. In fact, the patient's serological studies revealed her to be susceptible to infection; had the clinician not agreed to support a work transfer and had an infection-related adverse outcome occurred, liability issues may have arisen. Certainly, a return to work is reasonable for the documented IgG-positive patient or for susceptible patients after the epidemic has subsided.

## CASE 7

F.M. is a 37-yr-old G3P0111 white female at 15 weeks' gestation who presents with concerns about chemical exposures at work. For the past 6 months, she has been employed part time as a custodial worker in a research and development facility. Her job involves cleaning laboratory glassware and work surfaces with a solvent-based cleaning solution for 2–4 hr/day and some vacuuming and dusting of office spaces. Gloves are provided but seldom worn, and respirators are not available. She is no longer with her partner who was unemployed at the time of conception. Her wages are meager, and she cannot afford to leave her job. The patient's obstetric history includes a first trimester-induced abortion and Cesarean section delivery for fetal distress of a 32-week female infant. History-taking elicits no other apparent exposures or medical conditions of concern. Her only medications include prenatal vitamins and iron supplementation for moderate anemia. The physical examination is unremarkable except for a mild contact dermatitis of her hands.

According to the MSDS obtained by the patient from her employer, a primary constituent of the cleaning solution is 2-ethoxyethanol (EGEE). A review of the literature reveals this ethylene glycol ether to be a teratogen in a variety of animal species with an apparent NOAEL of 50 ppm (Chapter 19). It is also a potent testicular toxicant at higher doses and can cause CNS and hematopoietic effects (including macrocytic anemia). There is no evidence for mutagenicity. Like other organic solvents, EGEE is readily absorbed through the skin. The current OSHA 8-hr permissible exposure limit (PEL) is 200 ppm but is undergoing revision. Based on the animal NOAEL of 50 ppm for developmental effects, NIOSH's recent Recommended Exposure Limit (REL) for EGEE is 0.5 ppm (42).

Because of her part-time status and financial insecurity, F.M. wanted to avoid raising a complaint with her employer unless the threat to her health or the pregnancy was significant. Urine analysis for ethoxyacetic acid revealed an excessive concentration of 16 mg/g creatinine. The employer was contacted, and F.M. remained out of work until the cleaning solvent was replaced with a safer substitute 3 weeks later. After genetic counseling based on maternal age, F.M. consented to amniocentesis. Fetal karyotype revealed a trisomy 21 fetus. The patient chose to terminate the pregnancy and returned to work shortly thereafter.

This case illustrates the importance of biological monitoring in assessing exposure to occupational toxicants. According to NIOSH estimates (42), a urinary ethoxyacetic acid concentration of 5 mg/g creatinine corresponds to an inhalation exposure to the REL for EGEE (0.5 ppm) during an 8-hr workshift at moderate exercise intensity. With a half-life of 42 hr, sampling at the end of the work week provides an integrated weekly exposure estimate due to lung and skin absorption. Higher urinary concentrations could be due to air-borne exposures above the REL, dermal absorption, and/

or greater workloads. In this case, the nature of the patient's job tasks, lack of personal protective equipment, and dermatitis suggested a high probability of excessive skin absorption. Her overexposure was confirmed without having to rely on the cooperation of the employer. Instituting adequate engineering methods or expecting this worker to wear an air-supplied respirator, gloves, goggles, and impervious clothing while performing cleaning tasks during pregnancy were not reasonable control strategies. The company benefited by substitution of a chemical that OSHA is more stringently regulating as a reproductive and developmental toxicant. In this case, the fetus had a chromosomal anomaly most likely secondary to the patient's age. Although this patient chose to terminate the pregnancy, she felt considerable relief that a future pregnancy would occur in a better-controlled work environment.

### CASE 8

L.T. is a 19-yr-old G1P0 student who worked weekends delivering pizzas for a local franchise. She was involved in a motor vehicle accident during work hours and was brought to the emergency room semiconscious but with stable vital signs. Multiple x-ray examinations were performed including a head CT scan, posteroanterior and lateral chest films, and kidney-ureter-bladder, pelvic, and lumbosacral spine series, which revealed two broken ribs and a pelvic fracture. During the course of her hospitalization, L.T. mentioned that she was 3 weeks past her scheduled menses and might be pregnant. A pelvic ultrasound revealed an 8-week, viable intrauterine gestation. Her physician recommended a therapeutic abortion due to radiation hazards to the embryo.

This case illustrates a common misconception about the hazards of diagnostic x-ray procedures during pregnancy. Even the multiple examinations of this patient would likely result in embryonic doses far less than 5 rad and probably closer to 1 rad. Doses less than 5 rad would not be expected to produce embryonic malformations, growth deficits, or death, and the risk of nonthreshold effects (e.g., oncogenesis) is very low. Under these circumstances, it is inappropriate to recommend therapeutic abortion of a wanted pregnancy (Chapter 13).

While every effort should be made to ascertain pregnancy status before x-ray studies are performed and to defer elective procedures, the benefits of medically indicated diagnostic examinations far outweigh the risks to the conceptus. Radiation therapy to the abdomen or administration of [$^{131}$I] iodine for treatment of maternal thyroid conditions may result in much higher embryofetal exposures. In all cases where radiation exposure is of concern, an expert should calculate the estimated dose to the conceptus; this information provides a rational basis for patient counseling. If the absorbed dose to the embryofetus exceeds 5 rad, the patient must weigh the benefits of continuing the pregnancy. Certainly absorbed doses of more than 50 rad at any time during gestation have a high probability of inducing serious embryofetal effects (Chapter 13).

### SUMMARY

These cases illustrate some of the diverse issues that confront workers and clinicians concerned about occupational reproductive and developmental hazards. While each case has its unique aspects, they all point to the need for a well-coordinated, multidisciplinary, and advocacy-based approach. The knowledgeable primary care provider can play a vital role in identifying potential risks and mobilizing the resources necessary to address these problems effectively. In many cases, a change in the workplace catalyzed by the concerns of one patient leads to safer conditions for all workers.

### REFERENCES

1. Kline J, Stein Z, Susser M. Conception to birth. Epidemiology of prenatal development. New York: Oxford University Press, 1989:51.
2. Mosher W, Pratt W. Fecundity, infertility, and reproductive health in the United States, 1982. DHHS Pub. No. (PHS) 87–1990. Hyattsville, MD: National Center for Health Statistics, 1987.
3. Hendershot GE, Mosher WD, Pratt WF. Infertility and age: an unresolved issue. Fam Plann Perspect 1982;14:22–27.
4. Howe G, Westhoff C, Vessey M. Effects of age, cigarette smoking, and other factors on fertility. Findings in a large prospective study. Br Med J 1985;290:1697–1700.
5. Mishell DR Jr. Infertility. In: Droegemueller W, Herbst AL, Mishell DR, Stenchever MA, eds. Comprehensive gynecology. St. Louis: The CV Mosby Co., 1987;1038–1081.
6. Speroff L, Glass RH, Kase NG. Clinical gynecologic

endocrinology and infertility. 4th ed. Baltimore: Williams & Wilkins, 1989.

7. Paul ME, Himmelstein J. Reproductive hazards in the workplace: what the practitioner needs to know about chemical exposures. Obstet Gynecol 1988;71:921–938.

8. Sever LE, Hessol NA. Toxic effects of occupational and environmental chemicals on the testes. In: Thomas JA, McLachlan JA, Korach KS, eds. Endocrine toxicology. New York: Raven Press, 1985:211–248.

9. Mattison DR. Clinical manifestations of ovarian toxicity. In: Dixon RL, ed. Reproductive toxicology. New York: Raven Press, 1985:109–130.

10. Sommer B. Stress and menstrual distress. J Hum Stress 1978;4:5–10, 41–47.

11. Green BB, Daling JR, Weiss NS, Liff JM, Koepsell T. Exercise as a risk factor for infertility with ovulatory dysfunction. Am J Public Health 1986;76:1432–1436.

12. Harrington JM, Stein GF, Rivera RO, et al. The occupational hazards of formulating oral contraceptives: a survey of plant employees. Arch Environ Health 1978;33:12–15.

13. Bulgar WH, Kupfer D. Estrogenic action of DDT analogs. Am J Ind Med 1983;4:163–173.

14. National Research Council. Biological markers in reproductive toxicology. Washington, DC: National Academy Press, 1989.

15. Vermesh M, Kletzky OA, Davajan V, Israel R. Monitoring techniques to predict and detect ovulation. Fertil Steril 1987;47:259–264.

16. Finn MM, Gosling JP, Tallon DF, Joyce A, Meehan FP, Fottrell PF. Follicular growth and corpus luteum function in women with unexplained fertility, monitored by ultrasonography and measurement of daily salivary progesterone. Gynecol Endocrinol 1989;3:297–308.

17. Li T, Dockery F, Rogers AW, Cooke ID. How precise is histological dating of endometrium using the standard dating criteria? Fertil Steril 1989;51:759–763.

18. Working PK. Male reproductive toxicology: comparison of the human to animal models. Environ Health Perspect 1988;77:37–44.

19. Goyer RA. Lead toxicity:from overt to subclinical to subtle health effects. Environ Health Perspect 1990;86:177–181.

20. Winder C. Reproductive and chromosomal effects of occupational exposure to lead in the male. Reprod Toxicol 1989;3:221–233.

21. Harlan WR. The relationship of blood lead levels to blood pressure in the U.S. population. Environ Health Perspect 1988;78:2–13.

22. Davis JM, Svendsgaard DJ. Lead and child development. Nature 1987;329:297–300.

23. Lindbohm M-L, Sallmen M, Anttila A, Taskinen H, Hemminki K. Paternal occupational lead exposure and spontaneous abortion. Scand J Work Environ Health 1991;17:95–103.

24. Biller BMK, Coughlin JF, Saxe V, Schoenfeld D, Spratt DI, Klibanski A. Osteopenia in women with hypothalamic amenorrhea: a prospective study. Obstet Gynecol 1991;78:996–1001.

25. U.S. Department of Health and Human Services, Agency for Toxic Substances and Disease Registry (ATSDR). Toxicological profile for ethylene oxide. Atlanta: ATSDR,1990.

26. Hemminki K, Mutanen P, Saloniemi I, Neimi ML, Vainio H. Spontaneous abortion in hospital staff engaged in sterilizing instruments with chemical agents. Br Med J 1982;285:1461–1463.

27. Holmberg PC, Kurppa K, Riala R, et al. Solvent exposure and birth defects: an epidemiologic survey. Prog Clin Biol Res 1986;220:179–185.

28. Pastides H, Calabrese EJ, Hosmer DW Jr, Harris DR Jr. Spontaneous abortion and general illness symptoms among semiconductor manufacturers. J Occup Med 1988;30:543–551.

29. Huel G, Mergler D, Bowler R. Evidence for adverse reproductive outcomes among women microelectronic assembly workers. Br J Ind Med 1990;47:400–404.

30. Donald JM, Hooper K, Hopenhayn-Rich C. Reproductive and developmental toxicity of toluene: a review. Environ Health Perspect 1991;94:237–244.

31. Barlow SM, Sullivan R. Reproductive hazards of industrial chemicals. New York: Academic Press, 1982:276–282.

32. Ott MG, Skory LK, Holder BB, Bronson JM, Williams PR. Health evaluation of employees occupationally exposed to methylene chloride: metabolism data and oxygen half-saturation pressures. Scand J Work Environ Health 1983;(Suppl 1):31–38.

33. Connor J. Ribavirin pharmacokinetics. Pediatr Infect Dis J 1990;9(Suppl):S91–S92.

34. Hillyard IW. The preclinical toxicology and safety of ribavirin. In: Smith RA, Kirkpatrick W, eds. Ribavirin: a broad spectrum antiviral agent. New York: Academic Press, 1980:59–71.

35. Marks MI. Adverse drug reactions: United States experience. II. Pediatr Infect Dis J 1990;9(Suppl):S117–S118.

36. Harrison R. Reproductive risk assessment with occupational exposures to ribavirin aerosol. Pediatr Infect Dis J 1990;9(Suppl):S102–S105.

37. Harrison R, Bellows J, Rempel D, et al. Assessing exposures of health care personnel to aerosols of ribavirin—California. MMWR 1988;37:560–563.

38. National Institute for Occupational Safety and Health (NIOSH). A guide to industrial respiratory protection. Cincinnati: NIOSH, 1976:13.

39. Koren G. Studying the safety of ribavirin in human pregnancy. Pediatr Infect Dis J 1990;9(Suppl):S106–S107.

40. Kayman L. An industrial hygiene approach to controlling non-patient exposure to ribavirin aerosol. Pediatr Infect Dis J 1990;9(Suppl):S100–S101.

41. Centers for Disease Control. Risks associated with human parvovirus B19 infection. MMWR 1989;38:81–97.

42. U.S. Department of Health and Human Services, National Institute for Occupational Safety and Health (NIOSH). Criteria for a recommended standard. Occupational exposure to ethylene glycol monomethyl ether, ethylene glycol monoethyl ether, and their acetates. DHHS (NIOSH) publ no. 91–119. Cincinnati:NIOSH, 1991.

# 12

# Legal and Policy Issues

JOAN E. BERTIN, ELISABETH A. WERBY

Unlike the study of natural human diseases, occupational and environmental medicine focuses largely on potential health consequences from involuntary exposure to synthetic industrial toxicants. On the one hand, this distinction holds promise for improved regulation of toxic substances and disease prevention; on the other hand, it raises the contentious question of responsibility for adverse outcomes. Not surprisingly, emergence of these issues over the last two decades has prompted enactment of numerous laws designed to prevent and to remedy untoward health effects that result from hazardous exposures. These federal and state laws interact with each other and with pre-existing precedents to create a complex set of rules governing both the responsibilities of those who produce toxic agents and the rights of those who are injured by them.

The specter of developmental toxicity from exposure to occupational or environmental agents has been given unprecedented attention in recent years. Unfortunately, related questions of prevention and responsibility intersect with a contemporary political trend that seeks to abrogate the rights of women in the name of fetal health. This contradiction became the focus of a recent Supreme Court case addressing employer "fetal protection" policies that exclude all pregnant or fertile women from certain jobs. As discussed in Chapter 25, it is also reflected in recent attempts to establish drug or alcohol use during pregnancy as a form of "fetal abuse" subject to criminalization and incarceration.

Comprehensive care of the patient concerned about reproductive hazards goes beyond the realm of science to embrace legal and policy issues that impact on individual liberties and options. In the first section of this chapter, we discuss current occupational and environmental health laws, regulations, and case law with particular attention to the problem of reproductive harm. The second section discusses federal antidiscrimination law that protects the employment rights of women and examines the implications of the recent Supreme Court decision on employer "fetal protection" policies.

## RIGHTS AND REMEDIES FOR EXPOSURE TO TOXIC SUBSTANCES

### Regulatory Framework

The Occupational Safety and Health Act (OSH Act) of 1970 (1) marked the first significant federal recognition of the need to regulate exposure to toxic substances. Today, more than 12 federal laws under the jurisdiction of at least five federal agencies regulate community, home, and occupational exposures. Nearly one-half of the states have enacted parallel legislation as well.

Unfortunately, the potential of these laws

has been only partially realized. Hampered by bureaucratic delays, political pressures, and industry resistance, federal agencies have been slow to establish standards or otherwise to implement or to enforce the laws. Nonetheless, both federal and state regulations continue to hold promise for controlling exposures to toxic substances.

## Regulating the Work Environment: OSH Act

The OSH Act was enacted to "assure so far as possible every man and woman . . . safe and healthful working conditions." It resulted in the creation of three federal agencies to address health and safety issues: (*a*) the Occupational Safety and Health Administration (OSHA), a regulatory agency charged with setting occupational health and safety standards and assuring compliance; (*b*) the National Institute for Occupational Safety and Health (NIOSH), a research agency that evaluates workplace hazards and develops recommendations for OSHA standards; and (*c*) the Occupational Safety and Health Review Commission (OSHRC), a quasi-judicial board that reviews citations for violations of standards.

Unfortunately, the process of standard setting for toxic agents in the workplace has been slow. Of the more than 79,000 chemicals in the *Registry of Toxic Effects of Chemical Substances* compiled by NIOSH, OSHA has developed comprehensive substance-specific standards for only 28. OSHA's 1989 Air Contaminants Standard reduced or changed Permissible Exposure Limits (PELs) for an additional 428 substances. However, these new limits were not based on independent toxicity assessments by NIOSH; rather, for the most part, they constitute adoption by OSHA of pre-existing Threshold Limit Values (TLVs) established by the American Conference of Governmental Industrial Hygienists (ACGIH), a private group. The scientific basis for these TLVs has been recently challenged (2).

The OSH Act has been interpreted to afford protection from reproductive as well as other injuries caused by toxic insult (3). Yet, while at least 16% of the chemicals in NIOSH's *Registry* demonstrate some evidence of reproductive or developmental toxicity (4), only three—

dibromochloropropane (DBCP), lead, and ethylene oxide—have specific OSHA standards based, in part, on reproductive effects (5). In addition, limits for seven of the substances covered by the Air Contaminants Standard are based partially on reported reproductive toxicity in animals. These substances are acetonitrile, acetylsalicylic acid, captan, cyclohexylamine, hexafluoroacetone, phenylphosphine, and vinylidene chloride. Many other agents, such as vinyl chloride, benzene, and formaldehyde, are suspected reproductive toxicants but are regulated according to other adverse health effects (6).

The OSHA standard for DBCP was promulgated partially on evidence that it caused sterility in exposed male workers. This pesticide was phased out of production in the U.S. beginning in 1981. However, both lead and ethylene oxide remain in widespread use in industry. The standards for these chemicals include exposure limits, medical surveillance requirements, and provisions for counseling employees about potential reproductive and developmental effects. In addition, the Lead Standard provides for medical removal of workers, with wage and benefit protections, when employees have exceeded designated exposure levels or when exposures cannot be adequately controlled.

Under the OSH Act, a worker who is concerned about job exposures can file a confidential complaint with the regional OSHA office. The statute also prohibits employer harassment or dismissal of workers for filing OSHA complaints or otherwise exercising their rights under the Act. If there are reasonable grounds to suspect that an employer is in violation of a regulation, OSHA is obligated to inspect the workplace "as soon as practicable." Because few OSHA standards specifically address reproductive effects, however, failure to cite the employer is not necessarily synonymous with a clean bill of health. Private citizens may petition for promulgation or modification of a standard, but success on such petitions has been mixed (5).

## Laws Administered by the U.S. Environmental Protection Agency

Two statutes administered by the U.S. Environmental Protection Agency (EPA)—the

Toxic Substances Control Act (TSCA) of 1976 (7) and the Federal Insecticide, Fungicide and Rodenticide Act (FIFRA) (8)—represent efforts to regulate environmental toxic exposures and also have relevance in the occupational context. FIFRA is particularly significant for farm workers, whose employers are not subject to regulation by OSHA. Under TSCA, the EPA may take action on chemicals that are found in workplaces covered by the OSH Act, as well as elsewhere.

## REGULATING TOXIC CHEMICALS IN THE ENVIRONMENT: TSCA

Reflecting concern over the proliferation of toxic chemicals in U.S. commerce, TSCA was enacted to regulate new and existing chemicals that may pose "unreasonable risk" of injury to humans or to the environment. The statute authorizes the EPA to develop standards for the development of test data for these chemicals. Based on the test data, regulatory action may include labeling provisions, mandatory warnings, limitations on amounts and uses, or outright prohibition. In addition, the EPA can initiate emergency court action to control "imminent hazards" capable of serious or widespread injury.

Although the statute grants considerable discretion to the EPA Administrator in determining "unreasonable risk" and "imminent hazards," it is clear that these concepts include consideration of reproductive harm. Mutagenesis and teratogenesis are among effects to be considered in standards for development of test data. To this end, the EPA has issued guidelines for evaluating developmental toxicants (9) as well as proposed guidelines for assessing male and female reproductive risk (10, 11). Finally, the statute requires that the EPA initiate timely regulatory action upon notice that a substance may cause gene mutations, birth defects, or cancer.

Some aspects of TSCA offer considerable potential for action by citizens concerned about reproductive risks. Citizens may petition the EPA to issue or to change a rule pertaining to testing, use, or production of a chemical. Moreover, unlike the OSH Act, TSCA allows for citizen suits against persons alleged to be in violation of the statute. Finally, toxicology data-

bases and industrial chemical use inventories maintained by the EPA under TSCA are available to the public and may be useful in clinical assessment of patients.

## REGULATING PESTICIDES: FIFRA

FIFRA is primarily a registration and labeling law for pesticides. It requires premarket registration and labeling of all pesticides and issuance of "tolerance" limits for pesticides used on food crops. In addition, the statute establishes procedures for canceling registration of pesticides that may result in "unreasonable" adverse impacts on the environment.

Reproductive and developmental hazards are included in EPA's evaluation of pesticides under FIFRA. In the past, EPA has attempted to prevent these harms solely by labeling reproductive toxicants or by preventing fertile women from using the products in certain operations. Criticized as an inadequate response, even by the EPA's own internal analysis (12), the Agency appears to have adopted a different approach in recent years. For example, in 1987, EPA issued an Emergency National Suspension Order to end use of the herbicide, Dinoseb, after findings of acute toxicity in humans and teratogenic effects and testicular toxicity in experimental animals. The order was challenged by industry groups who persuaded the Administrator to permit continued use, with the proviso that fertile women be excluded from certain operations entailing potential exposure to the herbicide. This order was subsequently challenged in court by farm worker groups pressing to reinstate the suspension order and to ban the substance. The case was settled with an agreement to phase out use over a set period of time (13).

## Protection Through Information: "Right to Know" Laws

In the past decade, a number of laws have been promulgated that enhance public access to information about the nature, extent of use, and potential health effects of toxic chemicals. These "right to know" laws are valuable to clinicians, offering the potential for more effective and timely diagnosis and treatment of conditions resulting from toxic exposures. Although hazard notification may precipitate psychological stress, it may also encourage individuals to seek preventive medical care before clinical symptomatology occurs (14). In addition, enhanced access to information regarding exposures and risks may assist patients of both sexes in making decisions about childbearing. For example, some patients may choose to delay conception until they can transfer into safer jobs or reduce biological evidence of exposure to known toxicants, such as lead. Information about toxic exposures may also be useful in treating infertility and other reproductive disorders.

Right to know laws now exist in over 25 states and in a significant number of municipalities. Typical worker notification laws include provisions for disclosing the identity of hazardous substances, labeling, on-site worker training, and reporting procedures. Specific warnings regarding reproductive and developmental hazards may be required. Under some laws, state agencies are authorized to inspect businesses, and civil or criminal sanctions may be imposed for violations. Community right to know laws have a somewhat broader reach and often require a public agency to maintain records of potential hazards that are subject to public disclosure (15). Some states have enacted Toxic Use Reduction laws that move beyond mere notification of hazards to require reduction of toxic exposures at the source. The Massachusetts Toxics Use Reduction Act (16), for example, establishes a state institutional center to investigate alternative technologies.

With regard to occupational exposures, OSHA's 1983 Hazard Communication Standard (HCS) (17) establishes a uniform federal standard for information disclosure. It expressly preempts state occupational health notification laws, except OSHA-approved state regulatory plans. The Standard, which now applies to both manufacturing and nonmanufacturing sectors, establishes an informational program consisting of three interrelated parts:

(a) labeling of potentially dangerous products by manufacturers to alert downstream users of possible risks;
(b) provision of updated Material Safety Data Sheets (MSDSs) to downstream employers which, in turn, must be made readily available to employees; and

(c) worker training programs that address job-related hazards and preventive measures.

Reproductive hazards are included within the scope of the statute.

The HCS is performance oriented, i.e., it establishes general requirements for worker notification while allowing considerable discretion in the means of implementation. Preparation of MSDSs by individual suppliers without uniform reference standards has resulted in wide diversity in the format, language, and content of the data sheets. With the exception of certain known carcinogens, manufacturers are given broad discretion in determining what information to provide on MSDSs. Chemical ingredients not deemed hazardous by the manufacturer need not be disclosed. In addition, manufacturers are allowed to withhold information on trade secrets from the public. Trade secrets include product ingredients that, if revealed, might place the company at a disadvantage relative to its competitors. However, health professionals can obtain trade secret information if necessary for diagnosis, treatment, or surveillance. While a written request and signing of a nondisclosure statement are typically required, the information must be provided to the treating physician or nurse by telephone in medical emergencies.

Despite their limitations, MSDSs remain the primary written vehicles by which information regarding hazardous substances is transmitted to workers. Under the HCS, employers must maintain MSDSs for all hazardous chemicals used in the workplace and provide copies to employees upon request. Further, under OSHA's Access Rule (18), workers and their designated representatives are entitled to copies of biological and environmental monitoring exposure data and personal medical records maintained by the employer, even when exposures do not exceed permissible limits. If enforced, these rights are particularly valuable for diagnosis and treatment and may serve as evidence in compensation and tort cases. Unfortunately, however, these standards offer no provisions for exposed employees to transfer to safer jobs.

The Emergency Planning and Community Right to Know Act (EPCRA) (19), enacted as Title III of the Superfund Amendments and

Reauthorization Act (SARA) of 1986 (20), mandates community planning for release of hazardous substances into the environment. To assist in the planning process, owners and operators of facilities that manufacture or store hazardous chemicals must provide MSDSs to local emergency planning commissions. In addition, certain facilities are required to provide the EPA with information on routine toxic chemical emissions. The resulting Toxic Release Inventory (TRI) can be accessed through various computer services and sorted by geographic location. Thus, it provides a valuable starting point for clinicians attempting to identify some of the substances to which a patient has been exposed.

## Compensation for Injuries Due to Toxic Exposure

Neither the OSH Act nor other related federal laws give workers the right to sue employers for work-related harm. With some limited exceptions, the Workers Compensation system provides the exclusive remedy for illness or injury resulting from occupational exposures. Some states provide increased awards for willful or reckless acts such as violations of state or federal health and safety statutes or failure to warn of a known hazard (21). By and large, however, Workers Compensation is an inadequate remedy and frequently leaves victims of reproductive harm without compensation.

Victims of environmental contamination and workers in select circumstances may be entitled to sue for damages under common law, although proving that the exposure caused the harm is often a significant impediment to recovery. Nevertheless, the growing number of "toxic tort" actions, along with increasing judicial recognition of early presymptomatic markers of disease, are important trends for individuals seeking relief for reproductive and other injuries.

## WORKERS COMPENSATION

Enacted primarily between 1910–1920, state Workers Compensation laws reflected a compromise between the need to compensate victims of industrial accidents, on the one hand, and employers' desire for predictability and for

protection against excessive court judgments, on the other. As a quid pro quo for assurance of compensation regardless of fault, workers relinquished their right to sue employers for conditions related to employment. As discussed later in this chapter, there are some limited exceptions to this exclusivity bar.

For a number of reasons, the remedies provided by the Workers Compensation system are limited, particularly for occupational illnesses (as opposed to injuries). First, many workers remain unaware that they have a compensable condition, and those who do press claims often face complex and costly legal battles. When combined with residency requirements, statutes of limitations, and other obstacles imposed by many state compensation laws, it is no surprise that only approximately 3% of workers suffering from occupational diseases file a claim (22). Second, compared with 10% of workplace accident claims, nearly two-thirds of all occupational disease claims are controverted, primarily on the basis of causation. Overall, only 5% of workers severely disabled by occupational diseases are awarded compensation (22). Finally, although medical expenses are generally recoverable in full, many workers are awarded only a fraction of lost wages and are not entitled to compensation for lost fringe benefits or for pain and suffering. Indeed, the major sources of income for victims of occupational diseases have been social security and welfare (23).

Persons suffering reproductive harm from occupational exposures face additional hurdles. As a general rule, workers are entitled to disability benefits under Workers Compensation laws only if their medical conditions compromise their ability to work, resulting in wage loss. Some serious occupationally induced reproductive problems, such as infertility, do not impair job performance and, thus, do not meet these disability criteria. Because workers with these conditions are also barred from suing employers, they are essentially left without a remedy. In one infamous case, the court dismissed tort claims of male workers who alleged that their occupational exposure to DBCP caused sterility, mutagenesis, and carcinogenesis. Even though Workers Compensation provided no remedy for these nondisabling conditions, the employer was nevertheless protected by the exclusivity rule and was not liable in a common law tort action (24).

Unlike disability payments, medical expenses for reproductive injury are recoverable if occupational causation can be shown. For example, the medical costs associated with direct testicular injury, miscarriage, stillbirth, and any resulting psychological or psychiatric treatment will be covered in many states. Where the state scheme provides for medical evaluation of injury, the costs of tests to diagnose possible job-related injury, such as amniocentesis or ultrasound, should also be compensable.

Inasmuch as children of workers are not "employees," they are not entitled to Workers Compensation benefits for injuries induced by parental exposure to toxicants. The availability of tort remedies in these circumstances is uncertain. Some courts have held that state compensation schemes do not preclude tort actions against the employer by subsequently born children of workers injured as a result of the employer's negligence (25, 26). One court has taken the opposite view. It reasoned that the fetus is inseparable from the pregnant woman and held that the subsequently born child, injured in utero by the employer's negligence, was limited to remedies available to the mother. The court thus denied recovery in tort, while acknowledging that the current compensation scheme provided no alternative remedy (27). This decision has engendered considerable debate and stimulated efforts to amend state law to provide remedies in such circumstances.

## COMMON LAW REMEDIES

Common law tort remedies for injury or disease are potentially available to victims of community and home exposures; to workers not covered or otherwise barred by Workers Compensation statutes; and to workers who, in some states, can sue manufacturers and suppliers of the substances causing the harm (28). Tort suits may be based either on a negligence theory or on the basis of strict liability for manufacturing or distributing inherently dangerous products (29).

Despite the exclusivity bar under Workers Compensation schemes, most states permit workers to sue their employers for intentional acts resulting in occupational disease. The applicability of these statutes to situations involving reproductive harm remains largely untested. However, evidence that an employer knowingly concealed reproductive risks or failed to follow medical advice to reduce exposures would be compelling in any attempt to seek recovery for an injured worker who otherwise has no claim.

More than 40 states allow suits by or on behalf of children alleging prenatal injury, typically requiring that the child have been born alive. Some of these states permit recovery only for injuries sustained after the point of viability, although the trend is to allow suits for injuries from and even before conception (30). Depending on state law, parents may have a cause of action if there has been a prenatal injury resulting in miscarriage, stillbirth, or birth defects of which they were not adequately warned (6).

Traditionally, recovery in tort was available only on a showing of direct physical injury. In recognition of the unique nature of diseases associated with toxic exposures, however, an increasing number of courts have attempted to modify this stipulation. Some courts have dispensed with the physical injury requirement if presymptom medical surveillance indicates enhanced risk of disease (e.g., asbestosis); others have held that the requirement may be satisfied by subcellular changes or by mere ingestion of contaminants (31). These trends may be particularly relevant to cases involving subtle forms or early indicators of reproductive harm.

Further accommodation to the special problems of toxicant-induced illness is reflected in liberalization of statutes governing the time in which an action must be brought. Most states have amended restrictive statutes of limitation so that the clock does not begin to tick until the victim has or reasonably should have discovered the harm. Moreover, in SARA, Congress provided a federal commencement date for actions for personal injury and property damage arising from environmental pollutants released from a facility. The trigger is the date the plaintiff knew the injury was caused by the hazardous substance, and it replaces more restrictive state laws.

Despite these liberal trends, the problem of causation remains a significant obstacle to recovery in toxic tort, as well as in workers compensation cases. To prevail, a plaintiff must prove by a preponderance of the evidence that the injury was caused by a toxic exposure for which the defendant was responsible. Identifying the source of the exposure may be problematic, since hazardous substances are ubiquitous in air, drinking water, and food, as well as in workplaces. Pinpointing the responsible parties is also difficult, especially if, during a lengthy latency period, a worker has changed jobs, employers have gone out of business, and records are no longer available. Similar obstacles confront those suing manufacturers and industrial polluters. However, right to know legislation, if enforced and utilized, may supply some of the missing information critical to these cases.

Establishing the connection between exposure and illness typically requires expert testimony based on statistical evidence from epidemiological investigations, in vitro studies, or animal test data. The judicial response to use of this group-based information as proof of causation has been mixed. Nevertheless, in recognition of the special nature of toxic torts, most courts now place increasing reliance on statistical evidence (32).

Causation problems are particularly acute in cases involving allegations of harm to children from parental exposure to toxic substances. The effects of parental exposure on offspring may be subtle, interactive with environmental factors, and difficult to distinguish from background levels of risk. This situation may change as information disclosure laws yield critical information regarding the nature and extent of exposures and as research better describes toxicant-induced developmental effects.

## OTHER RELEVANT LAWS, LEGAL PRINCIPLES, AND CURRENT DEVELOPMENTS

Laws that may seem far afield to the practicing clinician may nonetheless impact on the medical advice that a patient is willing or is able to accept. In particular, laws pertaining to pregnancy may be relevant to the practicing obstetrician-gynecologist. A basic knowledge of women's legal rights is essential to making appropriate patient referrals for legal advice. In addition, clinicians may be asked to intercede on a patient's behalf in asserting these rights.

## Employment Discrimination

Women comprise approximately 45% of the U.S. workforce, and approximately 65% of all women with children under the age of 18 yr are in the labor force (33, 34). Employment is a necessity in many instances because women shoulder substantial financial responsibilities for themselves and their families. Moreover, employment is known to have health-enhancing effects during pregnancy and otherwise. For example, work-related benefits may provide the only source of medical insurance and access to prenatal care. Employment provides a higher standard of living and may represent escape from poverty for many women; housing, nutrition, and overall well-being generally improve as income rises. Paid employment also provides emotional satisfaction and rewards that are beneficial to health. Even employment that poses a risk of exposure to chemical or physical hazards may have these benefits, which must be factored into any risk-benefit calculation for women in the workforce (35).

Title VII of the Civil Rights Act (36) of 1964 prohibits discrimination in employment on the basis of sex, race, national origin, and religion. The statute specifically prohibits discrimination on the basis of pregnancy and childbearing capacity and provides that women affected by "pregnancy, childbirth, and related medical conditions shall be treated the same for all employment-related purposes...as others not so affected but similar in their ability or inability to work."

This section of the law, called the Pregnancy Discrimination Act, provides crucial benefits to many pregnant women and to new mothers. Under this provision, employers must assess women's ability to work in the same way they assess the ability of male employees to work. Employers may not assume that pregnant women cannot do certain jobs, and they may not require pregnant women or new mothers to provide greater proof of their ability than other workers. Thus, if an employer routinely accepts the treating physician's judgment about whether a worker is able to perform a job, the employer must do the same in the case of the pregnant employee.

The provision that requires employers to treat the pregnant worker "the same for all employment-related purposes" also means that pregnant workers are entitled to transfers, medical leaves, light duty assignments, or other job modifications, if these benefits are available to other workers with medical documentation. Other benefits, such as the entitlement to disability insurance and benefits, must also be accorded on a nondiscriminatory basis. States that provide partial wage replacement to workers who are temporarily incapacitated must also extend these benefits to pregnant and postpartum women when they are similarly temporarily incapacitated. Likewise, unemployment compensation benefits should be available to women who are unable to work during pregnancy because of an unacceptable level of health risk, if the same holds true for others out of work for health-related conditions.

The prohibition against sex discrimination also protects men from sex stereotyping that adversely affects their employment status. One pervasive stereotype is that males do not require protection from occupational reproductive hazards, and many employers proceed on the assumption that only women are at risk. However, as explained in other chapters, scientific data are accumulating that demonstrate the vulnerability of the male reproductive system to injury from occupational exposures and conditions; these exposures may affect fertility, the course of pregnancy, and potentially, the health of offspring. Under Title VII, an employer who recognizes the needs of women for benefits or job modifications to protect against reproductive injury must provide similar benefits to males and must accept the same kind of documentation that is required from a comparably situated woman worker. In addition, it is the right of couples to decide who will care for a newly born or adopted child. If women are granted child care leave by employers, men are also entitled to it on the same terms.

Thus, Title VII provides significant protection to working women when they become pregnant. Before enactment of this law, rules barring marriage and motherhood for female employees were common (37). Pregnant women were placed on mandatory maternity leave (38) and were denied accrued seniority and other benefits (39). Pregnancy was widely excluded from employment-related health insurance and disability plans (40, 41). Title VII eliminated many of these practices and made employment benefits, such as health insurance, available to large numbers of women. Pregnancy discrimination still occurs, but legal remedies are often available to women both to reclaim their jobs and to recover lost earnings for unlawful termination, denial of promotion, and other discriminatory acts, including harassment.

The knowledgeable clinician can provide invaluable service to patients and to their partners by being alert to their working conditions and to the possibility that legal remedies may exist that protect their health and employment rights. Patient advocacy in these matters may enable workers to continue to receive necessary income and the other benefits of employment when they might otherwise feel compelled to leave their jobs or to tolerate unacceptable levels of stress and anxiety from continued employment. Individuals aggrieved by discriminatory employment practices may file charges with the U.S. Equal Employment Opportunity Commission and state and local fair employment agencies. There are no costs or fees for such filings, and private legal counsel is not necessary. Nonprofit advocacy and educational organizations also provide advice and assistance to individuals complaining of employment discrimination.

## "Fetal Protection" Policies

An area of continuing dispute involves the employment rights of fertile women when the employer claims that the work environment poses a particular risk to the fetus. Many employers have adopted so-called "fetal protection" plans that are most prominent in historically male industries, such as the petrochemical and automotive industries (42). These policies often exclude all women of childbearing capacity and, in some cases, require women of all ages to submit proof of sterility to qualify for full employment rights. Some women have submitted to surgical sterilization to keep jobs central to their economic survival (43).

Women (and men) who work in hazardous workplaces do not do so *because* of the hazards but in spite of them. They are not thoughtless or selfish people who ignore the well-being of their children. Most accept the risks of employment, over which they have little or no control, precisely because it enables them to provide for their families. The work is often strenuous and may present numerous other obstacles as well. In predominantly male workplaces where the pay is highest (44), women often complain of isolation and sexual harassment (45). For unskilled women especially, no other employment provides comparable income and benefits (43).

"Fetal protection" policies have elicited heavy criticism from segments of the medical and scientific community, labor organizations, women's rights advocates, and environmentalists. Opposition to the policies is based, in part, on the contention that the plans rely upon and foster a distorted view of the science related to reproductive hazards. For example, some prominent scientists in the area of prenatal effects of lead exposure publicly repudiated use of their research in support of one company's policy. In a commentary "to assure that our research is interpreted fully and accurately and that it be placed in the proper biological context", they state:

> Considerable attention has been given to characterizing the impact of intrauterine exposure on children's growth and development. Much less attention has been devoted to assessing the effect of paternal exposure on infant outcome. In our studies we did not measure paternal exposure and therefore cannot rule this out as a contributing factor in our findings. . . . The limited data on paternal exposure should not be weighted equally with the positive findings on maternal exposure when drawing conclusions about the differential sensitivity of male and female workers. The position that a given level of paternal but not maternal exposure is acceptable is without logical foundation and insupportable on empirical grounds. . . . [We] do not believe that present data provide a sufficient scien-

tific basis for applying different lead exposure standards to male and female workers (46).

Other critics of the policy contend that the focus on fetal health and the assumption of fetal hypersusceptibility "willfully ignores a large body of data" demonstrating the effects of toxic chemicals on everyone exposed to them (47). One expert observed that only a small number of toxic chemicals have been shown to have more adverse effects on the conceptus than the adult, and concludes:

> These data suggest the importance of including reproductive and developmental endpoints in toxicity testing. However, it does not support the notion that any particular endpoint, including fetal development, is the most sensitive to toxicity. Rather, the data suggest that all endpoints need to be critically examined to define clearly the one most sensitive (47).

The same observer points to the potential for adverse health consequences if fertile or pregnant women lose decent employment, especially if their medical benefits go with it (35).

## LEGAL STATUS OF "FETAL PROTECTION" POLICIES

From a legal perspective, these arguments have been resolved by a recent decision of the Supreme Court of the United States, which held that "fetal protection" policies are prohibited by Title VII of the Civil Rights Act of 1964. The case, *United Automobile Workers (UAW) v. Johnson Controls* (48), involved a policy that restricted the employment rights of all women, without age restriction, unless they could prove their infertility. The primary occupational exposure in question was lead. One female plaintiff had been sterilized to retain her employment rights; another male plaintiff claimed that the company ignored the reproductive health effects of exposure to lead for men.

Johnson Controls Company adopted this policy even though OSHA, in its Final Standard for Occupational Exposure to Lead, had already rejected the contention forwarded by the Lead Industry Association and others that women should be barred from work in jobs involving lead exposure. Instead, OSHA concluded that lead was harmful to both males and females, and that both sexes required similar protection from its adverse effects (49).

The case has been called "the most important sex discrimination case in any court since 1964," the year that Congress passed Title VII. The Supreme Court held that employers may not resort to employment discrimination in an effort to eliminate a real or perceived risk to women or fetuses. The Court held that "Title VII plainly forbids illegal sex discrimination as a method of diverting attention from an employer's obligation to police the workplace." Justice Blackmun's majority opinion held that "fetal protection" policies like Johnson Controls' could *never* be justified under Title VII. The Court concluded that such policies do not further the kind of business interests that Title VII recognizes as providing a defense to blatant discrimination, because the policies are totally divorced from concerns related to job performance.

Recognizing that the policy at issue forced women workers "to choose between having a child and having a job," the Court rejected Johnson Controls' "professed moral and ethical concerns" as a justification for discrimination. The Court explained that "decisions about the welfare of future children must be left to the parents who conceive, bear, support and raise them rather than to employers who hire those parents." In a rebuke to both the lower courts and employers, the Court stated:

It is no more appropriate for the courts than it is for individual employers to decide whether a woman's reproductive role is more important to herself and her family than her economic role. Congress has left this choice to the woman as hers to make.

The Court also rejected the argument that any additional costs associated with employing women could justify discrimination. These costs might include both the expense of implementing workplace improvements and the costs of potential liability to the future children of workers. With regard to the latter, the Court observed:

. . . OSHA established a series of mandatory protections which, taken together, "should effectively minimize any risk to the fetus and newborn child". . . . If under general tort principles, Title VII bans sex-specific fetal-protection policies, the employer fully

informs the woman of the risk, *and the employer has not acted negligently*, the basis for holding an employer liable seems remote at best. [Emphasis added.]

The Court, thus, recognized the obligations imposed by OSHA, and inferentially by other federal and state regulatory bodies and by state tort law, that would subject employers to potential liability if they act in a negligent fashion. In this way, the Court indicated its intent that employers' duties to workers and their future children should be governed by these standards: the obligation to comply with safety and health laws and regulations, the duty not to be negligent, and the duty to warn.

## IMPLICATIONS OF THE SUPREME COURT'S RULING

The Supreme Court decision in the Johnson Controls case sends a clear message to employers and regulators that women are entitled to employment in all work environments and that their health needs must be considered in fashioning safety and health regulations and policies. The Supreme Court has plainly rejected the proposition that an employment health plan can protect fetuses more than it protects workers themselves.

The decision would apparently preclude any health and safety plan from making employment-related distinctions on the basis of sex or pregnancy, unless the plan distinguished among employees on the basis of their ability to perform the work. Thus, plans that require women to sign waivers or to provide medical certification to continue working, that discourage women from taking certain jobs, or that selectively recognize only health risks unique to women, would all likely be prohibited as a result of this decision. While the Court did not consider plans that provide benefits to women that are not available to men, this opinion and others indicate that an employer with such a plan might be liable to male employees for discrimination (50, 51). This important protection counters the tendency of some employers to ignore or to minimize reproductive risks for male workers.

The decision may mean that some women have to make hard choices that men have always made, to determine whether the benefits of employment are worth any risks involved. The alternative, however, was that women had no choice and, often, no job. Indeed, some women may make decisions that others deplore. The alternative presented by this case would have prevented all women from exercising any discretion in directing their own affairs, instead giving that power to employers.

The logical result of the Court's decision should be to stimulate employers to reduce exposures to levels that are safe for all workers, including pregnant women. Employers who cannot do so will be well advised to adopt nondiscriminatory health and safety policies that encompass all known risks. Any other course could subject them to continuing Title VII liability and to possible liability for violations of health and safety law.

Employers may also be vulnerable for failing to provide warnings to male workers with regard to reproductive risks that are documented in the scientific literature, even if not conclusively proven. The practice of providing warnings to women, sometimes on the basis of limited and unverified data, establishes a self-imposed duty of care that logically should extend to male workers. Inconsistency in carrying out this duty would enhance the likelihood of employer liability for harms that could be connected to a failure to warn male workers about reproductive risks.

Employer concern for tort liability might provide impetus to improve working conditions, and social concern for the well-being of pregnant working women should strengthen these efforts. Employers cannot discharge their legal duty to workers or their future children by extracting waivers or agreements from workers or applicants as a condition of employment. For example, any "agreement" between employers and workers that purported to excuse the employer from an obligation imposed by the OSH Act or regulations would undoubtedly be void.

An individual can assume certain risks, and consequently be precluded from recovery even for another's negligence, but only when the decision to do so is knowing and voluntary. Workers, however, do not act "voluntarily" if they have no real choice as to whether or not to relinquish their legal rights, as is the case if their entitlement to employment is at stake. Some courts have held that there is no "assumption of the risk" of hazardous employment if a safer method of performing the job has not been provided (52). It is also questionable whether workers "knowingly" assume certain risks, such as an increased risk of cancer or birth defects, if they cannot predict whether they will actually become affected (53).

The decision to accept certain risks to obtain or to retain desired employment is hardly an unreasonable one for which a worker is likely to be barred from recovery after demonstrating harm resulting from employer negligence. In the employment context, application of the "assumption of the risk" doctrine has long been discredited. Justice Frankfurter noted almost 50 yr ago:

> The notion of assumption of risk as a defense—that is, where the employer concededly failed in his duty of care and nevertheless escaped liability because the employee had "agreed to assume the risk" of the employers fault—rested, in the context of our industrial society, upon a pure fiction (54).

Thus, employer negligence that causes otherwise compensable injury will expose the employer to possible liability, notwithstanding any attempt to shift the responsibility to workers. Now that the Court has held that exclusion of women is impermissible, the concern for potential liability to the children of women workers can *only* be addressed by acting in a nonnegligent fashion, e.g., by reducing any recognized risks of employment. As noted in the *UAW* case, employers who do not act negligently and who take reasonable actions in relation to workplace hazards are unlikely to be liable for untoward consequences. If an employer cannot eliminate a known risk, workers should be informed about the nature of the risk. In addition, the employer may always offer reasonable alternatives, on a nondiscriminatory basis, to all workers facing irreducible health risks to minimize further both the impact of those risks on workers and the likelihood of liability. Such programs might include voluntary transfer options, voluntary medical or disability leave with benefits including guaranteed reinstatement, provision of medical counseling and referral to independent specialists, family planning information and services, and other services designed to assist employees in making responsible decisions. Such programs, adopted and administered in good faith, demonstrate the employer's reasonable and responsible efforts to address difficult risk evaluation issues. Reasonable conduct toward the parent, in all likelihood, is also sufficient to preclude liability to a future child.

As noted in earlier sections of this chapter, current federal regulation of potential reproductive toxicants is limited. This situation may make it difficult to determine safe exposure levels for some workplace toxicants. The Supreme Court's decision in the *UAW* case will hopefully refocus the attention of both scientists and regulators on problems of occupational reproductive harm and result in renewed enforcement efforts and additional standard setting to protect the health of workers and their offspring.

## REFERENCES

1. Occupational Safety and Health Act of 1970, 29 U.S.C. sec. 653, *et seq*.
2. Castleman BI, Ziem GE. Corporate influence on threshold limit values. Am J Ind Med 1988;13:531–559.
3. United Steelworkers of America v. Marshall, 647 F.2d 1189 (D.C. Cir. 1980), *cert. denied*, 453 U.S. 913 (1981).
4. Wells VE, Schnorr TM, Halperin WE. NIOSH selection of chemicals and study publications: setting priorities for reproductive research. Reprod Toxicol 1988;2:289–290.
5. U.S. Congress, Office of Technology Assessment. Reproductive health hazards in the workplace, OTA-BA-266. Washington, DC: U.S. Government Printing Office, 1985.
6. Working women's health concerns: a gender at risk? Bureau of National Affairs: Washington, DC, 1989.
7. Toxic Substances Control Act of 1976, 15 U.S.C. Sec. 2601 *et seq*.
8. Federal Insecticide, Fungicide and Rodenticide Act, 7 U.S.C. sec. 136 *et seq*.
9. U.S. Environmental Protection Agency. Guidelines for developmental toxicity risk assessment. 56 Fed Reg 63798–63826, 1991.
10. U.S. Environmental Protection Agency. Proposed guidelines for assessing male reproductive risk. 53 Fed Reg 24850, 1988.
11. U.S. Environmental Protection Agency. Proposed guidelines for assessing female reproductive risk. 53 Fed Reg 24834, 1988.
12. U.S. Environmental Protection Agency. Report of the teratology policy workgroup. Washington, DC: Environmental Protection Agency, 1985.
13. Love v. Thomas, 858 F. 2d 1347 (9th Cir. 1988), *cert.*
*denied sub nom. AFL-CIO v. Love*, 490 U.S. 1037 (1989).
14. Meyerowitz B, Sullivan C, Premeau C. Reaction of asbestos-exposed workers to notification and screening. Am J Ind Med 1989;15:463–475.
15. Hjelm C. Environmental law I: Worker and community right to know laws, 1987. Annual Survey of American Law, 1988.
16. Massachusetts Toxic Use Reduction Act, Chap. 265 of Acts of 1989.
17. Occupational Safety and Health Administration. Hazard Communication Standard, 29 C.F.R. Sec. 1910.1200 (1990).
18. Occupational Safety and Health Administration, Access Standard, 29 C.F.R. Sec. 1910.20 (1990).
19. Emergency Planning and Community Right to Know Act of 1986, 42 U.S.C. 11001 *et seq*.
20. Superfund Amendments and Reauthorization Act of 1986, Pub. L. 99–499, 42 U.S.C. 9601 *et seq*.
21. Larson A. Workers compensation law. Albany: Matthew Bender, 1990.
22. Locke L. Adapting workers compensation to the special problem of occupational disease. 9 Harv Environ Law Rev 249, 251 (1985).
23. Carle SD. A hazardous mix: discretion to disclose and incentives to suppress under OSHA's hazard communication standard. 97 Yale Law J 581, 585 n. 19 (1988).
24. Vann v. Dow Chemical, 561 F. Supp. 141 (W.D. Ark. 1983).
25. Adams v. Denny's, 464 So.2d 876 (La. App. 1985), *cert. denied*, 467 So.2d 530 (La. 1985).
26. Jarvis v. Providence Memorial Hospital, 444 N.W.2d 236 (Mich. App. 1989).
27. Bell v. Macy's, 261 Cal. Rptr. 447 (Cal. App., 1st Div. 1989).
28. Whitehead v. St. Joe Lead Co, 729 F.2d 238 (3d Cir. 1984).
29. Keeton W, Dobbs D, Keeton R, Owen D. The Law of Torts, 5th ed. St. Paul: West Publishing Co., 1984:¡68.
30. Note, Maternal tort liability. 22 Suffolk Univ Law Rev, 747 (1988).
31. Sterling v. Velsicol Chemical Corp, 885 F. 2d 1188 (6th Cir. 1988).
32. Gold S. Causation in toxic torts: burdens of proof, standards of persuasion, and statistical evidence. 96 Yale Law J 376, 377 (1986).
33. U.S. Dept of Commerce, Bureau of the Census. Statistical Abstract of the United States. Washington, DC: U.S. Government Printing Office, 1988.
34. Women's Bureau. Working mothers and their children. Facts on Working Women, no. 89–3. Washington, DC: U.S. Department of Labor, 1989.
35. Mattison DR. Risk assessment for developmental toxicity: airborne occupational exposure to ethanol and iodine. Risk: Issues in Safety and Health 1991;2:227–260.
36. Title VII of the Civil Rights Act of 1964, 42 U.S.C. 2000e.
37. *Phillips v. Martin-Marietta Corp*, 400 U.S. 542 (1971).
38. *Cleveland Bd of Ed v. LaFleur*, 414 U.S. 632 (1974).
39. Nashville Gas Co v. Satty, 434 U.S. 136 (1977).
40. *Geduldig v. Aiello*, 417 U.S. 484 (1974).
41. *Gilbert v. General Electric Co*, 429 U.S. 125 (1976).

42. Paul M, Daniels C, Rosofsky R. Corporate response to reproductive hazards in the workplace: results of the family, work, and health survey. Am J Occup Med 1989;16:267–280.

43. Bertin JE. Women's health and women's rights: reproductive health hazards in the workplace. In: Ratcliffe KS, Ferree MM, Mellow GO, et al., eds. Healing technology: feminist perspectives. Ann Arbor: Univ Michigan Press, 1989:289–303.

44. Norwood JL. Hearing before the Select Committee on Children, Youth, and Families, Work in America, Implications for Families. U.S. House of Representatives, 99th Cong., 2d Sess., April 17, 1986. Committee Reprint 5–59.

45. *Christman, et al. v. American Cyanamid Co.*, Civ. Action No. 80–0024P (N.D.W.Va.) Second Amended Complaint (1980).

46. Needleman HL, Bellinger D. Commentary: recent developments. Environ Res 1988;46:190–191.

47. Mattison DR. Exclusion of fertile women from the workplace: bad medicine, worse law. J Arkansas Med Soc 1990;86:491–492.

48. *International Union, UAW v. Johnson Controls*, U.S., 111 S. Ct. 1196 (1991).

49. U.S. Dept of Labor, Occupational Safety and Health Administration. Final standard for occupational exposure to lead, 29 C.F.R. sec. 1910.1025, 1989. Preamble to the Standard appears at 43 Fed Reg 52952, 1978.

50. *Newport News Shipbuilding and Drydock Co. v. EEOC*, 462 U.S. 669 (1983).

51. *California Federal Savings and Loan Association v. Guerra*, 479 U.S. 272 (1987).

52. Green v. Edmands Co, 639 F.2d 286 (5th Cir. 1981).

53. Comment: Employee assumption of risk: real or illusory choice. 52 Tenn Law Rev 35 (1984).

54. Tiller v. Atlantic Coast Line Railroad, 318 U.S. 54 (1943).

# IV

## Specific Toxicants

**PART A: PHYSICAL AGENTS**

# 13

·············································

# Ionizing and Nonionizing Radiations

ROBERT BRENT, MARVIN MEISTRICH, MAUREEN PAUL

The term "radiation" describes the transmission of energy from one body or source to another. In this broad sense, it encompasses diverse energy sources ranging (Fig. 13.1) from ionizing x-rays and γ rays to various forms of long-wavelength electromagnetic radiation (e.g., radar, microwaves), to ultrasound. The biological effects of these different forms of radiation vary considerably.

The effects of ionizing radiation have been studied more extensively than those of any other environmental hazard. This chapter reviews current knowledge regarding ionizing radiation and its effects on the adult germ cells and on pregnancy. A shorter section is devoted to nonionizing radiation, with emphasis on microwaves, magnetic resonance imaging, and ultrasound.

## IONIZING RADIATION

### Properties

Ionizing radiation is any form of radiation with sufficient energy to displace orbital electrons, resulting in the formation of electrically charged ions in matter. Both electromagnetic waves consisting of uncharged photons (x-rays, γ rays) and charged particles (α, β particles) can produce ionizations.

Each ionizing event reduces the energy of the particle or wave. Linear energy transfer (LET) refers to the energy lost per micrometer of track length and is dependent on the mass and charge of the particle. Heavy, charged α particles (e.g., radium 226, plutonium 239) produce dense paths of ionization along short distances; this high-LET radiation penetrates poorly but is hazardous if introduced internally. β Particles (e.g., strontium 90, iodine 131), with small mass and charge, and electromagnetic radiation from γ-and x-rays produce low-LET radiation with greater penetrating capabilities.

The principal unit of exposure to ionizing radiation is the roentgen (R), which is a measure of the amount of ionizations produced in air. The unit of absorbed radiation is the Gray (Gy) or rad (1 Gy = 100 rad). Exposure of typical tissues to 1 R yields approximately 1 rad of absorbed dose. However, different types of ionizing radiation can deposit the same total energy but produce different degrees of biological damage. The higher the LET, the greater the injury produced for a given absorbed dose. The dose equivalent, expressed in Seivert (Sv) or rem (1 Sv = 100 rem), is used to quantify the degree of biological effect. It is calculated by multiplying the absorbed dose (in rad or Gy) by a quality factor based on LET. The quality factor is 1 for x-rays and γ rays. Thus, for diagnostic x-rays (in soft tissues), an

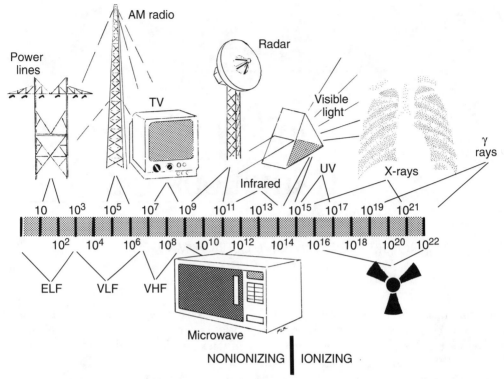

**Figure 13.1.**  The electromagnetic spectrum.

absorbed dose of 1 rad yields a dose equivalent of 1 rem. However, the quality factor for $\alpha$ particles is approximately 20; at equivalent energy depositions, $\alpha$ particles produce approximately 20 times the biological damage of $\gamma$ and x-rays.

Radionuclides emit ionizing radiation as a result of spontaneous transformations within their nuclei. This radioactivity is measured in curie (1 Ci = $3.7 \times 10^{10}$ disintegrations/sec) or becquerel (1 Bq = 1 disintegration/sec). The half-life of a radioactive substance describes the time necessary for one-half of its nuclei to decay spontaneously.

### Occurrence and Uses

Ionizing radiation exposures can be broadly classified into natural and human-made sources (Fig. 13.2) (1, 2). Natural background radiation represents the largest fraction of the annual effective dose equivalent to a member of the U.S. populace (approximately 3 mSv or 300 mrem). An average 0.6 mSv (60 mrem) per year comes from human-made sources, with the largest fraction due to medical x-rays. In the U.S., occupational sources account for only 0.3% of the annual dose equivalent (1).

In the workplace, external irradiation of the whole body is by far the most common type of exposure. However, internal deposition of radionuclides after ingestion, inhalation, or skin absorption can also occur.

According to estimates by the Environmental Protection Agency (EPA) for 1985 (3), over 1.7 million U.S. workers (excluding uranium miners and students) are nominally exposed to low-LET radiation, approximately 760,000 of whom receive measurable doses above background. The mean annual dose equivalent to all workers was 0.85 mSv (85 mrem) in 1985; the average dose to those measurably exposed was 1.9 mSv (190 mrem). These values have decreased by approximately 20% and 10%, respectively, since 1980. Table 13.1 provides a breakdown of measurable radiation exposures by occupational category.

Exposure to high-LET radiation is a concern in some occupational categories, such as miners exposed to air-borne radon decay prod-

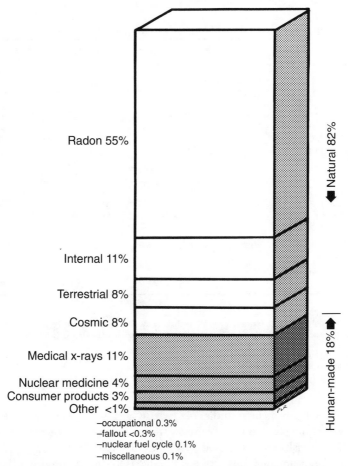

**Figure 13.2.** Sources of ionizing radiation to members of the United States population. Data from National Council on Radiation Protection and Measurements (NCRP). Ionizing radiation exposure of the population of the United States. NCRP report no. 93. Bethesda: NCRP, 1987:55.

ucts. An estimated 23,000 U.S. workers are exposed to high-LET radiation, with an average annual effective dose equivalent of approximately 5 mSv (500 mrem) (1).

## Reproductive and Developmental Effects

Exposure to ionizing radiation can produce a wide range of biological effects. The most critical molecular target is DNA, since alteration of the DNA may profoundly alter or kill the cell. Other important cellular effects include inhibition of cell division, chromosomal breakage, and oncogenic transformation. The degree of damage is influenced by several factors including the type of radiation, fractionation and dose

distribution, tissue sensitivities, and DNA repair capabilities. Rapidly dividing cells of the embryo or the reproductive germinal epithelium are particularly radiosensitive.

For regulatory purposes, radiation-induced health effects are divided into two broad categories (4). *Stochastic* effects refer to diseases, such as cancer or genetic disease, that can result from alterations produced in a single cell. A risk for induction of stochastic effects is presumed to exist even at low exposures. *Nonstochastic* effects require multicellular injury and appear to have a threshold dose below which deleterious effects do not occur. Most teratogenic effects are currently believed to be threshold phenomena.

Primary sources of data regarding radiation-

**Table 13.1.**
**Occupational Exposures to Low-LET Radiation, United States, 1985**

| Occupation | Number of Workers (thousands) | | Mean Annual Dose Equivalent (mSv)[a] | | Collective Dose Equivalent (person-Sv)[b] |
| | All | Exposed | All | Exposed | |
|---|---|---|---|---|---|
| Medicine | 734 | 267 | 0.4 | 1.1 | 280 |
| Industry | 274 | 101 | 0.6 | 1.5 | 148 |
| Nuclear fuel cycle | 205 | 107 | 2.2 | 4.2 | 450 |
| Government | 230 | 117 | 0.7 | 1.3 | 154 |
| Air transportation (flight crews)[c] | 114 | 114 | 3.5 | 3.5 | 400 |
| Miscellaneous | | | | | |
|   Education | 17 | 7 | 0.4 | 0.8 | 6 |
|   Security/Trans- portation | 165 | 49 | 0.08 | 0.3 | 13.7 |
| **TOTAL** (rounded) | 1739 | 762 | 0.85 | 1.9 | 1451.7 |
| Students | 68 | ? | 0.16 | ? | 11 |
| Uranium miners | 1.2 | 0.92 | .52 WLM[d] | .65 WLM[d] | 631 person-WLM[d] |

[a] 1mSv = 100 mrem.
[b] 1 person-Sv = 100 person-rem.
[c] A typical 5-hr transcontinental flight at 38,000 feet provides a whole body dose equivalent of 0.025 mSv (2.5 mrem) (2). Data from Environmental Protection Agency (EPA). Occupational exposure to ionizing radiation in the United States: 1985. Washington, DC: EPA, in preparation.
[d] One WLM (working level month) is an exposure to an average concentration of one working level (1.3 × 10$^5$ MeV of α energy from radon daughters per liter of air) for a working month of 170 hr.

induced reproductive effects include studies of atomic bomb survivors and patients therapeutically irradiated. Human risk estimates based on interspecies extrapolation and high-dose epidemiological studies remain tenuous for the usual low-dose exposures encountered in the environment or workplace.

## MALE REPRODUCTIVE EFFECTS

The human testis, and hence, the fecundity of the male, is extremely sensitive to ionizing radiation. For example, temporary azoospermia can occur after doses of x-rays as low as 0.3 Gy (30 rad) (5).

Although most occupational radiation exposures are below those expected to produce marked effects on testicular function, accidental exposures to higher levels do occur, as during nuclear reactor accidents. Testicular irradiation also results from therapeutic and diagnostic medical procedures. Childhood leukemia is the only condition for which the testis is the intended target in clinical radiotherapy. However, the scatter from radiation to nearby sites often results in doses to the testis in the 0.2- to

2.5-Gy (20–250 rad) range. For example, the testis receives about 2% of the dose to the tumor target from a 12 × 12 cm field whose edge is located 10 cm from the testis (6). For a prescription dose of 50 Gy (5000 rad) to such a field, the testicular dose can be 1 Gy (100 rad), which is sufficient to produce significant injury to the sensitive germinal epithelial cells.

Much of the information on targets for radiation effects in the human testis is extrapolated from studies of experimental animals and validated, where possible, in humans. Because most radiation-induced cell death occurs when cells attempt to divide, the radiation sensitivities of spermatogenic cells are largely dependent on their rates of proliferation. As expected, differentiating spermatogonia are very radiosensitive, having $LD_{50}$ values of 0.4 Gy (40 rad) or less. Radiation doses required to kill spermatocytes are higher than those for differentiating spermatogonia, and doses lethal to spermatids are still higher. The stem cell spermatogonia are slowly proliferating cells with a radiosensitivity intermediate between differentiating spermatogonia and spermatocytes. Other cells essential to male reproductive function (Sertoli and Leydig cells, epididymal cells) are generally minimally proliferative in the adult and, thus, are not functionally affected by moderate doses of radiation (7).

In most tissues, dose fractionation has a sparing effect because damage is repaired between doses. In the testis, however, irradiation causes the surviving stem cells to become more proliferative and, hence, more sensitive to subsequent doses. This phenomenon accounts for the greater sensitivity of the testis to fractionated or chronic exposures than to single doses of radiation within certain exposure ranges.

The long-term consequences of radiation damage to the testis are primarily related to effects on the stem cells. Stem cells that survive irradiation will proliferate, resulting in regeneration of the numbers of stem cells and in the appearance of colonies of differentiating spermatogonia. In rodents and, perhaps, in humans, the plateau to which sperm production recovers is related to stem cell survival. In humans, there is also a dose-dependent delay in initiation of recovery of sperm production (8).

There are three principal sources of data on which the quantitative responses of the human testes to irradiation are based: (a) studies of survivors of nuclear accidents or atomic explosions, (b) studies of prisoners experimentally exposed to single doses of x-rays to the testicles, and (c) follow-up of patients treated for malignant disease with radiotherapeutic procedures involving radiation scatter to the testes.

The investigation of the atomic bomb survivors performed 6–8 yr after exposure employed classical histopathological criteria rather than precise quantification of germ cells (9). Tubular sclerosis was the only endpoint showing a statistically significant and dose-related increase.

Rowley et al. (10) and Paulsen (11) reported quantitative histological counts of spermatogenic cells following experimental irradiations. They observed declines over a period of 100 days in the numbers of A spermatogonia (stem cells) and in the efficiency with which A spermatogonia differentiate into primary spermatocytes after 1 Gy (100 rad). An increase in the number of A spermatogonia and yield of spermatocytes occurred at approximately 200 days

postirradiation, returning to control levels in approximately 3 yr.

The effects of radiation on human sperm counts can be divided into four time phases. The first is the 8-week period after irradiation, during which the sperm are either spermatocytes or spermatids in the testis or spermatozoa in the epididymis and vas deferens. These cells are relatively radioresistant and, during the first 50–60 days after low doses of irradiation (less than 2 Gy), sperm production remains above 50% of control values (12). The second phase, beginning at 2 months after irradiation, is represented by a drastic reduction in sperm count. Oligospermia has been reported after 15 rad (12), and doses of ≥20 rad can produce azoospermia. A dose of approximately 35 rad results in a 50% incidence of azoospermia and a 100-rad dose results in a 90% incidence (Fig. 13.3). The time period for depletion of sperm in the ejaculate is consistent with the time required for radiosensitive spermatogonia to become sperm. Recovery begins during the third phase, and sperm production reaches control levels during the final phase. Recovery begins from 6 months following irradiation of the testes with single doses of 0.2 Gy (20 rad) to 24 months after 6 Gy (600 rad). Due to the greater sensitivity of the germinal epithelium to fractionated irradiation (5), approximately 24 months are required for initiation of recovery from azoospermia after fractionated doses of only 2.1 Gy (210 rad).

It is instructive to consider the percentages of men who remain azoospermic 2 yr after exposure. Sperm production recovers by this time in virtually all men exposed to single doses of less than 6 Gy (600 rad). In contrast, approximately 20% of men who receive 20–135 rad to the testis during fractionated (therapeutic) irradiation, as well as 85% of those who receive 210–312 rad, are still azoospermic 2 yr later. Men who receive more than 250 rad remain azoospermic for 2–14 yr, and some never recover sperm production. Thus, men in their reproductive years should be offered semen cryopreservation (sperm banking) before radiotherapeutic procedures in which scattered doses may approach this value or where additional chemotherapy (especially with alkylating agents) is planned (13).

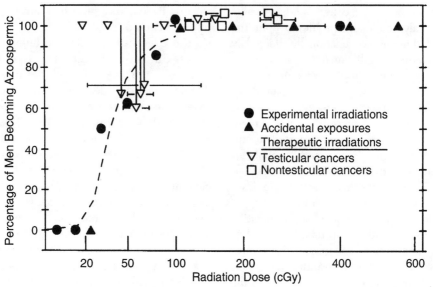

**Figure 13.3.**   Percentage of men who develop azoospermia at any time after various total doses of radiation from different sources. Data based on experimental irradiations are the most precise and a smooth curve was drawn using those points.

Although low doses associated with normal occupational exposure to radiation are not expected to affect sperm measures, one study (14) noted effects on workers who had estimated long-term exposure levels of 0.5–3.5 rad/yr. When compared to a control group, a higher percentage of the exposed workers had sperm concentrations of less than 40 million/ml and altered sperm motility and morphology. However, uncertainties regarding the dosimetry for estimating testicular dose and the effects of confounding variables raise questions regarding the validity of these conclusions.

In the clinical context, the most important semen measure for evaluation of radiation effects on male fertility appears to be sperm count. Baseline counts are essential to determine whether there were effects of radiation exposure. Even in normal fertile men, sperm concentrations range from less than 10 million/ml to more than 200 million/ml (15). In seminoma patients, Sandeman (16) reported that pretreatment sperm counts were below 20 million/ml in 77% compared to approximately 10% in the overall population. Shortly after irradiation, the percentage of morphologically normal sperm decreases. However, this parameter, as well as sperm motility, returns to control levels when sperm count recovers (17).

## FEMALE REPRODUCTIVE EFFECTS

The response of the female ovary to ionizing radiation is influenced by a number of factors including the stage(s) of growth and development of the germ cells, age and hormonal status, and characteristics of the exposure such as the type of radiation, dose rate, and fractionation. There are also marked differences in response between and even within species (18, 19). Identification of an appropriate and affordable experimental animal model from which to extrapolate data regarding human effects has been frustrating. The mouse and rat are poor models, since the synchronization of oogenesis in these species renders the ovaries more vulnerable to radiation exposure (20).

During embryofetal development, oogonia derived from the primordial germ cells actively proliferate, and then variable numbers enter meiotic prophase to become primary oocytes. The mitotically active cells are sensitive to destruction by radiation. However, due to species differences in synchronization, x-ray doses that result in significant depletion of oogonia in mice (20–30 R) and rats (100 R) have little effect in the rhesus monkey or human fetus (20, 21).

After birth, the oocytes remain arrested at

the diplotene stage of meiosis until shortly before ovulation. Approximately 90% of the total population of oocytes resides within single-layered primordial follicles, while the remainder are within growing or antral (Graffian) follicles. According to Baker (19, 20), radiation doses required to kill all oocytes in the mouse are 15 R for juvenile primordial follicles, 50 R for adult primordial follicles, and 2000 R for growing follicles. Doses are slightly higher in the rat. However, in the rhesus monkey, 5000 R is required to kill approximately 50% of adult primordial follicles, while only very high doses (7000–12,000 R) destroy all the oocytes (20, 22).

Studies of Japanese atomic bomb survivors followed for up to 18 yr postexposure reveal no impairment of fertility, even among women exposed to acute doses exceeding 1 Gy (100 rads) (23, 24). Among survivors exposed in utero 28 yr earlier, Blot et al. (25) found no dose-related effect for childless marriages, number of births, or the interval between marriage and first birth.

Among 182 cancer survivors who were treated with abdominal radiation during childhood, 12% experienced premature ovarian failure (26). The location of the gonads relative to the treatment field was the only risk factor for this complication. Ovarian failure occurred in 68% of patients who had both ovaries within abdominal radiotherapy fields (mean ovarian dose 3.2 Gy), 14% of patients whose ovaries were at the edge of the treatment field (approximately 2.9 Gy), and in none of the patients with one or both ovaries outside the field (approximately 0.54 Gy). In a retrospective cohort study of adult patients treated for cancer during childhood or adolescence, Byrne et al. (27) found that radiation treatment below the diaphragm (doses not provided) depressed fertility in both sexes by approximately 25%. In a subsequent study derived from the same cohort, patients who were treated with radiotherapy alone during adolescence were 3.7 times more likely to be menopausal by their early to mid 20s than were sibling controls (28).

Other reports of females exposed therapeutically to ovarian x-irradiation provide quantitative information about the doses necessary to induce temporary or permanent amenorrhea (29–31). The threshold for permanent sterilization of the human ovary decreases with increasing age, inasmuch as the number of oocytes in the ovaries of older women are already significantly depleted through the processes of ovulation and atresia. Ovarian doses in the range of 2.5–5.0 Gy (250–500 rad) induce permanent sterility in most women over the age of 40 yr, while the majority of younger women experience only temporary menstrual disturbances. A dose as high as 20 Gy (2000 rad) may be tolerated by young women, if it is fractionated over a period of several weeks (29). Doses ≤0.6 Gy (60 rad) are without effect in most age groups.

Ionizing radiation exposures encountered in the general environment or in the workplace are far below those expected to affect ovarian function. The same is true for usual ovarian doses from diagnostic x-rays, which range from approximately 0.02 mGy (2 mrad) for a P-A chest film to 2–5 mGy (200–500 mrad) for fluoroscopic studies or a lumbopelvic series (32).

## GENETIC EFFECTS

Radiation-induced mutations in parental germ cells can be of the chromosomal type (numerical or structural) or single gene mutations. The biological consequences of inherited mutations vary enormously. For example, unbalanced translocations and most autosomal aneuploidies result in embryo lethality. Some inherited balanced translocations may be associated with reduced fertility, enhanced susceptibility to cancer, or behavioral deficits. Autosomal dominant or X-linked disorders are readily discernible in first-generation progeny, while recessive mutations can cause effects at very low incidence in subsequent generations. In the human, these risks remain largely theoretical; epidemiological studies do not find an increase in genetic effects, probably because many induced mutations are lost before they appear in progeny.

Direct assessment of radiation-induced genetic effects in human populations is exceedingly difficult due to the background incidence of spontaneous mutations, complex multigenic effects on many human genetic disorders, and the inability to measure the effects of recessive mutations. Therefore, human risk estimates are based primarily on indirect evidence from experimental studies with mice. Extensive reviews of this complex subject are available (33–36).

Genetic risk can be estimated either by the number of genetic changes of any kind induced per unit of radiation delivered (direct method) or by the dose of radiation necessary to increase the occurrence of a specific genetic aberration to twice its background incidence in the population (doubling-dose method). Guidelines for human exposure to radiation rely heavily on the genetic doubling dose derived from the murine specific-locus test (37), which measures mutation rates at seven gene loci. Early estimates of the doubling dose for these radiation-induced mutations were approximately 0.5 Gy (50 rem), and remarkably similar doubling doses of approximately 20–50 rem were calculated for a variety of other endpoints (36). However, these estimates were based on single, acute exposures of murine germ cells to low-LET radiation, which is approximately three times more effective in inducing mutations than low-level, chronic irradiation (37). Applying this dose-rate factor, radiation protection agencies have set the minimum genetic doubling dose for humans at 1.0 Sv (100 rem) (33, 34). Based on accumulated murine data, some investigators have recently suggested much higher doubling doses of 1.4 Sv (140 rem) for acute exposure and 4.2 Sv (420 rem) for chronic exposure (38).

Children born to survivors of the atomic bomb explosions at Hiroshima and Nagasaki are the largest, most thoroughly monitored offspring of a population exposed to radiation. Six indicators of genetic effects were studied in this population: untoward pregnancy outcomes (stillbirth, major congenital defects, death within the first postnatal week); childhood mortality; sex chromosome aneuploidy; balanced chromosomal exchanges; protein mutations; and childhood cancer (39). There was no statistically significant effect of parental radiation exposure for any of these endpoints taken alone; however, analysis of all endpoints combined suggested a positive effect and an estimated genetic doubling dose of 1.7–2.2 Sv

(170–220 rem) (39). This value includes acute doses received by either parent and, hence, represents an average of the effects on male and female germ cells.

One recent case-control study (40) related the excess of childhood leukemia in the region of a British nuclear plant to low-dose occupational radiation exposure of the fathers. Paternal doses ≥0.01 Sv (1 rem) in the 6 months before conception, or total preconceptual doses ≥0.1 Sv (10 rem), were associated with a six- to eight-fold increased risk of leukemia in offspring. However, the much larger atomic bomb studies challenge the biological plausibility of these findings, revealing no excess of leukemia among children of parents who received significantly higher doses of radiation before conception (41).

The Committee on the Biological Effects of Ionizing Radiations recently published revised estimates of the effects of low-LET radiation on various human genetic disorders (Table 13.2) (34). These estimates assume a minimum human doubling dose of 1 Sv (100 rem) for chronic exposure. Risks are based on an average population exposure (above background levels) of 0.01 Sv (1 rem) per 30-yr generation (i.e., 0.01 Sv to each parent over a 30-yr childbearing period or an average of 0.33 mSv/yr). The majority of severe autosomal dominant disorders emerge in first-generation offspring; this excess parental radiation dose would add, at most, 5–20 additional cases to the spontaneous background incidence of 2500 cases per million liveborns. The incidence of recessive disease might increase very slowly over many generations. Assuming a background incidence of major congenital anomalies of 2–3% in liveborns, the excess 0.01 Sv parental dose would result in a risk of 10 additional cases in $10^6$ first-generation offspring and a risk of 10–100 cases per $10^6$ offspring after many generations (i.e., at equilibrium).

While genetic risk is small, it may be prudent to delay conception for a period of 3–6 months after appreciable exposure to ionizing radiation. In male mice, the stem spermatogonia are 2–20 times less sensitive to the induction of mutations by single, acute doses of irradiation than are later germ cell stages. Waiting at least 3 months before con-

**Table 13.2.**
**Estimated Human Genetic Risks of 0.01 Sv (1 rem) of Ionizing Radiation per Generation**[a]

| Disease Classification | Current Incidence (per $10^6$ livebirths) | Additional Cases (per $10^6$ livebirths/0.01 Sv/generation) | |
| --- | --- | --- | --- |
| | | First Generation | Equilibrium |
| Autosomal Dominant | | | |
|   Clinically severe | 2500 | 5–20 | 25 |
|   Clinically mild | 7500 | 1–15 | 75 |
| X-linked | 400 | <1 | <5 |
| Recessive | 2500 | <1 | Very slow increase |
| Chromosomal | | | |
|   Unbalanced translocations | 600 | <5 | Very little increase |
|   Trisomies | 3800 | <1 | <1 |
| Congenital abnormalities | 20,000–30,000 | 10 | 10–100 |

[a]From National Research Council, Committee on the Biological Effects of Ionizing Radiations. Genetic effects of ionizing radiation. In: Health effects of exposure to low levels of ionizing radiation, BEIR V. Washington, DC: National Academy Press, 1990:70, with permission.

ception ensures that the fertilizing sperm was a stem cell at the time of radiation exposure. Experiments in female mice exposed to high-dose radiation also suggest that the risk of transmitting mutations to offspring is considerably reduced several months after exposure (42). After high-dose radiotherapy, genetic risks are not significant enough to advise against conception, but the pregnancy should be carefully monitored.

## PRENATAL EFFECTS

There have been many experiments and observations about the effects of radiation on the developing embryo. Nevertheless, we have a great deal to learn about radiation teratogenesis. The subject is summarized briefly here and reviewed extensively elsewhere (43–45).

The effects of radiation depend, in part, on the stage of gestation at which exposure occurs. Before implantation, the conceptus has a decreased sensitivity to the teratogenic and growth-retarding effects of irradiation and a greater susceptibility to radiation-induced lethal effects (Figs. 13.4 and 13.5) (46, 47). During early organogenesis, the embryo is very sensitive to the growth-retarding, teratogenic, and lethal effects of irradiation but has the ability to recover somewhat from the growth-retarding effects in the postpartum period (48). During early fetal development, the conceptus has diminished susceptibility to multiple organ teratogenesis but retains central nervous sys-

tem (CNS) sensitivity; it is growth retarded at term and recovers poorly from the growth deficit postnatally. During the later fetal stages, the conceptus is not grossly deformed by radiation but can sustain permanent cell depletion of various organs and tissues if the radiation exposure is high enough. Many mechanisms have been postulated to account for the embryopathic effects of radiation including cell death, mitotic delay, disturbances of cell migration, and others. The same pathogenic mechanisms may not be primarily operative at all stages of gestation. Radiation-induced cell death may be minimally important at one stage of gestation because of the embryo's ability to replace the dead cells. At another stage, cell lethality may be a primary factor, because the embryo has lost this ability.

Other radiation-induced effects that have been invoked to explain embryopathological conditions are cytogenetic abnormalities and somatic mutations. Cytogenetic abnormalities may be responsible for preimplantation death in the irradiated mammalian zygote (46, 49). If one uses the radiation mutation rate in mammalian cells (37, 38) for estimating potential teratogenicity, it is obvious that point mutations do not account for even a small proportion of radiation-induced teratogenicity.

While some radiation-induced effects are immediately obvious, others can be ascertained only in the postpartum or adult period. Examples include neuronal depletion, infertility, tissue hypoplasia, neoplasia, or shortening of life

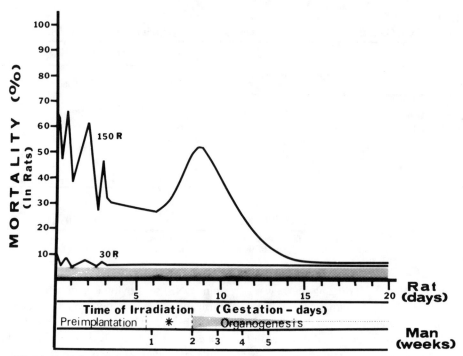

**Figure 13.4.** The lethal effect of radiation in rats is greater on the first day. It appears that the $LD_{50}$ shifts at different times of the day during early gestation, possibly because the cells are dividing synchronously; therefore, the zygote will vary in its radiosensitivity, depending on the stage of the cell cycle. Note that the embryo becomes somewhat resistant in the implantation stage and then becomes sensitive to the lethal effect of radiation during early organogenesis. A 30-rad dose on the first day apparently does increase the resorption rate. The superimposition of the lethality curve for rats onto the human embryonic development timetable may not be appropriate and is for purposes of comparison only, but it allows one to estimate roughly the stages at which the human embryo might be most readily killed by high doses of radiation.

span (50). For several reasons, neurophysiological and behavioral changes in adult organisms irradiated in utero are the most difficult to evaluate. First, it is not easy to eliminate postnatal environmental effects as contributing factors. Second, reported findings are frequently neither reproducible nor dose related. Third, it may not be possible to correlate behavioral alterations with neuroanatomic changes. Finally, animal behavior tests may have minimal application to the human situation.

## Human Radiation Teratogenesis

Growth retardation and CNS effects, such as microcephaly or eye malformations, are the cardinal manifestations of intrauterine radiation effects in humans. Numerous studies (51–59) indicate that microcephaly is the most common malformation observed in humans randomly exposed to high doses of radiation during pregnancy. In reports by Goldstein and Murphy

(51–53), 25% of embryos exposed to more than 1 Gy (100 rad) of radiation became microcephalic or hydrocephalic children. Almost all the microcephalic children were mentally retarded. Many were growth retarded, and three had various abnormalities of the eyes. The unique finding was that no visceral, limb, or other malformation was identified unless the child exhibited growth retardation, microcephaly, or readily apparent eye malformations. Dekaban (54) reported that infants born to women who received therapeutic radiation between 3 and 20 weeks' gestation (protracted exposure of approximately 2.5 Gy) were microcephalic, mentally retarded, or both. All of the malformed infants exhibited growth retardation, and some had eye, genital, and skeletal abnormalities.

From a sample of 1265 subjects exposed in utero at Hiroshima, 183 were analyzed by Miller (55) and by Wood et al. (56, 57). Of the 78 fetuses irradiated before 16 weeks' gesta-

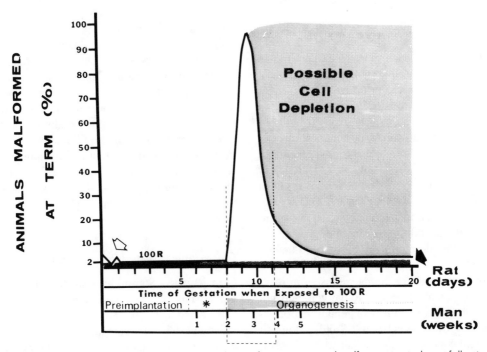

**Figure 13.5.** This graph depicts the relative incidence of gross congenital malformations in the rat following an exposure of 100 rad. The *solid arrow* on the right side of the ordinate points to the 2% control incidence of congenital malformations seen in this species. The incidence of malformations before the ninth day is the same as in the controls. The *open arrow* on the left side of the ordinate points to a slight increase in malformations on the first day. (This was inserted because of the work of Russell in a particular strain of mice.) A very large increase in malformations occurs during the early organogenetic period, which corresponds to the third and fourth weeks of human pregnancy. This high incidence of gross malformations falls off rapidly as organogenesis diminishes. Note that organogenesis to some degree (CNS) continues to term. Although gross malformations may not be produced during the late fetal stages with 100 rad, an irreversible cell loss occurs. The asterisk (*) is placed at the stage of implantation to indicate that, although malformations are not readily produced at this stage, growth retardation can be induced.

tion, 32% were microcephalic and 14% were mentally deficient. Of the 105 fetuses irradiated at 16 weeks or older, 7% were microcephalic and 4% were mentally deficient. Most microcephalic offspring who were also mentally deficient exhibited short stature, while those of normal intelligence did not. The incidence of microcephaly rose with increasing exposure. Severe mental retardation was not observed in any patient who received less than 0.5 Gy (50 rad) in utero.

In a summary of the data on microcephaly, Blot (60, 61) noted no increased risk for microcephaly in the population exposed to less than 1.5 Gy (150 rad) in Nagasaki, but he did report an increased risk in the Hiroshima population exposed to doses as low as 10–19 rad. It is possible that the decreased head size observed at lower doses in Hiroshima was due to causes

other than radiation. In experimental animals, 10–20 rad of low-LET radiation does not increase the incidence of microcephaly (44).

In a reanalysis of the Japanese atomic bomb survivor data using revised dosimetry, Schull et al. (62, 63) report a linear dose-related increase in severe mental retardation and neonatal seizures after exposures between 8 and 15 weeks postconception. The increases are statistically significant above 0.5 Gy (50 rad) and exhibit a possible threshold at 10–20 rad. Analyses of IQ and school performance among atomic bomb survivors prenatally exposed during this interval reveal dose-related decreases, with an estimated loss of 0.2–0.3 IQ points per rad (34, 62). Using a linear model, loss of IQ points from usual doses encountered during diagnostic or occupational radiation would be too low to be detected (64).

The most sensitive exposure window for induction of mental retardation (8–15 weeks postconception) corresponds to the time of most rapid cell proliferation and migration of immature neurons from periventricular areas to the cerebral cortex (62). Mental retardation is not observed in subjects exposed before 8 weeks or after 26 weeks postconception. Before 8 weeks, the cerebral neuronal precursors are relatively radioresistant, while depletion of other cell types (e.g., glial cells) can result in small head size without mental retardation. The late fetal period is characterized by continued cellular differentiation and accelerated growth and development of the cerebellum (34, 64).

Irradiation of the human fetus from diagnostic exposures below 5 rad has generally not been observed to cause congenital malformations or growth retardation (65, 66), but not all epidemiological studies are negative (67). Animal data support the contention that gross congenital anomalies will not be increased in a human pregnant population exposed to 20 rad or less (Table 13.3). The fractionated or protracted doses characteristic of most human radiation exposures are likely to be less effective in producing malformations than acute exposures. It is possible that subtle functional or

biochemical changes may be produced at low radiation levels with low incidence.

Although there is a threshold (more than 25 rad) for the induction of abortion during and after early organogenesis (Table 13.3), there are data neither to support nor to refute the possibility that abortion in the preimplantation period may be a stochastic phenomenon. Exposures of 10 rad on the first day of mammalian development produce no apparent increase in abortions, but very large-scale studies would be necessary to detect small increases at low doses.

## Oncogenic Effect of Prenatal Radiation

Over 30 yr ago, Stewart et al. suggested that the human embryo was more sensitive than the child or adult to the leukemogenic effects of radiation; they later concluded that other cancers also occur more frequently in persons exposed in utero to diagnostic radiological procedures (primarily pelvimetry) (68–70). The present estimate is that a 0.01–0.02 Gy (1–2 rad) in utero radiation exposure increases the chance of leukemia developing in offspring by a factor of 1.5–2.0 over the natural incidence. In contrast, the doubling dose for leukemia induction in an adult population is approxi-

**Table 13.3.**
**Estimation of the Risks of Radiation in the Human Embryo Based on Human Epidemiological Studies and Mouse and Rat Radiation Embryological Studies**

| Embryonic Age (days) | Minimal Lethal Dose (rad) | Approximate LD$_{50}$ (rad) | Minimum Dose (rad) for Permanent Growth Retardation in the Adult | Minimum Dose (rad) for Increased Incidence Mental Retardation | Minimum Dose for Recognized Gross Anatomic Malformation (rad) | Minimum Dose for Induction of Genetic, Carcinogenic and Minimal Cell Depletion Phenomena (rad) |
|---|---|---|---|---|---|---|
| 1–5 | 10 | <100 | No effect in survivors | | | Unknown |
| 18–28 | 25–50 | 140 | 20–50 | 20–50 Severe CNS anatomic malformations more likely than mental retardation | 20 | Unknown |
| 36–50 | 50 | 200 | 25–50 | 50[a] | 50 | Unknown |
| 50–150 | >50 | >100 | 25–50 | 50[a] | [b] | Unknown |
| To term | >100 | Same as mother | >50 | 100 | | Unknown |

[a]Recent information published by Yamazaki and Schull (62) suggest an increased risk at lower exposures.
[b]Anatomic malformations of a severe type cannot be produced this late in gestation except in the genitourinary system and tissue hypoplasia in specific organ systems, such as the brain and testes.

mately 0.3 Gy (30 rad). Numerous other studies (71–74) indicate a 1.3- to 3-fold higher incidence of leukemia in children exposed to diagnostic radiation in utero, although some studies fail to substantiate this association (66).

Identification and control of confounding factors make interpretation of radiation carcinogenesis studies difficult. Increased risks of childhood malignancies have been associated with a number of other factors including tobacco smoke exposure (75) and birthweight (76). Questions arise as to whether the increased risk of malignancy is due to the low-dose diagnostic radiation exposure or to some other characteristic of the pregnancies that prompts x-ray examination and is itself associated with an increased childhood cancer risk.

Studies of atomic bomb survivors have failed to find an association between in utero radiation exposure and childhood leukemia. In a study of 1300 people, some of whom were exposed to the atomic bomb while in utero, Kato (77) observed no increased evidence of malignancy in the first 24 yr of follow-up. In the longest follow-up study to date (78), two cases of cancer (Wilms tumor and liver cancer) developed before 15 yr of age among 1630 Japanese children exposed to atomic bomb radiation in utero; neither case involved leukemia. Prenatal radiation exposure was associated in this study with an increased frequency of adult tumors that occurred earlier than usual during adult life.

In summary, most investigators agree that low doses of radiation present a carcinogenic risk to the embryo and to the adult and that there may be different risks per rad at different stages of development. However, findings of an increased cancer risk among children exposed in utero to low-dose diagnostic radiation must be reconciled with the fact that high-dose animal and human studies (77–79) have not found marked increases in cancer incidence, which one would expect if the embryo were as sensitive to radiation-induced carcinogenesis effects as Stewart et al. (70) suggest. The multiplicity of factors involved and the difficulties in their identification and control cannot be overemphasized. Until more is understood about the mechanisms of radiation-induced carcinogenesis during different stages of development,

doubt will remain concerning the magnitude of the role of in utero radiation in induction of leukemia and other malignancies.

Assuming that the leukemogenic effects of low-level radiation are real, let us examine how difficult it would be to use this information to counsel a patient who has received a dose of 0.02 Gy (2 rad) during pregnancy. According to Stewart and colleagues, the risk of leukemia following this exposure in utero is 1:2000 vs. 1:3000 in unexposed controls over a 10-yr period. (In fact, the hypothetic incremental risk for 2 rad of in utero radiation is 1:6000 over a 10-yr period. It is the combination of the control risk plus the incremental radiation risk that results in a 1:2000 risk for these patients.) If a clinician were inclined to recommend therapeutic abortion because the probability of developing leukemia is 50% greater than controls, 1999 exposed nonleukemic subjects would be aborted for every leukemic "saved." Moreover, the provider would be placed in a serious dilemma, because there are other situations in which the risk of leukemia is greater.

## Radioisotopes and the Embryo

No occupational reproductive studies involving radioisotope exposure are available; therefore, this section explores effects of medically administered radioisotopes.

The number and type of medical radionuclide procedures have changed considerably in the last two decades. In the U.S., the frequency of all diagnostic nuclear medicine procedures increased from 16/1000 population in 1972 to 32/1000 population in 1982 (80). Over the years, a number of procedures have been introduced and others have been eliminated. For example, ultrasonography has supplanted the use of nuclear medicine procedures to localize the placenta.

The precise estimation of the hazards of a particular isotope depends on accurate dosimetry, i.e., determination of the total dose absorbed by the fetus or a particular fetal tissue and the dose rate.

Administration of most radiopharmaceuticals results in extremely low fetal exposures. Iodine, however, is an exception, especially if the patient is being treated for thyroid malignancy or hyperthyroidism. Iodine 131, administered as the inorganic ion or bound to protein, is commonly used for uptake studies and radioactive scanning. The fetal thyroid absorbs and incorporates iodides readily by the 10th week of gestation and continues to do so thereafter (Table 13.4). Fetal thyroid avidity for iodides is greater than that of the maternal thyroid (81). Ordinarily, the whole-body dose to the embryo from $^{131}$I is insignificant when compared with the thyroid dose. If large doses of $^{131}$I are administered, significant embryonic or fetal exposure can occur because of the accumulation of $^{131}$I in the bladder adjacent to the uterus.

Total fetal thyroid destruction can result from therapeutic (ablative) doses of $^{131}$I administered to pregnant women. Although there are no reports of immediate deleterious fetal effects from tracer doses of radioactive iodine, a theoretical concern about the induction of thyroid cancer cannot be disregarded. The use of radioactive iodine should be avoided during pregnancy, unless it is essential for the medical care of the mother and there is no substitute. Even if administered during the first 5–6 weeks of gestation, when the fetal thyroid has not yet developed, the total dose to the embryo should be estimated.

Inorganic radioactive potassium, sodium, phosphorus, cesium, thallium, selenium, chromium, iron, and strontium cross the placenta readily. Radioactive phosphorus and strontium administered in large doses to animals result in embryonic abnormality and death (82). These isotopes are used in less than 1% of procedures; only radioactive phosphorus or gold is utilized therapeutically.

Most new isotope agents are bound to some complex macromolecule or macroaggregate. These newer agents cross the placenta in minuscule amounts and deliver extremely low doses to the embryo. Total body dose is considerably lower with technetium 99m ($^{99m}$Tc) bound to macromolecules than with protein-labeled $^{131}$I, and there is less concern about the fetal thyroid as a target organ.

## Counseling the Pregnant Woman

The hazards to the embryo of usual occupational radiation exposure or those encountered during diagnostic roentogenology (2–500 mrad) are minimal when compared with spontaneous mishaps that can befall human pregnancies (Tables 13.3 and 13.5). In spite of the fact that doses of 1–3 rad can produce cellular effects and that diagnostic exposure during pregnancy has been associated with malignancy in childhood, the maximum theoretical risk to human embryos exposed to doses of 5 rad or less is extremely small. In our experience, when the data and risks regarding low-dose radiation are appropriately explained, patients invariably choose to continue wanted pregnancies. It is inappropriate to recommend therapeutic abortion for risks with probabilities of occurrence far below the expected spontaneous incidence in the embryo or fetus.

There is ample evidence to indicate that high-dose external exposures (e.g., abdominal radiation therapy) can deleteriously affect the fetus. In these cases, clinicians should consult with either the radiotherapist or a qualified medical physicist to determine the total dose delivered to the embryo. If the conceptus absorbs 0.50 Sv (50 rem) or more at any time during gestation, there is a significant possibility of damage. If the dose absorbed during the early organogenetic period amounts to several hundred rem, there is a reasonable probability that the embryo will abort. As one proceeds into the second and third trimesters, the chance of abortion and malformations declines, but irreparable damage to the CNS can occur. The risk of 0.50–1.0 Gy (50–100 rad) acute external radiation from the 8th-15th weeks postconception presents a substantial risk for mental retardation to the surviving fetus (54, 59, 62).

For each radionuclide procedure, the dose

**Table 13.4.**
**Thyroidal Radioiodine Dose of the Fetus[a]**

| Gestation Period | Fetal/Maternal Ratio (thyroid gland) | Dose to Thyroid (fetus) (rad/uCi)[b] |
|---|---|---|
| 10–12 weeks | | 0.001 (precursors) |
| 12–13 weeks | 1.2 | 0.7 |
| 2nd trimester | 1.8 | 0.7 |
| 3rd trimester | 7.5 | |
| Birth imminent | | 8.0 |

[a]Data from Book S, Goldman M. Thyroidal radioiodine exposure of the fetus. Health Phys 1975;29:874–877.
[b]Dose of $^{131}$I ingested by mother.

**Table 13.5.**
**Risk of 0.5 Rem (5 mSv) (Maximum Permissible Exposure for Women Radiation Workers with Reproductive Potential)**

|  | 0 rem | Additional Risk of 0.5 rem (5 mSv) |
|---|---|---|
| Risk of spontaneous abortion | $150,000/10^6$ | 0 |
| Risk of major congenital malformations | $30,000/10^6$ | 0 |
| Risk of severe mental retardation | $5000/10^6$ | 0 |
| Risk of childhood malignancy/10-yr period | $7000/10^6/10$ yr | $166/10^6/10$yr (68) or $2.5/10^6/10$ yr ($ABCC^a$ data) |
| Risk of early- or late-onset genetic disease | $100,000/10^6$ | Risk in next generation is negligible |
| Total risk (using Stewart data) (68) | $285,700/10^6$ | $166/10^6$ (55–57) |
| Ratio of total risk to additional risk of radiation |  | 1721/1 |
| Total risk (using $ABCC^a$ data) | $285,700/10^6$ | $2.5/10^6$ $(ABCC)^a$ |
| Ratio of total risk to additional risk of radiation |  | 114,280/1 |

$^a$ABCC = Atomic Bomb Casualty Commission.

to the embryo must be calculated individually and is dependent on the form of the isotope, the site of administration, and the nature of the disease. Often, the embryonic dose will be less than the maternal dose, because the nature of the isotope preparation prevents its transfer across the placenta. Even when the fetal thyroid absorbs significant dosage (more than 50 mSv or 5 rem), the total fetal exposure may be quite low. In the majority of instances, the exposure will be too low to present a significant risk to the embryo (83).

When counseling patients concerning the risks of a particular exposure to radiation, the following information should be evaluated:

(a) Stage of pregnancy at the time of the exposure;
(b) Menstrual history;
(c) Previous pregnancy history;
(d) History of congenital malformations;
(e) Other potentially harmful environmental exposures during the pregnancy;
(f) Age of the pregnant woman and partner;
(g) For diagnostic or therapeutic radiation exposures: type of radiation procedure; dates and number of procedures performed;
(h) For other environmental or occupational radiation exposures: type and frequency of radiation exposure; results of personal dosimetry monitoring;

(i) Calculation of the embryonic exposure by a medical physicist or competent radiologist;
(j) Status of the pregnancy: wanted or unwanted.

In addition to the technical data on risk estimates, other factors may influence patient decisions including age, number of children in the family, the religious and ethnic background of the family, and the desirability of the pregnancy. A summary of essential information should be documented in the medical record. It is important to emphasize that the patient has been informed, that even normal pregnancy poses a significant risk of problems, and that a decision to continue the pregnancy does not mean that the counselor is guaranteeing a normal outcome.

## Protection from Ionizing Radiation

Minimization of exposure to ionizing radiation is the best way to prevent untoward health effects. In the medical care setting, the pregnancy status of patients should be known before any type of abdominal x-ray or radionuclide study is planned. Elective procedures should be delayed until the postpartum period. Conversely, essential radiological studies take priority over the small risks of diagnostic radiation to the embryo-fetus. When patients of reproductive age require high-dose therapeutic radiation, every effort should be made to achieve the desired treatment goal with the least impact on gonadal function. Appropriate shielding, limitation of treatment fields, and fractionated dosing are important protective measures. If permanent sterilization is an unavoidable possibility, patients can be offered the option of cryopreservation of germ cells or other in vitro technologies.

Apart from medical radiological procedures, ionizing radiation exposure of U.S. citizens and workers is regulated by a number of federal agencies (3). The Nuclear Regulatory Commission (NRC) licenses all users of radioactive source or byproduct materials, except for military applications by the Departments of Defense or Energy. Regulation of occupational exposures incurred during mining and milling operations is shared by the NRC and the Mine Safety and Health Administration (MSHA). The Occupational Safety and Health Administration (OSHA) is responsible for the protection of most other radiation workers, including those utilizing accelerators, x-ray systems, and other electronic products. Protection of the public falls primarily to the EPA (e.g., drinking water, discharges, air-borne emissions) and the NRC (e.g., releases from nuclear power plants).

Federal regulations governing radiation exposures are designed to prevent the occurrence of nonstochastic effects and to minimize the risks of stochastic effects. To accomplish these objectives, the 1987 radiation protection guidance (RPG) developed by the EPA for regulatory agencies (84) sets forth specific exposure limits while simultaneously emphasizing the ALARA principle, i.e., that exposures be kept "as low as reasonably achievable."

The current occupational limit for ionizing radiation exposure to the whole body is 50 mSv (5 rem)/yr. The RPG and NRC (85) also stipulate that the total dose to the embryo-fetus due to occupational exposure of a declared pregnant woman not exceed 5 mSv (500 mrem), with avoidance of substantial variations in dose rate. In keeping with this latter point, the National Council on Radiation Protection and Measurements (NCRP) (86) recommends that, once pregnancy is recognized, occupational exposure to the conceptus should not

exceed 0.5 mSv (50 mrem) in any one gestational month. In conferring a degree of protection during the prenatal period that exceeds that provided other workers, these measures have raised concerns about job discrimination against fertile or pregnant women (87).

The whole-body radiation limit for individual members of the general public is currently set by the 1960 RPG at 5 mSv (500 mrem)/yr, exclusive of medical exposures and natural background radiation. When individual doses are not measured, the RPG stipulates that average exposures should not exceed 1.7 mSv (170 mrem)/yr. Although not based on new findings of increased risk, recommendations have been made to lower the limit for the general public to 1 mSv (100 mrem) (86, 88) and to decrease the annual occupational limit to 20 mSv (2 rem) (88).

Occupational radiation protection requires an integrated approach involving worker education, environmental and personnel monitoring, and engineering controls. Common monitoring devices include pocket dosimeters and film or thermoluminescent badges. In many facilities, radiation safety officers are available to assist clinicians in the interpretation of workers' monitoring results.

Three key concepts govern radiation protection—time, distance, and shielding (32). For a point source of x-rays or γ rays, the exposure rate is inversely proportional to the square of the distance from the source (inverse square law); therefore, doubling the distance quarters the exposure. Examples of distance controls include the use of long-handled tongs to manipulate radioactive materials and minimizing the time spent at the immediate bedside of patients undergoing radiological procedures or treatments. The appropriate choice of shielding depends on the type and energy of the radiation involved. Electromagnetic ionizing radiation can be highly penetrating and requires high-density shielding materials such as concrete or lead. β-Radiation can be shielded by relatively lightweight materials such as plastic, aluminum, or thick rubber gloves (32). In occupational settings, measures to prevent internal deposition of radionuclides are similar to those used for toxic chemicals and include ventilation, enclosure of work processes, protective clothing and devices, and adequate hygiene practices.

## NONIONIZING RADIATION

Nonionizing radiation includes the portion of the electromagnetic spectrum where the energy of the emitted photons is insufficient to ionize atoms or molecules. As shown in Figure 13.1, the higher wave frequency (shorter wavelength) region of the nonionizing radiation spectrum includes ultraviolet, visible, and infrared light. Radiofrequency (RF) radiation occurs at wave frequencies between $0-3 \times 10^{12}$ hertz (Hz or cycles per second); radiofrequencies from $3 \times 10^{8}-3 \times 10^{11}$ Hz (300 MHz to 300 GHz) are called microwaves. RF radiation is used in telecommunications systems and in industrial operations such as welding of metals; processing of plywood and plastics; and drying of foods, veneers, paper, and other products. The low frequency (long wavelength) region of the electromagnetic spectrum includes 60 Hz, the frequency of electrical power transmission systems in the U.S. These low-frequency energies are usually referred to as "electromagnetic fields" rather than radiation per se.

While nonionizing radiation is incapable of ionization, the absorbed electromagnetic energy (except at very low frequencies) is dissipated primarily in the form of heat. Biological effects attributable to cellular heating are well-documented. Possible nonthermal biological responses (e.g., neuroendocrine effects, alteration of cell membrane ion fluxes) are currently under investigation (89).

Thermal effects induced by nonionizing radiation are influenced by a number of factors, including the strength of the electromagnetic field. The incident energy at the surface of the body or organ is termed the power density and is expressed in milliwatts per square centimeter ($mW/cm^2$). The specific absorption rate (SAR) is the rate of energy absorption per unit body mass and is expressed in watts per kilogram (W/kg) (90). Hazardous biological effects of RF radiation are associated with whole-body SARs greater than 4 W/kg (89, 90).

Heating efficiency is also influenced by the characteristics of the electromagnetic waves. Low-frequency (less than 15 MHz), long-wavelength (more than 20 m) radiation associated with power lines and television and radio transmissions pass through the body without giving up appreciate amounts of energy. Somewhat higher radiofrequencies, including those used in medical diathermy (27.5 MHz) and industrial heaters and sealers (approximately 10–40 MHz), penetrate and readily heat internal structures. Microwave ovens generate 2450–MHz waves that can produce hyperthermia above the 24 mW level with a penetration of several centimeters. Microwaves with frequencies greater than 10,000 MHz have little organ penetration but can cause significant hyperthermia at the skin surface (91).

The susceptibility of a specific tissue to heating depends on its water content, dielectric properties, and vascularity. Greater amounts of heat are produced in tissues with high water content (e.g., muscle) than in those with low water content (e.g., fat and bone). Environmental factors that promote or inhibit heat dissipation are also important modulating influences (92).

## Radiofrequency/Microwave Radiation

The eyes, testes, and the developing embryo are most vulnerable to the thermal effects of RF/microwave radiation. Chapter 16 reviews the effects of heat on spermatogenesis and embryogenesis; specific data regarding RF radiation-induced effects on reproduction have been reviewed by the EPA (93) and others (89, 91, 92). In general, experimental animal studies show a threshold for induction of birth defects at maternal core temperatures of 41–42°C. RF radiation is teratogenic at high SARs (greater than 15 W/kg) that approach lethal levels for pregnant animals. Specific absorption rates ≤10 W/kg appear to have no effect on organ weight, litter size, teratology, or growth. Fortunately, usual industrial and environmental exposures to RF radiation are well below thresholds for induction of developmental effects.

There is no conclusive evidence of genetic damage after RF radiation exposure (89, 93). One recent study of paternal occupational RF exposure found no association with teratogenesis (94). There is also no evidence to support induction of malignancy through prenatal exposure. RF/microwave radiation of sufficient intensity can damage the testes by thermal action. In experimental animals, temporary effects on sperm production are evident when radiation-induced testicular temperatures exceed 37°C, with permanent sterility induced over 45°C (93). Exposure of rats to microwave radiation at an SAR as low as 5.6 W/kg produced a temperature of 41°C and temporary infertility (95). There has been only one small case-control study of workers occupationally exposed to microwave radiation for a mean duration of 8 yr. Slight but statistically significant decreases were reported in sperm concentration, percent motile sperm, and proportion with normal morphology (96). Loss of libido was also claimed. In most cases, these conditions resolved by 3 months after cessation of exposure.

Based on a hazardous effect level of 4 W/kg, the NCRP (97) recommends an occupational exposure limit of one-tenth this level, or an SAR of 0.4 W/kg, for radiofrequencies between 300 kHz and 100 GHz. The limit is decreased to 0.08 W/kg for members of the general public. Complex new exposure limits were recently developed by the American National Standard Institute (ANSI)(90).

The best means of controlling exposure to RF/microwave radiation is through engineering measures. Thin metal shields or wire screens are 100% effective in shielding radiation from microwave ovens and other devices. Leakage can be avoided by installation of effective seals on door hinges and other vulnerable parts. Where leakage is a possibility in industrial settings, monitoring of personnel is recommended. Even if leakage does occur, the flux of electromagnetic waves is diminished in relation to the square root of the distance from the source. Potentially high RF areas in the general environment (e.g., the immediate vicinity of radar installations) should be fenced off and clearly designated as controlled access areas.

## Magnetic Resonance Imaging

There has been a dramatic revolution in diagnostic imaging in the past two decades with the introduction of computer tomography (CT scans), ultrasonography, and magnetic resonance imaging (MRI). While there is general consensus that ultrasound and MRI present less risk at diagnostic exposure levels than radiographic procedures, much less is known about the reproductive effects of these newer modalities.

MRI procedures utilize three forms of electromagnetic fields: static magnetic fields, time-varying (pulsed) magnetic fields, and signal-producing RF radiations. The patient is first placed in a very strong static magnetic field, which aligns the hydrogen nuclei of water and other nuclei with magnetic spin with the magnetic field to produce a net magnetic moment. The subject is then exposed to RF energy, which is absorbed by certain protons in the patient (depending on the magnetic field in specific areas and the RF frequency). When the RF frequency is turned off, the protons that were excited return to their ground state by radiating their absorbed RF energies; these are collated and reconstructed into an interpretable image (98).

Unlike the CT scan or diagnostic radiography, the embryo cannot be readily shielded during MRI. Thus, most MRI procedures involving examination of the torso of a pregnant woman will expose the embryo to a complex set of electromagnetic fields.

The bioeffects of low-frequency electromagnetic fields have been extensively studied over the last decade and were recently reviewed (99, 100). Reported in vitro effects that could theoretically influence embryonic development include loss of ionized calcium from nerve membranes, altered permeability of endothelial cells, alteration of the blood-brain barrier, interference with nerve conduction, and alterations in cell metabolism and proliferation.

Delgado et al. (101) found that pulsed magnetic fields (PMF) increased developmental abnormalities in chick embryos. In a multilaboratory replication of the Delgado experiments, both positive and negative findings were reported; the combined data showed a small but statistically significant increase in developmental alterations among PMF-exposed embryos vs. sham-exposed controls, when assessed at 48 hr postincubation. However, not all conditions were fully uniform among laboratories, and the investigators did not determine whether there were malformations or changes in survival at the time of hatching (102). Other studies revealed no differences between control embryos and those exposed to magnetic fields (103). Studies of mammalian embryos have also yielded conflicting results, with some investigators reporting small increases in resorptions or malformations after magnetic field exposure and others finding no effects (100). In these experiments, the biological effects observed are highly dependent on the frequency and intensity of the fields, as well as on other exposure characteristics (99, 100).

As explained previously, RF radiation can produce hyperthermia, which is the most likely explanation for its reproductive and teratogenic effects. However, RF energies used in MRI have a limited power deposition rate; it is estimated that the temperature of an exposed uterus will not rise more than $0.2°C$, which would have no biological effect on the developing embryo or fetus.

Few studies have assessed reproductive risks specific to MRI during pregnancy (104–107). Heinricks et al. (105, 107) exposed pregnant mice during early organogenesis to 0.35-tesla (T) static fields, a RF of 15 MHz, and the associated gradient magnetic field. There were no induced skeletal anomalies (the primary focus of the project). Significant reduction in length was reported after 16 hr of exposure at higher field strengths (2.3 T; RF 100 MHz). Studies that attempted to separate magnetic field effects from RF radiation suggest that the combination is more effective, but this is only a preliminary finding (105). Lengthy exposures over hours or days have little relevance to the usual utilization of MRI techniques in humans.

In line with U.S. Food and Drug Administration guidelines, current medical MRI scanners employ static magnetic fields with flux densities less than 2.5 T and time-varying magnetic fields of less than 3 T/sec. Whole-body RF SARs do not exceed 0.4 W/kg, and thermal effects are not to be expected.

There are sporadic reports of MRI use during known pregnancies for the evaluation of congenital malformations (108, 109). In 1987, a National Institutes of Health (NIH) Consensus Development Conference recommended that women in their first trimester of pregnancy avoid MRI procedures unless the clinical condition could not be managed utilizing other diagnostic techniques (110). However, the developing CNS is still sensitive to embryotoxic agents in the second trimester and, at that time, the fetal CNS has poor repairability.

In the case of ionizing radiation exposure during pregnancy, we have vast amounts of quantitative animal and human data on which to estimate the risk. Furthermore, we can usually estimate the embryonic exposure. With MRI exposure, we have limited and controversial animal data following long exposures and minimal ability to estimate exposure, except within broad ranges. There really are insufficient data for the clinician to perform an accurate risk-benefit analysis. With an inadvertent exposure in a wanted pregnancy, however, the present accumulated data would not warrant an interruption of pregnancy. More careful monitoring, counseling, and support of the patient are certainly appropriate.

## Ultrasound

The introduction of ultrasound technology has revolutionized the field of medicine and reduced the necessity for many x-ray examinations. Obstetric and gynecological ultrasounds account for over half of the ultrasound imaging volume in the U.S. (111).

Ultrasound is a form of mechanical energy that produces oscillations in an elastic medium (water, tissue) at frequencies above the threshold for human hearing (16,000–20,000 Hz). Reflection of sound energy by internal structures forms the basis of sonographic imaging techniques; however, some energy is also absorbed. The dose to a specific tissue depends on the ultrasound frequency, attenuation by intervening tissues, and the duration of exposure.

Most medical diagnostic applications of ultrasound utilize frequencies of 1–10 MHz at very low intensities $(0.0001–0.5 \text{ W/cm}^2)$ (112); 3.5–5.0 MHz is the usual frequency range for obstetric examinations. With pulse-echo ultrasound, exposure occurs only when the pulse is "on," which is a fraction of the total time necessary to perform a clinical examination. In contrast, therapeutic applications of ultrasound involve frequencies of 0.75–3.0 MHz intentionally delivered at power levels sufficient to cause tissue heating (113).

Ultrasound is also applied extensively in industry in cutting, welding, brazing, and other material processing operations, as well as in materials testing, measurement, and structural analysis. Ultrasound-induced cavitation (violent disruption of gas bubbles within a liquid) is exploited to accelerate mixing, cleaning, emulsification, and chemical reactions (113).

Biological effects are induced at ultrasound energies sufficient to cause hyperthermia or cavitation. Other nonthermal effects on cellular structure or function have been observed in in vitro systems, but their biological significance for humans is unknown (113). Fortunately, the low frequencies and brief exposure times used in obstetrical ultrasound procedures produce negligible tissue heating (112, 114). Even continuous fetal monitoring with Doppler devices does not cause appreciable temperature elevations (112). In mammals, the risk of occurrence of cavitation from exposure to ultrasound intensities and pulse durations characteristic of diagnostic sonography is apparently very low (115). Conversely, the intense cavitation produced in industrial cleaning tanks can be hazardous to areas of the worker's body in direct contact with the liquid medium (113).

## REPRODUCTIVE AND DEVELOPMENTAL EFFECTS

Studies of potential reproductive and developmental effects of ultrasound have been extensively reviewed (112, 113, 116–119). Diagnostic ultrasound energies do not appear to be mutagenic, and the majority of studies have not found increases in cytogenetic abnormalities (120). The American Institute of Ultrasound in Medicine identified over 300 reports addressing developmental effects (117). Most mammalian studies have involved exposure of rats or mice to energy levels far exceeding those used in medical diagnostics. Embryo lethality and teratogenic effects are noted at levels producing hyperthermia. The majority of low-intensity studies have not shown fetotoxic ef-

fects (118, 121); however, in two studies, exposure of mice to 1 MHz ultrasound at intensities of 0.5–5.5 W/cm$^2$ (122) or to 0.12 W/cm$^2$ continuous exposure (123) resulted in reduced birthweight and perinatal mortality, respectively. The latter intensity was closer to, but still exceeded, levels used in diagnostic procedures.

Human data accumulated over 25 yr reveal no consistent adverse effects from prenatal diagnostic ultrasound examinations (116, 119). Studies assessing malformations, birthweight, postnatal hearing deficits, and carcinogenesis have been uniformly negative. Lyons et al. (124) found no significant effect of in utero ultrasound exposure on height or weight at birth and up to 6 yr of age. Stark et al. (125) found no association between prenatal ultrasound exposure and a variety of indicators of neurological development, including IQ. A higher risk of dyslexia was observed among children exposed to ultrasound in utero than in unexposed groups. Possible confounding by birthweight makes interpretation of this finding problematic; however, the results warrant further research.

In some investigations, lower pregnancy rates occurred among women whose follicular development was monitored by ultrasound before donor insemination compared with unmonitored women (126, 127). However, in a recent investigation of women undergoing ovulation induction, Abdul-Karim et al. (128) found no effect of periovulatory ultrasound exposure on pregnancy rate or conceptus viability. Additional research in this area is also needed.

## RECOMMENDATIONS

Available animal and human data indicate that diagnostic exposure to ultrasound presents negligible risks to the developing embryo and that the benefits of indicated examinations far outweigh the risks (129). The practice of routine prenatal ultrasound screening remains controversial. In 1984, a National Institutes of Health (NIH) task force recommended prenatal ultrasound examinations only for specific medical indications (130). Although no studies have assessed effects of therapeutic ultrasound during gestation, the induced hyperthermia contraindicates its use.

The high-intensity ultrasound used in industrial operations is unlikely to produce adverse reproductive or developmental effects, as only a very small fraction of ultrasound energy passes from air to skin. High-power ultrasound in liquid media (e.g., cleaning tanks) allows for good acoustic coupling to the human body; however, only the upper extremities in contact with the liquid are at risk. In addition, effective screens are available to protect against occupational ultrasound exposure.

## SUMMARY

The term radiation evokes emotional responses both from lay persons and professionals, many of whom are unfamiliar with radiation biology or the quantitative nature of the risks. Frequently, microwave, magnetic fields, ultrasound, and ionizing radiation risks are confused.

Although it is impossible to prove the absence of risk for any environmental hazard, it appears that exposure to microwave radiation below maximal permissible levels presents no measurable risk to workers or to the embryo. Ultrasound exposure at usual diagnostic frequencies and intensities also appears quite innocuous. Continued surveillance and research into potential risks of these low-level exposures should continue; but, at present, ultrasound not only improves obstetric care but also reduces the necessity of diagnostic x-ray procedures.

The data with regard to the reproductive risks of MRI exposures in pregnant women are scant. There are minimal and conflicting animal data. With usual clinical exposures, we do not have enough information to infer that there is a substantial risk to the embryo. Wanted pregnancies should, therefore, be continued after inadvertent exposures.

Embryonic and fetal exposures to isotopes present variable risks, depending on the isotope and the exposure, and need to be individually assessed. The calculations and risk assessment are frequently quite complicated and should be performed by an appropriate expert.

In the field of ionizing radiation, we have better comprehension of the biological effects and the quantitative maximum risks than for any other environmental hazard. Impairment of spermatogenesis occurs at exposures of 0.1–0.15 Gy (10–15 rad); with the exception of high doses, recovery of testicular function usually occurs in time. Doses required to cause ovulatory dysfunction or sterility are age dependent. Accumulated data indicate that doses less than 5 rad do not increase the incidence of gross congenital malformations, growth retardation, or abortion; however, one cannot definitively exclude risks to the embryo at lower doses. Whether there exists a threshold exposure for genetic, carcinogenic, cell-depleting, and life-shortening effects has not been determined. Certainly, maximal risks attributed to low-dose exposures are thousands of times smaller than the spontaneous risks of malformations, abortion, or genetic disease.

Decisions regarding continuation of pregnancy after irradiation belong to the well-informed patient. There is no medical justification based on risk estimates for recommending termination of a wanted pregnancy in women exposed to 0.05 Gy (5 rad) or less of ionizing radiation.

Exposures to ionizing radiation in the workplace and environment should be kept as low as reasonably achievable through an integrated system of control measures. In the medical setting, judicious use of x-ray procedures is warranted, and presumably safer modalities such as ultrasound should be used whenever possible.

## REFERENCES

1. National Council on Radiation Protection and Measurements (NCRP). Ionizing radiation exposure of the population of the United States. NCRP report no. 93. Bethesda: NCRP, 1987.
2. National Council on Radiation Protection and Measurements (NCRP). Exposure to the population in the United States and Canada from natural background radiation. NCRP report no. 94. Bethesda: NCRP, 1987.
3. U.S. Environmental Protection Agency (EPA). Occupational exposure to ionizing radiation in the United States: 1985. Washington, DC: U.S. EPA, in press.
4. International Commission on Radiological Protection (ICRP). Recommendations of the international commission on radiological protection. ICRP publication no. 26. Oxford: Pergamon Press, 1977.
5. Meistrich ML, van Beek MEAB. Radiation sensitivity of the human testis. Adv Radiat Biol 1990;14:227–268.
6. Shapiro E, Kinsella TJ, Makuch RW, et al. Effects of fractionated irradiation on endocrine aspects of testicular function. J Clin Oncol 1985;3:1232–1239.

7. Delic JI, Henry JH, Morris ID, Shalet SM. Dose and time relationships in the endocrine response of the irradiated adult rat testis. J Androl 1986;7:32–41.

8. Meistrich ML. Critical components of testicular function and sensitivity to disruption. Biol Reprod 1986;34:17–28.

9. Jordan S, Hasegawa CM, Keehn RJ. Testicular changes in atomic bomb survivors. Arch Pathol 1966;82:542–554.

10. Rowley MJ, Leach DR, Warner GA, Heller CG. Effect of graded doses of ionizing radiation on the human testis. Radiat Res 1974;59:665–678.

11. Paulsen CA. The study of irradiation effects on the human testis including histologic, chromosomal and hormonal aspects. Terminal Report, Atomic Energy Commission contract no. AT(45–1–22–25), 1973.

12. Heller CG. Effects on the germinal epithelium. In: Langham WM, ed. Radiobiological factors in manned space flight: report of the Space Radiation Study Panel of the Life Sciences Committee. Washington, DC: National Academy of Sciences, 1967:134–133.

13. da Cunha MF, Meistrich ML, Fuller L, et al. Recovery of spermatogenesis after treatment for Hodgkin's disease: limiting dose of MOPP chemotherapy. J Clin Oncol 1984;2:571–577.

14. Popescu HI, Lancranjan I. Spermatogenesis alteration during protracted irradiation in man. Health Phys 1975;28:567–573.

15. Meistrich ML, Brown CC. Estimation of the increased risk of human infertility from alterations in semen characteristics. Fertil Steril 1983;40:220–230.

16. Sandeman TF. The effects of x-irradiation on male human fertility. Br J Radiol 1966;39:901–907.

17. MacLeod J, Hotchkiss RS, Sitterson BW. Recovery of male fertility after sterilization by nuclear radiation. JAMA 1964;187:637–641.

18. Baker TG. Radiosensitivity of mammalian oocytes with particular reference to the human female. Am J Obstet Gynecol 1971;110:746–761.

19. Baker TG. Effects of ionizing radiation on mammalian oogenesis: a model for chemical effects. In Dixon RL, ed: Reproductive toxicology. New York: Raven Press, 1985:21–34.

20. Baker TG. Comparative aspects of the effects of radiation during oogenesis. Mutat Res 1971;11:9–22.

21. Baker TG. The sensitivity of rat, monkey, and human oocytes to x-irradiation in organ culture. In: Sikov MR, Mahlum DD, eds. Radiation biology of the fetal and juvenile mammal. Washington, DC: U.S. Atomic Energy Commission, 1969:955–961.

22. Baker TG. The sensitivity of oocytes in post-natal rhesus monkeys to x-irradiation. J Reprod Fertil 1966;12:183–192.

23. Seigel D. Frequency of live births among survivors of the atomic bombs, Hiroshima and Nagasaki. Radiat Res 1966;28:278–288.

24. Blot WJ, Sawada H. Fertility among female survivors of the atomic bombs of Hiroshima and Nagasaki. Am J Hum Genet 1972;24:613–622.

25. Blot WJ, Shimizu Y, Kato H, Miller RW. Frequency of marriage and live birth among survivors prenatally exposed to the atomic bomb. Am J Epidemiol 1975;106:128–136.

26. Stillman RJ, Schinfield JS, Schiff I, et al. Ovarian failure in long-term survivors of childhood malignancy. Am J Obstet Gynecol 1981;139:62–66.

27. Byrne J, Mulvihill JJ, Myers MH, et al. Effects of treatment of fertility in long-term survivors of childhood or adolescent cancer. N Engl J Med 1987;317:1315–1321.

28. Byrne J, Fears TR, Gail MH, et al. Early menopause in long-term survivors of cancer during adolescence. Am J Obstet Gynecol 1992;166:788–793.

29. Lushbaugh CC, Casarett GW. The effects of gonadal irradiation in clinical radiation therapy: a review. Cancer 1976;37:1111–1120.

30. Ash P. The influence of radiation on fertility in man. Br J Radiol 1980;53:271–278.

31. Damewood MD, Grochow LB. Prospects for fertility after chemotherapy or radiation for neoplastic disease. Fertil Steril 1986;45:443–459.

32. Shapiro J. Radiation protection: a guide for scientists and physicians. 3rd ed. Cambridge: Harvard University Press, 1990.

33. United Nations Scientific Committee on the Effects of Atomic Radiation (UNSCEAR). Genetic effects of radiation. In: Ionizing radiation: sources and biological effects. Report A/41/16. New York: United Nations, 1986: Suppl 16:7–164.

34. National Research Council, Committee on the Biological Effects of Ionizing Radiations (BEIR). Health effects of exposure to low levels of ionizing radiation, BEIR V. Washington, DC: National Academy Press, 1990.

35. Abrahamson S. The genetic impact of low-level ionizing radiation: risk estimates for first and subsequent generations. In: National Council on Radiation Protection and Measurements (NCRP). Some issues important in developing basic radiation protection recommendations. Bethesda: NCRP, 1987:89–102.

36. Searle T. Radiation—the genetic risk. Trends Genet 1987;3:152–157.

37. Russell WL, Russell LB, Kelly EM. Radiation dose rate and mutation frequency. Science 1958;128:1546–1550.

38. Neel JV, Lewis SB. The comparative radiation genetics of humans and mice. Annu Rev Genet 1990;24:327–362.

39. Neel JV, Schull WJ, Awa AA, et al. The children of parents exposed to atomic bombs: estimates of the genetic doubling dose of radiation for humans. Am J Hum Genet 1990;46:1053–1072.

40. Gardner MJ, Snee MP, Hall AJ, et al. Results of case-control study of leukemia and lymphoma among young people near Sellafield nuclear plant in West Cumbria. Br Med J 1990;300:423–429.

41. Yoshimoto Y, Neel JV, Schull WJ, et al. Malignant tumors during the first 2 decades of life in the offspring of atomic bomb survivors. Am J Hum Genet 1990;46:1041–1052.

42. Russell WL. Factors that affect the radiation induction of mutations in the mouse. An Acad Brasillira de Ciencias 1967;39:65–75.

43. Brent RL. Irradiation in pregnancy. In: Sciarra JJ, ed. Davis' Gynecology and Obstetrics, vol 2. New York: Harper & Row 1972:1–32.

44. Brent RL. Radiations and other physical agents. In: Wilson JG, Fraser FC, eds. Handbook of teratology, vol 1. New York: Plenum Press, 1977;153–223.

45. Brent RL. Radiation teratogenesis. Teratology 1980;21:281–298.

46. Brent RL, Borden BT. The indirect effect of irradiation of embryonic development. III. The contribution of ovarian irradiation, oviduct irradiation, and zygote irradiation to fetal mortality and growth retardation in the rat. Radiat Res 1967;30:759–773.

47. Russell LB, Russell WL. The effects of radiation on the preimplantation stages of the mouse embryo. Anat Rec 1950;108:521.

48. Russell LB, Russell WL. An analysis of the changing radiation response of the developing mouse embryo. J Cell Comp Physiol 1954;43:103–149.

49. Russell LB, Saylors CL. The relative sensitivity of various germ-cell stages of the mouse to radiation-induced nondysfunction, chromosome losses and deficiencies. In: Sobels FH, ed. Repair from genetic radiation. New York: Pergamon Press, 1963:313–332.

50. Brent RL, Bolden BT. The long–term effects of low-dosage embryonic irradiation. Radiat Res 1961;14:453–454.

51. Goldstein L, Murphy DP. Microcephalic idiocy following radium therapy for uterine cancer during pregnancy. Am J Obstet Gynecol 1929;18:189–195, 281–283.

52. Goldstein L, Murphy DPL. Etiology of ill health in children born after maternal pelvic irradiation. II. Defective children born after postconceptional maternal irradiation. Am J Roentgenol 1929;22:322–331.

53. Murphy DP, Goldstein L. Micromelia in a child irradiated in utero. Surg Gynecol Obstet 1930;40:79–80.

54. Dekaban AS. Abnormalities in children exposed to x-irradiation during various stages of gestation: tentative timetable of radiation injury to the human fetus. J Nucl Med 1968;9:471–477.

55. Miller RW. Delayed radiation effects in atomic bomb survivors. Science 1969;166:569–574.

56. Wood JW, Johnson KG, Omori Y. In utero exposure to Hiroshima atomic bomb. An evaluation of head size and mental retardation-twenty years later. Pediatrics 1967;39:385–392.

57. Wood J, Johnson K, Omori Y, et al. Mental retardation in children exposed in utero to the atomic bomb in Hiroshima and Nagasaki. Am J Public Health 1967;57:1381–1390.

58. Plummer G. Anomalies occurring in children exposed in utero to the atomic bomb in Hiroshima. Pediatrics 1952;10:687–692.

59. Yamazaki J, Wright S, Wright P. Outcome of pregnancy in women exposed to the atomic bomb in Nagasaki. Am J Dis Child 1954;87:448–463.

60. Blot W. Growth and development following prenatal and childhood exposure to atomic radiation. J Radiat Res 1975;16(suppl):82–88.

61. Blot WJ, Miller RW. Mental retardation following in utero exposure to the atomic bombs of Hiroshima and Nagasaki. Radiology 1973;106:617–619.

62. Yamazaki JN, Schull WJ. Perinatal loss and neurological abnormalities among children of the atomic bomb: Na-gasaki and Hiroshima revisited, 1949 to 1989. JAMA 1990;264:605–609.

63. Dunn K, Yoshimaru H, Otaki M, Annegers JF, Schull WJ. Prenatal exposure to ionizing radiation and subsequent development of seizures. Am J Epidemiol 1990;131:114–123.

64. Miller RW. Effects of prenatal exposure to ionizing radiation. Health Phys 1990; 59:57–61.

65. Kinlen LJ, Acheson FD. Diagnostic irradiation, congenital malformations, and spontaneous abortion. Br J Radiol 1968;41:648–654.

66. Tabuchi A. Fetal disorders due to ionizing radiation. Hiroshima J Med Sci 1964;13:125–173.

67. Jacobsen L, Mellemgaard L. Anomalies of the eyes in descendants of women irradiated with small x-ray loses during age of fertility. Acta Ophthalmol (Copenh) 1968;46:352–54.

68. Stewart A, Webb D, Hewitt D. A survey of childhood malignancies. Br Med J 1958;1:1495–1508.

69. Kneale GW, Stewart AM. Prenatal x-rays and cancers: further tests of data from the Oxford survey of childhood cancers. Health Phys 1986;51:369–376.

70. Gilman EA, Kneale GW, Knox EG, Stewart AM. Pregnancy x-rays and childhood cancers: effects of exposure age and radiation dose. Radiol Prot 1988;8:3–8.

71. Lilienfield AM. Epidemiological studies of the leukemogenic effects of radiation. Yale J Biol Med 1966;39:143–164.

72. Diamond EL, Schmerler H, Lilienfield AM. The relationship of intrauterine radiation to subsequent mortality and development of leukemia in children: a prospective study. Am J Epidemiol 1973;97:283–313.

73. Monson RR, MacMahon B. Prenatal x-ray exposure and cancer in children. In: Boice JD Jr, Fraumeni JF Jr, eds. Radiation carcinogenesis: epidemiology and biological significance. New York: Raven Press, 1984:97–105.

74. Harvey EB, Boice JD Jr, Honeyman M, Fannery JT. Prenatal x-ray exposure and childhood cancer in twins. N Engl J Med 1985;312:541–545.

75. Stjernfeldt M, Berglund K, Lindsten J, Ludvigsson J. Maternal smoking during pregnancy and risk of childhood cancer. Lancet 1986;1:1350–1352.

76. Daling JR, Starzyk P, Olshan AF, Weiss NS. Birthweight and incidence of childhood leukemia. J Natl Cancer Inst 1984;72:1039–1041.

77. Kato H. Mortality in children exposed to the A-bombs while in utero. Am J Epidemiol 1971;93:435–442.

78. Yoshimoto Y. Cancer risk among children of atomic bomb survivors: a review of RERF epidemiologic studies. JAMA 1990;264:596–600.

79. Upton AC, Odell TT JR, Sniffen EP. Influence of age at time of irradiation on induction of leukemia and ovarian tumors in RF mice. Proc Soc Exp Biol Med 1960;104:769–772.

80. National Council on Radiation Protection and Measurements (NCRP).Exposure of the U.S. population from diagnostic medical radiation. NCRP report no. 100. Bethesda: NCRP, 1989.

81. Book S, Goldman M. Thyroidal radioiodine exposure of the fetus. Health Phys 1975;29:874–877.

82. Sikov MR, Noonon TR. Anomalous development induced

duced in embryonic rat by the maternal administration of radiophosphorus. Am J Anat 1958;103:137–162.

83. Brent RL. The effects of ionizing radiation, microwaves and ultrasound in the developing embryo: clinical interpretations and applications of the data, vol. 14. In: Lockhart JC, ed. Current problems in pediatrics. Chicago: Year Book Medical Publishers, 1984:1–87.

84. U.S. Environmental Protection Agency. Federal radiation protection guidance for occupational exposures. Fed Reg 1987;52:2822–2834.

85. Nuclear Regulatory Commission. Final rule. Standards for protection against radiation. 10 CFR Part 20, 1991.

86. National Council on Radiation Protection and Measurements (NCRP). Recommendations on limits for exposure to ionizing radiation. NCRP report no. 91. Bethesda: NCRP, 1987.

87. Martins BI. NRC, NCRP, ICRP and recommendations on prenatal radiation exposure [Letter]. Health Phys 1989;56:572–573.

88. International Commission on Radiological Protection (ICRP). 1990 recommendations of the International Commission on Radiological Protection. Ann ICRP 1991;21:1–201.

89. Michaelson SM. Biological effects of radiofrequency radiation: concepts and criteria. Health Phys 1991;61:3–14.

90. Peterson RC. Radiofrequency/microwave protection guides. Health Phys 1991;61:59–67.

91. Brent RL. The effects of embryonic and fetal exposure to x-ray, microwaves and ultrasound. Clin Obstet Gynecol 1983;26:484–510.

92. Wilkening GM, Sutton CH. Health effects of non-ionizing radiation. Med Clin North Am 1990;74:489–507.

93. Elder JA, Cahill DF. Biological effects of radiofrequency radiation. Report no. EPA-600/8–83–026F. Research Triangle Park, NC: Environmental Protection Agency, 1984.

94. Logue JN, Hamburger S, Silverman PM, Chiacchierini RP. Congenital anomalies and paternal occupational exposure to shortwave, microwave, infrared, and acoustic radiation. J Occup Med 1985;27:451–452.

95. Berman E, Carter HB, House D. Tests of mutagenesis and reproduction in male rats exposed to 2450 MHz (CW) microwaves. Bioelectromagnetics 1980;1:65–76.

96. Lancranjan I, et al. Gonadic function in workmen with long-term exposure to microwaves. Health Phys 1975;29:381–383.

97. National Council on Radiation Protection and Measurements (NCRP). Biological effects and exposure criteria for radiofrequency electromagnetic fields. NCRP report no. 86. Bethesda: NCRP, 1986.

98. Bottomly PA. NMR imaging techniques and applications: a review. Rev Sci Instrum 1982;53:1319–1337.

99. Anderson LE. ELF: exposure levels, bioeffects, and epidemiology. Health Phys 1991;61:41–46.

100. Juutilainen J. Effects of low frequency magnetic fields on embryonic development and pregnancy. Scand J Work Environ Health 1991;17:149–158.

101. Delgado JMR, Monteagudo JL, Garcia MQ, et al. Teratogenic effects of weak magnetic fields. IRCS Med Sci 1981;9:392.

102. Berman E, Chacon L, House D, et al. Development of chick embryos in a pulsed magnetic field. Bioelectromagnetics 1990;11:169–187.

103. Maffeo S, Brayman AA, Miller MW, et al. Weak low frequency electromagnetic fields and chick embryogenesis: failure to reproduce positive findings. J Anat 1988;157:101–104.

104. Marx JL. Imaging technique passes muster. Science 1987;238:888–889.

105. Heinricks WL, Heinricks S, Flannery M, et al. Magnetic resonance spectroscopy (MRS): embryotoxicity in balb/c pregnant mice [Abstract]. Presented at the Society for Gynecologic Investigation 33rd Annual Meeting, Toronto, 1986.

106. Foster MA, Knight CH, Rimmington JE, et al. Fetal imaging by nuclear magnetic resonance: a study in goats. Radiology 1983;149:193–195.

107. Heinricks WL, Fong P, Flannery M, et al. Midgestational exposure of pregnant balb/c mice to magnetic resonance imaging conditions. Magn Reson Imaging 1988;6:305–313.

108. Smith FW, MacLennan F. NMR imaging in human pregnancy: a preliminary study. Magn Reson Imaging 1984;2:57–64.

109. Turner RJ, Hankins GDV, Weinreb JC, et al. Magnetic resonance imaging and ultrasonography in the antenatal evaluation of conjoined twins. Am J Obstet Gynecol 1986;155:645–649.

110. National Institute of Child Health and Human Development. Antenatal diagnosis: report of a consensus development conference. NIH publication no. 79–1973. Bethesda: National Institute of Health, 1979.

111. Johnson JL, Abernathy DL. Diagnostic imaging procedure volume in the United States. Radiology 1983; 146:851–854.

112. National Council on Radiation Protection and Measurements (NCRP). Biological effects of ultrasound: mechanisms and clinical implications. NCRP report no. 74. Bethesda: NCRP, 1983.

113. Hill CR, ter Harr G. Ultrasound. In: Suess MJ, ed. Nonionizing radiation protection. Copenhagen: World Health Organization, 1982:199–228.

114. Soothill PW, Nicolaides KH, Rodeck CH, Campbell S. Amniotic fluid and fetal tissues are not heated by obstetric ultrasound scanning. Br J Obstet Gynaecol 1987;94:675–677.

115. Carstensen EL. Acoustic cavitation and the safety of diagnostic ultrasound. Ultrasound Med Biol 1987; 13:597–606.

116. Reece EA, Assimakapoulos E, Xue-Zhong Z, Hagry Z, Hobbins JC. The safety of obstetric ultrasonography: concern for the fetus. Obstet Gynecol 1990;76:139–146.

117. Sikov MR. Report of the Bioeffects Committee of the American Institute of Ultrasound in Medicine. Effect of ultrasound on development. Part 1: introduction and studies in inframammalian species. J Ultrasound Med 1986;5:577–583.

118. Sikov MR. Report of the Bioeffects Committee of the American Institute of Ultrasound in Medicine. Effect of ultrasound on development. Part 2: studies in mamma-

lian species and overview. Ultrasound Med 1986; 5:651–661.

119. Ziskin MC, Petitti DB. Epidemiology of human exposure to ultrasound: a critical review. Ultrasound Med Biol 1988;14:91–96.

120. Miller MW. Does ultrasound induce sister chromatid exchanges? Ultrasound Med Biol 1985;11:561–570.

121. Carstensen EL, Gates AH. The effects of ultrasound on the fetus. J Ultrasound Med 1984;3:145–147.

122. O'Brien WD Jr. Dose-dependent effect of ultrasound on fetal weight in mice. J Ultrasound Med 1983;2:1–8.

123. Curto KA. Early postpartum mortality following ultrasound radiation. In: White D, Barnes R, eds. Ultrasound in medicine, vol. 2. New York: Plenum Press, 1975:529–530.

124. Lyons EA, Dyke C, Toms M, Cheang M, Math M. In utero exposure to diagnostic ultrasound: a 6-year follow-up. Radiology 1988;166:687–690.

125. Stark CR, Orleans M, Haverkamp AD, Murphy J. Short and long term risks after exposure to diagnostic ul-trasound in utero. Obstet Gynecol 1984;63:194–200.

126. Williams SR, Rothschild I, Wesolowski D, Austin C, Speroff L. Does exposure of preovulatory oocytes to ultrasonic radiation affect reproductive performance? J in Vitro Fert Embryo Transf 1988;5:18–21.

127. Demoulin A, Bologne R, Hustin J, Lambotte R. Is ultrasound monitoring of follicular growth harmless? Ann NY Acad Sci 1985;442:146–152.

128. Abdul-Karim RW, Terry FM, Badawy SZA, Sheehe PR. Effect of ultrasound monitoring of follicular growth on the conception rate. J Reprod Med 1990;35:147–151.

129. Brent RL, Jensh RP, Beckman DA. Medical sonography: reproductive effects and risks. Teratology 1991;44:123–146.

130. U.S. Department of Health and Human Services, Public Health Service, National Institutes of Health: Diagnostic ultrasound imaging in pregnancy. NIH publication no. 84–667. Washington, DC: US Government Printing Office, 1984.

# Video Display Terminals

## MAUREEN PAUL

Reports of adverse pregnancy outcomes among users of video display terminals (VDTs) have captured considerable media attention over the last decade and prompted research efforts and legislative initiatives to protect pregnant women from exposure to VDTs. With millions of VDTs in use in U.S. workplaces, clinicians caring for women during pregnancy undoubtedly encounter frequent questions about the safety of these devices. Should I decrease my hours of VDT use or transfer from the job altogether? Is it true that I am exposed to radiation from these machines? Is there anything I can do to minimize my risk during pregnancy? The purpose of this chapter is to help clinicians answer these common questions through a review of accumulated data on VDTs and pregnancy and provision of reasonable recommendations regarding VDT use.

## WHAT IS A VIDEO DISPLAY TERMINAL?

A VDT is simply a computer that most commonly uses a cathode ray tube (CRT) to display written information. The CRT of a VDT is similar to a vacuum tube used in a television set. The basic function of the CRT is to generate a beam of electrons that impinges on a phosphor-coated screen, converting the energy of the moving electrons into light.

As shown in Figure 14.1, operation of a CRT depends on a number of important components (1). Electrons are emitted by a cath-ode at the rear of the tube. A series of anodes creates an intense electric field that accelerates and focuses the electron beam. Magnetic coils arranged outside of the tube are called "deflection devices." When electric current flows through the coils, magnetic fields are induced that move the beam up and down the screen (vertical deflection) or across it (horizontal deflection). The flyback transformer is the source of electric current to the horizontal deflection system, the term "flyback" referring to the rapid return of a beam that has reached the far right of the screen back to the left margin. The CRT screen is coated with fluorescent material known as "phosphor." When electrons strike the phosphor, their kinetic energy is transformed primarily into visible light. Finally, the screen is encased in a glass envelope that contains a shielding material such as lead oxide.

## ARE THERE RADIATION HAZARDS ASSOCIATED WITH VDTs?

VDTs are potential sources of ionizing and nonionizing radiations (Chapter 13). In terms of possible reproductive effects, the emissions that are of greatest interest include x-rays and low frequency electromagnetic fields.

### X-rays

X-rays are produced when the fast-moving electrons suddenly decelerate as they strike the inside of the fluorescent screen. This ionizing

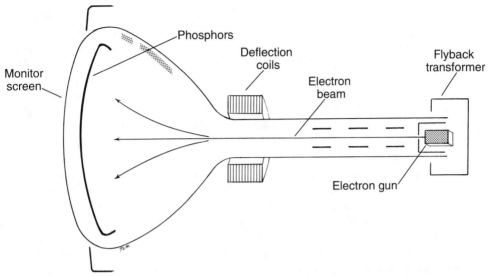

**Figure 14.1.** Basic components of a video display terminal. See text for details.

radiation is almost completely absorbed by the glass envelope of the CRT. Measurements of x-ray emissions from thousands of VDT units throughout the world have been indistinguishable from background levels and well below occupational exposure limits (1). Under low background conditions, Pomroy and Noel (2) found that exposure rates of emitted radiation from several VDT models were below $3 \times 10^{-9}$ Roentgens (R) per hour, providing an annual dose equivalent to the gonads of less than 0.0015 millirems (mrem). This dose equivalent is markedly below that received from other natural background sources of radiation. Hirning and Aitken (3) estimated the total first trimester x-ray dose to the fetus from a hypothetical VDT emitting radiation at the maximum allowable exposure rate for electronic products (0.5 mR/hr) to be 6 mrad. The recommended occupational limit for during pregnancy is 500 mrad. The few VDTs that were found to emit x-rays exceeding regulatory limits were withdrawn from the market over 10 yr ago (4).

In light of these considerations, clinicians can assure their patients that x-ray emissions from VDTs do not pose a health hazard during pregnancy. Use of a lead apron is not warranted. Because aging of machines is not expected to affect radiation emissions, it is not necessary to test x-ray emissions periodically from VDTs that meet government regulations (5).

## Low Frequency Electromagnetic Fields

Very low radiofrequency (VLF) fields in the principal frequency range of 15–22 kilohertz (kHz) are emitted by the flyback transformer and horizontal deflection coil. The vertical deflector system is the main source of extremely low frequency (ELF) fields ranging from approximately 45–80 Hz; 50- or 60-Hz fields also originate from the transformer that powers the machine. All electrical or electronic devices produce electromagnetic fields at these ELF powerline (50 or 60 Hz) frequencies. However, unlike the continuous fields characteristic of most electrical devices, VDTs produce primarily pulsed (time-varying) VLF and ELF fields (1).

Testing of emissions from VDTs involves separate measurements of the electric and magnetic field components. Field strength significantly decreases with distance from the machine. While measurements taken at 30 cm from the screen have traditionally been considered representative of an operator's exposure, most VDT users sit approximately 50 cm from their screens, where field exposures are lower (6). VLF emissions have been measured for numerous VDT models, while ELF testing has been more limited.

In the VLF range, typical electric field strengths at 30 cm in front of the screen range from nondetectable to 5 volts/meter (V/m); magnetic field strengths are generally below 100 milliamperes/meter (mA/m) (1, 5, 6). Measurements of VLF electric and magnetic field strengths at the same distance from the flyback transformer (toward the rear of units) may be as high as 150 V/m and over 1000 mA/m, respectively (5, 7). While the frontal emissions are well within recommended limits, exposure to an operator sitting close to the back or sides of an adjacent machine may exceed these limits.

In the ELF range, reported values 30 cm in front of VDT screens range from 1–10 V/m for the electric field and 30–600 mA/m for the magnetic field (5, 6). There are no established occupational limits for exposure to ELF electromagnetic fields. However, measured ELF emissions in front of VDTs are similar to ambient levels found in homes and laboratories (typically 1–10 V/m and 10–1000 mA/m); they are weaker than fields emanating from many common household appliances, although these household exposures are usually of short duration (5, 6).

For many years, it was believed that weak pulsed electromagnetic fields were incapable of producing adverse developmental effects. Then, in 1982, Delgado and colleagues (8) observed a marked increase in malformation rates in chick embryos exposed to low levels of pulsed magnetic fields (PMFs). In a well-controlled, multilaboratory replication of the Delgado experiments known as the Henhouse Project, chick malformation rates were increased in five of six laboratories but reached statistical significance in only two laboratories. When the data from all six laboratories were pooled, the difference in the incidence of abnormalities was small, but highly statistically significant (9). Not all studies have been positive, but accumulated data suggest that low frequency magnetic fields can affect avian development, at least under some experimental conditions (10). However, the relevance of the chick embryo as a model for human development is questionable, and few experiments used the sawtooth-shaped magnetic pulses characteristic of VDT emissions. Laboratory studies of rodents exposed during pregnancy to low frequency sawtooth magnetic fields have yielded conflicting results. Some show increased rates of resorption or malformations, while others are negative (6, 10, 11).

The contention that PMFs may affect development in animals is supported by in vitro research that demonstrates effects of PMFs on cell function including increased rates of cell proliferation, effects on membrane signal transduction, and altered synthesis of protein and essential macromolecules (12, 13). In addition, limited epidemiological data suggest that residential exposure to powerline frequency magnetic fields may increase the risk for childhood cancer (14, 15) and that there may be a seasonal pattern of fetal loss among women using electrically heated beds (16). While these latter studies involve continuous fields of different intensities than the predominant emissions from VDTs, they contribute to a growing body of evidence that electromagnetic fields may exert biological effects. Certainly, more experimental work is needed in this important area, particularly regarding the relevant exposure parameters and biological mechanisms of action.

Until more definitive information is available, it is prudent for workers to limit unnecessary exposure to electromagnetic fields. Because the strength of these fields drops off considerably with distance from the source and the strongest fields are emitted from the rear of a VDT machine, sitting 50 cm from the screen and not closer than 1 m from the back or sides of adjacent machines effectively accomplishes this goal (5).

## DO VDTs CAUSE ADVERSE PREGNANCY OUTCOMES?

### Cluster Reports: Initial Concern

Public concern about possible hazards to pregnancy from VDT use first arose in 1980 when offices of the *Toronto Star* reported that four of seven pregnant women who had used VDTs delivered infants with dissimilar congenital defects. Subsequently, numerous other small "clusters" of spontaneous abortions or birth defects were reported among VDT operators in North America and Europe (17).

A cluster is an aggregation of untoward health events that occurs close together in space and/or time. Clusters are extremely anxiety producing. However, due to small sample sizes and other methodological problems, investigations of clusters often raise more questions than they answer.

Most VDT-prompted cluster investigations have confirmed abnormally high incidences of miscarriages or birth defects among small populations of office workers, but none have specifically incriminated VDTs. Furthermore, given the relatively high frequency of spontaneous abortion in the general population and the millions of women workers using VDTs, the random occurrence of clusters would not be unusual (17). Concern about these clusters, however, generated more than a decade of epidemiological research into the potential pregnancy hazards of VDTs.

## Epidemiological Studies of VDTs and Pregnancy Outcome

### METHODOLOGICAL CONSIDERATIONS

Marcus (18) has recently reviewed a number of important methodological issues pertinent to the study of VDTs and pregnancy outcome. Foremost among these is the definition of exposure, i.e., what is it about VDT work that might induce miscarriage or birth defects? Three factors have been postulated: electromagnetic radiation emissions, psychosocial stress, and ergonomic factors related to prolonged stationary postures. Unfortunately, most epidemiological studies to date have ascertained exposure to VDTs by hours of use but have failed to measure these three variables specifically. This omission can result in misclassification of exposure. For example, if stress is the "true" exposure related to adverse pregnancy outcome and subjects instead are grouped according to use or nonuse of VDTs, the "VDT-exposed" group will likely include some women with low stress levels (truly unexposed) and the "VDT-unexposed" group will include some highly stressed workers (truly exposed). As long as this misclassification is random (e.g., absent a bias that selects most of the highly stressed women into the VDT-exposed group), the result is an underestimation of risk. In other words, this type of error decreases the ability to detect a true association between use of VDTs and pregnancy outcome.

Negative results of studies that define exposure according to VDT use should, therefore, be viewed with caution.

Marcus also identifies two types of bias that should be carefully addressed in these studies: recall bias and diagnostic bias. Many of the studies assessing the reproductive effects of VDTs are of the case-control design. In these studies, recall bias occurs if women with adverse pregnancy outcomes recall their hours of VDT use "better" than women who had normal births. The effect of this bias is to elevate the risk of VDT use falsely, so that it is important to consider this bias whenever a positive association is found in a case-control investigation. Diagnostic bias occurs when there is a difference in the gestational age at which pregnancy is diagnosed between VDT users and nonusers. If pregnancy is diagnosed earlier in VDT users, there is greater opportunity for spontaneous abortion to occur, leading to increased miscarriage rates among users as compared with nonusers.

Confounding is an important consideration in all epidemiological studies. A confounder is a variable related to the exposure of interest, and it is also an independent cause or correlate of the health outcome under study. For example, maternal age is a significant risk factor for spontaneous abortion and may also be independently related to VDT use. Failure to control for confounders may lead to erroneous conclusions about the cause of an adverse outcome. Fortunately, most VDT-reproduction studies have controlled for known confounders.

With millions of women using VDTs throughout the world, even a small increase in risk of an adverse pregnancy event would have enormous public health significance. However, detection of a small increase in risk requires very large population sizes. For example, in a prospective cohort study, at least 22,000 subjects would be required to detect a 10% increased risk of clinically recognized miscarriages among VDT users (19). The required sample size would be far greater for detection of total major malformations and would be quite infeasible for any one specific malformation, given the rare occurrence of specific defects in the general population. These statistical considerations make it unlikely that a human epidemiological study will ever be designed that unequivocally disproves a small effect of VDT use on pregnancy outcome (19).

## SPECIFIC EPIDEMIOLOGICAL STUDIES

There are a number of published epidemiological studies assessing the association between VDT use and pregnancy outcome. As mentioned above, many of these are case-control studies. In a case-control investigation, subjects are grouped according to outcome (e.g., cases = women who spontaneously aborted; controls = women with livebirths), and data are gathered about the exposure of interest (e.g, hours of VDT use) and potential confounding variables. The odds ratio compares the frequency of VDT use among cases as compared with controls. Other studies are historical cohort investigations. With this study design, historical data are used to categorize women by VDT exposure and to assess their subsequent birth outcomes. A relative risk is calculated that compares the frequency of the abnormal outcome of interest in the exposed group with the frequency in the unexposed group.

Kurppa and colleagues (20) in Finland used population-based registry data to study the association between VDT use and congenital anomalies. Cases were women who delivered infants with congenital malformations; controls were women who delivered liveborn infants without malformations, matched for time of delivery and health care district. Subjects were interviewed shortly after delivery about their general work conditions during pregnancy, although no specific questions were asked about VDT use. An industrial hygienist and two occupational health experts used occupational title and interview data to estimate potential exposure to VDTs. Logistical regression methods were used to control for important confounders. The adjusted odds ratio for all malformations pooled was 0.9 (C.I. 0.6–1.3) when women with first-trimester VDT use were compared to women not exposed. The elevated odds ratio of 1.6 (0.7–3.9) for cardiovascular defects was not statistically significant, although the sample size was too small to assess risks for specific anomalies adequately. The

authors concluded that their study did not support a teratogenic risk for operators of VDTs.

McDonald et al. (21) extracted data from a large Montreal survey of work in pregnancy to design a case-control study of the VDT question. The study design is explained in detail in Chapter 15. Briefly, over 56,000 women were interviewed about present and past pregnancies and about their work conditions during gestation. Women employed at least 30 hr/week during pregnancy were asked about hours of VDT use. In an individual analysis, the observed number of spontaneous abortions for women with different degrees of VDT use was compared with the number expected based on all working women (O/E ratio). Separate analyses were performed for present and past pregnancies and for year of conception, because VDT use increased each year. In a subsequent grouped analysis to control for recall and diagnostic bias better, the researchers compared O/E ratios for spontaneous abortion in 42 occupational groupings categorized according to the percentage of pregnant women who used VDTs for 15 or more hr/week. Variables controlled in the analyses included maternal age, number of prior miscarriages, and smoking.

There was no evidence of an association between spontaneous abortion and VDT use in previous pregnancies for any year of conception. In current pregnancies, only women with intermediate use of VDTs (7–29 hr/week) had a statistically significant increase in the O/E ratio (O/E = 1.25; CI 1.07–1.46). Ratios were similar in the occupational groupings despite wide ranges in VDT use. Recall bias is a likely explanation for the findings in current pregnancies, because nonusers of VDTs had a lower risk of spontaneous abortion than all working women (suggesting under-reporting of VDT use after a normal birth), and the only significant increased risk was noted among part-time, not full-time, users. McDonald and colleagues also assessed the relationship between use or nonuse of VDTs and congenital malformations in this study. No increased rate of defects was noted among VDT users, either for total malformations or for specific types of anomalies.

In a historical cohort study using Swedish national registry data, Ericson and Kallen (22) studied pregnancy outcomes among three cohorts of white collar workers classified by occupational title into high, medium, and low probabilities of VDT use. Observed rates of hospitalized spontaneous abortions and significant malformations were compared with expected frequencies based on national rates adjusted for maternal age (for both outcomes) and parity and delivery unit (for malformations). There was no statistically significant increase in either outcome for women in the highest exposure group.

To explore the possibility that the negative findings were due to misclassification of exposure, these same researchers designed a case-control study within the three cohorts of women (23). Cases were defined as women with pregnancies occurring in 1980–1981 that resulted in hospitalized spontaneous abortion or "birth defects" (defined as perinatal deaths, severe malformations, or birthweight less than 1500 g). Controls were women with pregnancies absent these characteristics. Information about hours of VDT use, other occupational exposures, and smoking during pregnancy was collected by mailed questionnaire. The overall response rate was 93%. There was no significant association between work with VDTs more than 20 hr/week and spontaneous abortion. For their broadly defined birth defects category, the crude odds ratio was 2.0 (CI = 1.2–3.2) for VDT exposure over 10 hr/week and 2.3 (CI = 1.4–3.9) for exposure over 20 hr/week. As stress and smoking were strongly linked to VDT work in this study, the effect of VDT use on all adverse outcomes combined (spontaneous abortion and "birth defects") was analyzed after stratification for these potential confounders. The crude odds ratio of 1.4 (CI = 1.1–1.8) associated with VDT work of more than 10 hr/week decreased to 1.2 (CI = 0.6–2.3) and became statistically nonsignificant after stratification for stress and smoking. The authors suggest that recall bias played a role in this study, since chemical exposures unlikely to cause embryofetal toxicity (e.g., handling self-copying paper) were reported more often by case women than controls.

Four U.S. studies have examined the relationship between VDT work and spontaneous abortion. In an historical cohort study, Brix and Butler (24) interviewed 728 female clerical and administrative support workers employed by the state of Michigan who had been pregnant at least once between 1980 and 1985. Information was obtained about their reproductive histories, relevant confounders, and work conditions, including hours of VDT use. Crude analysis revealed no association between hours of VDT exposure and spontaneous abortion. Using an observed-to-predicted model while controlling for known risk factors through logistical regression, the researchers noted a modest excess risk of miscarriage for women using VDTs more than 20 hr/week (OR = 1.25), but the results did not achieve statistical significance. However, the sample size for full-time users was small. The investigators also very crudely assessed stress in past pregnancies using job title and found no association with spontaneous abortion.

In 1988, Goldhaber et al. (25) published results of a case-control study that generated considerable media attention and public concern. They identified a large cohort of pregnant women receiving care at three Kaiser Permanente clinics in the San Francisco Bay area during a period in 1981–1982 when the pesticide malathion was sprayed in the area. A case-control study was then embedded within the cohort to investigate the reproductive effects of a number of environmental exposures, including the aerial spraying and VDT work. Medical records and computerized hospital discharge data were used to identify pregnancies resulting in fetal loss before 28 weeks of gestation, reportable birth defects, and normal livebirths. In 1984, the researchers collected exposure information through mailed questionnaires and telephone interviews to attain an overall response rate of approximately 85%. Questions were asked about employment during each trimester of pregnancy, including hours of VDT use per trimester. Logistical regression methods were used to adjust for known confounders. Because full-time VDT users had their pregnancies diagnosed slightly earlier than nonusers, gestational age at pregnancy diagnosis was included in the model for spontaneous abortion.

Analysis revealed no excess risk for miscarriage among women using VDTs 20 or fewer hr/week during the first trimester when compared with other working women not using VDTs. However, a statistically significant 80% increased risk for spontaneous abortion was noted in the group using VDTs more than 20 hr/week. The effect of VDT exposure was also examined after classifying subjects into four occupational categories using Census Bureau codes. A significant dose-response relationship was observed in only one of the occupational groups (administrative support/clerical), although the number of full-time VDT users was small in the other three categories. Analysis of the birth defects data in this study revealed a 40% increased risk for use of VDTs 5 or more hr/week, although numbers were small and results did not reach statistical significance (26).

Because most women in the Kaiser Permanente clinics tended to stay within the system for the duration of their pregnancies, major strengths of this study involved objective verification of outcome and little loss to follow-up. Unlike prior investigations, both hospitalized and nonhospitalized spontaneous abortions were included. However, exposure assessment was again based on hours of VDT use. The fact that women were asked to recall VDT exposure more than 2 yr after their pregnancies raises the issue of recall bias. However, if this bias were operative, one would expect self-reports of other environmental exposures also to be increased among women with adverse outcomes; this was not the case for other exposures such as malathion.

In a large case-control study designed primarily to assess the association between solvent exposure and spontaneous abortion, Windham et al. (27) also collected limited information on VDT use during pregnancy by telephone interview. Cases included women in Santa Clara County, California, who had spontaneous abortions confirmed by review of medical records and pathology reports; controls were women matched for hospital and last menstrual period who had livebirths. After controlling for a variety of confounders, the odds ratio for spontaneous abortion and VDT use (less than or greater than 20 hr/week) was 1.2 and did not reach statistical significance. Slightly higher, but still nonsignificant, odds ratios were found for early pregnancy loss for both categories of VDT use. Among the subset of study participants who were members of the Kaiser Permanente Health Plan, there was a modest association between spontaneous abortion and VDT use greater than 20 hr/week (OR = 2.1, CI = 1.1–3.8). However, no dose-response effect was noted, and analysis by occupational category did not reveal a greater risk for clerical workers, as did Goldhaber et al. This study also found no significant relationship between VDT use and the risk of delivering low birthweight or growth-retarded infants.

The long-awaited study by the National Institute for Occupational Safety and Health (NIOSH) was published in 1991 (28). This occupational cohort study was specifically designed to address weaknesses in exposure ascertainment that characterized previous investigations. The cohort was comprised of two types of telephone operators in the communications industry: directory assistance operators who used only VDTs, and general telephone operators who used only non-CRT devices known as light-emitting diodes or neon glow tubes. These two groups otherwise shared similar observable work characteristics including salary, hours of work (full time), ergonomic conditions (sitting at their machines 7 hr daily), and other stress-related variables (e.g., high volume of calls, computer-based and supervisory monitoring). Through interviews, married operators were identified whose pregnancies resulted in livebirth, stillbirth, or spontaneous abortion during the 1983–1986 study period; information about alcohol consumption, smoking, and medical conditions was also collected for each pregnancy. Personnel and payroll records were used to assess objectively the hours of VDT use during the first and second trimesters of pregnancy. Low frequency electromagnetic field emissions were measured 30 cm from the sides and at the operator's position of 48 randomly selected VDTs, 24 light-emitting diodes, and 24 neon glow tubes. Measured x-ray emissions were below background for all machines tested. The directory assistance operators used only two models of VDTs during the study period. All the non-CRT devices were manufactured by the same company. The researchers used multiple regression analysis to evaluate the effect of VDT use on the incidence of spontaneous abortion while controlling for other confounders and special statistical methods to adjust for nonindependence of multiple pregnancy outcomes in the same woman. The sample size of 882 pregnancies was adequate to detect a 1.5-fold increased risk for spontaneous abortion with approximately 85% power (29).

In this well-designed study, there was no association between occupational VDT use and clinically recognized spontaneous abortion. This remained true when VDT use was categorized as a dichotomous variable (yes/no) or by hours of use during the first trimester or first 28 weeks of pregnancy, and when separate analyses were performed for overall fetal loss, early and late miscarriages, and for only those losses reported to a physician. Overall rates of spontaneous abortion for users and nonusers were within expected rates for the general population (14.8% and 15.9%, respectively).

Mean VLF electric and magnetic field emissions were significantly higher for VDT units than for non-VDT devices (the latter not exceeding background levels) both 30 cm in front of the machines and at the operator's abdomen (approximately 50 cm). While mean frontal emissions for ELF electric fields also differed significantly between VDT and non-VDT devices, ELF magnetic field measurements at the operator's abdomen did not. One of the two VDT models emitted higher electromagnetic fields than the other; however, no increased risk for miscarriage was associated with the model of VDT used.

There are a number of important points to consider about this study. First, unlike other studies to date, this investigation objectively quantifies degree of use of VDTs and controls for psychosocial stress and ergonomic factors through comparison of two cohorts with remarkably similar working conditions. Because of these similarities, the study is not designed to evaluate the association between spontaneous abortion and psychosocial stress or ergonomic factors. However, it is probably fair to assume that work characterized by a high volume of calls, frequent monitoring, and stationary postures for 7 hr/day involves significant stress. The observation that miscarriage rates for VDT users working under these conditions are within generally accepted normal rates is reassuring. Second, the researchers addressed

the issue of recall bias by comparing self-reports of pregnancy outcome with information on birth certificates for a subset of the study population that had a livebirth subsequent to a spontaneous abortion. Correlation between self-reports and vital record data was similar for the two types of operators, arguing against recall bias as an explanation for the negative findings. Third, because only two VDT models were used by operators in the study, questions arise as to how representative the electromagnetic field emissions are of other devices on the market. If these fields play a role in adverse pregnancy outcome, measured values low in comparison to other models might explain the negative findings. However, comparison of the mean field values in this study with means from other reports assessing a variety of VDT models reveals that the NIOSH values are typical or somewhat higher (30). Finally, the study was primarily designed to assess the association between spontaneous abortion and occupational VDT use, not electromagnetic field exposure. While mean abdominal exposures to ELF magnetic fields did not significantly differ for users of VDT and non-VDT devices, measured values were generally very low compared to other common sources of ELF magnetic fields found in homes and workplaces (5, 6).

## SUMMARY AND RECOMMENDATIONS

After nearly a decade of study, the preponderance of the epidemiological evidence does not support a significant association between use of VDTs and spontaneous abortion. The limited number of studies on teratogenic effects of VDTs has found no association with total malformations, but no study has had sufficient power to evaluate specific anomalies adequately.

In vitro assays and experimental animal studies suggest that low frequency electromagnetic fields are biologically active and may affect development. The relevance of these data for humans is not yet certain. Until more is understood about this complex area, it is prudent for workers and citizens to limit chronic exposure to low frequency fields to the extent possible.

Under most circumstances, women do not need to curtail or to discontinue use of VDTs during pregnancy. However, given the potential for exposure to low frequency electromagnetic fields and the physical and psychosocial stressors associated with many VDT-related occupations, clinicians can use the following information to make reasonable recommendations to patients:

1. Electromagnetic fields are strongest at the back and sides of VDTs, and their intensity decreases considerably with distance. Exposure is minimal if VDT operators sit 50 cm from the screen and at least 1 m from the back or sides of adjacent VDTs. Because power frequency fields are emitted from all electrical devices, turning off VDTs, printers, and other electrical office equipment when not in use also reduces exposure.

2. The glass screen of a VDT effectively absorbs ionizing radiation. In keeping with federal regulations, VDTs manufactured after 1983 are also shielded to prevent excessive emissions of radiofrequency radiation. There are currently no requirements for shielding of low frequency electromagnetic field emissions from VDTs. However, employers can minimize the electric field component by providing special screen filters or linings for the outer cases of the VDTs with grounded material such as copper, silver, or nickel (31). Unfortunately, reducing magnetic fields is technically more difficult and costly because these emissions readily penetrate common shielding materials. Researchers are exploring ways to use special metals or field cancellation techniques to address the problem of magnetic field exposure. Some major manufacturers have recently marketed new lines of computers with reduced VLF magnetic field emissions. In addition, new VDT technologies have been introduced that are not based on conventional cathode ray tubes. Some computers, for example, use plasma or liquid crystal displays (e.g., laptops) that do not emit VLF fields. However, these alternative technologies are not yet refined; the screens are harder to read, and they are not adapted for all computer systems. In addition, they do emit ELF magnetic fields (31).

3. Prolonged VDT work may cause considerable musculoskeletal discomfort or repetitive strain injuries, such as tenosynovitis or carpal tunnel syndrome (32). These conditions may be exacerbated by pregnancy. Ergonomic stressors related to VDT work can be reduced by proper design of the operator's work station. While a detailed description is beyond the scope of this chapter, the basic components of a model VDT work station are presented in Figure 14.2.

4. Adequate rest breaks are important to prevent eye fatigue and musculoskeletal problems associated with VDT use. Operators should be provided at least a 15-minute break for every 2 hr of VDT work.

## REFERENCES

1. Bergqvist UOV. Video display terminals and health: a technical and medical appraisal of the art. Scand J Work Environ Health 1984;10 (Suppl 2):1–87.
2. Pomroy C, Noel L. Low-background radiation measurements on video display terminals. Health Phys 1984;46:413–417.
3. Hirning CR, Aitken JH. Cathode-ray tube x-ray emission standard for video display terminals. Health Phys 1982;43:727–731.
4. Bureau of Radiologic Health, Division of Compliance. An evaluation of radiation emissions from video display terminals. HHS Publication FDA 81–8153. Washington, DC: Bureau of Radiologic Health, 1981.
5. Marriott IA, Stuchly MA. Health aspects of work with visual display terminals. J Occup Med 1986;28:833–848.
6. Kavet R, Tell RA. VDTs: field levels, epidemiology, and laboratory studies. Health Phys 1991;91:47–57.
7. Marha K, Charron D. The distribution of a pulsed very low frequency electric field around video display terminals. Health Phys 1985;49:517–521.
8. Delgado JMR, Leal J, Monteagudo JL, Gracia MG. Embryological changes induced by weak, extremely low frequency electromagnetic fields. J Anat 1982;134:533–551.
9. Berman E, Chacon L, House D, et al. Development of chicken embryos in a pulsed magnetic field. Bioelectromagnetics 1990;11:169–187.
10. Juutilainen J. Effects of low-frequency magnetic fields on embryonic development and pregnancy. Scand J Work Environ Health 1991;17:149–158.
11. Berman E. Proceedings of the NICHD workshop on the reproductive effects of video display terminal use: the developmental effects of pulsed magnetic fields on animal embryos. Reprod Toxicol 1990;4:45–49.
12. Tenforde TS, Kaune WT. Interaction of extremely low frequency electric and magnetic fields with humans. Health Phys 1987;53:585–606.
13. Cleary SF. In vitro studies: low frequency electromag-

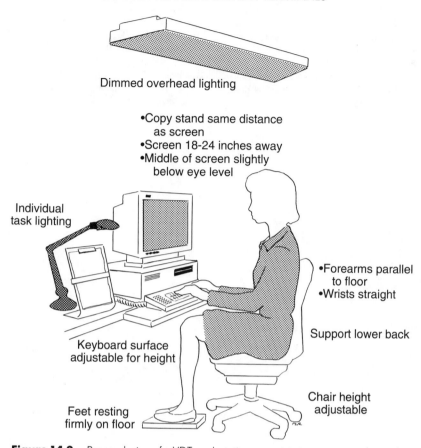

Dimmed overhead lighting

•Copy stand same distance
  as screen
•Screen 18-24 inches away
•Middle of screen slightly
  below eye level

Individual
task lighting

•Forearms parallel
  to floor
•Wrists straight

Support lower back

Keyboard surface
adjustable for height

Feet resting
firmly on floor

Chair height
adjustable

**Figure 14.2.** Proper design of a VDT work station can minimize ergonomic hazards.

netic fields. Presented at the NIOSH Scientific Workshop on the Health Effects of Electromagnetic Radiation on Workers, Cincinnati, OH, January 30–31, 1991.

14. Savitz DA, Wachtel H, Barnes FA, John EM, Tvrdik JG. Case control study of childhood cancer and exposure to 60 Hz magnetic fields. Am J Epidemiol 1988;128:10–20.

15. Savitz DA, John EM, Kleckner RC. Magnetic field exposure from electric appliances and childhood cancer. Am J Epidemiol 1990;131:763–773.

16. Wertheimer N, Leeper E. Fetal loss associated with two seasonal sources of electromagnetic field exposure. Am J Epidemiol 1989;129:220–224.

17. Abenhaim L, Lert F. Methodological issues for the assessment of clusters of adverse pregnancy outcomes in the workplace: the case of video display terminal users. J Occup Med 1991;33:1091–1096.

18. Marcus M. Proceedings of the NICHD workshop on the reproductive effects of video display terminal use: epidemiologic studies of VDT use and pregnancy outcome. Reprod Toxicol 1990;4:51–56.

19. Rigau-Perez JG. Proceedings of the NICHD workshop on the reproductive effects of video display terminal use: summary of final discussion. Reprod Toxicol 1990;4: 67–69.

20. Kurppa K, Holmberg PC, Rantala K, Nurminen T, Saxen L. Birth defects and exposure to video display terminals during pregnancy: a Finnish case-referent study. Scand J Work Environ Health 1985;11:353–356.

21. McDonald AD, Cherry NM, Delorme C, McDonald LC. Visual display units and pregnancy: evidence from the Montreal survey. J Occup Med 1986;28:1226–1231.

22. Ericson A, Kallen B. An epidemiological study of work with video screens and pregnancy outcome: I. A registry study. Am J Ind Med 1986;9:447–457.

23. Ericson A, Kallen B. An epidemiological study of work with video screens and pregnancy outcome: II. A case-control study. Am J Ind Med 1986;9:459–475.

24. Brix K, Butler R. Spontaneous abortions among VDT operators. Presented at the American Public Health Association Annual Meeting, Las Vegas, Nevada, October 1986.

25. Goldhaber MK, Polen MR, Hiatt RA. The risk of miscarriage and birth defects among women who use visual display terminals during pregnancy. Am J Ind Med 1988;13:695–706.

26. Goldhaber MK. The risk of miscarriage and birth defects among women who use visual display terminals during pregnancy. Reprod Toxicol 1990;4:57–60.

27. Windham GC, Fenster L, Swan SH, Neutra RR. Use of video display terminals during pregnancy and the risk of spontaneous abortion, low birthweight, or intrauterine growth retardation. Am J Ind Med 1990;18:675–688.

28. Schnorr TM, Grajewski BA, Hornung RW, et al. Video display terminals and the risk of spontaneous abortion. N Engl J Med 1991;324:727–733.

29. Schnorr TM. The NIOSH study of reproductive outcomes among video display terminal operators. Reprod Toxicol 1990;4:61–65.

30. Schnorr TM, Grajewski BA, Murray WE. Video display terminals and spontaneous abortions [Letter]. N Engl J Med 1991;325:812–813.

31. Office Technology Education Project. VDTs, radiation, and pregnancy. Boston: Office Technology Education Project, 1990.

32. Bammer G. How technologic change can increase the risk of repetitive motion injuries. Semin Occup Med 1987;2:25–30.

# 15

## Ergonomics

### MARIAN C. MARBURY

M.G. is a 32-yr-old gravida 1, para 0 female at 30 weeks' gestation. Her pregnancy is uncomplicated except for moderate ankle edema that worsens at work and improves on weekends. She works as a cashier at a convenience store, is on her feet for 8 hr per shift, works a rotating shift, and has to lift 40-lb boxes for restocking at night. She is concerned about her working conditions, because she has heard that physically stressful work can lead to preterm birth. Her company has no disability policy. She could take an unpaid leave but needs both the income and the health insurance that come with her job. Her manager is willing to consider suggestions for job modifications made by an obstetrician, as long as they are concrete and specific.

This hypothetical case history raises a number of questions faced by clinicians caring for pregnant working women. What is the relationship between physically stressful work and pregnancy outcome? Are physically stressful working conditions a problem for otherwise low-risk pregnancies? What does "physically stressful" mean, anyway? What job modifications might be useful in this case?

Unfortunately, complete answers to these questions are not currently available. While the American Medical Association Advisory Panel on Reproductive Hazards in the Workplace has published guidelines on how far into pregnancy various job tasks can be performed by low-risk women (1), the scientific basis for these guidelines is lacking. Nonetheless, intense interest in these issues has stimulated a number of studies

in the past decade. This chapter critically reviews the epidemiological literature on occupational ergonomic stressors and pregnancy outcome and makes recommendations where there is sufficient evidence. The primary outcomes addressed are spontaneous abortion, gestational age, and birthweight; while other important effects are biologically plausible, such as pregnancy-induced hypertension, the available literature is too sparse to support any conclusions.

### ERGONOMIC STRESSORS: DEFINITION

Ergonomics is the study of the relationship between workers and the psychological and physical aspects of the workplace, including equipment, facilities, tools, job demands, and work methods. Ergonomic stress arises when there is an imbalance between the worker and the work environment, resulting in excessive demand on the worker. Ergonomic stressors may be crudely categorized as either physical exertions or work organization. Physical exertions involve high-energy expenditure or biomechanical forces transmitted within the musculoskeletal system; physical exertions include heavy or frequent lifting, prolonged standing or sitting, work with heavy machinery, and climbing stairs or ladders. Work organization involves such factors as hours worked, shift work, machine-paced work, and speed of work. In this chapter, psychological stress will not be addressed, as it entails a different set of considerations and has been difficult to quantify.

## POSSIBLE MECHANISMS FOR THE EFFECT OF ERGONOMIC STRESSORS ON PREGNANCY OUTCOME

The physiological factors that regulate gestational age and birthweight are not well understood. Gestational age is ultimately determined by the onset of labor, while fetal weight is also influenced by the adequacy of placental perfusion.

Fuchs and Stubblefield (2) have proposed a model that provides a physiological basis for an effect of ergonomic exposures on both birthweight and gestational age. They postulate that a wide variety of factors, including heavy physical work and fatigue, cause stress. Stress results in the release of catecholamines, that, in turn, increase blood pressure and uterine irritability and decrease placental function. Uterine irritability causes cervical changes that contribute to the onset of labor. Decreased placental function also reduces progesterone production, leading to an increase in prostaglandin synthesis, which also promotes cervical changes.

Physically stressful work might also adversely influence birthweight through its effect on the circulatory system. During exercise, the release of norepinephrine and epinephrine from the adrenal medulla and the stimulation of vasodilating sympathetic fibers cause an increase in circulation to skeletal muscles (3). At the same time, exercise is associated with visceral vasoconstriction (4). Animal studies suggest that uteroplacental blood flow is decreased as a result. Briend (5) hypothesized that, because fetal nutrition is dependent on placental blood flow, prolonged exercise would result in fetal deprivation. However, more recent studies have demonstrated that blood flow within the uterus is preferentially redistributed to cotyledons in response to vasoconstriction. Thus, while myometrial flow is substantially reduced, cotyledonary flow decreases only slightly, permitting continued adequate oxygenation (6).

Briend (5) also suggests that prolonged standing reduces placental perfusion. Standing reduces venous return and plasma volume and activates the sympathetic nervous system. During pregnancy, growth of the uterus is associated with an exaggerated lumbar lordosis. As the sacrolumbar spine is projected forward, compression of the aorta and vena cava decreases blood volume. Prolonged standing, especially in forward flexed postures, could, therefore, further aggravate the decrease in uteroplacental blood flow.

## REVIEW OF THE EVIDENCE

### Methodological Issues

Three types of study designs have been used to address the relationship between ergonomic exposures and pregnancy outcomes: cross-sectional, case-control, and prospective cohort. The advantages and disadvantages of each design are reviewed in Chapter 9. This section highlights a few methodological issues as they apply to studies of ergonomic stressors and pregnancy outcomes.

### EXPOSURE ASSESSMENT

In studies of ergonomic stressors, job titles are often used as indirect measures of ergonomic exposures. This method may result in misclassification of exposure status; i.e., women whose work does not actually involve exposure to the ergonomic stressor of concern will be classified with women of the same job title whose work does entail exposure. If the misclassification is random with respect to outcome, it reduces the apparent association between the exposure and outcome. Job title may also be correlated with other characteristics that affect pregnancy outcome, such as socioeconomic status.

Direct assessment of exposure usually involves administering standardized questionnaires to study participants to ascertain their exposure to a variety of ergonomic stressors. Questions might be asked regarding the amount of lifting the job entails, the number of hours spent standing, and other factors. The validity of the information depends on the subjects' ability to recall and quantify accurately factors that are likely to be quite variable over time. If the questionnaire is administered after delivery, recall bias may also occur. More objective methods, such as keeping logs of daily activities or videotaping work practices, have not yet been attempted in studies of ergonomic stressors and pregnancy outcomes.

The further removed that the actual exposure is from the exposure variable, the greater the opportunity for misclassification. In addition, if the exposure variable is vaguely defined, specific ameliorative measures will not be obvious.

## DEFINITION OF OUTCOME

The outcomes most commonly studied in relation to ergonomic stressors are spontaneous abortion, birthweight, and gestational age. The definition and ascertainment of each of these endpoints may vary among studies.

Spontaneous abortion is usually defined as the nondeliberate interruption of an intrauterine pregnancy before the 28th week since the last menstrual period (7), although investigators have differed in the number of weeks used as a cutoff. As discussed in Chapter 9, the method of ascertaining spontaneous abortions (e.g., interviews, hospital record review) may significantly affect the estimate of abortion frequency and risk factors.

While data on birthweight are usually of high quality, analyses of birthweight have varied among studies in two important ways. First, birthweight has been treated either as a dichotomous variable (≤2500 g vs. >2500 g) or as a continuous variable. When treated as a dichotomous variable, statistical analysis focuses on whether there are differences in the proportions of low birthweight babies between exposure groups. This approach necessitates the use of a larger sample size and will not detect those exposures that cause a shift in the distribution of birthweight (e.g., maternal smoking). When birthweight is treated as a continuous variable, the statistical analysis focuses on differences in mean birthweight between exposure groups. Because this analysis is more sensitive and requires a smaller sample size, it is generally preferable.

Second, not all studies have taken into account the effect of gestational age on birthweight. Birthweight may be low either because of premature birth or intrauterine growth retardation, reflecting two different pathological mechanisms. Studies that fail to make this crucial distinction are difficult to interpret.

Gestational age as an outcome has also been treated both as a dichotomous and a continuous variable. As a dichotomous variable, preterm birth is usually defined as birth occurring before 37 completed weeks of gestation (8). Again, this statistical analysis has less power to detect subtle effects than one based on comparing mean gestational ages among exposure groups.

## CONFOUNDING FACTORS

Many factors are known to influence both birthweight and gestational age. For example, parity, social class, maternal stature, preeclampsia, maternal hypertension, and smoking have been associated with low birthweight (9). Maternal age, smoking, social class, and a history of perinatal loss have been associated with preterm delivery (10). Clearly, some of these factors are also associated with employment status. For example, women of higher parity are less likely to be employed outside of the home (11).

In evaluating the relationship between ergonomic exposures and pregnancy outcomes, socioeconomic status (SES) is the confounding factor of greatest potential importance. At least in developed countries, there is a strong association between SES and the probability of being employed in physically stressful work: lower paying jobs are much more likely to be physically demanding. Lower SES has also been consistently associated with adverse pregnancy outcomes, although the nature of this association is not clear. Because of the complex interrelationships among ergonomic exposures, SES, and pregnancy outcomes, studies that are either confined to one stratum of SES or that assess exposure-outcome relationships within strata of SES are more informative than other studies. It is unlikely that confounding by SES can be fully controlled by simply including indicator variables for SES (e.g., educational status) in multivariate models.

### Studies of Employment and Pregnancy Outcome

Research done in Great Britain in the 1950s suggested that employment outside of the home during pregnancy resulted in an increase in the incidence of preterm birth (12–14) and stillbirth (13). However, more contemporary studies from Israel (15), France (16), Great Britain (17), Australia (18), and the United

States (11, 19) have found that the pregnancy outcomes of employed women are either as favorable or better than the outcomes of nonemployed women. Several explanations have been suggested for this favorable association including the socioeconomic advantages related to wage earning, increased access to medical care of employed women, and the superior health status necessary for employment relative to the general population.

The one study not consistent with these results is an analysis of data from the Collaborative Perinatal Project by Naeye and Peters (20). Although the analysis was performed in the 1980s, the data were collected from 1959–1966. In this study, job title was used to classify women into one of three categories: not employed outside the home, employed in a sedentary job, and employed in a standing job. Birthweight was reportedly 150–400 g less in women employed outside the home after 28 weeks' gestation, except for those who were primiparous and worked in sedentary jobs. While this study has been cited as evidence that employment outside of the home may deleteriously affect fetal health, the failure of the analysis to control simultaneously for multiple confounding factors, the noncontemporary nature of the sample, and the inconsistency of the results with other studies cast doubt on the generalizability of these results to today's workforce.

Nonetheless, the question remains whether leaving work at some point before term is beneficial. While limited evidence suggests that this is advantageous in developing countries where working conditions are more arduous (21), the question has not been appropriately addressed in studies from developed nations. This question cannot be answered simply by examining the relationship between outcome and duration of employment during pregnancy because women may leave work before delivery either by choice or because of pregnancy complications. Prospective studies, in which date of and reasons for termination are carefully documented, will be essential in resolving this issue.

## Studies of Ergonomic Exposures and Spontaneous Abortion

Very few studies have examined the association between ergonomic stressors and spontaneous abortion. Of the seven studies described below, only the Montreal survey (22, 23) was specifically concerned with characterizing the effect of ergonomic stressors. Hemminki et al. (24) used the computerized census and medical records data systems available in Finland to study the relationship between occupation and pregnancy outcome in an industrialized town. Seamstresses in a textile factory had a higher spontaneous abortion rate than other employed women (OR = 3.0), and the risk increased further if the husband worked in a metallurgical factory (OR = 3.8). No information was obtained on individual exposures, but the authors noted that both piece work and noise were common in the textile industry. Similarly, Heidam (25) noted an increased risk of spontaneous abortion among factory workers (OR = 1.3) and speculated on the potential contribution of shiftwork and noise to the increase.

Axelsson et al. (26) conducted a retrospective cohort study of 782 women who had been employed in a university laboratory over an 8-yr period. A questionnaire containing specific questions on heavy lifting, stress, shiftwork, other occupational exposures during pregnancy, and pregnancy outcome was sent to all the women; data on pregnancy outcome were verified by medical records. A strong association between spontaneous abortion and shiftwork was noted (RR = 3.2), but no association was found with stress or heavy lifting. In another study in which chemical exposures were the primary exposures of interest, Figa-Talamanca (27) surveyed 4121 women working in 24 factories. A question was included on working position (standing, sitting, or both) out of concern that it might be a confounding factor. The spontaneous abortion rate did not vary with posture.

Taskinen et al. (28) conducted a nested case-control study of women employed in the pharmaceutical industry. Forty-four women who had a spontaneous abortion were each age-matched with three controls. Information about occupational exposures during the first trimester, including heavy lifting and work position, was gathered for each subject by a questionnaire filled out by the factory nurse or physician. A strong association was found between continuous heavy lifting and spontaneous abortion (OR = 5.7); however, the association is based on just six exposed cases.

Results of these studies are inconsistent: two did not find an association with working position (27, 28); one found a relationship with shiftwork, but not with heavy lifting (26); and one found an association with continuous heavy lifting (28). Their information is limited by relatively small sample sizes and their primary focus on other occupational, rather than ergonomic, factors.

Klebanoff et al. (29) assessed the relationship between ergonomic stressors and spontaneous abortion in a high SES population: 1284 female medical residents and 1481 partners of male medical residents. Questionnaires were sent to all women and a random sample of men who graduated from medical school in 1985. Questions were asked about all pregnancies and, specifically, about the first pregnancy to begin during residency and about some job aspects. Although information on individual stressors was not specifically ascertained, residency is generally characterized by prolonged standing, long hours, and stress. Using survival analysis to adjust for the higher rate of induced abortions among women residents, the investigators found no significant difference in the rate of spontaneous abortions between the two groups.

The Montreal survey represents the largest study of reproductive outcomes performed to date (22, 23). Between 1983 and 1984, 56,012 women were interviewed at the time of hospitalization about their present and past pregnancies and about their employment conditions during those pregnancies. Specific data were obtained on perceptions of the work environment (heat, cold, noise, vibration), work demands (lifting heavy weights, physical effort, standing ≥6 hr/day, working >40 hr/week), and work organization (rotating shift, assembly line work, piece work). Individual and grouped analyses were performed. In the individual analyses, the observed number of spontaneous abortions for women with a specific exposure was compared to the number expected based on nonoccupational confounding factors. (This O/E ratio can be interpreted as a relative risk.) However, because of the potential for recall

bias and bias due to the shorter time between exposure and outcome for women with spontaneous abortions compared to women with normal deliveries, the investigators also performed grouped or ecological analyses. Although ecological analysis is less susceptible to bias, it is also less sensitive and more likely to underestimate any association.

In the first analysis of this dataset, the investigators considered all pregnancies of women who had been employed during gestation, including 30,964 that had just ended and 26,298 prior pregnancies (22). Spontaneous abortion was not associated with heat or work organization factors. Evidence for an increased risk of spontaneous abortion with lifting heavy weights, standing, noise, and vibration was inconsistent. The most consistent risk factors were physical effort, working >40 hr/week, and cold. In the grouped analyses, spontaneous abortion was associated with lifting heavy weights in current pregnancies, and lifting heavy weights, physical effort, and working long hours in past pregnancies.

In a second analysis of this dataset, the investigators confined their attention to the 22,613 previous pregnancies of women employed at least 30 hr/week during gestation (23). The same ergonomic exposures (except those involving work organization) were examined on both an individual and ecological basis. Increased O/E ratios, basically consistent across occupational groups and for early, mid, and late spontaneous abortions, were found for lifting heavy weights more than 15 times a day (O/E = 1.5); other physical effort (O/E = 1.4); standing more than 8 hr/day (O/E = 1.2); working ≥46 hr/week (O/E = 1.2); changing shiftwork (O/E = 1.3); and exposure to noise (O/E = 1.2), vibration (O/E = 1.1), and cold (O/E = 1.2). Because of possible correlations between these factors, they were examined simultaneously in a regression; the resulting O/E ratios were lower but still significant. The grouped analysis gave higher estimates of relative risk than the individual analysis, suggesting that these results are not simply due to recall bias.

Because of its large size and comprehensive assessment of ergonomic exposures, the Montreal study represents the best information to date on the relationship of these exposures to spontaneous abortion. Nonetheless, in the absence of a clear underlying biological mechanism, further confirmatory work is needed.

## Studies of Ergonomic Stressors and Late Outcomes of Pregnancy

The literature on ergonomic stressors and late outcomes of pregnancy literally doubled in 1989–1990, reflecting an increasing recognition of the importance of the issue (Table 15.1). This section focuses specifically on associations with birthweight and gestational age.

Of the 18 studies described in Table 15.1, six used job title in some way to infer subjects' ergonomic exposures. As described previously, Naeye and Peters (20) used job titles to place women into one of three categories. Mean birthweight, not controlled for gestational age, was lower in women who worked outside the home after the 28th week of gestation, particularly for women employed in standing positions. These findings were not confirmed in studies using somewhat different classification schemes (described in Table 15.1) by Meyer and Daling (30) and Zuckerman et al. (19).

In a prospective cohort study of 1206 employed women, Teitelman et al. (31) defined three categories of activity level based on job title: sedentary, standing, and active. Active jobs were defined as those involving continuous or intermittent walking with active range of motion, such as janitors and physicians. The relative risk for preterm birth was 2.7 for women in standing jobs compared with women in active jobs, and their mean gestational age was 2.5 days shorter. When confounding was controlled, apparent differences in the low birthweight rate were not statistically significant.

Clearly, these studies are not consistent: two studies had positive findings and two had negative. Of the two positive studies, one found a relationship between standing and birthweight, and the other found a relationship between standing and gestational age. All four studies used different methods of categorizing exposure, and women who were in Teitelman's "active" category (and had better outcomes) would have been included in the standing category by the other studies. Resolution of the discrepancies between these studies is not possible, but the limitations of using job title for exposure assessment are apparent.

Two studies linked job title with other sources of information to categorize exposure. Homer et al. (32), in an analysis of data from the National Longitudinal Survey of Labor Market Experience Youth Cohort, linked the job titles of 772 women to the Job Characteristics Scoring System developed by Robert Karasek. The physical exertion variable in this system is based on the question, "Does your job require lots of physical effort?"; values are rated on a four-point scale. This system was used to categorize job titles into two categories of physical exertion. Women in the highest physical exertion category were at higher risk for having a preterm low birthweight baby (RR = 5.1), a low birthweight baby (RR = 2.7), a preterm infant (RR = 2.0), and babies of lower mean birthweight (160 g).

Ramirez et al. (33) examined the association between physical activity and preterm birth in a case-control study of active duty U.S. Army primigravidas. Physical activity assessment was based on the physical demand assessment of all military occupational specialties, which, in turn, was based on the maximum upper body strength required to perform the job in combat conditions. The relative risk for preterm birth increased from 1.4 for women in the medium demand category to 1.8 for those in the very heavy demand category.

In the remaining studies described in Table 15.1, data on exposure were obtained by means of an interviewer- or self-administered questionnaire. Direct comparisons among these studies is hindered by differences in the way exposures were assessed or defined, in definition of outcomes examined, and in the extent to which potential confounding variables were controlled.

Table 15.2 summarizes the literature on gestational age in relationship to the three ergonomic exposure variables most commonly assessed: standing, heavy lifting, and physically strenuous work. Many studies have also considered the combined effect of different exposures, and these results are in the "composite score" column. Table 15.3 is similar, but considers effects on birthweight. These

**Table 15.1.**
**Studies of Ergonomic Stressors and Outcomes of Late Pregnancy[a]**

| Study (reference) | Measure of Exposure | Results |
|---|---|---|
| **Job title Used to Infer Exposure**<br>Cross-sectional survey of 7722 pregnancies from Collaborative Perinatal Project, 1959–1966; U.S. (20) | Job title used to infer one of three maternal work categories: not employed, sedentary job, standing job | Birthweight[b] 150–400 g lower (depending on other factors) for women working outside of the home, particularly in jobs involving standing; no difference in gestation, head circumference, birth length |
| Case-control study based on birth certificates; cases = 2911 women giving birth to babies weighing <2500 g; controls = 2911 women with babies weighing 2500–3700 g; U.S. (30) | Mother's usual occupation on birth certificate used to infer activity level (housewife, sitting >75%, sitting 25–75%, standing >75%) | No relationship between LBW and activity level |
| Cross-sectional survey of 1507 women attending an inner city prenatal clinic; U.S. (19) | Job title used to infer one of three maternal work categories: not employed outside the home, employed in standing position, other work histories | No association between working in standing position and gestational age, birthweight, or head circumference |
| Case-control study; cases = 604 Army primigravidas giving birth at ≤37 weeks'; controls = 6070 women with term or post-term deliveries; U.S. (33) | Occupational physical demand, based on an analysis of maximum upper body strength required for each job in combat conditions | OR for PTB increased from 1.4 for jobs with median demands to 1.8 for jobs with very heavy demands |
| Prospective cohort study of 1206 women; U.S. (31) | Job title used to define three groups: standing, active, sedentary | Adjusted OR for PTB = 2.7 for women standing >3 hr/day, and mean gestational age lower; LBW and mean birthweight not different after confounding controlled |
| Cross-sectional study of 772 women taking part in a national survey who had given birth before interview and worked during recent pregnancy; U.S. (32) | Job title linked with Karasek's Job Characteristics Scoring System to assess degree of physical exertion associated with job title | Women working in high exertion jobs were more likely to deliver a preterm LBW baby (OR = 5.1); a LBW baby (OR = 2.7); a PTB baby (OR = 2.0); and birthweight was 160 g less |
| **Exposure Assessed Through Questionnaire**<br>Case-control study; cases = 175 women giving birth <37 weeks'; controls = 313 women giving birth at 37 + weeks'; U.S. (49) | Questionnaire: paid employment; hr/week; standing/moving around on job; frequency of lifting and weight lifted; sports and physical activities | No relationship between physical activity at work and PTB; exercise during pregnancy had a beneficial effect (OR = 0.5) |
| Cross-sectional study of 1928 working women; France (34) | Questionnaire: five sources of stress (standing >5 hr/day, work on industrial machine, physical exertion, mental stress, "environment") used to calculate occupational fatigue score | PTB directly related to occupational fatigue score (OR = 5.1[c], contrasting women with score of 4–5 to those with 0); mental stress and environment contribute most strongly |

**Table 15.1.**
**Studies of Ergonomic Stressors and Outcomes of Late Pregnancy[a] (continued)**

| Study (reference) | Measure of Exposure | Results |
|---|---|---|
| Cross-sectional study of 621 hospital workers at seven hospitals; France (39) | Questionnaire: four working groups; three ergonomic stressors (heavy cleaning tasks, carrying heavy loads, lengthy periods of standing); cumulative score of all three | Score of 2 or more conditions associated with PTB (OR = 3.5) and LBW (OR = 1.6)[c] NS; also associated with increased hospitalization during pregnancy and sick leave frequency |
| Cross-sectional study of 2387 women who worked first trimester of pregnancy; France (40) | Questionnaire: two working groups; four stressors (standing position, heavy load carrying, assembly line work, physically demanding work); cumulative score of all 4 | Women with 3–4 stressors had higher PTB compared to women with none (OR = 2.1)[c]; risk of LBW[b] babies higher if score 3–4 (OR = 2.0)[c] or job involved considerable physical effort (OR = 1.6)[c] |
| Cross-sectional study of 22,761 women employed at conception who remained in same conditions up to 28 weeks' or when left; Canada (36) | Questionnaire: 60 occupational working groups; stressors—lifting weights, other physical effort, prolonged standing, long work week, assembly line work, piece work, shiftwork, environmental conditions; also used Mamelle's occupational fatigue score | Lifting weights and working ≥46 hr/week associated with PTB (RR = 1.3 for both) and LBW[b] (1.3 for lifting; 1.2 for working ≥46 hr); LBW[b] also associated with changing shift (RR = 1.4) and noise (RR = 1.1); no association with standing ≥8 hr/day; Mamelle's occupational fatigue score weakly, but significantly, related to both PTB and LBW[b] |
| Cross-sectional study of 22,761 women; reanalysis of (36), controlling birthweight for gestational age; Canada (46) | Questionnaire: 60 occupational working groups; stressors—lifting weights, other physical effort, prolonged standing, long work week, assembly line work, piece work, shiftwork, environmental conditions; also used Mamelle's occupational fatigue score | Lower mean birthweight associated with lifting heavy weights and changing shiftwork; composite score not significantly associated with birthweight |
| Case control study; cases = 189 women giving birth <37 weeks'; controls = 189 women matched for age and parity, urban/rural residence; Finland (50) | Questionnaire: stressors—shiftwork, standing/moving, heavy physical loading, vibration, noise, temperature | No association between occupational factors and PTB |
| Cross-sectional study of 1475 working women whose babies were the control group in a case-control study; Finland (41) | Physical load score calculated from description of activities using a standardized evaluation method; scores then collapsed into four categories | Increased risk for shorter gestations among women in highest mean (OR = 2.2)[c] and short term (OR = 1.5)[c] physical load category, but not when analyses restricted to women in lower SES; also at higher risk for SGA babies (OR = 2.7)[c] |
| Prospective study of 3906 working women; Sweden (51) | Questionnaire: four categories of heavy lifting at work, as reported during the first trimester | No overall association seen between heavy lifting and PTB or LBW or mean birthweight; some indication of a decrease in birthweight associated with heavy lifting among women who worked past 32 weeks |

**Table 15.1.**
**Studies of Ergonomic Stressors and Outcomes of Late Pregnancy[a] (continued)**

| Study (reference) | Measure of Exposure | Results |
|---|---|---|
| Prospective study of 15,786 low to middle class urban women; Guatemala (42) | Questionnaire: employment in work force; office or manual; sitting, standing, or walking position; level of physical intensity (sedentary, moderate, intense); number of hours worked; activity score summarized joint effects | Risk of SGA babies higher among manual workers (OR = 1.3) and among those who stood (OR = 1.2) or walked (OR = 1.3); risk of SGA/PTB higher among manual workers (OR = 2.6); standing associated with PTB (OR = 1.6); high activity score also associated with SGA and SGA/PTB babies |
| Prospective cohort study of 1507 women; United Kingdom (45) | Questionnaire given at three times during pregnancy; stressors: hours of work, energy expended at work and housework (kcal estimated), hours of paid housework, posture | No association between any measures of maternal work stress, including posture, and birthweight adjusted for gestational age or gestational age alone |
| Prospective cohort study of 2741 women; Philippines (43) | Questionnaire during third trimester asking about activity at work and home; stressors; standing, energy expenditure, physical stress | No association between stressors and birthweight or gestational age for employed women; standing and physical stress associated with decreased gestational age and birthweight among nonemployed women |
| Cross-sectional survey of 989 female medical residents compared to 1239 wives of male residents; U.S. (44) | Major exposure: medical resident during pregnancy; also inquired about hours of work, number of nights on call | Residents at higher risk for preterm labor (OR = 2.0)[c] but not PTB (OR = 0.9) or SGA babies compared to nonresidents; working >100 hr/week doubled risk of PTB |

[a]SGA = small for gestational age; LBW = low birthweight; PTB = preterm birth; NS = not statistically significant; OR = odds ratio; RR = relative risk
[b]Birthweight not controlled for gestational age
[c]Prevalence odds ratio calculated from the data

tables graphically demonstrate the inconsistency of results in the current literature, with the apparent exception of an association between a composite score and preterm birth.

Mamelle et al. (34) conducted one of the earliest investigations that used questionnaires to assess individual ergonomic demands. Immediately after delivery, 1928 women who had been employed during pregnancy were interviewed about lifestyle and occupational activity during pregnancy. The occupational data were used to define five sources of fatigue: posture (sitting or standing), work on an industrial machine, physical exertion, mental stress, and environment. Each source was then scored either 0 or 1, depending on whether certain elements were present. Some sources were more clearly defined than others. For example, posture received a score of 1 if the work involved standing >3 hr/day. In contrast, environment received a score of 1 if the job involved either manipulation of chemical substances or if two of three elements (significant noise level, cold temperature, or very wet atmosphere) were present. Although varying in the magnitude of the risk, each source was found to be significantly associated with the risk of a preterm birth. When combined into an overall occupational fatigue score, the proportion of women having a preterm birth varied from 2.3% when the score was 0, to 11.1% when the score was 4 or 5. When the relationship between preterm birth and all of the sources were examined simultaneously, mental stress and environment

**Table 15.2.**
**Studies of Ergonomic Stressors and Gestational Age[a]**

| Study (reference) | Standing | Heavy Lifting | Physically Strenuous | Composite Score |
|---|---|---|---|---|
| Berkowitz et al. (49) | — | — | NA | NA |
| Saurel-Cubizolles et al. (39) | NA | NA | NA | + |
| Saurel-Cubizolles and Kaminski (40) | — | — | — | + |
| McDonald et al. (36) | — | + | — | + |
| Mamelle et al. (34) | + | — | + | + |
| Mamelle and Munoz (35) | — | — | — | + |
| Hartikainen-Sorri and Sorri (50) | — | NA | — | NA |
| Launer et al. (42) | + | NA | NA | +[b] |
| Ahlborg et al. (51) | NA | — | NA | NA |
| Nurminen et al. (41)[c] | NA | NA | NA | + |
| Klebanoff et al. (44) | NA | NA | — | NA |
| Barnes et al. (43)[d] | ± | NA | ± | — |

[a]All studies assessed preterm birth (gestational age <37 weeks), except as noted; NA = not assessed.
[b]No association was found between birth and the composite activity score, but the score was associated with premature, small-for-gestational-age babies.
[c]Dichotomized gestational age into < or >280 days.
[d]Standing and physical stress were associated with decreased gestational age among women not working outside the home, but not employed women.

**Table 15.3.**
**Studies of Ergonomic Stressors and Birthweight[a]**

| Study (reference) | Standing | Heavy Lifting | Physically Strenuous | Composite Score |
|---|---|---|---|---|
| Saurel-Cubizolles et al. (39)[b,c] | — | NA | NA | — |
| Saurel-Cubizolles and Kaminski (40)[b,c] | — | — | + | + |
| Launer et al. (42)[d] | + | NA | NA | + |
| Ahlborg et al. (51)[b,e] | NA | — | NA | NA |
| Nurminen et al. (41)[d] | NA | NA | NA | + |
| Armstrong et al. (46)[e] | NA | + | NA | — |
| Rabkin et al. (45)[e] | — | NA | NA | — |
| Klebanoff et al. (44)[d] | NA | NA | — | NA |
| Barnes et al. (43)[f] | ± | NA | ± | — |

[a]NA = not assessed.
[b]Outcome was low birthweight (≤2500 g).
[c]Did not control for gestational age.
[d]Outcome was small for gestational age (≤10th percentile weight, ≥37 weeks age); Launer also examined preterm, small for gestational age (≤10th percentile weight, <37 weeks age).
[e]Outcome was mean birthweight.
[f]Standing and physical stress were associated with decreased birthweight among economically inactive women, but not women working outside of the home.

emerged as the two most important factors. However, since 90% of women who had these two sources also had a third source, the investigators concluded that, in identifying a strenuous job, the number of sources was as informative as the specific sources.

The investigators also examined the interaction between physical stress and "medical factors" (previous preterm delivery, spontaneous abortion, stillbirth, or perinatal death, and/or pathology during the first 5 months of pregnancy that might or might not be related to prematurity). Compared to women who had no medical factor or work-related physical stress (RR = 1.0), the relative risk of preterm delivery was 1.4 for women who only had a medical factor, 2.1 for women with only physical stress, and 2.8 for women with both.

To examine the reliability of the occupational fatigue score, Mamelle and Munoz (35) conducted a case-control study of 200 women who delivered before 37 weeks' gestation and 400 women who delivered at term. The authors report partial confirmation of their initial findings. Examined individually, posture and physical exertion were not related to preterm birth, environment was related but not significantly, and work on a machine and mental stress were significantly related. The cumulative fatigue score was again related to the risk of preterm birth, with women scoring 1 or 2 having a moderately increased risk (OR = 1.5) and women scoring 3 or higher having the highest risk (OR = 1.9), compared to women with scores of 0.

In the Montreal survey (36), McDonald et al. constructed a cumulative fatigue index based on essentially the same criteria as Mamelle. The composite score also demonstrated a statistically significant association with preterm birth, but of a much less magnitude: there was a 7% increase in risk among women with a score of 2, and a 16% increase with a score of 3 or more.

The utility of this scoring system is unclear. For epidemiological studies of the relationship between ergonomic stressors and pregnancy outcomes, it appears to be inadequate: divergent aspects of work are pooled together in a single source, each source is assumed to have an independent and additive effect, and joint effects between various sources cannot be examined (37). These factors, along with the vague definitions of stressors, also make it impossible to identify priorities for possible job modifications during pregnancy. Whether such a scoring system could be clinically useful in identifying women at high risk of preterm birth remains to be demonstrated. Other prenatal scoring systems designed to detect women at risk for preterm birth have not proven to have high predictive value when applied prospectively to populations different than the one in which it was developed (38).

Other investigators have also used a composite score approach in studies of physical work stress and preterm birth. Saurel-Cubizolles et al. (39) studied 621 women who worked in hospitals for at least 13 weeks during pregnancy. Questionnaires were administered by hospital personnel to women returning to work at the end of postnatal leave. Three working conditions were combined into a composite score: heavy cleaning tasks, carrying heavy loads, and prolonged standing. In the overall sample, the preterm delivery rate was 6% among women with a score of 0, 5% with a score of 1, 18% with a score of 2, and 30% with a score of 3. The association between the composite score and preterm birth was especially strong among the ancillary staff who are responsible for housekeeping.

In a later study of 2387 women employed during the first trimester, Saurel-Cubizolles and Kaminski (40) examined the effects of prolonged standing, carrying heavy loads, assembly line work, and physically demanding work, individually and combined into a cumulative score. Only assembly line work was individually associated with increased risk of preterm birth. Again, however, the cumulative score was strongly associated: the proportion of preterm births was 4% among those with a score of 0, 5.1% with a score of 1 or 2, and 8.2% with a score of 3 or higher. Women were divided into two occupational groups: production, service, and shop workers; and professional, administrative, and clerical workers. The relationship between the cumulative score and preterm birth was apparent in the first group; but the latter group contained only 39 women with scores of 3 or 4, and none had a preterm birth.

Other investigators have used different approaches to assess the cumulative effect of multiple sources of physical stress. Nurminen et al. (41) evaluated the physical load of each woman's job based on a standardized method that reflects energy expenditure. Because few women delivered prematurely, gestational age less than 280 days was evaluated. Mothers in the highest physical load category had a higher risk (OR = 1.4) than those in the lowest category, and mothers whose short-term physical load was high were also at greater risk (OR = 1.2). When the analyses were restricted to women in the two lower socioeconomic classes, this increased risk was no longer apparent.

In a prospective study of 15,786 Guatemalan women, Launer et al. (42) used an activity score based on type of work, position, physical intensity level, and number of hours of work to assess the relationship between physical demands and preterm birth. After adjusting for monthly income and maternal weight and height, working in a standing position was associated with an increased risk of preterm birth

(RR = 1.6), and working in a walking position was associated with a two-fold risk of preterm small-for-gestational-age (SGA) infants. The activity score was linearly related to the proportion of preterm SGA babies, with women in the highest demand category having the highest proportion. This same trend was apparent, but not statistically significant, for preterm birth.

Results of an investigation of Filipino women were more equivocal. Barnes et al. (43) divided their population of 2741 women into categories of working outside the home, economically active at home, and economically inactive. Within each category, the effects of three stressors were assessed: physical stress, defined as spending any time in activity requiring more than 0.06 kcal/kg/min; energy expenditure, expressed as kcal/kg/min estimated from all activities both inside and outside of the home; and standing. No stressor was associated with gestational age among working women; physical stress was associated with decreased gestational age among economically inactive women, and standing had a negative impact on women economically active at home. An explanation for these inconsistent results is not immediately apparent. Nonetheless, the assessment of stressors both in and out of the workplace is an important step forward in exposure assessment.

Despite general agreement among studies, the question remains as to whether investigators have succeeded in truly disentangling the effects of SES from the effects of physically stressful work. In the studies that have examined the association between physically demanding work and preterm birth within SES strata (36, 39, 40), only the study by McDonald et al. (36) had sufficient women in the higher SES strata with physically demanding work to assess the relationship. This study reported an association between heavy lifting and preterm birth in all occupational sectors, although only the sectors representing lower SES had sufficient numbers individually to reach statistical significance. In the two studies by Saurel-Cubizolles et al. (39, 40), the relationship between physically demanding work and preterm birth was apparent in the lower SES strata but lacked sufficient numbers of women with phys-

ically stressful work in the higher strata to permit any evaluation.

The only investigation to focus on the effects of ergonomic stressors in a high SES population is Klebanoff et al.'s (44) study of pregnancy outcomes of female residents and wives of male residents. The investigators reported no differences in the proportion of preterm births between the female residents and residents' wives. Women in the surgical specialties were at higher risk (OR = 1.6) than other residents, but this was not statistically significant. The risk of preterm birth was twice as high for residents who worked more than 100 hr/week compared to those who worked less. Although the investigators concluded that working long hours (<100 hr) in a stressful occupation did not have an effect on the outcome of pregnancy in a healthy, higher SES population, they also reported that female residents were twice as likely to experience premature labor as were wives of male residents. To explain this finding, they suggested that attending obstetricians might be more likely to diagnose early labor in a group of women perceived to be at high risk, that female residents might be more likely to report symptoms, or that preterm labor due to work-related stress might be reversible. However, a likely alternative explanation is that residents who experience premature labor are treated much more aggressively and, therefore, successfully. Thus, while their conclusion that women medical residents are not at increased risk for premature birth is supported by their data, the results may not be generalizable to women in other stressful occupations.

In summary, while no individual study is persuasive regarding the association of physically stressful work and preterm delivery, the literature as a whole suggests that such an association exists. Whether this association varies by social class is not yet clear. Resolving this question would undoubtedly provide scientific insight into the underlying nature of the association. For clinical practice, the question is less pressing, inasmuch as the majority of patients who have physically stressful work will also be of lower SES.

In contrast to the data on preterm delivery, the data on birthweight are more contradictory. As with preterm delivery, no individual ergonomic stressor has been found to be consistently associated with effects on birthweight, although studies examining specific stressors are sparse (Table 15.3). Seven studies used a composite score or some other assessment of overall activity level: three found an effect on birthweight and four did not.

Of the three studies that found an association between physically stressful work and birthweight (40–42), one (40) did not control for the effect of gestational age. Because this study also found a strong association between the composite score and preterm birth, it is not possible to judge the extent to which the decrease in birthweight was secondary to the decrease in gestational age. The prospective study of Guatemalan women by Launer and co-workers (42) found that women who worked in standing or walking positions were at higher risk of delivering SGA babies (OR = 1.2 and 1.3, respectively) and that there was a direct relationship between physical activity score and the proportion of both SGA and SGA/preterm births. Although the study seems to be methodologically sound, the described nutritional status of this study population appears to be poorer than that of the general U.S. population. In addition, the definition of SGA was based on norms from a well-nourished population, and fully 20% of the women gave birth to babies meeting this definition. Thus, while the conclusions of the study may well be valid for the Guatemalan study population, they are not necessarily generalizable to developed countries. In the third study to report an association between decreased birthweight and physically stressful work, Nurminen et al. (41) found an increased risk of SGA babies among women in the highest mean (OR = 2.4) and highest short-term (OR = 1.8) physical work load categories, when analyses were restricted to women in nonagricultural, lower SES categories. However, there was only a 55-g difference in the median birthweight between the highest and lowest work load categories.

This weak, but positive, evidence of an association between birthweight and physical exertion has not been confirmed in other studies. Rabkin et al. (45) conducted a prospective study of 1507 women, of whom 626 worked >30 hr/week and 202 worked part-time. Questionnaires were administered at the initial prenatal visit and at 17, 28, and 36 weeks' gestation. An activity measure considered the nature of paid employment, the usual posture at work, the starting and stopping time, commuting time and mode, amount of time spent performing childcare and housework, and the nature and duration of leisure activities. Estimates of energy requirements in kcal/min were also used as indices of exposure. Overall, no association was found between mean birthweight and any measure of exposure. Although the study was relatively small, it had sufficient power to detect an 80-g difference in birthweight. Similar results were reported by Barnes et al. (43) for Filipino women working outside of the home, although they did find a decrease in birthweight associated with standing and physical stress among nonworking women.

The initial report from the Montreal survey (36) found an association between birthweight and several ergonomic stressors, but the effect of gestational age was not considered. A further analysis (46), in which birthweight was controlled for gestational age, confirmed the association between birthweight and both lifting heavy weights and shift work, but the association with working more than 45 hr/week and the cumulative fatigue index was no longer apparent.

Although not containing an explicit measure of physical exertion, the investigation by Klebanoff et al. (44) is a fourth important study that did not find an association between physically strenuous work and birthweight. In their comparison of the pregnancy outcomes of female medical residents and wives of male residents, there was no difference in the proportion of women delivering SGA infants or babies weighing less than 2500 or 1500 g at birth, or in the mean birthweight of the babies. There was also no difference in the proportion of SGA babies between residents who worked >100 hr/week and those who worked less.

Thus, in contrast to the relatively consistent data between ergonomic exposures and preterm delivery, the evidence for an association with birthweight is both limited and variable.

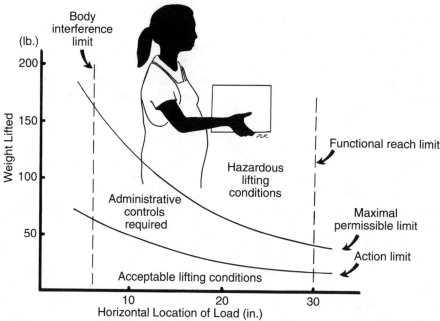

**Figure 15.1.** Maximum weight vs. horizontal location of load (distance from load to body centerline) for infrequent lifts from floor to knuckle height. Modified from National Institute for Occupational Safety and Health (NIOSH): Work practices guide for manual lifting. Cincinnati: NIOSH, 1981:125.

The weight of the evidence suggests that, if there is an adverse effect of ergonomic exposures on birthweight, it is likely to be small.

## ERGONOMIC STRESSORS AND MATERNAL HEALTH

Women undergo a number of well-described physiological changes during pregnancy that may make them more susceptible to an adverse impact of ergonomic stressors. However, there is no available evidence to support unequivocal prohibitions; the impact of ergonomic stressors will vary considerably, depending on the individual woman's physical fitness and strength as well as her overall health status.

In general, the impact of ergonomic stressors on maternal health and/or comfort is likely to be greatest during the third trimester. Lifting of heavy loads is likely to present a particular stress. For pregnant and nonpregnant workers alike, biomechanical analysis has shown that the degree of stress on the lumbar spine caused by lifting is directly related to the distance from the body that the load is lifted (48), with greater distance causing greater stress (Fig. 15.1). As the abdomen increases in size,

pregnant women must bend over more and reach out further to pick up a load. In addition, because of the increased oxygen uptake and cardiorespiratory demands during late pregnancy, the maximum amount of weight a woman can lift may decrease.

Another important change during later pregnancy is increasing spinal lordosis accompanied by a shift in the center of gravity from the instep of the foot to the base of the big toe. The resulting compensatory change in posture requires the erector spinae muscles to contract statically, leading to low back discomfort during prolonged standing. Venous stasis, a common problem during pregnancy, may also be exacerbated by prolonged standing, resulting in lower extremity edema and varicosities. Prolonged sitting can also lead to low back discomfort and pressure on the suprapopliteal region, further exacerbating venous stasis.

## SUMMARY AND RECOMMENDATIONS

The need for more research on the effect of ergonomic stressors on pregnancy outcome is clear. Nonetheless, sufficient scientific evidence exists to support certain conclusions and recommendations. First, employment outside the home per se is not a risk factor for adverse pregnancy outcome. This, in itself, should be reassuring information for pregnant women in the labor force.

Second, clinicians must elicit in some detail the number and type of ergonomic stressors to which pregnant patients are exposed. Simply knowing the job title is insufficient, as jobs with the same title can vary widely in their exposures. Questions should address the number of hours spent standing, the frequency of lifting and the approximate weight lifted, the woman's perception of the physical strenuousness of her job, work on a machine, the number of hours worked, and the amount of shift work. The clinician should also ascertain the degree of physical energy expenditure at home. Important questions here include the number and ages of children at home and the extent to which help is available for household tasks.

The purpose of this history is two-fold: to identify women who may need job modifications during the third trimester for their health, safety, and comfort, and to identify women who may be at high risk for preterm labor. In general, job modifications for maternal health and safety should be based on an assessment of the individual woman's needs and her adaptation to the work environment. Restrictions that do seem justified during the third trimester include work requiring balance (e.g., climbing ladders) and lifting weights that either are bulky, and thus, awkward, or that are close to the woman's prepregnant lifting capacity.

The lumbosacral discomfort that often develops in women with sedentary jobs can be alleviated by use of a chair with a back rest that supports both the lumbar and sacral areas and a footrest that reduces pressure on those areas. Ideally, the work surface would be of a height that work can be performed either sitting or standing to allow frequent change of posture (e.g., a high stool matched to a high workbench). Fatigue can often be alleviated by decreasing work loads or increasing the number of work breaks. More frequent work breaks or modifying the working position may also be necessary for women who experience edema or develop varicosities from prolonged standing.

Although the scientific data are not yet conclusive as to which or how many exposures are necessary to increase the risk of preterm delivery, a woman whose job involves two or more specific ergonomic exposures or whose work is physically strenuous overall should be considered at potential risk. This risk should be evaluated in the context of other known risk factors (e.g., a history of preterm delivery). If other risk factors are absent and the woman is healthy, it may be sufficient to warn her of the symptoms of preterm labor, explore possible job modifications, and perhaps check for cervical dilation more frequently during the third trimester. If there are other factors that place her at high risk, explore ways to limit exposure to ergonomic stressors through job modifications, job transfers, or disability leave. If these options are not available, then seeing her frequently during the second half of pregnancy and placing her in a preterm birth prevention class may be sufficient. It is important to recognize that the choices are not clear-cut; removing a woman from her job, with consequent loss of income and insurance, may well be more damaging to her and her child's health than to remain employed under close surveillance.

## REFERENCES

1. American Medical Association Council on Scientific Affairs. Effects of pregnancy on work performance. JAMA 1984;251:1995–1997.
2. Fuchs F, Stubblefield PG. Preterm birth: causes, prevention, and management. New York: Macmillan Publishers, 1984.
3. Guyton AC, Cowley AW Jr, Young DB. Integration and control of circulatory function. Int Rev Physiol 1976;9:341–385.
4. Rowell LB. Human cardiovascular adjustments to exercise and thermal stress. Physiol Rev 1974; 54:75–159.
5. Briend A. Maternal physical activity, birth weight and perinatal mortality. Med Hypotheses 1980;6:1157–1170.
6. Lotgering FK, Gilbert RD, Longo LD. Exercise in pregnancy in the experimental animal. In: Mittelmark RA, Wiswell RA, Drinkwater BL, eds. Exercise in pregnancy 2nd ed. Baltimore: Williams & Wilkins, 1991:157–173.
7. World Health Organization. Spontaneous and induced abortion. Technical Report series no. 461. Geneva: World Health Organization, 1970.
8. World Health Organization. Manual of the international statistical classification of diseases, injuries and causes of death. Volume 1, 9th rev. Geneva: World Health Organization, 1975.

9. Alberman E. Low birthweight. In: Bracken MB, ed. Perinatal epidemiology. New York: Oxford University Press, 1984:86–98.

10. Van den Berg BJ, Oechsli FW. Prematurity. In: Bracken MB, ed. Perinatal epidemiology. New York: Oxford University Press, 1984:69–85.

11. Marbury MC, Linn S, Monson RR, et al. Work and pregnancy. J Occup Med 1984;26:415–421.

12. Douglas JWB. Some factors associated with prematurity. J Obstet Gynaecol Br Emp 1957;64:16.

13. Stewart AM. A note on the obstetric effects of work during pregnancy. Br J Prev Soc Med 1955;9:159–161.

14. Illsley R, Billewicz WZ, Thomson AM. Prematurity and paid work during pregnancy. Br J Prev Soc Med 1954;8:153–156.

15. Gofin J. The effect on birthweight of employment during pregnancy. J Biosoc Sci 1979;11:259–267.

16. Saurel MN, Kaminski M. Pregnant women at work. Lancet 1983;1:475.

17. Murphy JF, Dauncey M, Newcombe R. Employment in pregnancy: prevalence, maternal characteristics, perinatal outcome. Lancet 1984;2:1163–1168.

18. Najman JM, Morrison J, Williams GM, Andersen MJ, Keeping JD. The employment of mothers and the outcomes of their pregnancies: an Australian study. Public Health 1989;103:189–198.

19. Zuckerman BS, Frank DA, Hingson R, Morelock S, Kayne HL. Impact of maternal work outside the home during pregnancy on neonatal outcome. Pediatrics 1986;77:459–464.

20. Naeye RL, Peters EC. Working during pregnancy: effects on the fetus. Pediatrics 1982;69:724–727.

21. Manshade JP, Eeckels R, Manshade-Desmet V, Vlietinck R. Rest versus heavy work during the last weeks of pregnancy: influence on fetal growth. Br J Obstet Gynaecol 1987;94:1059–1067.

22. McDonald AD, Armstrong B, Cherry NM, et al. Spontaneous abortion and occupation. J Occup Med 1986;28:1232–1238.

23. McDonald AD, McDonald JC, Armstrong B, et al. Fetal death and work in pregnancy. Br J Ind Med 1988;45:148–157.

24. Hemminki K, Kyyronen P, Niemi M-L, Koskinen K, Sallmen M, Vainio H. Spontaneous abortions in an industrialized community in Finland. Am J Public Health 1983;73:32–37.

25. Heidam LZ. Spontaneous abortions among dental assistants, factory workers, painters, and gardening workers: a follow up study. J Epidemiol Commun Health 1984;38:149–155.

26. Axelsson G, Lutz C, Rylander R. Exposure to solvents and outcome of pregnancy in university laboratory employees. Br J Ind Med 1984;41:305–312.

27. Figa-Talamanca I. Spontaneous abortions among female industrial workers. Int Arch Occup Environ Health 1984;54:163–171.

28. Taskinen H, Lindbohm M-L, Hemminki K. Spontaneous abortions among women working in the pharmaceutical industry. Br J Ind Med 1986;43:199–205.

29. Klebanoff MA, Shiono PH, Rhoads GG. Spontaneous and induced abortion among resident physicians. JAMA 1991;265:(21):2821–2825.

30. Meyer BA, Daling JR. Activity level of mother's usual occupation and low infant birth weight. J Occup Med 1985;27:841–847.

31. Teitelman AM, Welch LS, Hellenbrand KG, Bracken MB. Effect of maternal work activity on preterm birth and low birth weight. Am J Epidemiol 1990;131:104–113.

32. Homer CJ, Beresford SA, James SA, Siegel E, Wilcox S. Work-related physical exertion and risk of preterm, low birthweight delivery. Paediatr Perinat Epidemiol 1990;4:161–174.

33. Ramirez G, Grimes RM, Annegers JF, Davis BR, Slater CH. Occupational physical activity and other risk factors for preterm birth among U.S. army primigravidas. Am J Public Health 1990;80:728–730.

34. Mamelle N, Laumon B, Lazar P. Prematurity and occupational activity during pregnancy. Am J Epidemiol 1984;119:309–322.

35. Mamelle N, Munoz F. Occupational working conditions and preterm birth: a reliable scoring system. Am J Epidemiol 1987;126:150–152.

36. McDonald AD, McDonald JC, Armstrong B, Cherry NM, Nolin AD. Prematurity and work in pregnancy. Br J Ind Med 1988;45:56–62.

37. Punnett L, Marbury M. Re: Occupational working conditions and preterm birth: a reliable scoring system [Letter]. Am J Epidemiol 1989;129:451.

38. Main DM, Gabbe SG. Risk scoring for preterm labor: where do we go from here? Obstet Gynecol 1987;157:789–793.

39. Saurel-Cubizolles MJ, Kaminski M, Llado-Arkhipoff J, et al. Pregnancy and its outcome among hospital personnel according to occupation and working conditions. J Epidemiol Commun Health 1985;39:129–134.

40. Saurel-Cubizolles MJ, Kaminski M. Pregnant women's working conditions and their changes during pregnancy: a national study in France. Br J Ind Med 1987;44:236–243.

41. Nurminen T, Lusa S, Ilmarinen J, Kurppa K. Physical workload, fetal development and course of pregnancy. Scand J Work Environ Health 1989;15:404–414.

42. Launer LJ, Villar J, Kestler E, De Onis M. The effect of maternal work on fetal growth and duration of pregnancy: a prospective study. Br J Obstet Gynaecol 1990;97:62–70.

43. Barnes DL, Adair LS, Popkin BM. Women's physical activity and pregnancy outcome: a longitudinal analysis from the Philippines. Int J Epidemiol 1991;20:162–172.

44. Klebanoff MA, Shiono PH, Rhoads GG. Outcomes of pregnancy in a national sample of resident physicians. N Engl J Med 1990;323:1040–1045.

45. Rabkin CS, Anderson HR, Bland JM, Brooke OG, Chamberlain G, Peacock JL. Maternal activity and birth weight: a prospective population-based study. Am J Epidemiol 1990;131:522–531.

46. Armstrong BG, Nolin AD, McDonald AD. Work in pregnancy and birthweight for gestational age. Br J Ind Med 1989;46:196–199.

47. Tafari N, Naeye RL, Gobezie A. Effects of maternal

undernutrition and heavy physical work during pregnancy on birthweight. Br J Obstet Gynecol 1980;87:222–226.

48. National Institute for Occupational Safety and Health. Work practices guide for manual lifting, DHHS (PHS) no. 81–122. Cincinnati: National Institute for Occupational Safety and Health, 1981.

49. Berkowitz GS, Kelsey JL, Holford TR, Berkowitz RL.

Physical activity and the risk of spontaneous preterm delivery. J Reprod Med 1983;28:581–588.

50. Hartikainen-Sorri A-L, Sorri M. Occupational and sociomedical factors in preterm birth. Obstet Gynecol 1989;74:13–16.

51. Ahlborg G, Bodin L, Hogstedt C. Heavy lifting during pregnancy—a hazard to the fetus? A prospective study. Int J Epidemiol 1990;19:90–97.

# 16

## Atmospheric Variations, Noise, and Vibration

HOWARD HU, MITCHELL BESSER

In recent years there has been growing interest in the human reproductive effects of exposure to physical agents encountered in occupational or community settings. While the effects of some physical factors such as x-irradiation are generally well-characterized, less is known about the biological activity of others. In this chapter, several types of physical exposures and environments are discussed: atmospheric variations, including heat and hot environments and hypobaric (high altitude) and hyperbaric (diving and pressurized) environments; noise; and vibration. The reproductive effects of some of these exposures have been studied at length; others have not, remain controversial, and require further study.

### HEAT AND HOT ENVIRONMENTS

Internal temperature in the human body is regulated within narrow limits. Protection from excessive heat is provided predominantly by sweat production and evaporation. Less important mechanisms include evaporative cooling from the lungs and physiological diversion of blood flow from muscles and other deep sites of heat production to the cooler surfaces of the body, where heat is dissipated by convective exchange with air.

Heat and hot environments can stress this thermoregulatory system and pose a physical hazard in almost any climate or workplace, especially during the summer. Occupations and activities requiring heavy exertion increase the potential for problems by adding metabolically generated heat to the background heat load. In addition, humidity and still air can greatly increase the heat stress of an environment by impeding evaporative and convective cooling. These conditions are common in tropical climates and in some industries such as canning, textiles, and laundering.

During gestation, augmentation of maternal cutaneous blood flow serves to dissipate excess heat generated by increased metabolic demands. At rest, fetal temperature is approximately 0.5°C higher than maternal temperature, creating a gradient that facilitates fetomaternal heat transfer across the placental bed (1). A rise in maternal core body temperature can reverse the gradient, resulting in increased fetal temperatures. Exercise studies demonstrate that fetal temperature changes generally parallel those in the pregnant woman, although a lag period is observed at the onset and cessation of exercise (1). Protracted heat exposure sufficient to increase significantly the maternal core temperature raises concerns about developmental effects.

In the male, the testes are suspended in the scrotum at a temperature 2–3°C cooler than the body cavity. Spermatogenesis occurs most effectively in this environment. Testicular heating, with its attendant alterations in sperm production, has been studied as a cause of infertility.

## Effects on Pregnancy

### EXPERIMENTAL ANIMAL STUDIES

In laboratory animals, heat exposure is clearly teratogenic. The risk of an adverse outcome depends on the timing of exposure and the degree and duration of temperature elevation. Unfertilized ova are not affected by small elevations in temperature, whereas the embryonic stage of development is extremely sensitive to hyperthermic exposures (2–4). Edwards et al. (5) showed that hyperthermia in the first trimester induces multiple congenital malformations in guinea pigs. They postulated that the rapidly proliferating cells in the first trimester are most affected by heat, inducing abnormal development in multiple organ systems. Animals exposed to heat later in gestation, when cell proliferation has slowed, are not similarly affected.

Other studies suggest specific heat parameters necessary for induction of adverse pregnancy outcomes. Cockroft and New (6) determined that rat neural tissue is particularly sensitive to temperatures greater than 40°C. Shiota (7) induced teratogenesis by increasing core temperature by 4.0°C for 5 min, 3.5°C for 10 min, 3.0°C for 20 min, or 2.5°C for 60 min. Edwards et al. (5) showed that, for each degree of temperature elevation above 2.5°C, there was significantly greater impairment of brain development.

### HUMAN STUDIES

#### Fever and Pregnancy

Several human studies that focus primarily on fever during pregnancy suggest that maternal core temperature elevations greater than 38.9°C present a risk of abnormal fetal development. Febrile episodes occurring during the period of neural tube closure (days 20–28 postconception) have been associated with a significantly increased incidence of CNS-related defects compared to control groups without fever during pregnancy (8–10). Studies of influenza epidemics in Europe in the 1950s and 1960s reveal a two- to three-fold increase in congenital anomalies among infants born to women with sustained febrile episodes in the first trimester of pregnancy (11, 12). Exposures between gestational weeks 4–7 resulted in structural and functional abnormalities in the neonate including CNS, facial, and limb abnormalities; mental deficiency; hypotonia; and seizures. For hyperthermic exposures between weeks 7–16, functional abnormalities were predominant with hypotonia and mental deficiency most common. No infants exposed to high temperatures after 16 weeks' gestation had malformations, although some mild growth deficiency was noted. In all of these studies, temperature elevations were significant and sustained for more than 1 day. None of the studies noted an increased risk of stillbirth or preterm delivery.

Other investigations have not found an association between hyperthermia and adverse pregnancy outcomes. The Collaborative Perinatal Project collected data on 50,000 pregnant women (13). One hundred sixty-five women had documented febrile episodes greater than 38.9°C for 1–3 days in the first trimester of pregnancy, and 13 women had "high fevers" without documentation. When this group of 178 women was matched against a control group without hyperthermia in pregnancy, there were no differences in the incidence of neurological abnormalities, congenital anomalies, spontaneous abortions, stillbirths, preterm births, or growth-retarded infants. Other prospective and retrospective studies failed to find a significant association between hyperthermia due to influenza in early pregnancy and abnormal pregnancy outcomes (14, 15).

#### Heat/Hot Environments

Although there are anecdotal accounts linking hot tub and sauna use in pregnancy with congenital anomalies, there are insufficient data to indicate a significant association. Reports conflict as to whether reasonable hot tub or sauna use causes body temperature to reach 38.9°C. Harvey et al. (16) found that few female test subjects were able to stay in a hot tub, and none in a sauna, until vaginal temperatures reached 38.9°C. Minimum time intervals to increase vaginal temperature to 38.9°C were 15 min in a hot tub set to 39°C and 10 min in a hot tub set to 41.1°C. Sohar et al. (17), testing men and women in a sauna set to 80–90°C, showed that the average increase in rectal temperature was only 0.9°C after 20 min. However, 22% of the volunteers had temperatures above 39°C after this time period. Data from Finland, where women use the sauna throughout pregnancy, show no associated increase in the incidence of anencephaly or other congenital anomalies (18–20).

No reports suggest that normal exercise in pregnancy induces sufficient maternal hyperthermia to be embryocidal or teratogenic (21).

There is a single report of increased fetal malformations among women working in laundries; however, no description of the degree, duration, or gestational timing of temperature exposure is provided (22). There are no data suggesting that firefighters are exposed to sufficient heat for long enough periods to raise body temperature and to induce fetal malformations (23).

## SUMMARY AND RECOMMENDATIONS

There are many opportunities for pregnant women to be exposed to heat and hot environments. However, few studies specifically address the epidemiological relationship between this physical hazard and pregnancy outcome. A physiological model exists in which rapidly proliferating embryonic tissues might be adversely affected by hyperthermic conditions involving elevation of core temperature beyond 39°C. Evidence from animal studies clearly indicates that elevation of core temperature of sufficient degree and duration during specific gestational age intervals induces spontaneous abortion, fetal malformation, and postnatal developmental abnormalities. Some human studies of pregnancy complicated by significant febrile episodes suggest an association with adverse developmental outcomes; others, however, do not.

Fortunately, thermoregulatory mechanisms protect humans from deleterious hyperthermic imbalance under most environmental and occupational circumstances. However, if heat stress is severe enough to elevate core temperature to 39°C, concerns arise not only about developmental effects, but also about direct effects on the pregnant woman, including heat exhaustion and heat stroke (24). Even at lesser heat extremes, pregnant workers whose jobs involve prolonged standing or strenuous work may be intolerant of hot, humid environments. Reduction of cardiac output created by decreased venous return, coupled with peripheral vascular dilation to dissipate the heat generated by both the fetus and the employee's own increased metabolic rate, may lead to dizziness or syncope in these settings.

In view of these considerations, it is prudent to avoid excessive heat exposure during pregnancy. Patients with significant febrile illnesses should be encouraged to take antipyretic medications. Hot tub and sauna use should be restricted to 15 min, a seemingly safe interval.

Pregnant women potentially exposed to excessive heat in occupations should minimize the possibility of heat imbalance through avoidance of heavy exertion and appropriate work practices (24). Industrial hygiene guidelines developed by the National Institute for Occupational Safety and Health (NIOSH) to guard against core temperature elevation and the general health hazards of heat are probably sufficient to protect against reproductive effects as well. These guidelines include monitoring of hot workplaces using a special thermometer that takes into account heat transfer, humidity, and wind velocity; medical surveillance by a physician; use of appropriate ventilation and other engineering controls and protective clothing and equipment; and worker education (24, 25).

Women who have experienced hyperthermic episodes during early pregnancy can be reassured that adverse outcomes are unlikely. α-Fetoprotein screening and ultrasound can be performed during the second trimester for further reassurance.

### Male Reproductive Effects

In the male, each testis is suspended in the scrotum by a vascular pedicle, the spermatic cord, which contains the spermatic artery and venous pampiniform plexus. These vessels interdigitate, producing a countercurrent heat exchange that reduces heat flow to the testis. Temperature reduction in the testis is also mediated by the cremasteric muscle, which contracts or relaxes in relation to scrotal temperature, and by the thin-walled scrotum which has little insulating connective tissue and subcutaneous fat. A normal body-scrotal temperature gradient is carefully maintained, with the testis approximately 2–3°C cooler than the body cavity.

Data from studies on chronic disorders and acute exposures suggest that heat and hot environments can affect sperm production and male fertility to the extent that testicular temperature is raised. Human and animal experiments in which the testes are exposed to controlled amounts of temperature elevation corroborate this impression.

## EXPERIMENTAL HYPERTHERMIA

Animal studies indicate that heat exposures sufficient to induce hyperthermia cause testicular atrophy, seminiferous tubule degeneration, abnormal spermatogenesis, and azoospermia. These changes are reversible, with recovery 6 weeks after cessation of exposure (26).

In human hyperthermia experiments, reductions in sperm concentration and sperm motility are consistently seen. Changes in sperm concentration occur 3–7 weeks after temperature exposure, and recovery is noted 4–11 weeks after exposure ceases. In studies involving longer durations of heat exposure, the recovery interval is prolonged, lasting as long as 6 months (27).

## CHRONIC DISORDERS

Semen studies in men with chronic testicular heat exposure due to cryptorchidism and retractile testes reveal decreased sperm counts and sperm motility and increased numbers of abnormal forms (28, 29). Testosterone production is normal (30). In animal studies in which the testes are transferred from the scrotum to the peritoneal cavity, degeneration of the seminiferous tubules is noted. Spermatogenesis is arrested with no development of mature spermatozoa. Return of the testes to the scrotum results in normalization of spermatogenesis (31). Varicocele formation, which is often accompanied by testicular hyperthermia, is also associated in some reports with abnormal semen analysis and infertility (32, 33).

In paraplegic men in wheelchairs, Brendley (34) noted a chronic 0.9°C elevation of scrotal temperature relative to nonparalyzed men. Semen analyses in the paraplegic men revealed normal counts but absent sperm motility.

There are no human data to suggest that cytogenetic aberrations or congenital defects result from elevated intratesticular temperature.

## ACUTE HEAT EXPOSURES

### Fever

Acute or intermittent elevations in testicular temperature during the course of fever have been found to impact on sperm parameters and male fertility. MacLeod (35) analyzed serial semen samples from patients with chickenpox and staphylococcal pneumonia who had febrile courses lasting 3 days to 3 weeks with temperatures in excess of 37.9°C. These analyses revealed a fall in sperm count and motility and an increase in abnormal forms after 40 days, a nadir lasting 30 days, and normalization after 20–30 days. However, the possibility of confounding by the effects of antibiotics or the infectious agents themselves could not be excluded.

### Clothing

The relative impact of jockey shorts and boxer shorts on semen production is unclear. Brendley (34) measured scrotal temperatures in a subject wearing boxer shorts and Jockey shorts; boxer shorts resulted in scrotal temperatures 0.5°C cooler than Jockey shorts. Zorgniotti et al. (36) found no significant difference in the semen analyses of men wearing boxer or Jockey shorts.

### Occupational/Environmental Heat Exposures

Semen analyses from men exposed to elevated temperatures while performing summer outdoor labor reveal significant reductions in sperm concentration and sperm motility (37, 38). The lower the subject's pre-exposure sperm count and motility, the greater the proportional reduction. Fertility was also noted to be reduced, with fewer children born to the wives of these men during the spring season (37). Several studies suggest that there are circannual rhythms in human sperm counts unrelated to exposure to hot climates (39, 40). A statistically significant high-amplitude seasonal variation has been noted, with highest values in the winter and spring and lowest values in the summer and fall. Others refute these findings, claiming no significant seasonal variation in sperm analysis (41).

## SUMMARY AND RECOMMENDATIONS

Both chronic and acute heat exposures to the testes can affect spermatogenesis. Chronic disorders that elevate testicular temperature, such as cryptorchidism, retractile testis, and possibly varicocele, induce abnormalities in sperm parameters and reduce fertility. After acute febrile and occupational hyperthermic exposures, the most consistent abnormalities noted are decreases in sperm count and motility. These findings are more pronounced in men with pre-exposure semen analysis values in the low-normal range. Underwear appears to have little effect on spermatogenesis.

A 3- to 7-week interval between heat exposure and a fall in sperm count is consistent with the clearance of unaffected sperm from the epididymis and arrest of normal sperm generation in the seminiferous tubules. Complete recovery after 4–11 weeks is consistent with a 64-day cycle for sperm regeneration from spermatogonia. Histological studies reveal limited, if any, thermal damage to the testosterone-producing Leydig cells.

Semen analyses should be performed on men exposed to high temperatures at work who are experiencing fertility problems. If abnormal, patients are counseled about ways to minimize heat exposure, and semen parameters are followed monthly for signs of recovery. As previously mentioned, NIOSH guidelines are available for monitoring and controlling heat exposures in the workplace.

## HYPOBARIC (HIGH ALTITUDE) ENVIRONMENTS

Individuals living and working at high altitudes and aircraft personnel working in cabins that are pressurized to 5000–8000 ft experience exposure to hypobaric (low-pressure) and hypoxic environments. Although the percentage of oxygen remains at 21% at high altitudes, decreased pressure reduces the gradient for oxygen absorption, leading to a fall in arterial $PO_2$. At 18,000 feet, the partial pressure of oxygen is half that at sea level. Concern regarding the effect of high-altitude exposure on reproductive function has focused primarily on fertility and pregnancy outcomes. Most studies have examined the role of chronic exposure (i.e., living at high altitude); a few have considered the effects of brief periods of exposure.

### Female Reproductive Effects

#### MENSTRUATION

A number of animal and human studies suggest that a change from low to high altitude can disrupt menstrual function. Rats transported from sea level to 14,000 feet for 90 days were observed to have disruption of oestrus cycles that resolved after return to sea level (42). Five of 10 college women taken from sea level to 14,000 feet reported menstrual changes over 10 weeks; three described a reduction in menstrual flow, and two noted decreased cycle lengths. These changes resolved within 2 months of returning to sea level. The other five subjects noted no change in their menstrual function (43).

Studies have also been performed on female mountain climbers and flight attendants; however, hypobaric exposures in these situations are confounded by the stresses of climbing and the changes in sleep cycles and time zones experienced by airline personnel. Six of seven Himalayan mountain climbers ascending to greater than 25,000 feet noted changes in menses, with three describing shorter cycles, two lighter flow, and one heavier flow. Changes resolved in all of the climbers within 4 months of returning to sea level (44). Iglesias et al. (45) interviewed 200 flight attendants routinely exposed to cabin pressure equivalent to an altitude of 500 feet. Fifty percent had menstrual problems before starting the job. Among these women, half experienced no change in their condition; the rest were evenly distributed between worsening and improvement of their previous problems. Of the women who started to fly without a menstrual disorder, approximately 50% developed menstrual problems. The most common problems described by the flight attendants were menorrhagia, more frequent periods, irregular periods, and dysmenorrhea. When questioned about changes in menses while in flight, 52% noted no change in blood flow, 28% described heavier flow, and 20% reported lighter flow. No variation in menses could be attributed to differences in age or sexual activity among the subjects (44, 46).

## FERTILITY

The effects of high altitude on female fertility remain controversial. Population studies in Nepal (47, 48) and Peru (49) suggest that women living at higher altitudes have a significantly lower completed fertility rate than women living at lower altitudes. Opinions differ as to the role of cultural factors in this difference (47, 48). Studies in Bolivia (50, 51) show no variation in crude fertility rates when comparing populations at low and high altitudes. Fertility differences noted in other studies have been attributed to methodological problems.

## PREGNANCY OUTCOMES

The effects of high altitude on pregnancy are clearer than they are for fertility. While acute exposure to altitude during pregnancy is apparently benign, chronic exposure is associated with decreased fetal growth. Studies of a Colorado population at 10,000 feet indicate that reduced birthweight is due to retardation of fetal growth after 30 weeks' gestational age (52–55). At each gestational age interval after 30 weeks, a progressive decrease in fetal size is observed at increased altitude (54). Unger et al. (52) stratified the Colorado population into altitude groups and found that babies born at sea level weighed, on average, 346 g more than babies born above 10,000 ft. Infants of women smokers living at high altitude weighed 550 g less than babies born at sea level (53).

Unger et al. (52) found that the rate of low birthweight (less than 2500 g) was 6.8% at sea level and 13% above 10,000 ft. There was no difference in the incidence of preterm birth. For preterm and term babies born at altitude,

there was no increase in perinatal morbidity or mortality. These findings have been confirmed in a high altitude population in the Peruvian Andes (56, 57). Yip (58), controlling for socioeconomic and ethnic factors, analyzed data from 1978–1981 for all U.S. births to college educated, white, married women between 20 and 39 yr old. At altitudes above 10,000 ft, there was a 10% reduction in mean birthweight and a three-fold increase in the incidence of low birthweight compared to births at less than 1500 ft. Decreases in birthweight were clearly due to fetal growth retardation because the length of gestation remained unaffected. It appears that low birthweight at higher altitudes may not be as disadvantageous as low birthweight at lower altitudes. This may reflect a lower normative range for birthweight at higher altitudes.

Growth retardation has been attributed to the hypoxic environment at altitude. Moore et al. (53) found a direct correlation between birthweight and maternal arterial $PO_2$ and hemoglobin concentrations. Another study found that infants born at 15,000 ft weighed 15% less than those delivered at sea level, but the placentas weighed 12% more. The authors suggest that the larger placenta represents a response to the hypoxic environment at altitude, providing better fetal oxygenation (56). Significantly increased cord and neonatal hematocrits noted in babies born at altitude may also represent an adjustment to the hypoxic environment (57).

Acute changes of altitude during gestation do not appear to have an adverse effect on pregnancy outcome. Studies of exposure to commercial jet travel with cabin pressures comparable to 8000 ft show that pregnant women have small increases in heart rate and blood pressures within the normal range. Respiratory rate and $PCO_2$ remain unchanged. Arterial $PO_2$ falls by 25%. Fetal monitoring during flight reveals no change in fetal heart rate or variability (59, 60).

Barry and Bia (61) warn that the decrease in arterial $PO_2$ noted at altitude and in aircraft cabins could be detrimental to women with certain medical conditions. Women with profound anemias may become symptomatic at altitude, and those with sickle cell disease may experience a crisis from the hypoxic environment. Supplemental oxygen is recommended for these women during flight. They also suggest that pregnant women avoid altitudes greater than 15,000 ft because no adequate data exist for exposure to these heights.

## Male Reproductive Effects

Some human and animal studies on altitude exposure describe semen changes that might impact on male fertility. Human volunteers taken from sea level to 14,000 ft for 4 weeks were found to have statistically significant reductions in sperm count and motility and increased numbers of abnormal forms. These changes appeared after 1 week at altitude and normalized after returning to sea level (62). Male rats exposed intermittently over 4 weeks to altitude chambers at 21,500 ft were found to have reduced testicular weights, increased numbers of abnormal sperm forms, and poorer mating performance compared to rats at sea level (63).

On the other hand, studies on Peruvian populations chronically exposed to altitude revealed normal semen analyses and urinary gonadotropin levels among high altitude (14,000 ft) residents (64). Serum gonadotropins, testosterone, and prolactin levels were measured in Nepalese sherpas living at 4500 ft, 8500 ft, and 14,000 ft. Small elevations in luteinizing hormone (LH) levels were noted in the sherpas living at the highest altitude, but all other hormonal studies did not differ among the three groups (65).

## Summary and Recommendations

During pregnancy, chronic exposure to hypobaric environments is clearly associated with intrauterine growth retardation, especially among women who smoke. Growth retardation is not accompanied by an increase in perinatal morbidity or mortality despite a two- to three-fold increase in low birthweight babies. No increase in premature births is noted.

Commercial air travel and acute exposure to altitudes less than 15,000 ft pose no adverse effects on maternal or fetal well-being. Pregnant women with medical problems that might be exacerbated by hypoxic environments should be carefully counseled. Avoidance of high altitudes or supplemental oxygen during flight may be necessary for these women.

There is limited evidence that acute exposure to hypobaric environments is associated with irregular menstrual cycles. There is no consistent association with a decrease in female fertility.

In males, acute exposures to high altitude induce reversible changes in semen parameters in some studies. Men chronically exposed to hypobaric environments, however, do not demonstrate any differences in semen analysis. Hormone studies suggest that, except for a modest rise in LH, other hormones are unchanged in men living at altitude. A reduction in male fertility has been observed in animals acutely exposed to altitude. This effect has not been studied in humans.

## HYPERBARIC ENVIRONMENTS

The ambient air pressure exceeds 1 atmosphere absolute (ATA), the atmospheric pressure found at sea level, in underwater diving and occupations including caisson operations and underwater tunneling. (*Caissons* are tubular steel structures submerged in a river or sea bed or water-bearing ground. They are used for construction or repair of bridges and piers and in excavation work. The pneumatic type of caisson has a closed top and is entered through an airlock; the bottom is open, allowing workers to excavate the ground, and water is excluded by the maintenance of a pressurized [hyperbaric] environment. In *tunneling* operations, compressed air is used to keep out water and to aid in supporting the structure.) Pressures encountered generally range from 2–5 ATA, although commercial divers often submerge to depths greater than 100 m at 11 ATA pressure. (A 10-m increase in depth below seawater adds 1 ATA pressure.) With the growing popularity of recreational scuba diving, men and women of reproductive age are increasingly likely to be exposed to hyperbaric environments.

In general, concerns about systemic and reproductive effects from exposure to hyperbaric environments arise from the phenomenon of nitrogen bubble formation that occurs when ascending too rapidly from depth. These toxic effects are known as "the bends" or "decompression sickness."

Attempts to avoid nitrogen bubble formation led to the development of depth and time charts that dictate allowable time periods at various depths and appropriate decompression stops that permit nitrogen levels to equilibrate and divers to ascend unharmed. However, these charts were not devised to account for the altered physiology of pregnancy.

## Effects on Pregnancy

The risk of hyperbaric exposure during pregnancy is unclear. One mechanism for maternal and fetal morbidity is nitrogen bubble formation.

Pregnancy produces changes in the cardiovascular, renal, hematological, and respiratory systems. Nitrogen is absorbed by adipose tissue, which is increased during gestation. The placenta is very permeable to nitrogen, allowing for rapid equilibration of the gas between the pregnant woman and fetus (66). The patent ductus arteriosus and foramen ovale of the fetus offer the opportunity for nitrogen bubbles to bypass the pulmonary bed. In the event of decompression sickness, bubbles could embolize developing embryonic or fetal structures, inducing spontaneous abortion or malformations. These complex physiological changes of pregnancy make the construction of appropriate depth and time charts difficult.

Human and experimental animal studies have sought to determine fetal and maternal risks relative to the degree of exposure to hyperbaric conditions, the gestational age at the time of exposure, and the occurrence of decompression sickness.

### EXPERIMENTAL ANIMAL STUDIES

Investigations of laboratory animals exposed to hyperbaric conditions during pregnancy have shown conflicting results. Studies in rats and sheep (67, 68) during early gestation and near term found that exposure to pressures as high as 7 atmospheres with depth times causing maternal decompression sickness did not result in fetal wastage or anomalies. In other studies (69–71), animals experiencing decompression sickness without treatment had significantly

higher rates of fetal wastage and anomalies than those treated with hyperbaric oxygen or gradual ascent. Animals treated with hyperbaric oxygen had anomaly rates no different from nondived controls.

Investigations of physiological changes in pregnant animals during diving have been revealing, yet also contradictory. Nemiroff et al. (67), studying sheep near term, monitored maternal and fetal circulation during dives (to 165 ft) that exceeded U.S. Navy Dive Table no-decompression limits. He found that 8 of 12 ewes, but no fetuses, developed bubbles in their circulation. None of the affected ewes showed signs of decompression sickness. Chen (unpublished data cited in 67) exposed rats to dives that induced severe decompression sickness and death. Autopsies revealed no bubbles in the fetal circulation. Powell and Smith (72) monitored second and third trimester sheep and goats, finding that both the maternal and fetal circulations had bubbles. Bubbles were noted in the fetal circulation even when the pregnant animals showed no signs of decompression sickness.

### HUMAN STUDIES

There are no prospective controlled studies in humans describing the dangers of scuba diving during pregnancy. Bolton (73) conducted a retrospective survey using mailed questionnaires. Two hundred eight female divers responded, including 136 who dived during pregnancy and 72 who did not. Of the women who dived during pregnancy, 39% did so in the first trimester, 41% in the second trimester, and 20% in the third trimester. Seventy-nine percent restricted their diving to within no-decompression limits at depths less than 100 ft. Women who dived during pregnancy reported more infants with major and minor congenital anomalies (5.5%) than women who did not dive (0%). Of note, the incidence of major and minor congenital anomalies among the diving women was not significantly different from the rate expected in the general population (7%). There was no increased incidence of spontaneous abortion, ectopic pregnancy, stillbirth, low birthweight infants, neonatal death, or other neonatal problems.

Turner and Unsworth (74) reported a case of an anomalous fetus born to a woman who made 20 uncomplicated nondecompression dives to less than 100 ft between 40 and 50 days from her last menstrual period. The infant was born with arthrogryposis, micrognathia, short neck, and penis adherent to the scrotum. Bangasser (personal communication cited in 67) found no increase in maternal or fetal complications in 72 women who dived during gestation.

There are no reports of adverse pregnancy outcomes after occupational exposures to hyperbaric environments.

## Male Reproductive Effects

Little is known regarding the effects of hyperbaric environments on male reproductive function. Two studies on male rats exposed to 2–3 ATA and one investigation on rats exposed chronically to 21 ATA found no significant changes in testicular histology (75, 76). Another study found shortened duration of spermatozoan motility in rats exposed to greater than 3 ATA (77). Fryer et al. (78) found evidence of disorganization and patchy epithelial necrosis upon electron microscopic examination of testicular tissue from mice exposed to 50 ATA. These changes disappeared 2 weeks after exposure. No reports have been published on humans.

## Summary and Recommendations

There are currently no prospective studies in humans during any stage of gestation to define clearly the risk of hyperbaric exposure during pregnancy. Retrospective studies indicate that pregnant women who dive, especially in the first trimester, have a higher rate of anomalous offspring than nondivers. However, these studies are subject to recall bias, and malformation rates among divers are no higher than in the general population. Animal studies suggest that bubble formation may occur in the fetus in the absence of overt signs of maternal decompression sickness. Fetal anatomy imposes risk of bubble embolization to peripheral structures, resulting in compromised embryogenesis and intrauterine growth. In some studies inducing maternal decompression sickness, fetal effects were not observed if hyperbaric oxygen was administered.

At present, standards for hyperbaric exposure comparable to the U.S. Navy Dive Tables have not been developed for pregnancy. Given the current state of knowledge in this area, diving and other hyperbaric exposures cannot be recommended as safe for the pregnant woman. Hyperbaric exposure is not known to have significant effects on male reproductive function, but studies are limited.

## NOISE

Noise is a common feature of the modern environment and is well established as a risk factor for hearing loss. More recent efforts have focused on assessment of indirect noise-induced health effects and on identification of the most hazardous types of noise.

Noise is defined as unwanted sound. Like any sound, noise is caused by a fluctuation of the ambient pressure that propagates in the elastic media, air. In this sense, it can be distinguished from vibration that is caused by oscillation in solid media. The *decibel* (dB) scale is commonly used to measure "loudness" and represents the magnitude of the pressure change converted into a logarithmic scale. *Frequency* is the rate at which the pressure fluctuations repeat in a sinusoidal fashion; it is expressed in units of cycles per second or Hertz (Hz). The range of human hearing lies roughly between 20 and 20,000 Hz.

Noise can be divided into two broad classes: continuous and impulsive. In many industrial situations, impulsive noises are superimposed on a background of continuous noise. Some typical noise readings are depicted in Figure 16.1.

The recent finding that sound is well transmitted into the fetal environment has heightened concern about effects on the conceptus (79). There is a theoretical basis for anticipating that noise can affect reproductive physiology and fetal development. Through effects on the autonomic and reticular nervous systems, noise may elicit a number of physiological responses including changes in cardiovascular volume, heart rate, blood pressure, and endocrine function (80). Teratogenic effects seen in animals may be due, in part, to fetal hypoxia resulting from noise-induced increases in maternal catecholamines with reduced utero-

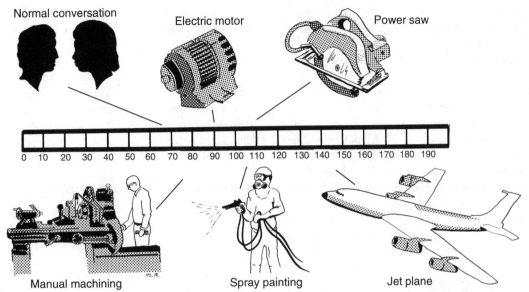

**Figure 16.1.** Some typical sound levels (dBA) in general and occupational environments.

placental blood flow (81, 82). However, experimental noise exposure has not been consistently associated with alterations in stress hormone levels and uteroplacental blood flow in humans (83, 84).

## Effects on Pregnancy

### EXPERIMENTAL ANIMAL STUDIES

Increased fetal heart rate and fetal activity are well known to occur in response to sound (85). External sound, particularly of low frequency, is transmitted into the uterine environment more readily than has been previously appreciated (79, 86). For frequencies below 500 Hz, maternal tissues attenuate sound by only 10–15 dB.

Noise is associated with embryofetal toxicity in some animal studies. Increased resorption rates and decreased numbers of live fetuses per litter were observed in female mice exposed to 100 dB of noise during early pregnancy (87). Exposure of mice to semicontinuous 126 dB low-frequency noise, intermittent 110 dB midfrequency noise, or semicontinuous very high-frequency (18–20 kHz) 113-dB noise produced similar effects, as well as decreased pregnancy rates and reduced fetal weights (88). Effects have been noted with noise exposure limited to either the preimplantation or postimplantation period (89).

Studies that have focused on possible late stage effects have yielded inconsistent results. Some studies report intrauterine growth retardation, fetal mortality, and altered behavioral attributes; others show no significant effects. Interpretation of these studies is hampered by differences in test conditions as well as by the difficult task of extrapolating to humans from endpoints typically assessed in experimental animal studies (79).

Lower levels of noise may also have an effect. The human cochlea and peripheral sensory end organs complete their normal development by the 24th week of gestation, although CNS auditory maturation continues into postnatal life (90). Studies on newborn animals reveal a critical period late in fetal development when the cochlea is very sensitive to damage from noise exposure (91). It is possible that noise levels that are too low to be perceived as psychologically annoying to adults may have subtle effects on the fetus.

### HUMAN STUDIES

As pointed out by Meyer et al. (92), exposure assessment of noise in human epidemiological studies is made difficult by the problem of distinguishing the perception of noise from actual sound. The effect of the same noise stimulus on any two individuals can be markedly different depending upon individual interpretation and response to the signal, previous acclimation, cultural differences, and other factors.

To date, many of the epidemiological studies on noise and reproduction have been community-based surveys examining the possible effects of airport noise on birth outcomes. Several investigators have reported a slightly higher frequency of birth defects (e.g., anencephaly and spina bifida) and lower birthweight among families residing near airports in comparison to controls (93–96). While investigators have used in-depth interviewing techniques to control for potential confounders, the ecological nature of these investigations limits the degree to which an etiological association can be inferred.

One recent occupational case-control study on birth outcomes found that women with an estimated exposure to noise in the workplace averaging 80 dB over an 8-hr shift had an increased risk for threatened abortion, pregnancy-induced hypertension, and shortened gestational length (97). The same researchers noted no increased risk of congenital malformations (98). In another recent study, children with high-frequency hearing loss were more likely to have been born to women who were exposed consistently to noise in the range of 85–95 dB during pregnancy, especially if the noise was of low frequency (99). This case-control study had a number of potential weaknesses, however, including reliance on retrospective noise evaluations and several sources of potential bias. An investigation of 22,761 livebirths that related outcomes to self-reported maternal occupational exposures revealed a slight increased risk of low birthweight among noise-exposed women in manufacturing and health care jobs (100).

## Adult Reproductive Effects

Little has been written about the effects of noise on menstrual cycles or female fertility. One study of rats exposed to "white noise" at 95 dB found disturbances in menstrual cycling that seemed to be mediated by hormonal levels (101). A human case-control study found that involuntary infertility was significantly associated with a self-reported history of excessive occupational noise exposure (102).

Similarly, little research has been directed at the effects of noise on male reproductive function. In a clinical series of 93 men under evaluation for infertility, no association was found between sperm count, motility, morphology, or seminal fluid chemistry and self-reported exposure to noise (103).

## Summary and Recommendations

Limited evidence suggests that physiological responses to noise exposure may affect reproductive function. Moreover, transmission of external sound, particularly of low frequency, to the fetal environment has been found to occur readily. Animal studies suggest that semicontinuous loud noise of low or high frequency leads to increased fetal resorption rates and growth retardation. Human studies have been limited largely to ecological investigations of communities exposed to airport noise and case-control studies of pregnancy outcomes in relation to self-reported noise exposure. Some of these investigations have suggested an increased risk of threatened abortion, pregnancy-induced hypertension, and lower birthweight and high-frequency hearing loss among children. Conclusions are difficult to draw, however, because of the crude design of the studies.

Limits for occupational noise exposure set by the Occupational Safety and Health Administration (OSHA) are designed to protect only against hearing loss. Employers are required to reduce workplace noise levels to 90 dB (for an 8-hr workday) through implementation of engineering and administrative controls and to provide hearing protectors when noise levels cannot otherwise be minimized (104).

Current data are not sufficient to establish a noise exposure that will protect against adverse reproductive effects. One group of Canadian researchers concerned about the effects of low-frequency noise on the fetal auditory system suggests that pregnant women avoid occupational noise exposures over 85 dB (99). Better validated recommendations await further research in this area.

## VIBRATION

Vibration refers to the mechanical oscillation of a surface around its reference point. Vibration is distinguished from sound in that the surface is solid (as opposed to air or liquid), and the oscillations are usually uniform rather than intermittent and varying in frequency.

## Whole-body and Segmental Vibration

An estimated 8 million workers in the U.S. are exposed to occupational vibration as either whole-body vibration or segmental vibration to a specific body part. Truck, tractor, bus, and other vehicle operators are subject to chronic, whole body, low-frequency vibration transmitted through the seats or floors of their workposts. Grinders and chain-saw, chipping hammer, and other pneumatic-tool operators are exposed to higher frequency, segmental vibration.

Little is known about the general health effects of vibration in the occupational setting. Some epidemiological studies, including one conducted by NIOSH, suggest an association between long-term employment in jobs involving whole-body vibration and changes in bone structure, gastrointestinal symptoms, prostatitis, and nerve conduction velocity (105). Chronic exposure to segmental vibration through the use of vibratory hand tools is well known to elicit a Raynaud's phenomenon (24). The pathophysiological mechanism seems to involve vascular injury and arterial vasospasm.

Very little has been published on the possible reproductive effects of occupational exposure to vibration in either women or men. A few reports linking industrial vibration exposure to menstrual disorders have been published in Bulgaria (106, 107). It is not known whether the phenomenon of vascular pathology associated with segmental vibration can extend to reproductive organs exposed to either whole-body or regional vibration. This topic deserves further study.

## Vibratory Acoustic Stimulation

During the course of antenatal testing, some pregnant women are exposed to a form of vibration through the use of vibratory acoustic stimulation (VAS) devices. These instruments use an electronic artificial larynx to produce a broadband vibration at various frequencies. Obstetrical researchers are exploring fetal heart rate in response to VAS as an indicator of fetal health status. The stimulus from a VAS device is produced by surface-to-surface contact and, thus, can technically be thought of as a vibration; however, the device operates at frequencies between 10,000 and 15,000 Hz with multiple harmonics, thereby generating a stimulus with the features of noise (108). These devices are applied to the maternal abdomen for intervals ranging from 5 sec to 1 min. In a recent study of 16 women at term, Nyman et al. (109) recorded mean intrauterine sound pressure levels of 115 dB during VAS stimulation.

Studies assessing potential risks of VAS use are very limited. Sherer et al. (110) reported a case in which external VAS testing of a healthy, term fetus was followed by severe and prolonged fetal bradycardia, necessitating cesarean section delivery. At delivery, a tight nuchal cord was found; Apgar scores were 7 (1 min) and 10 (5 min). Ohel et al. (111) reported normal auditory acuity in a small group of 2-day-old neonates exposed in utero to VAS stimulation. Recently, Arulkumaran et al. (112) found no evidence of hearing loss at 7 yr of age in 465 children, the majority of whom had been exposed once to VAS testing at term. These findings, however, do not necessarily extend to VAS exposures that are more frequent or that occur at earlier gestational ages.

## Summary and Recommendations

Very little is known about the impact of exposure to physical vibration on reproductive health. The association of Raynaud's phenomenon with the use of vibratory hand tools raises the issue of whether whole body vibration and/or vibration localized to the abdomen can affect pregnancy or the reproductive organs. The recent use of VAS devices has introduced an iatrogenic source of vibration exposure during pregnancy. While the exposure is brief and occurs late in fetal development, neither the efficacy nor safety of VAS devices has been well established.

## REFERENCES

1. Lotgering FK, Gilbert RD, Longo LD. Maternal and fetal responses to exercise during pregnancy. Physiol Rev 65:1–36.

2. Woody CO, Ulberg LC. Viability of one-cell sheep ova as affected by high environment temperature. J Reprod Fertil 1964;7:275–280.

3. Bellve AR. Viability and survival of mouse embryos following parental exposure to high temperature. J Reprod Fertil 1972;30:71–81.

4. Ulberg LC, Sheehan LA. Early development of mammalian embryos in elevated ambient temperatures. J Reprod Fertil 1973;19(Suppl):155–161.

5. Edwards MJ, Mulley R, Ring S, Wanner RA. Mitotic cell death and delay of mitotic activity in guinea-pig embryos following brief maternal hyperthermia. J Embryol Exp Morph 1974;32:593–602.

6. Cockroft DL, New DAT. Abnormalities induced in cultured rat embryos by hyperthermia. Teratology 1978;17:277–284.

7. Shiota K. Induction of neural tube defects and skeletal malformations in mice following brief hyperthermia in utero. Biol Neonate 1988;53:86–97.

8. Pleet H, Graham JM, Smith DW. Central nervous system and facial defects associated with maternal hyperthermia at four to fourteen weeks gestation. Pediatrics 1981;68:785–789.

9. Smith MSR, Edwards MJ, Upfold JB. The effects of hyperthermia on the fetus. Dev Med Child Neurol 1986;28:803–813.

10. Layde PM, Edmonds LD, Erickson JD. Maternal fever and neural tube defects. Teratology 1980;21:105–108.

11. Hakosalo J, Saxen L. Influenza epidemic and congenital defects. Lancet 1971;2:1346–1347.

12. Coffey VP, Jessop WJE. Maternal influenza and congenital deformities. Lancet 1959;2:935–938.

13. Clarren SK, Smith DW, Harvey MAS, Ward RH, Myrianthopoulos NC. Hyperthermia—a prospective evaluation of a possible teratogenic agent in man. J Pediatr 1979;95:81–83.

14. Hardy JMB, Azarowicz EN, Mannini A, Medearis DN, Cooke RE. The effect of Asian influenza on the outcome of pregnancy, Baltimore 1957–1958. Am J Public Health 1961;51:1182–1188.

15. Doll R, Hill AD, Sakula J. Asian influenza in pregnancy and congenital defects. Br J Prev Soc Med 1960;14:167–172.

16. Harvey MAS, McRorie MM, Smith DW. Suggested limits to the use of the hot tub and sauna by pregnant women. Can Med J 1981;125:50–53.

17. Sohar E, Shoenfeld Y, Shapiro Y, Ohry H, Cabili S. Effects of exposure to Finnish sauna. Israel J Med Sci 1976;12:1275–1282.

18. Saxen L, Holmberg PC, Nurminen M, Kuosma E. Sauna and congenital defects. Teratology 1982;25:309–313.

19. Rapola J, Saxen L, Granroth G. Anencephaly and the sauna. Lancet 1978;1:1162.

20. Granroth G, Hakama M, Saxen L. Defects of the central nervous system in Finland. Variations in time and space, sex distribution and parental age. Br J Prev Soc Med 1977;31:164–170.

21. Lotgering FK, Gilbert RD, Longo LD. The interactions of exercise and pregnancy: a review. Am J Obstet Gynecol 1984;149:560–568.

22. McDonald AD. Maternal health in early pregnancy and congenital defects. Br J Prev Soc Med 1961;15:154–166.

23. Evanoff BA, Rosenstock L. Reproductive hazards in the workplace: a case study of women firefighters. Am J Ind Med 1986;9:503–515.

24. Hu H. Other physical hazards. In: Levy BS, Wegman DH, eds. Occupational health—recognizing and preventing work-related disease. Boston: Little, Brown and Company, 1988:263–79.

25. National Institute for Occupational Safety and Health. Criteria for a recommended standard: occupational exposure to hot environments. DHHS publication nos. 86–113. Washington, DC: National Institute for Occupational Safety and Health, 1986.

26. Venkatachalam PS, Ramanthan KS. Effect of moderate heat on the testes of rats and monkeys. J Reprod Fertil 1962;4:51–56.

27. Mieusset R, Grandjean H, Mansat A, Pontonnier F. Inhibiting effect of artificial cryptorchidism on spermatogenesis. Fertil Steril 1985;43:589–594.

28. Nistal M, Paniagua R. Infertility in adult males with retractile testis. Fertil Steril 1984;41:395–403.

29. Weisman AI. Azoospermia due to testicular non-descent (semen studies on adult crytorchids). Hum Fertil 1941;6:45–47.

30. Lipshultz L. Cryptorchidism in the subfertile male. Fertil Steril 1976;27:609–620.

31. Moore CR. Experimental studies on the male reproductive system. J Urol 1951;65:497–506.

32. Greenberg SH. Varicocele and male fertility. Fertil Steril 1977;28:699–706.

33. Cockett ATK, Urry RL, Dougherty KA. The varicocele and semen characteristics. J Urol 1979;21:435–436.

34. Brendley GS. Deep scrotal temperature and the effect on it of clothing, air temperature, activity, posture and paraplegia. Br J Urol 1982;54:49–55.

35. MacLeod J. Effect of chickenpox and of pneumonia on semen quality. Fertil Steril 1951;2:523–533.

36. Zorgniotti A, Reiss H, Toth A, Sealfon A. Effect on clothing on scrotal temperature in normal men and patients with poor semen. Urology 1982;19:176–178.

37. Levine RJ. Differences in the quality of semen in outdoor workers during summer and winter. N Engl J Med 1990;323:12–17.

38. Levine RJ, Bordson BL, Matthew RM, Brown M, Stanley JM, Starr TB. Deterioration of semen quality during summer in New Orleans. Fertil Steril 1988;49:900–903.

39. Saint-Pol P, Beuscart R, Leroy-Martin B, Hermand E, Jablonski W. Circannual rhythms of sperm parameters of fertile men. Fertil Steril 1989;51:1030–1033.

40. Tjoa WS, Smolensky MH, Hsi BP, Steinberger E, Smith KD. Circannual rhythm in human sperm count revealed by serially independent sampling. Fertil Steril 1982;38:454–459.

41. Mortimer D, Templeton HA, Lenton EA, Coleman RA.

Annual patterns of human sperm production and semen quality. Arch Androl 1983;10:105.

42. Donayre J. The oestrus cycles of rats at high altitude. J Reprod Fertil 1969;18:29–32.

43. Harris CW, Shields JL, Hannon JP. Acute altitude sickness in females. Aerospace Med 1966;37:1163–1167.

44. Kramer PO, Drinkwater BL, Folinsbee LJ, Bedi JF. Ocular functions and incidence of acute mountain sickness in women at altitude. Aviat Space Environ Med 1983;54:116–120.

45. Iglesias R, Terres A, Chavarria A. Disorders of the menstrual cycle in airline stewardesses. Aviat Space Environ Med 1980;51:518–520.

46. Farrell BL, Allen MF. Physiologic/psychologic changes reported by USAF female flight nurses during flying duties. Nurs Res 1973;22:31–34.

47. Laurenson IF, Benton MA, Bishop AJ, Mascie-Taylor CGN. Fertility at low and high altitude in central Nepal. Soc Biol 1985;32:65–70.

48. Bangham CRM, Sacherer JM. Fertility of Nepalese sherpas at moderate altitudes: comparison with high-altitude data. Ann Human Biol 1980;7:323–330.

49. Abelson AE. Altitude and fertility. Hum Biol 1976;48:83–92.

50. Godoy RA. Human fertility and land tenure in highland Bolivia. Soc Biol 1984;31:290–297.

51. Dutt JS. Altitude and fertility: the confounding effect of childhood mortality—a Bolivian example. Soc Biol 1980;27:101–113.

52. Unger C, Weiser JK, McCullough RE, Keefer S, Moore LG. Altitude, low birthweight and infant mortality in Colorado. JAMA 1988;259:3427–3432.

53. Moore LG, Rounds SS, Jahnigen D, Grover RF, Reeves JT. Infant birthweight is related to maternal arterial oxygenation at high altitude. J Appl Physiol 1982;52:695–699.

54. McCullough RE, Reeves JT, Liljegren RL. Fetal growth retardation and increased infant mortality at high altitude. Arch Environ Health 1977;32:36–39.

55. Grahn D, Kratchman J. Variations in neonatal death rate and birthweight in the U.S. and possible relations to environmental radiation, geology and altitude. Am J Hum Genet 1963;15:329–352.

56. Kruger H, Arias-Stella J. The placenta and the newborn infant at high altitudes. Am J Obstet Gynecol 1970;106:586–591.

57. Ballew C, Haas JD. Hematologic evidence of fetal hypoxia. Am J Obstet Gynecol 1986;155:166–169.

58. Yip R. Altitude and birthweight. J Pediatr 1987;111:869–876.

59. Parer JT. Effects of hypoxia on the mother and fetus with emphasis on maternal air transport. Am J Obstet Gynecol 1982;142:957–961.

60. Huch R, Baumann H, Fallenstein F, Schneider KTM, Holdener F, Huch A. Physiologic changes in pregnant women and their fetuses during jet air travel. Am J Obstet Gynecol 1986;154:996–1000.

61. Barry M, Bia F. Pregnancy and travel. JAMA 1989;261:728–731.

62. Donayre J, Guerra-Garcia R, Moncloa F, Sobrevilla LA. Endocrine studies at high altitude. IV. Changes in the semen of men. J Reprod Fertil 1968;16:55–58.

63. Altland PD, Highman B. Sex organ changes and breeding performance of male rats exposed to altitude: effect of exercise and physical training. J Reprod Fertil 1968;15:215–222.

64. Sobrevilla LA, Romero I, Moncloa F, Donayre J, Guerra-Garcia R. Endocrine studies at high altitude. III. Acta Endocrinol 1967;56:369–375.

65. Bangham CRM, Hackett PH. Effects of high altitude on endocrine function in the sherpas of Nepal. J Endocrinol 1978;79:147–148.

66. Longo LD, Delivoria-Papadoopoulos M, Power GG, Hill EP, Forster RE. Diffusion equilibrium of inert gases between maternal and fetal placental capillaries. Am J Physiol 1970;219:561–569.

67. Nemiroff MJ, Willson JR, Kirschbaum TH. Multiple hyperbaric exposures during pregnancy in sheep. Am J Obstet Gynecol 1981;140:651–655.

68. Bolton-Klug ME, Lehner CE, Lamphier EH, Rankin JHG. Lack of harmful effects from simulated dives in pregnant sheep. Am J Obstet Gynecol 1983;146:48–51.

69. Gilman SC, Bradley ME, Greene KM, Fischer GJ. Fetal development: effects of decompression sickness and treatment. Aviat Space Environ Med 1983;54:1040–1042.

70. Willson JR, Blessed WB, Blackburn PJ. Hyperbaric exposure during pregnancy in sheep: staged and rapid decompression. Undersea Biomed Res 1983;10:11–15.

71. Lehner CE, Rynning C, Bolton ME, Lamphier EH. Fetal death during decompression studies in sheep. Undersea Biomed Res 1982;9(Suppl):46–47.

72. Powell MR, Smith MT. Fetal and maternal bubbles detected non-invasively in sheep and goats following hyperbaric decompression. Undersea Biomed Res 1985;12:59–67.

73. Bolton ME. Scuba diving and fetal well-being: a survey of 208 women. Undersea Biomed Res 1980;7:183–189.

74. Turner G, Unsworth I. Intrauterine bends? Lancet 1982;1:905.

75. Nakada T, Saito H, Ota K, Saegusa T, Chikenji M, Matsushita T. Serum testosterone, testicular connective tissue protein and testicular histology in rats treated with hyperbaric oxygen. Int Urol Nephrol 1986;18:439–447.

76. Nakada T, Ota K, Saegusa T, Saito H. The influence of hyperbaric oxygenation on rat testes. Invest Urol 1976;14:93–94.

77. Bar-Sagie D, Mayevsky A, Bartoov B. Effects of hyperbaric oxygenation on spermatozoan motility driven by mitochondrial respiration. J Appl Physiol 1981;50:531–537.

78. Fryer P, Gross J, Halsey MJ, Monk S, Wardley-Smith B. Sperm maturation associated with subfertility following hyperbaric exposure of mice. Undersea Biomed Res 1986;13:413–423.

79. National Research Council; Committee on Hearing, Bioacoustics, and Biomechanics; Assembly of Behavioral and Social Sciences. Prenatal effects of exposure to high-level noise. Report of Working Group 85. Washington, DC: National Academy Press, 1982.

80. Kryter K. Nonauditory effects of environmental noise. Am J Public Health 1972;60:389–398.

81. Geber W. Developmental effects of chronic maternal audiovisual stress on the rat fetus. J Embryol Exp Morph 1966;16:1–16.

82. Geber W. Cardiovascular and teratogenic effects of chronic intermittent noise stress. In: Physiological effects of noise. Welch BL, Welch AS, eds. New York: Plenum Press, 1970.

83. Follenius M, Brandenberger G, Lecornu C, Simeoni, M, Reinhardt B. Plasma catecholamine and pituitary adrenal hormones in response to noise exposure. Eur J Appl Physiol 1980;43:254–261.

84. Hartikainen-Sorri A-L, Kirkinen P, Sorri M, Anttoner H, Tuimala R. No effect of experimental noise exposure on human pregnancy. Obstet Gynecol 1991;77:611–615.

85. Yao QW, Jakobsson J, Nyman M, et al. Fetal responses to different intensity levels of vibroacoustic stimulation. Obstet Gynecol 1990;75:206–209.

86. Gerhardt KJ, Abrams RM, Oliver CC. Sound environment of the fetal sheep. Am J Obstet Gynecol 1990;162:282–287.

87. Kimmel CA, Cook RO, Staples RE. Teratogenic potential of noise in mice and rats. Toxicol Appl Pharmacol 1976;36:239–245.

88. Nawrot PS, Cook R, Staples RE. Embryotoxicity of various noise stimuli in the mouse. Teratology 1980;22:279–189.

89. Cook RO, Nawrot PS, Hamm CW. Effects of high-frequency noise on prenatal development and maternal plasma and uterine catecholamine concentrations in the CD-1 mouse. Toxicol Appl Pharmacol 1982;66:338–348.

90. Lenoir M, Pujol R, Bock RG. Critical periods of susceptibility to noise-induced hearing loss. In Salvi RJ, Henderson D, Hamernik RP, Colletti V, eds. Basic and applied aspects of noise-induced hearing loss. New York: Plenum Press, 1986:227–234.

91. Lenoir M, Pujol R. Sensitive period for acoustic trauma in the rat pup cochlea: histological findings. Acta Otolaryngol 1980;89:317–322.

92. Meyer RE, Aldrich TE, Easterly DE. Effects of noise and electromagnetic fields on reproductive outcomes. Environ Health Perspect 1989;81:193–200.

93. Jones FN, Tauscher J. Residence under an airport landing pattern as a factor in teratism. Arch Environ Health 1978;33:10–12.

94. Edmonds L, Layde P, Erickson J. Airport noise and teratogenesis. Arch Environ Health 1979;34:243–247.

95. Knipschild P, Meijer H, Salle H. Aircraft noise and birthweight. Int Arch Occup Environ Health 1981; 48:131–136.

96. Schell L. Environmental noise and human prenatal growth. Am J Phys Anthropol 1981;56:63–70.

97. Nurminen T, Kurppa K. Occupational noise exposure and course of pregnancy. Scand J Work Environ Health 1989;15:117–124.

98. Kurppa K, Rantala K, Nurminen T, Holmberg PC, Starck J. Noise exposure during pregnancy and selected structural malformations in infants. Scand J Work Environ Health 1989;15:111–116.

99. Lalande NM, Hetu R, Lambert J. Is occupational noise exposure during pregnancy a risk factor of damage to the auditory system of the fetus? Am J Ind Med 1986; 10:427–435.

100. McDonald AD, McDonald JC, Armstrong B, Cherry NM, Nolin AD, Robert D. Prematurity and work in pregnancy. Br J Ind Med 1988;45:56–62.

101. Greifahn B. Noise-induced reactions during menstrual cycle. (Engl abstract). Eur J Appl Physiol 1974:32: 171–182.

102. Rachootin P, Olsen J. The risk of infertility and delayed conception associated with exposures in the Danish workplace. J Occup Med 1983;25:394–402.

103. Effendy I, Krause W. Environmental risk factors in the history of male patients of an infertility clinic. Andrologia 1987;19:262–265.

104. 29 CFR 1910.95. Washington, DC: US Government Printing Office, 1989.

105. Helmkamp JC, Talbott EO, Marsh GM. Whole body vibration—a critical review. Am Ind Hyg Assoc J 1984;45:162–172.

106. Pramatarov A, Balev L. Menstruation disorders and the effect of vibration of motor vehicles on female conductors in Sofia urban transportation. Akush Ginekol (Sofiia) 1969;8:31–37 (in Bulgarian).

107. Marinova G, Svetoslavova E, Mateeva E. Industrial vibrations and their repercussions on the basic functions of the genital system in women. Akush Ginekol (Sofiia) 1976;15:74–78 (in Bulgarian).

108. Gagnon R. Stimulation of human fetuses with sound and vibration. Semin Perinatol 1989;13:383–402.

109. Nyman M, Arulkumaran S, Hsu TS, Ratnam SS, Till O, Westgren M. Vibroacoustic stimulation and intrauterine sound pressure levels. Obstet Gynecol 1991;78: 803–806.

110. Sherer DM, Menashe M, Sadovsky E. Severe fetal bradycardia caused by external vibratory acoustic stimulation. Am J Obstet Gynecol 1988;159:334–335.

111. Ohel G, Harawitz E, Linder N, et al. Neonatal auditory acuity following in utero vibratory acoustic stimulation. Am J Obstet Gynecol 1987;157:440–441.

112. Arulkumaran S, Skurr B, Tong H, Kek LP, Yeoh KH, Ratnam SS. No evidence of hearing loss due to fetal acoustic stimulation test. Obstet Gynecol 1991;78:283–285.

# 17

.................................................

# Metals

RICHARD K. MILLER, DAVID BELLINGER

Interest has been heightened recently concerning metal exposures and public health policy, especially involving reproduction and development. Concerns about the developmental effects of lead have resulted in new guidelines to prevent environmental exposure. Dietary exposure to mercury due to contamination of both fresh and salt waters remains an important public health issue. Cigarette smoking, a source of exposure to cadmium and other toxicants, has received unprecedented attention in recent years, leading to its prohibition in public spaces and workplaces. Yet these three metals are not the only metals of concern. Exotic metals are now commonly used in manufacturing, especially in the electronics industry. Tellurium was a rarity only 20 yr ago; today, it is found in a wide range of consumer products from black glass to photocopy dyes to microchips.

As with all exposures, the concerns for metal exposures can be divided into three categories: (a) occupational exposure, (b) consumer use, and (c) environmental exposure. Inappropriate use or poor handling may result in unfortunate toxic exposures. For example, a few years ago, babies were demonstrating neurobehavioral toxicity for unexplained reasons. The only common thread was the use of cloth diapers from the same laundry service. It was discovered that phenylmercury, used as a disinfectant, was not adequately rinsed from the diapers. The residual phenylmercury was then easily absorbed through infants' skin when they urinated in the diapers (1).

This chapter concentrates on the three metals of greatest concern today: lead, mercury, and cadmium. Quite often, an apparent single metal exposure will be discovered to be an exposure to a cluster of metals. Information on other metals is available in recent publications (1, 2–4) and the book's Appendix.

External monitoring of worker exposure is an essential part of any occupational evaluation. However, air-borne exposure limits established by regulatory bodies are not necessarily set with reproductive and developmental toxicity in mind. The emergence of biological markers of exposure allows for better estimation of doses reaching the reproductive tissues or conceptus. In addition, with the advent of newer clinical diagnostic tools such as ultrasound, Doppler technology, chorionic villous sampling, DNA adducts, sperm evaluation, hormonal evaluations, and molecular biological technology, it is possible to begin assessing early effects on the male/female, the pregnant woman, and the conceptus (5). Eventual integration of these methods into the risk assessment process will be an important step in protecting worker health. In addition, advances in fetal therapy may hold promise for correction and treatment of exposure-related deficits (6).

In this chapter, air-borne exposure limits are listed where appropriate for each metal. Biomarkers of exposure or reproductive/

developmental toxicity are utilized where available to assess risk for an individual patient better. However, with few exceptions (e.g., methylmercury and lead), the correlations are still primitive for most metals.

## LEAD

Lead's reproductive toxicity has been recognized for well over a century. Lead salts were once used as abortifacients. Early clinical experience and the results of limited epidemiological studies of lead and reproductive function were summarized in 1944 as follows:

> It is generally agreed that if pregnancy does occur it is frequently characterized by miscarriage, intrauterine death of the fetus, premature birth and, if living children are born, they are usually smaller, weaker, slower in development and have a higher infant mortality (7).

More recent epidemiological studies generally confirm these observations and establish with greater clarity the dose-response and dose-effect relationships underlying them, particularly at the lower lead levels typical of current occupational and community exposures.

## Occurrence: Sources and Properties

Since the mid-1970s, dramatic reductions in organolead compounds added to gasoline have resulted in decreased occupational exposures to tetraethyl- and tetramethyl-lead. However, exposure to inorganic lead remains a significant occupational and environmental hazard (Table 17.1).

Lead is unusual among environmental pollutants in that there are numerous sources and pathways of environmental exposure, resulting in a relatively high level of background exposure. Consequently, there is a modest margin of safety between the "average" body burden in the population and that considered toxic.

Virtually all lead exposure is "anthropogenic," i.e., due to human activities. The major nonoccupational sources and pathways of exposure include paint, water, food, dust/soil, and air. Lead in paint is the most important source of high-dose exposure, especially for children, and will remain so well into the future. Although the allowable level of lead in paint was reduced to 0.06% net weight in 1977, an

**Table 17.1.**
**Summary Data on Lead**

| | |
|---|---|
| Exposure Limits[a] | |
| As fumes and dust | $0.05$ mg/m$^3$ (OSHA) |
| Blood | OSHA advises $<30$ µg/dl in workers who wish to bear children[b] |
| Water | .05 ppm (EPA) |
| Toxicity | Neuropathies |
| | Hypertension |
| Embryo/fetus/newborn | Developmental delays in humans |
| | Birth defects in animals: cleft palate, hydronephrosis, skeletal, CNS |
| | Stillbirths |
| Reproduction | Male—infertility (azoospermia) |
| | Dose-related decrease in testosterone |
| | Disruption of CNS-gonadal axis |
| | Sperm—abnormal forms, motility |
| | Female—pregnancy loss (high doses) |
| Human data | Excellent |
| Animal data | Excellent |

[a]OSHA = Occupational Safety and Health Administration; EPA = U.S. Environmental Protection Agency.
[b]Recent data show adverse effects on the adult cardiovascular system and children's development at lower lead levels.

enormous reservoir of leaded paint remains in U.S. homes. The Agency for Toxic Substances and Disease Registry (ATSDR) (8) estimates that 52% of all residential housing units (42 million) contain more than 0.7 mg/cm$^2$ lead (99% of pre-1940 units, 70% of 1940–1959 units, and 20% of 1959–1970 units). Renovating such housing without proper precautions may result in hazardous exposures for those conducting the renovations as well as for residents (9).

The U.S. Environmental Protection Agency (EPA) estimates that 42 million people in the U.S. receive drinking water containing lead at concentrations greater than 20 µg/liter. Most of the lead in water can be traced to household plumbing, not to the source water or to the distribution system. Factors that contribute to increased levels include lead pipe service connections, use of lead solder to join copper pipes, and water that is "plumbosolvent" (due to temperature, pH, or mineral content). The greatest water lead hazards are found in homes more than 50 or less than 5 yr old.

The contributions of lead in air and food to total exposure have declined due to reductions in the amount of lead added to gasoline and to changes in canning methods. However, residence in proximity to a stationary lead source (e.g., smelter, refinery, battery factory) may still involve significant air-borne exposures. In addition, consumption of certain imported canned foods or the use of lead or lead-glazed ceramic utensils, vessels, or dishes may result in substantial exposures (10). Medicinal or cosmetic preparations favored by certain ethnic or cultural groups may also be heavily contaminated by lead.

Lead in household dust and soils is particularly hazardous to children. Lead in these media derive from deposition of air-borne lead and deteriorated leaded paint from interior and exterior surfaces of structures.

The contributions of these various pathways are cumulative and together represent the "background" exposure to which any occupational exposure adds. Lead poisoning, generally recognized as the oldest occupational disease, currently accounts for the majority of cases of elevated heavy metal exposure reported to the New York State Heavy Metals registry (11). An estimated 827,000 workers in the U.S. are exposed to lead (12). "Carry-home" of leaded dust on workclothes can result in substantial exposure to family members as well (13). Occupations and hobbies or cottage industries that involve the greatest exposures to lead are listed in Table 17.2.

Certain behavioral habits may increase an individual's lead burden. Consumers of cigarettes or alcohol, for example, tend to have higher blood lead levels (14–16).

In the last National Health and Nutrition Examination Survey (NHANES II), the mean blood lead concentration among women in the U.S. who were 18–45 yr old was 10–12 μg/dl. Among men of comparable age, the mean level was 14–18 μg/dl (17). The EPA Clean Air Scientific Advisory Committee recently cited 10 μg/dl as the maximum acceptable blood lead level for sensitive populations, identified as fetuses and young children (18). The Centers for Disease Control (CDC) recently revised the intervention

**Table 17.2.**
**Occupational and Recreational Sources of Lead Exposure**

Occupations
   Primary and secondary smelting
   Scrap metal handling
   Storage battery manufacturing
   Metal foundry work
   Cable and wire manufacturing
   Polyvinyl chloride plastics manufacturing
   Automobile radiator repair
   Construction trades (especially deleaders)
   Ceramics industry
   Iron/steel structure demolition
   Ship breaking
   Lead mining and milling
   Printing industries
   Metal welding and cutting
   Automobile repair and spray painting
   Firing range instruction
   Electrical components manufacturing
   Paint manufacturing
   Rubber products manufacturing
Hobbies and Cottage Industries
   Jewelry-making and repair
   Pottery making (glaze mixing)
   Stained glass window construction
   Electronics
   Glassblowing
   Print making
   Home remodeling/renovation
   Antique/furniture restoration
   Shot making and riflery
   Urban gardening
   Liquor distillation

blood lead level downward, from 25 μg/dl to 10 μg/dl (19). Extrapolating from updated NHANES II data, however, the ATSDR (8) estimated that in 1984 approximately 4 million women of childbearing age and 400,000 newborns had blood lead levels exceeding 10 μg/dl. There are increasing data to support classifying adult males and females as sensitive populations as well (20, 21). The prevalence of unacceptable exposures among workers remains particularly high (22).

## Toxicology

### METABOLISM

Inhalation and ingestion are the major routes of lead exposure, and urinary and fecal excretion are the major pathways of elimination. Various kinetic models of body lead burden have been proposed (23, 24). Most include three major compartments differing in exposure averaging time: (*a*) blood, a short-term storage site (half-life of approximately 28 days) involving both red cell and plasma components; (*b*) soft tissue sites such as brain, liver, and kidney; and (*c*) bone, a long-term storage site (half-life of decades) involving cortical and trabecular components.

Lead is readily transferred across the placenta. The correlation between maternal venous blood lead level at delivery and the concentration of lead in umbilical cord blood is 0.6–0.9, with the cord blood lead level generally lower by 10–20% (25, 26). Transfer begins at least as early as the 12th to 14th week of pregnancy (27); and, as in adults, lead accumulation in the fetus is greatest in bone, liver, and brain.

Clarification of the kinetics of lead in the maternal-fetal unit is a major research need. A number of indices are used to estimate fetal lead exposure including maternal venous blood lead level in the first trimester or at delivery, placental lead level, and umbilical cord blood lead level. However, the best measure of exposure remains unclear, and relationships among the various markers are not well understood (28). These indices most likely provide complementary rather than redundant information about the parameters of prenatal exposure (e.g., timing, dose, duration).

It is possible that hormonal mechanisms regulating the mobilization of stored maternal calcium to fulfill requirements of fetal skeletal ossification and, later, of lactation, also mobilize lead stored in long-term bone compartments (29, 30). Postmenopausal bone demineralization may also result in mobilization of lead from bone stores (21). If pregnancy does induce significant mobilization of stored lead, a woman's lifetime lead burden—not simply her exposure immediately before or during pregnancy—may be relevant to fetal exposure. This conjecture has yet to be validated but warrants careful study.

## MECHANISMS OF ACTION

The molecular mechanisms of lead's reproductive toxicity are poorly understood. They may include interference with protein synthesis, in-

hibition of various membrane and mitochondrial enzymes, and impairment of the heme biosynthetic pathway. The consequences of these molecular actions may be organ specific. For example, lead's impact on heme biosynthesis affects erythropoiesis and other heme-dependent neural, renal/endocrine, and hepatic processes (e.g., cellular energetics, neurotransmitter function, detoxification of xenobiotics, biosynthesis of vitamin D).

In the past decade, considerable evidence has accumulated documenting lead's interference with intracellular calcium distribution and a variety of calcium-dependent signaling and regulatory mechanisms. One mechanism of lead's developmental toxicity may involve competition between lead and calcium in activating critical regulatory enzymes (31). For example, brain protein kinase C is inhibited at picomolar concentrations of lead, making it more sensitive to lead than to calcium (32).

On a histopathological level, lead interferes with the development of cerebral growth (33) and synaptic connectivity (34), perhaps via its effects on the morphoregulator neural cell adhesion molecule and its role in synaptic elaboration and selection (35).

## REPRODUCTIVE HEALTH EFFECTS

### Females

High-dose lead exposure is associated with impaired fertility (36). In rodents, lead at high doses suppresses the prepubertal surge of follicle-stimulating hormone (FSH) thought to be essential for normal ovarian development (37). In nonhuman primates, lead-related follicular atresia has been reported (38), along with suppression of luteal function, as reflected by decreased circulating progesterone levels (39). Lead induces persistent changes in the primate menstrual cycle, including less frequent cycles, fewer days of menstrual bleeding, and greater variability in intercycle intervals (40). Whether the effects of lead are due to direct ovarian toxicity, a central neuroendocrine dysfunction in the hypothalamo-pituitary-ovarian axis, or both, is unclear. A series of rodent studies by Wiebe et al. (41, 42) demonstrate lead effects on ovarian gonadotropin-receptor binding and steroid metabolism. Some effects were cross-generational, appearing as alterations of ovarian function in offspring of exposed females.

Although older studies suggest an association between high-dose occupational exposure to lead and spontaneous fetal loss (36), a recent study of women living near a large lead smelter in Mitrovica, Yugoslavia, found no increase in risk over a blood lead range of 5–40 µg/dl (43). High tissue lead levels have been reported in stillbirths (28, 44), but it is not known whether this observation is the cause, a correlate, or an effect of the stress resulting in fetal death (45, 46).

Several case studies of women with lead poisoning (blood lead levels greater than 50 µg/dl) during pregnancy have been reported in the recent medical literature (47–50). In general, their infants were of low birthweight or small-for-gestational-age. Developmental follow-up was reported for periods of 13 months to 4 ½ yr. While in some reports the children's development was described as "within normal limits," more detailed evaluations in other studies revealed developmental delays of varying magnitude, especially in the acquisition of language (51).

Recent epidemiological studies of low-level in utero lead exposure (maternal venous or umbilical cord blood lead levels less than 30 µg/dl) and birth outcome present a mixed picture. The most consistent finding to date is an inverse relationship between maternal blood lead level and duration of gestation (52–56). For instance, in a cohort of 861 women living near a large lead smelter in Australia, the relative risk of preterm delivery (less than 37 weeks' gestation) was 4.4 among women with first trimester lead levels greater than 14 µg/dl, using women with levels ≤8 µg/dl as the reference group (52). In a disadvantaged U.S. cohort, each log unit increase in maternal blood lead level was associated with a 0.6-week reduction in gestation (approximately 1.8 weeks over the 1- to 25-µg/dl range), even though the cohort was restricted to pregnancies beyond 34 weeks' gestation (53). However, several other studies have not observed a gestational age reduction with increasing exposure to lead (25, 45, 57, 58).

Evidence linking low-level in utero lead exposure to impaired fetal growth is similarly mixed. In some studies, greater exposure is associated with reduced birthweight (46, 59–61), a higher prevalence of low birthweight or intrauterine growth retardation (58), reduced head circumference (60–63), and reduced length (46, 59). Decreased growth in the first postnatal year has also been reported among infants with prenatal and early postnatal blood lead levels persistently greater than 8 µg/dl (64). Not all studies have observed a lead-associated reduction in birthweight, however (45, 52, 58).

Although lead is teratogenic at high doses in several animal models (65), the teratogenicity of low-level in utero lead exposure in humans is uncertain. A recent case report suggests a link between high exposure limited to early pregnancy (less than 12 weeks' gestation) and a common pattern of malformations (the VACTERL association) similar to the urorectocaudal pattern observed in animals (66). In a cohort of more than 4000 women, Needleman et al. (67) reported that the risk of a minor congenital anomaly was 2.4 times greater among infants with cord blood lead levels ≥15 µg/dl than among infants with lead levels less than 1 µg/dl. The association was not specific to any particular anomaly or pattern of anomalies. This finding has not been replicated (45, 52), although no study has matched the statistical power of the Needleman study.

In the same cohort of women studied by Needleman et al., an increased prevalence of pregnancy hypertension and elevated blood pressures during labor was reported among women whose infants had higher cord blood lead levels (in the 0- to 35-µg/dl range) (68).

The developmental toxicity of in utero lead exposure came under intensive investigation in the 1980s in a set of ongoing prospective studies in North America, Europe, and Australia (46, 56, 69–79). In several of the cohorts under study, in utero levels of 10–20 µg/dl were associated with modest behavioral and cognitive delays, with delay persisting for periods ranging from 6 months (91) to 4 or 5 yr (72, 80). In other cohorts, however, no developmental correlates of in utero exposure have been found (76–78). Striking differences among cohorts in terms of sociodemographic characteristics and in levels of postnatal lead exposure may account for some of the discrepancies (81).

These cohorts have not yet been followed long enough to determine whether school performance is associated with in utero exposure to lead. In one study of children from the upper socioeconomic strata, the significant cognitive delays displayed through age 2 yr by children with cord blood lead levels greater than 10 µg/dl appeared to attenuate by age 5 yr (72). Subgroup analyses revealed, however, that an association between preschool performance and prenatal lead exposure was still evident among children with higher concurrent exposures (≥10 µg/dl), as well as among boys and children below the median socioeconomic status (71).

## Males

Little attention has been devoted to evaluating the impact of lead on male reproductive function. The implications of this neglect extend well beyond the science of lead toxicity to bear as well on a complex of social, legal, and economic principles. As discussed in Chapter 12, corporate exclusionary policies that restrict women from certain lead-related jobs on the basis of unacceptable reproductive risk have recently been the focus of Supreme Court action. While decreasing significant lead exposures among women may be justified on scientific and medical grounds, permitting them among men is based on an unsubstantiated assumption of safety (82).

In experimental animal studies, lead exposures inducing blood levels of 35 µg/dl and higher produce altered spermatogenesis and decreased synthesis and activity of steroidogenic hormones (83). Lead crosses the blood-testis barrier and is found in human seminal fluid (84) and testicular tissues (85), as well as in the hypothalamus and pituitary (86). Several studies of clinically lead-poisoned or heavily exposed workers (i.e., blood lead levels ≥40–50 µg/dl) have reported a variety of changes in male germ cell structure and function including teratospermia, asthenospermia, and hypospermia (87–89). In general, however, the available studies of lead and male reproductive function suffer from small sample sizes, poor

characterization of lead exposure histories, biased selection of cases or controls, and confounding by chelation therapy, medical conditions, or other toxicant exposures.

As with females, the mechanism of lead's reproductive toxicity among males is poorly understood (90). Observations such as altered luteinizing hormone dynamics, decreased FSH, and decreased serum testosterone suggest a central defect in hypothalamo-pituitary function (91, 92); while other effects, such as decreased spermatogenesis and peritubular fibrosis, suggest direct gonadotoxicity (89). It may be that testicular dysfunction reflects acute exposure, while impact at the hypothalamo-pituitary level reflects chronic exposure (93). The marked inconsistency in findings highlights the need for rigorous large-scale population studies across a range of doses, particularly the low to moderate doses currently considered "acceptable" for workers and the general public.

Studies of the contribution of paternal lead exposure to pregnancy outcome are scarce. Increased rates of chromosomal aberrations and sister chromatid exchange have been reported in lead-exposed workers (94, 95). Animal data suggest that preconception exposures to the male can result in impaired implantation (96) and decreased birthweight (97). A recent study of low-dose exposure in male rats reported decreased fertility and impaired neurological development in offspring (98). Evidence of a weak association between paternal lead exposure and strabismus in offspring has also been reported (99). In a recent case-control study of male workers biologically monitored for inorganic lead, blood lead levels greater than 30 µg/dl during the year before conception were associated with a significantly increased risk of spontaneous abortion in the workers' wives (100). These data point to the importance of evaluating paternal exposures in future investigations of lead and adverse pregnancy outcome.

## Clinical Assessment

The clinical evaluation of couples experiencing problems with fertility or pregnancy includes a thorough history and physical examination to identify potential sources and signs of lead exposure and appropriate biological exposure monitoring. Table 17.3 depicts blood lead levels at which various biological effects are seen in adults. Unfortunately, intervention at the onset of symptoms may not afford adequate protection because lead levels at which reproductive outcomes occur are well below those producing overt systemic toxicity.

Accordingly, periodic biological monitoring of lead absorption is a primary way to identify individuals with excessive exposure. Blood lead is the most practical index available to clinicians for this purpose and, thus, the most frequently employed. Erythrocyte protoporphyrin (EP) concentrations are run concurrently by most laboratories and reflect lead-induced heme enzyme inhibition. Interpretation of EP values during pregnancy is complicated by the elevated EP levels found in iron-deficiency states. The utility of EP in screening for blood lead elevation is limited by the fact that, even in children, its sensitivity is adequate only for detecting blood lead levels of 50 $\mu$g/dl and higher (101).

Blood lead has distinct drawbacks as an exposure monitor, especially in an adult population. Because the residence time of lead in blood is only about 1 month, blood lead is a relatively poor index of total body lead burden. Individuals with high cumulative absorption but little recent exposure may have blood lead

**Table 17.3.**
**Relationship between Blood Lead Levels and Various Biological Effects[a]**

| Biological Effect | Blood Lead Levels ($\mu$g/dl) |
|---|---|
| Gastrointestinal colic | >80 |
| Acute encephalopathy | >80 |
| Anemia | >80 |
| Chronic renal disease | >60 |
| Altered spermatogenesis | >35 |
| Peripheral neuropathy | >30 |
| Increased EP[b] | >20–25 |
| Inhibition of ALA-D[c] | >20 |
| Increased blood pressure | ? threshold |
| Developmental delays in offspring | ? threshold |

[a]Modified from Goyer RA. Lead toxicity: from overt to subclinical to subtle health effects. Environ Health Perspect 1990;86:178.
[b]EP = erythrocyte protoporphyrin.
[c]ALA-D = Delta-aminolevulinic acid dehydratase.

levels well within the normal range, yet still be at risk. The lead mobilization test, which measures lead diuresis in response to a challenge dose of CaNaEDTA, may be more helpful in assessing an individual's body lead burden and candidacy for a full course of chelation therapy. However, its use in pregnancy is not recommended.

The development of noninvasive in vivo methods for measuring the large fraction of body burden sequestered in bone represents a significant advance in exposure assessment (102). K-line x-ray fluorescence (XRF) methods have already proven useful in evaluating lead biokinetics in retired or treated workers. An L-line XRF method is being developed for use with children and pregnant women (103). Its use may clarify the extent to which pregnancy-induced lead mobilization and redistribution affects transfer of lead to the fetus (29).

The Occupational Safety and Health Administration (OSHA) lead standard (104), promulgated in 1978, was one of the few occupational regulations to address reproductive concerns specifically. The standard requires medical consultation, at company expense, when: (a) the concentration of lead in workroom air exceeds an "action level" of 30 $\mu$g/m$^3$ (8-hour time-weighted average) for more than 30 days/yr, or (b) any male or female employee desires medical advice concerning the reproductive effects of lead. While blood lead levels of 50 $\mu$g/dl are generally regarded as excessive, the standard specifically recommends 30 $\mu$g/dl as the limit for "males and females who wish to bear children" and for pregnant women. When biological monitoring reveals excessive blood lead levels, or when the examining physician determines that the worker has a medical condition that increases the risk of health impairment from exposure to lead, the practitioner can implement "medical removal protection." Medical removal protection allows for transfer of an employee from exposure above the action level without loss of wages, benefits, or seniority for as long as the physician deems necessary. While the employer may designate the initial examiner, the worker does have a right under the standard to a second medical opinion by a physician of his or her choice.

Although the OSHA standard was quite successful in reducing occupational lead exposure, it now requires revision in light of current scientific and medical evidence of the adverse impact of lead on both male and female workers. Given placental permeability to lead, the fetal and newborn exposures recommended under this standard greatly exceed those currently considered permissible in young children (less than 10 µg/dl). In addition, the current standard does not apply to the construction and agricultural industries despite the high exposures that may be routinely incurred in these trades (9). Moreover, not all workers who are entitled to participate in biological monitoring programs under the current OSHA standard are given the opportunity to do so (105). One prominent occupational health physician has recommended that the OSHA Permissible Exposure Limit for lead in the workplace air be reduced to 20 µg/m³ and that any worker whose blood lead level reaches 20 µg/dl be removed until it has fallen to 10 µg/dl (106).

## Prevention and Treatment

Because of limited treatment options, primary prevention of exposure remains the most effective approach to reduce the reproductive and developmental morbidity associated with lead. Ideally, couples at risk for excessive lead exposure should be screened in the preconception period and advised to delay pregnancy until elevated blood lead levels are corrected and sources of exposure controlled. Selective lead screening during the prenatal period may identify women with lead burdens sufficiently high to warrant consideration of pregnancy termination, screening of family members, and other measures. Because the vast majority of women have much lower lead levels that are not amenable to intervention, however, routine prenatal screening would serve largely to identify individuals whose environments should be investigated for lead hazards.

Chelation therapy is generally contraindicated during pregnancy unless there are overriding concerns about maternal health impairment from lead poisoning. Chelation may induce temporary acute increases in blood lead levels, and currently available agents promote excretion of essential trace metals as well as

lead. Animal studies show these agents to be teratogenic, due most likely to the zinc deficiency state they produce (107, 108). Successful chelation in the week before delivery has been reported (45, 47); however, chelation may do little to reduce fetal lead burden because neonatal blood lead concentrations more closely resemble the women's prechelation lead levels than their postchelation levels. Greater delay in fetal than maternal elimination of lead appears to occur with maternal intoxication (109).

In some cases, screening identifies a patient whose elevated lead exposure is attributable to some modifiable aspect of the workplace, environment, or personal behavior. For instance, couples may be undertaking home renovations in anticipation of the birth of a child, or a hobby may involve the use of lead glazes, paints, or solder. A patient may work in an occupation amenable to better control of lead exposure through engineering methods or through the use of personal protective equipment. Outside of the workplace, however, an individual's lead burden most likely represents the cumulative effect of several minor, and perhaps unidentifiable, sources, making successful intervention difficult. Even after removal from a known source of lead exposure, reduction of body lead burden in the absence of chelation can require months or even years.

Counseling is an important aspect of the management of all patients with excessive blood lead levels. In some cases, the patient may wish to consider pregnancy termination to avoid the risks of potentially serious growth and neurobehavioral complications in offspring. At lesser blood levels (10–40 µg/dl), pregnant women should be advised about the nature of more subtle developmental delays found in studies to date. At the present time, it is unknown whether the problems induced by low-level in utero lead exposure persist into the childhood years.

Women with excessive lead burdens who choose to continue pregnancy should be carefully followed. Serial ultrasounds are indicated to ascertain fetal growth and development. Patients should be counseled about the symptoms of preterm labor and undergo frequent cervical checks in the third trimester. In addition to identifying and ameliorating known sources of lead exposure, providers should encourage patients to reduce their use of cigarettes and alcohol. Deficiencies of iron, calcium, and zinc are associated with increased lead absorption and possible toxicity (110) and should be corrected. Maternal blood lead levels should be followed throughout the pregnancy, and an umbilical cord blood sample analyzed for lead at delivery. Close involvement of the pediatric service in patient management is essential to assure appropriate evaluation and treatment of the infant. Rehabilitation therapy and postnatal environmental lead abatement may significantly decrease potential long-term morbidity from prenatal lead exposure.

## MERCURY

### Occurrence

Mercury (Hg) permeates our existence. Between 2700–6000 tons of Hg are released each year from the earth's crust. In addition, approximately 10,000 tons are generated in mining (particularly gold) and manufacturing processes using Hg (e.g., pulp and paper and caustic soda production) (3). Additional sources of Hg are fossil fuels, combustion, fungicides, production of cement, smelting of sulfur ores, and refuse incineration (111). The release of Hg from dental amalgams has also generated recent concern.

Yet, it is important to distinguish the form of mercurial exposure. There are inorganic (vapor and metallic) forms as well as organic Hg. In the global cycle for Hg, emitted Hg vapor is converted to soluble forms ($Hg^{++}$) that are deposited into soil and water via precipitation. Usually Hg vapor has an atmospheric residence time of 0.4–3.0 yr, while soluble Hg has a residence time of only a few weeks.

The first stop in the aquatic bioaccumulation process is the conversion of inorganic to methylated forms of Hg. Methylmercury (MeHg) can be formed either nonenzymatically or via microbes. MeHg rapidly binds to proteins and bioaccumulates in the food chain, especially in swordfish, shark, tuna, freshwater bass, trout, pike, and walleyes. The bioaccumulation in fish compared to water can be 10,000- to 100,000-fold. The levels of selenium in the water can reduce the uptake of MeHg (111).

As noted in Table 17.4, most individuals are primarily exposed to MeHg through the diet. Yet, water and air can contribute significantly to the daily intake of total Hg depending upon the level of contamination. In most foodstuffs, Hg is in the inorganic form and below the level of detection (20 μg/kg wet weight). Fish and fish products from polluted waterways can have levels greater than 1200 μg/kg (111). The consumption of 200 g of fish containing 500 μg Hg/kg provides an intake of 100 μg Hg, principally as MeHg. This amount of MeHg is one-half of the World Health Organization's (WHO) recommended tolerable weekly intake (111).

Practically all MeHg in the diet is absorbed and distributed to all tissues within 4 days. The blood to hair ratio in humans is approximately 1:250. Cord blood MeHg levels are generally greater than maternal blood levels. The red

**Table 17.4.**
**Estimated Daily Intake and Retention (μg/day) of Total Mercury and Mercury Compounds in the General Population *Not* Occupationally Exposed**[a]

| Exposure | Elemental Mercury Vapor | Inorganic Mercury Compounds | Methylmercury |
|---|---|---|---|
| Air | 0.030[b] (0.024)[c] | 0.002 (0.001) | 0.008 (0.0064) |
| Food | | | |
| Fish | 0 | 0.600 (0.042) | 2.4 (2.3) |
| Nonfish | 0 | 3.6 (0.25) | 0 |
| Drinking water | 0 | 0.050 (0.0035) | 0 |
| Dental amalgams | 3.8–21.0 (3–17) | 0 | 0 |
| Total | 3.9–21.0 (3.1–17) | 4.3 (0.3) | 2.41 (2.31) |

[a]Modified from World Health Organization (WHO). Environmental health criteria 101, methylmercury. Geneva: WHO, 1990.
[b]Estimated average daily intake.
[c]Estimated amount retained in the body of an adult.

blood cell to plasma distribution ratios are about 20:1 in humans, monkeys, and guinea pigs, compared to 7:1 for mice and greater than 100:1 for rats.

MeHg is converted to inorganic Hg in humans. The rate of Hg excretion is proportional to the body burden and fits a single compartment model with a biological half-time of 50 (39–70) days in fish-eaters. Interestingly, lactating females have a significantly shorter half-life for Hg.

Mean values for total Hg are: whole blood, 8 μg/liter; hair, 2 μg/g; urine, 4 μg/liter; and placenta, 10 μg/kg. In fish-eaters who consume 200 μg Hg/day, the Hg blood levels can be approximately 200 μg/liter with hair levels being approximately 50 μg/g (111).

## Toxicology

### METHYLMERCURY

Use of mercurial fungicides and the inappropriate disposal of Hg by industry can lead to substantial environmental exposure to both inorganic and organic Hg. In terms of reproductive and developmental toxicity, the organic mercurials, especially MeHg, are of principal concern.

### Studies in Human Populations

The two largest human populations studied for the toxicity of MeHg were in Minamata and Niigata, Japan, and in Iraq. The Japanese expo-sure resulted from consumption of contaminated fish from Minamata Bay due to industrial inorganic Hg pollution, while the Iraqi exposure was due to the consumption of grain contaminated with a MeHg fungicide (111–114). It was quite evident that the newborns and children were more affected by the exposures than were the adults.

As noted in Figure 17.1, a dose-dependent appearance of toxic symptoms, including death, has been observed in adults exposed to MeHg. Both blood and hair analyses can be used as biomarkers of exposure. However, the hair has the advantage of providing a history of exposure based upon the length of the hair. A single hair specimen can establish when during pregnancy the MeHg exposure occurred. Because of the long half-life for Hg, exposure persists long after ingestion stops.

Severe damage to the developing CNS can be caused by prenatal exposure to MeHg. Based upon the dose-response curves (Fig. 17.2), the conceptus is much more sensitive to the neurotoxic actions of MeHg than is the mother (114). Equally important, the pregnant woman may be more sensitive to MeHg than is the nonpregnant female adult (111, 114).

MeHg is fetotoxic in mice (single exposure 2.5–7.5 mg/kg), teratogenic in rats, and produces behavioral alterations in monkey offspring (50–70 μg/kg/day before and during pregnancy) (115–118). Spermatogenesis in mice is affected at 1 mg/kg MeHg. Recent

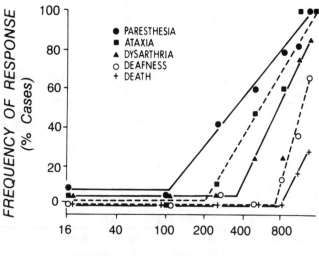

**Figure 17.1.** The frequency of signs and symptoms of methylmercury poisoning in adult victims in Iraq compared with maximal hair concentration of Hg. From Clarkson TW. The role of biomarkers in reproductive and developmental toxicology. Environ Health Perspect 1987;74: 103–107, with permission.

FREQUENCY OF RESPONSE
(% Cases)

- ● PARESTHESIA
- ■ ATAXIA
- ▲ DYSARTHRIA
- ○ DEAFNESS
- + DEATH

MAXIMUM HAIR CONC. (ppm)

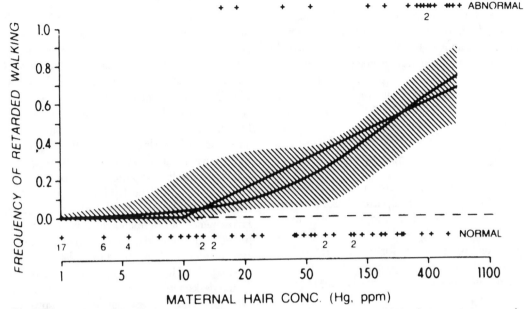

**Figure 17.2.** Relationships between the maximal maternal hair concentrations of Hg during pregnancy and the frequency of cases of motor retardation (retarded walking) in offspring from the Iraqi study. The *shaded area* denotes nonsimultaneous 95% confidence limits for the smooth curve. Normal and abnormal (retarded walking) outcomes are plotted above and below the corresponding maternal hair values. From: World Health Organization (WHO), Environmental health criteria 101, methylmercury. Geneva: WHO, 1990:90, with permission. Calculations based on Cox et al. (158).

quantitative and qualitative assessments in nonhuman primates have been compared with humans who have been exposed to different concentrations of MeHg (118). It is remarkable how well the behavioral and neuropathological effects agree across species at the higher concentrations of MeHg. Neurobehavioral functioning is also similar across species at lower exposure levels; however, due to a lack of human pathological data at lower exposure levels, no neuropathological correlations can be established at this time.

In human adults, no adverse effects have been detected with long-term daily Hg intake (3–7 $\mu$g/kg body weight), corresponding to hair levels of 50–125 $\mu$g/g. Issues relating to the increased susceptibility of pregnant women to MeHg require further evaluation (111).

In the Iraqi outbreak, the lowest level of MeHg in maternal hair associated with severe neurological effects in offspring was 404 $\mu$g/g. The highest no-observed effect level for severe effects was 399 $\mu$g/g (111). Fish-eating populations studied to date have not demonstrated such severe effects.

Psychomotor retardation in offspring (history of seizures, abnormal reflexes, delayed achievement of developmental milestones) was noted below maternal hair levels associated with severe effects (118). When the data were extrapolated, motor retardation was greater than background frequency at maternal hair levels of 10–20 $\mu$g/g (111; Fig. 17.2). Boys (but not girls) of mothers with hair levels during pregnancy of 23.9 $\mu$g/g demonstrated abnormal muscle tone or reflexes. Four-year-old children whose mothers had maternal hair levels from 6–86 $\mu$g/g (2nd highest was 19.6 $\mu$g/g) demonstrated developmental retardation according to the Denver Test.

### Risk Estimates

According to the WHO (111), "The general population does not face a significant health risk from methylmercury. Certain groups with a high fish consumption may attain a blood methylmercury level (about 20 $\mu$g/liter, corresponding to 50 $\mu$g/g of hair) associated with a low (5%) risk of neurological damage to adults."

The fetus is at particular risk. Recent evidence demonstrates that, at peak maternal hair Hg levels above 70 μg/g, there is a high risk (greater than 30%) of neurological disorders in offspring. A prudent interpretation of the Iraqi data implies that a 5% risk may be associated with a peak Hg level of 10–20 μg/g in maternal hair.

## OTHER ORGANOMERCURIALS

Liver damage, renal damage, and intestinal complaints have been reported in subjects exposed to phenylmercury and other substances. In 13 workers exposed in a phenylmercury manufacturing facility for 11–23 yr, no evidence of toxicity was apparent with urinary excretion concentrations of 85–100 μg Hg/liter (1).

Phenylmercury is rapidly metabolized to inorganic Hg, which accumulates in and is excreted by the kidney. The rate of urinary excretion of Hg appears to be a predictor of early mild effects on the kidney (1).

Phenylmercury compounds are teratogenic in animals and are potent spermicides in humans. Six thousand infants were exposed to phenylmercury in diapers. Many of these infants developed acrodynia (119). These infants had increased excretion of γ-glutamyl transpeptidase (renal brush border enzyme) which correlated with increased urinary excretion of Hg. Estimated threshold values were 4 μg Hg/kg/24 hr for enzymuria and 14 μg Hg/kg/24 hr for diuresis.

## MERCURY VAPOR/AMALGAMS/ INORGANIC MERCURY

The principal exposure to Hg vapor in the general population is via dental amalgams, which release Hg vapor into the mouth. When fillings are removed, an acute increase in Hg release is noted. The rate of Hg release is enhanced by stressing the surfaces during chewing and brushing. The Hg released from dental amalgams is deposited in body tissues and excreted via the kidney. Increased urinary Hg levels are noted. Estimated release rates from amalgams are consistent with Hg content in autopsy tissue in the general population (120).

Occupational exposure to Hg vapor can result in renal, pulmonary, and psychomotor toxicity (1). Current studies of female dentists/dental workers have not demonstrated a Hg-associated increase in birth defects or pregnancy losses (4, 121, 122). Only limited information is available concerning the effects of occupational exposures to Hg (vapor/inorganic) on reproduction. Menstrual disorders (hypermenorrhea/dysmenorrhea) have been associated with work in Hg plants, especially for women employed longer than 3 yr (4, 123). The Hg levels in the factory fluctuated between trace and 0.08 mg/m$^3$. Hypermenorrhea/dysmenorrhea were also reported in dental workers and women working in Hg rectifier stations. In these plants, it was reported that Hg was on the workers' hands and on the desks, tables, and floors in the work areas (4). Apparently, substantial Hg exposure was occurring.

In contrast to direct exposures in women, a recent epidemiological study concerning paternal exposure to Hg vapor in a chloralkali plant suggested that urinary Hg levels greater than 50 μg/liter were associated with a two-fold risk of spontaneous abortion in the workers' wives (124).

In contrast to organic mercurials, inorganic Hg does not easily transit the placenta but is concentrated by the placenta itself (125). Even with such placental concentration, a recent study in sheep (126) demonstrated the release of Hg from dental fillings with the appearance of Hg in the fetus. Transfer of Hg to the newborn lamb via breast milk was also noted.

## Prevention and Treatment

In the occupational setting, monitoring of the workplace and of the employee to minimize exposure to Hg is essential, but unfortunately, is not routinely instituted. Occupational exposure limits for Hg are listed in Table 17.5. In the monitoring process, it is important to monitor for the appropriate form of Hg.

Environmental exposure can occur via air, water, or food. Of particular concern are dietary modifications to reduce cholesterol-containing foods. Fish has been recommended as an alternative. Unfortunately, the bioaccumulation of MeHg in the food chain, especially in swordfish, shark, tuna, and freshwater fish grown in con-

**Table 17.5.**
**Summary Data on Mercury**

| | Methylmercury (MeHg) | Mercury Vapor | Mercury Amalgams |
|---|---|---|---|
| Exposure limits[a] | | | |
|   Hair (WHO) | 5 ppm ($\mu$g/g) | | |
|   Air (OSHA) | 0.01 mg/m$^3$ | 0.05 mg/m$^3$ | |
|     STEL | 0.03 mg/m$^3$ | | |
|     IDLH level | 10 mg/m$^3$ | 28 mg/m$^3$ | |
| Estimated unstimulated Hg release, daily uptake | | | 1.15 ± 0.45 $\mu$g |
| Estimated stimulated Hg release, daily uptake | | | 7.72 ± 6.98 $\mu$g |
| Toxicity—see text for dose-response relationship | | Nephrotic syndrome | None identified |
|   CNS damage | | Lung damage | |
|   Pregnant female more sensitive than nonpregnant | | Gingivostomatis | |
|   female or male | | Psychomotor | |
|   Human and animal data consistent | | abnormalities | |
| | | Sensory neuropathies | |
| Embryo/fetus/newborn | | | |
|   CNS damage | | Infants more suscepti- | None identified |
|   More sensitive than adult | | ble than older children/ | |
|   Passes rapidly into the conceptus and mother's milk | | adults | |
|   Human and animal data consistent | | No useful human infor- | |
| | | mation | |
| Reproduction | | Menstrual irregularities | |
| Principal source | | | |
|   Dietary (in fish—shark, swordfish, tuna) | | Environmental: air | Silver/mercury tooth |
|   Fungicide—contaminated foodstuffs and pulp | | Occupational: gold | fillings |
|   processing | | mining | |
| Human data | | | |
|   Excellent | | Good for general toxi- | Fair |
| | | city | |
| | | Poor for reproductive/ | |
| | | developmental | |
| Animal data | | | |
|   Excellent | | Fair | Fair |
| Recommendations | | | |
|   Minimize consumption of fish containing high | | Minimize exposures and | Avoid removal of large |
|   levels of MeHg (especially shark, swordfish) to once | | monitor manufacturing | numbers of amalgams |
|   per month | | settings to meet expo- | during pregnancy |
| | | sure limits | |

[a]WHO = World Health Organization; OSHA = Occupational Safety and Health Administration; STEL = Short-term exposure limit; IDLH = Immediately dangerous to life or health.

taminated waters such as bass, trout, pike, and walleyes, can lead to substantive exposures. The recommendation is to limit swordfish and shark meals to no more than one per month. Consumption of freshwater fish depends on whether or not they are grown in contaminated regions. Your state department of health can provide information about local water conditions. The WHO advises monitoring of hair levels for MeHg in individuals (especially women of childbearing age) who consume more than 100 g fish/day. Extensive removal of amalgam tooth fillings should be postponed if possible until after delivery and nursing.

Chelation therapy has been used in the treatment of acute inorganic mercurial intoxication with success. For pregnant patients who have been chronically exposed to low concentrations of Hg, chelation therapy has not been established as useful or safe.

## CADMIUM

### Occurrence

Cadmium (Cd) is widely available in the environment and is common in the workplace because of its use in nickel-cadmium batteries, paints, electroplating, smelting, and mining, especially of zinc and lead. Besides inhalation via fumes, ingestion of shellfish, liver, and kidney can be major dietary sources. Shellfish (oysters, scallops, mussels) can have Cd levels from 100–1000 µg/kg. It is estimated that the total daily intake from food, water, and air in North America and Europe is approximately 10–40 µg/day (127). The half-life of Cd in the body is approximately 30 yr. Gastrointestinal absorption of Cd is poor (5–8%) compared with inhalation (128).

Cigarette smoking is another major source of Cd exposure for the general population. A cigarette contains 1–2 µg of Cd of which approximately 10% is inhaled. Thus, smoking 1–2 packs of cigarettes per day will double the daily intake of Cd. Cigarette smoking during pregnancy is significantly associated with increased levels of Cd in the human placenta (125). Absorption of Cd is increased by low dietary calcium and low serum ferritin, while zinc and selenium appear to decrease Cd absorption.

Typically, Cd is transported in the blood bound to red blood cells and albumin. Small amounts of cadmium-metallothionein (Cd-MT) may also circulate. Metallothionein is a 61 amino acid protein (approximately 6500 daltons) with 20 cysteines. It normally binds Cd, Hg, zinc, and copper, and the protein can be induced by increasing the amounts of these metals. Cd bound to metallothionein intracellularly is apparently nontoxic and can serve as a sink to store Cd and to reduce its toxicity. In rodents, extracellular Cd-MT is nephrotoxic, but not placental toxic (129).

## Toxicology

Adult toxicity from Cd exposure is dependent upon amount and length of exposure. Chronic pulmonary disease has been noted in Cd-exposed workers. Nephrotoxicity is typically noted in workers having 200–300 µg/g of Cd in the renal cortex. This tubular necrosis results in the release of $\beta_2$-microglobulin in the urine. The WHO (130) reports that workroom air exposures of 50 µg Cd/$m^3$ for more than 10 yr can produce nephrotoxicity. In nephrotoxic, Cd-exposed patients, Thun et al. (131) demonstrated a significant increase in systolic pressure. Increased cerebrovascular disease has been noted in Cd-exposed patients. In animal

carcinogenicity studies, Cd produces tumors, lung carcinomas, and sarcomas at the site of injection (132). Interestingly, there was also a low incidence of carcinoma of the prostate following direct injection (133). Workers exposed to Cd (plus other metals and cigarette smoke) had increased risks for lung and prostate cancers (134, 135). According to Goyer (127), the risk of prostate cancer appears debatable.

There are no epidemiological studies in women that demonstrate that Cd affects fertility or the rate of spontaneous abortions. In the Fuchu area of Japan, environmental contamination from a mine resulted in Itai-Itai (ouch, ouch) disease, especially in postmenopausal women. However, animal studies implicate Cd in oocyte toxicity, producing persistent estrus (136).

In animal studies, the male is particularly susceptible to the toxic effects of Cd when it is given parenterally. Doses of 1.1–2.2 mg Cd/kg produce selective testicular damage (137). Damage to the vascular endothelium and obstruction of the microcirculation in the testes results in necrosis of spermatogenic cells. There is also a concentration of Cd in the seminiferous tubules, especially in rete-testis fluid (138).

Human data are anecdotal at best. Autopsy data from four Cd workers previously employed in poorly ventilated working conditions demonstrated elevated levels of Cd in the testis (18–94 µg/g wet weight) compared to three non-Cd-exposed men (0.30–0.34 µg/g). In these four cases, the testes were macroscopically normal but had only occasional spermatozoa. Some questions were raised about the role of intercurrent disease processes (emphysema) in producing these effects, since mitosis was still occurring in the spermatocytes. However, Cd may be implicated because of its long half-life and the specificity of its effects on spermatids and spermatocytes (4).

When injected into rodents during early gestation, Cd is highly teratogenic, resulting in facial malformations (cleft palate, anophthalmia, microphthalmia, exencephaly), undescended testes, hydrocephalus, and resorptions (139–142). Neonatal injections of Cd in rodents have also been associated with extensive CNS hemorrhages and necrosis, as well as hydrocephalus (142, 143). Significant amounts of Cd are detected in the day 8 embryo within 24 hr following administration (144). These teratological and pharmacokinetic responses during organogenesis are substantially different from the responses noted late in gestation. Some of the differences are attributed to the dominance of the visceral yolk sac early in gestation in the rodent, which may provide better access of Cd to the conceptus compared to later in gestation when the chorioallantoic placenta is performing the dominant transport role (144).

Single injections of Cd late in gestation to mice and rats produce fetal lethality and placental necrosis within 18–24 hrs, but not observable CNS teratogenesis (142, 145–147); comparable injections on day 12 of gestation do not produce this high incidence of fetal loss (148). The effects observed after maternal administration of Cd are not due to a direct effect on the fetus, but rather to an effect on the placenta (146). While direct fetal injections of Cd in utero produce a dose-related incidence of hydrocephalus, this effect is not observed following maternal administration of Cd (149). Administration of metallothionein-Cd did not produce the fetal lethality or placental necrosis in the pregnant rat, but did cause significant maternal nephrotoxicity (129).

Thus, it appears that Cd does not produce direct fetal toxicity but, in fact, protects the fetus by concentrating the Cd in the placenta itself (150, 151). There are reductions in uteroplacental blood flow by 12 hr (152); however, the initial insult appears to be directly on the placenta, with increased mitochondrial calcium levels and ultrastructural changes occurring within 4–6 hr (152). These effects can be prevented by the immediately prior administration of zinc (153). In addition, Cd inhibits the transfer of zinc (141) and cobalamin (144) from mother to conceptus in the rat.

The human placenta also highly concentrates Cd (151). In particular, levels of Cd in the placentae of cigarette smokers are higher than in nonsmokers, while levels of lead, zinc, and copper are not significantly different (125,

151). In in vitro studies utilizing the perfused human placenta, plasma Cd concentrations that cause placental necrosis in rodents produce similar effects in the human placenta (154). Further, a dose-related decrease occurs in the production and release of human chorionic gonadotropin (154). As in the rodent, the human placenta retains the Cd and releases very little to the fetal side (155). The actual tissue concentrations of Cd that produce placental toxicity (156) are at least 10-fold lower than the doses reported to produce nephrotoxicity in the human (128).

Even though little Cd crosses to the conceptus, Brill et al. (4) reported higher blood levels of Cd in newborns with respiratory disease than in normal infants. Rodent newborns treated with Cd in utero from days 12–15 had reduced pulmonary function with labored breathing, reduced lung weight, and inhibited surfactant production, and increased neonatal death (157). The lungs had reduced cellular glycogen, fewer lamellar bodies, and delayed epithelial differentiation of the alveoli. Fetuses treated directly with Cd later in gestation (day 19) exhibited no such pulmonary problems, but rather CNS damage. These clinical and animal studies raise interesting questions about the role of Cd in respiratory distress syndrome and CNS development.

## Recommendations

There are substantial animal data to indicate that Cd is toxic to the testis and also to the embryo and to the placenta, as well as teratogenic (Table 17.6). In humans, Cd can be nephrotoxic and appears to induce Itai-Itai disease at a higher incidence in postmenopausal women. However, there are no epidemiological studies to demonstrate a relationship between occupational exposure and a teratogenic effect of Cd in the human. Based on available animal and in vitro data, patients demonstrating Cd-induced nephrotoxicity and/or chronic pulmonary disease may also be at risk for reproductive and developmental toxicity. The use of a variety of chelating agents have been investigated experimentally; however, none are approved for use in acute or chronic Cd toxicity (127).

**Table 17.6.**
**Summary Data on Cadmium**

| Exposure limits[a] | |
|---|---|
| As dust | $0.2 \text{ mg/m}^3$ (OSHA) |
| | $0.6 \text{ mg/m}^3$ (ceiling limit) (OSHA) |
| | $0.05 \text{ mg/m}^3$ (ACGIH) |
| As fumes | $0.1 \text{ mg/m}^3$ (OSHA) |
| | $0.3 \text{ mg/m}^3$ (ceiling limit) (OSHA) |
| | $0.05 \text{ mg/m}^3$ (ACGIH) |
| Toxicity | Carcinogen |
| | Renal tubular dysfunction |
| | Itai-Itai syndrome |
| | Severe bony deformities |
| | Chronic renal disease |
| | Lung carcinomas (inhalation exposure) |
| | Associated with essential hypertension |
| Embryo/fetus/newborn | Birth defects (in animals) |
| | Placental toxicity (in human and animal placentae) |
| | Implantation failure/pregnancy loss (in animals) |
| Reproduction | Testicular toxicity (in animals) |
| | Ovarian toxicity (in animals) |
| Human data | Poor for reproductive/developmental issues |
| Animal data | Good for reproductive/developmental issues |

[a]OSHA = Occupational Safety and Health Administration; ACGIH = American Conference of Governmental Industrial Hygienists.

## REFERENCES

1. Clarkson TW, Friberg L, Nordberg GF, Sager PR. Biological monitoring of toxic metals. New York: Plenum Press, 1988.
2. Clarkson TW, Nordberg GF, Sager PR, eds. Developmental and reproductive toxicity of metals. New York: Plenum Press, 1983.
3. Schardein JL. Chemically induced birth defects. New York: Marcel Dekker, 1985.
4. Barlow S, Sullivan F. Reproductive hazards of industrial chemicals. New York: Academic Press, 1982.
5. National Research Council. Biomarkers of toxicity during reproduction and development. Washington, DC: National Academy Press, 1989.
6. Miller RK. Fetal drug therapy: principles and issues. Clin Obstet Gynecol 1991;34:241–250.
7. Cantarow A, Trumper M. Lead poisoning. Baltimore: Williams & Wilkins, 1944:85.
8. U.S. Agency for Toxic Substances and Disease Registry. The nature and extent of childhood lead poisoning among U.S. children: a report to Congress. Washington, DC: U.S. Department of Health and Human Services, July, 1988.
9. Marino P, Franzblau A, Lilis R, Landrigan P. Acute lead poisoning in construction workers: the failure of current protective standards. Arch Environ Health 1989; 44:140–145.
10. Avila MH, Romieu I, Rios C, Rivero A, Palazuelos E. Lead glazed ceramics as major determinants of blood lead levels in Mexican women. Environ Health Perspect 1991;94:117–120.
11. Baser M, Marion D. A statewide case registry for surveillance of occupational heavy metals absorption. Am J Public Health 1990;80:162–164.
12. U.S. Centers for Disease Control. Surveillance for occupational lead exposure-United States, 1987. MMWR 1989;38:642–646.
13. Baker E, Folland D, Taylor T, et al. Lead poisoning in children of lead workers: home contamination with industrial dust. N Engl J Med 1977;296:260–261.
14. Grandjean P, Olsen N, Hollnagel H. Influence of smoking and alcohol consumption on blood lead levels. Int Arch Occup Environ Health 1981;48:391–397.
15. Rabinowitz M, Needleman H. Environmental, demographic, and medical factors related to cord blood lead levels. Biol Trace Element Res 1984;6:57–67.
16. Baghurst P, McMichael A, Vimpani G, Robertson E, Clark P, Wigg N. Determinants of blood lead concentrations of pregnant women living in Port Pirie and surrounding areas. Med J Austral 1987;146:69–73.
17. Mahaffey K, Annest J, Roberts J, Murphy R. National estimates of blood lead levels: United States, 1976–1980. Association with selected demographic and socioeconomic factors. N Engl J Med 1982;307:573–579.
18. U.S. Environmental Protection Agency Clean Air Science Advisory Committee. Review of the OAQPS lead staff paper and the ECAO air quality criteria document supplement. EPA-SAB-CASAC-90–002, 1990.
19. U.S. Centers for Disease Control. Preventing lead poisoning in young children: a statement by the Centers for Disease Control. Washington, DC: U.S. Department of Health and Human Services, 1991.
20. Victery W, Tyroler H, Volpe R, Grant L. Summary of discussion sessions: symposium on lead-blood pressure relationships. Environ Health Perspect 1988;78:139–155.

21. Silbergeld E, Schwartz J, Mahaffey K. Lead and osteoporosis: mobilization of lead from bone in postmenopausal women. Environ Res 1988;47:79–94.

22. Maizlish N, Rudolph L, Sutton P, Jones J, Kizer K. Elevated blood lead in California adults, 1987: results of a statewide surveillance program based on laboratory reports. Am J Public Health 1990;80:931–934.

23. Rabinowitz M, Wetherill G, Kopple J. Kinetic analysis of lead metabolism in healthy humans. J Clin Invest 1976;58 260–270.

24. Marcus A. Multicompartment kinetic models for lead. Environ Res 1985;36:441–489.

25. Angell N, Lavery J. The relationship of blood lead levels to obstetric outcome. Am J Obstet Gynecol 1982;142:40–46.

26. Zetterlund B, Winberg J, Lundgren G, Johansson G. Lead in umbilical cord blood correlated with the blood lead of the mother in areas with low, medium or high atmospheric pollution. Acta Paediatr Scand 1977;66:169–175.

27. Barltrop D. Transfer of lead to the human foetus. In: Barltrop D, Burland W, eds. Mineral metabolism in pediatrics. Oxford: Blackwell Scientific Publications, 1969:135–151.

28. Baghurst P, Robertson E, Oldfield R. Lead in the placenta, membranes, and umbilical cord in relation to pregnancy outcome in a lead-smelter community. Environ Health Perspect 1991;90:315–320.

29. Silbergeld EK. Lead in bone: implications for toxicology during pregnancy and lactation. Environ Health Perspect 1991;91:63–70.

30. Hu H. Kowledge of diagnosis and reproductive history among survivors of childhood plumbism. Am J Public Health 1991;81:1070–1072.

31. Bondy S. Intracellular calcium and neurotoxic events. Neurotoxicol Teratol 1989;11:527–531.

32. Markovac J, Goldstein G. Picomolar concentrations of lead stimulate brain protein kinase C. Nature 1988;334:71–73.

33. Logdberg B, Berlin M, Schutz A. Effects of lead exposure on pregnancy outcome and the fetal brain of squirrel monkeys. Scand J Work Environ Health 1987;13:135–145.

34. McCauley P, Bull R, Tonti A, et al. The effect of prenatal and postnatal lead exposure on neonatal synaptogenesis in rat cerebral cortex. J Toxicol Environ Health 1982;10:639–642.

35. Regan C. Lead-impaired neurodevelopment. Mechanisms and threshold values in the rodent. Neurotoxicol Teratol 1989;11:533–537.

36. Rom W. Effects of lead on the female and reproduction: a review. Mt Sinai J Med 1976;43:542–552.

37. Petrusz P, Weaver C, Grant L, Mushak P, Krigman M. Lead poisoning and reproduction: effects on pituitary and serum gonadotropins in neonatal rats. Environ Res 1979;19:383–391.

38. Vermande-VanEck G, Meigs J. Changes in the ovary of the Rhesus monkey after chronic lead intoxication. Fertil Steril 1960;11:223–234.

39. Franks P, Laughlin N, Dierschke D, Bowman R, Meller P. Effects of lead on luteal function in rhesus monkeys. Biol Reprod 1989;41:1055–1062.

40. Laughlin N, Bowman R, Franks P, Dierschke D. Altered menstrual cycles in rhesus monkeys induced by lead. Fund Appl Toxicol 1987;9:722–729.

41. Wiebe J, Barr K. Effect of prenatal and neonatal exposure to lead on the affinity and number of estradiol receptors in the uterus. J Toxicol Environ Health 1988;24:451–460.

42. Wiebe J, Barr K, Buckingham K. Effect of prenatal and neonatal exposure to lead on gonadotropin receptors and steroidogenesis in rat ovaries. J Toxicol Environ Health 1988;24:461–476.

43. Murphy M, Graziano J, Popovac D, et al. Past pregnancy outcomes among women living in the vicinity of a lead smelter in Kosovo, Yugoslavia. Am J Public Health 1990;80:33–35.

44. Wibberley D, Khera A, Edwards J, Rushton D. Lead levels in human placentae from normal and malformed births. J Med Genet 1977;36:339–345.

45. Ernhart C, Wolf A, Kennard M, Erhard P, Filipovich H, Sokol R. Intrauterine exposure to low levels of lead: the status of the neonate. Arch Environ Health 1986;41:287–291.

46. Rothenberg S, Schnaas L, Mendez C, Hidalgo H. Effects of lead on neurobehavioral development in the first thirty days of life. In: Smith M, Grant L, Sors A, eds. Lead exposure and child development: an international assessment. Lancaster, UK: Kluwer Academic Publishers, 1989:387–395.

47. Singh N, Donovan C, Hanshaw J. Neonatal lead intoxication in a prenatally exposed infant. J Pediatr 1978;93:1019–1021.

48. Timpo A, Amin J, Casalino M, Yuceoglu A. Congenital lead intoxication. J Pediatr 1979;94:765–767.

49. Sensirivatana R, Supachadhiwong O, Phancharoen S, Mitrakul C. Neonatal lead poisoning: an unusual clinical manifestation. Clin Pediatr 1983;22:582–584.

50. Ghafour S, Khuffash F, Ibrahim H, Reavey P. Congenital lead intoxication with seizures due to prenatal exposure. Clin Pediatr 1984;23:282–283.

51. Bellinger D, Needleman H. Prenatal and early postnatal exposure to lead: developmental effects, correlates, and implications. Int J Ment Health 1985;14:78–111.

52. McMichael A, Vimpani G, Robertson E, Baghurst P, Clark P. The Port Pirie cohort study: maternal blood lead and pregnancy outcome. J Epidemiol Commun Health 1986;40:18–25.

53. Dietrich K, Krafft K, Bier M, Succop P, Berger O, Bornschein R. Early effects of fetal lead exposure: neurobehavioral findings at 6 months. Int J Biosoc Res 1986;8:151–168.

54. Moore M, Goldberg A, Pocock S, et al. Some studies of maternal and infant lead exposure in Glasgow. Scott Med J 1982;27:113–122.

55. Huel G, Boudene C, Ibrahim M. Cadmium and lead content of maternal and newborn hair: relationship to parity, birth weight, and hypertension. Arch Environ Health 1981;36:221–227.

56. Rothenberg S, Schnaas L, Cansino-Ortiz S, et al. Neu-

robehavioral deficits after low level lead exposure in neonates: the Mexico City pilot study. Neurotoxicol Teratol 1989;11:85–93.

57. Graziano J. Reproductive effects of lead: Yugoslavian study report. Paper presented at Conference on Lead Research: implications for environmental health. Research Triangle Park, NC, January 1989.

58. Bellinger D, Leviton A, Rabinowitz M, Allred E, Needleman H, Schoenbaum S. Weight gain and maturity in fetuses exposed to low levels of lead. Environ Res 1991;54:151–158.

59. Bornschein R, Grote J, Mitchell T, et al. Effects of prenatal lead exposure on infant size at birth. In: Smith M, Grant L, Sors A, eds. Lead exposure and child development: an international assessment. Lancaster, UK: Kluwer Academic Publishers, 1989:307–319.

60. Ward N, Watson R, Bryce-Smith D. Placental element levels in relation to fetal development for obstetrically "normal" births: a study of 37 elements. Evidence for effects of cadmium, lead and zinc on fetal growth, and for smoking as a source of cadmium. Int J Biosoc Res 1987;9:63–81.

61. Ward N, Durrant S, Sankey R, Bound J, Bryce-Smith D. Elemental factors in human fetal development. J Nutr Med 1990;1:19–26.

62. Baghurst P, Robertson E, McMichael A, Vimpani G, Wigg N, Roberts R. The Port Pirie Cohort Study: lead effects on pregnancy outcome and early childhood development. Neurotoxicology 1987;8:395–402.

63. Routh D, Mushak P, Boone L. A new syndrome of elevated blood lead and microcephaly. J Pediatr Psychol 1979;4:67–76.

64. Shukla R, Bornschein R, Dietrich K, et al. Fetal and infant lead exposure: effects on growth in stature. Pediatrics 1989;84:604–612.

65. Gerber G, Leonard A, Jacquet P. Toxicity, mutagenicity and teratogenicity of lead. Mutat Res 1980;76:115–141.

66. Levine F, Muenke M. VACTERL association with high prenatal lead exposure: similarities to animal models of lead teratogenicity. Pediatrics 1991;87:390–392.

67. Needleman H, Rabinowitz M, Leviton A, Linn S, Schoenbaum S. The relationship between prenatal lead exposure and congenital anomalies. JAMA 1984;251:2956–2959.

68. Rabinowitz M, Bellinger D, Leviton A, Needleman H, Schoenbaum S. Pregnancy hypertension, blood pressure during labor, and blood lead levels. Hypertension 1987;10:447–451.

69. Ernhart C, Morrow-Tlucak M, Wolf A, Super D, Drotar D. Low level lead exposure in the prenatal and early preschool periods: intelligence prior to school entry. Neurotoxicol Teratol 1989;11:161–170.

70. Bellinger D, Leviton A, Waternaux C, Needleman H, Rabinowitz M. Longitudinal analyses of prenatal and postnatal lead exposure and early cognitive development. N Engl J Med 1987;316:1037–1043.

71. Bellinger D, Leviton A, Sloman J. Antecedents and correlates of improved cognitive performance in children exposed in utero to low levels of lead. Environ Health Perspect 1990;89:5–11.

72. Bellinger D, Sloman J, Leviton A, Needleman H, Rabinowitz M, Waternaux C. Low-level lead exposure and children's cognitive function in the preschool years. Pediatrics 1991;87:219–227.

73. Dietrich K, Krafft K, Bornschein R, et al. Low-level fetal lead exposure effect on neurobehavioral development in early infancy. Pediatrics 1987;80:721–730.

74. Dietrich K, Succop P, Bornschein R, et al. Lead exposure and neurobehavioral development in later infancy. Environ Health Perspect 1990;89:13–19.

75. McMichael A, Baghurst P, Wigg N, Vimpani G, Robertson E, Roberts R. Port Pirie cohort study: environmental exposure to lead and children's abilities at the age of four years. N Engl J Med 1988;319:468–475.

76. Cooney G, Bell A, McBride W, Carter C. Neurobehavioral consequences of prenatal low level exposures to lead. Neurotoxicol Teratol 1989;11:95–104.

77. Cooney G, Bell A, McBride W, Carter C. Low level exposures to lead: the Sydney Study at four years. Dev Med Child Neurol 1989;31:640–649.

78. Moore M, Bushnell I, Goldberg A. A prospective study of the results of changes in environmental lead exposure in children in Glasgow. In: Smith M, Grant L, Sors A, eds. Lead exposure and child development: an international assessment. Lancaster, UK: Kluwer Academic Publishers, 1989:371–378.

79. Grant L, Davis M. Effects of low-level lead exposure on paediatric neurobehavioral development: current findings and future directions. In Smith M, Grant L, Sors A, eds. Lead exposure and child development: an international assessment. Lancaster, UK: Kluwer Academic Publishers, 1989:49–115.

80. Dietrich KN, Succop PA, Berger OG, Hammond PB, Bornschein RL. Lead exposure and the cognitive development of urban preschool children: the Cincinnati lead study cohort at age 4 years. Neurotoxicol Teratol 1991;13:203–211.

81. Davis M, Svensgaard D. Lead and child development. Nature 1987;329:297–300.

82. Needleman H, Bellinger D. Commentary: recent developments. Environ Res 1988;46:190–191.

83. Winder C. Reproductive and chromosomal effects of occupational exposure to lead in the male. Reprod Toxicol 1989;3:221–233.

84. Saaranen M, Suistoma U, Kantola M. Saarikoski S, Vanha-Perttula T. Lead, magnesium, selenium, and zinc in human seminal fluid; comparison with semen parameters and fertility. Human Reprod 1987;2:475–479.

85. Tipton IH, Cook MJ. Trace elements in human tissue. Health Phys 1963;9:103–145.

86. Stumpf WE, Sar M, Grant LD. Autoradiographic localization of $^{210}$Pb and its decay products in rat forebrain. Neurotoxicology 1980;1:593–606.

87. Lancranjan I, Popescu H, Gavenescu O, Klepsch I, Serbanescu M. Reproductive ability of workmen occupationally exposed to lead. Arch Environ Health 1975;30:396–401.

88. Chowdhury AP, Chinoy NJ, Gautam AK, et al. Effect of lead on human semen. Adv Contracept Deliv Syst 1986;2:208–210.

89. Assennato G, Paci C, Baser M, et al. Sperm count suppression without endocrine dysfunction in lead-exposed men. Arch Environ Health 1987;42:124–127.

90. Al-Hakkak Z, Zaid Z, Ibrahim D, Al-Jumaily I, Bazzaz A. Effects of ingestion of lead monoxide alloy on male mouse reproduction. Arch Toxicol 1988;62:97–100.

91. Cullen M, Kayne R, Robins J. Endocrine and reproductive dysfunction in men associated with occupational inorganic lead intoxication. Arch Environ Health 1984;39:431–440.

92. Gustafson A, Hedner P, Schutz A, Skerfving S. Occupational lead exposure and pituitary function. Int Arch Occup Environ Health 1989;61:277–281.

93. Rodamilans M, Osaba M, To-Figueras J, et al. Lead toxicity on endocrine testicular function in an occupationally exposed population. Hum Toxicol 1988;7:125–128.

94. Grandjean P, Wulf H, Niebuhr E. Sister chromatid exchange in response to variations in occupational lead exposure. Environ Res 1983;32:199–204.

95. Al-Hakkak Z, Hamany H, Murad A, Hussain A. Chromosome aberrations in workers at a storage battery plant in Iraq. Mutat Res 1986;171:53–60.

96. Johannson L, Wide M. Long-term exposure of the male mouse to lead: effects on fertility. Environ Res 1986;41:481–487.

97. Stowe HD, Goyer RA. The reproductive ability and progeny of F1 lead-toxic rats. Fertil Steril 1971;22:775–760.

98. Silbergeld E, Akkerman M, Fowler B, Albuquerque E, Alkondon M. Lead: male-mediated effects on reproduction and neurodevelopment. The Toxicologist 1991;11:81 (abstract 239).

99. Hakim R, Stewart W, Canner J, Tielsch J. Occupational lead exposure and strabismus in offspring: a case-control study. Am J Epidemiol 1991;133:351–356.

100. Lindbohm M-L, Salimen M, Anttila A, Taskinen H, Hemminki K. Paternal occupational lead exposure and spontaneous abortion. Scand J Work Environ Health 1991;17:95–103.

101. Mahaffey K, Annest J. Association of erythrocyte protoporphyrin with blood lead level and iron status in the Second National Health and Nutrition Examination Survey, 1976–1980. Environ Res 1986;41:327–338.

102. Hu H, Milder F, Burger D. X-ray fluorescence: issues surrounding the application of a new tool for measuring burden of lead. Environ Res 1989;49:295–317.

103. Rosen JF, Markowitz ME, Bijur PE, et al. Sequential measurements of bone lead content by L x-ray fluorescence in CaNa$_2$ EDTA-treated lead-toxic children. Environ Health Perspect 1991;93:271–277.

104. U.S. Occupational Safety and Health Administration. Occupational exposure to lead: final standard. Fed Reg 1978;43:52952–52960.

105. Rudolph L, Sharp D, Samuels S, Perkins C, Rosenberg J. Environmental and biological monitoring for lead exposure in California workplaces. Am J Public Health 1990;80:921–925.

106. Landrigan P. Lead in the modern workplace. Am J Public Health 1990;80:907–908.

107. Brownie C, Noden D, Krook L, Haluska M, Aronson A. Teratogenic effect of calcium edetate (CaEDTA) in rats and the protective effects of zinc. Toxicol Appl Pharmacol 1986;82:426–443.

108. Thomas D, Chisolm J. Lead, zinc and copper decorporation during calcium disodium ethylenediamine tetraacetate treatment of lead-poisoned children. J Pharmacol Exp Ther 1986;82:426–443.

109. Mayer-Popken O, Denkhaus W, Konietzko H. Lead content of fetal tissues after maternal intoxication. Arch Toxicol 1986;58:203–204.

110. Mahaffey KR. Nutritional factors in lead poisoning. Nutr Rev 1981;39:353–362.

111. World Health Organization (WHO). Environmental health criteria 101, methylmercury. Geneva: WHO, 1990.

112. Amin-Zaki L, Elhassani S, Majeed MA, Clarkson TW, Doherty RA, Greenwood M. Intra-uterine methylmercury poisoning in Iraq. Pediatrics 1974;54:587–595.

113. Amin-Zaki L, Elhassani S, Majeed MA, et al. Perinatal methylmercury poisoning in Iraq. Am J Dis Child 1976;130:1070–1076.

114. Marsh DO, Clarkson TW, Cox C, Myers GJ, Amin-Zaki L, Al-Tikriti S. Fetal methylmercury poisoning. Arch Neurol 1987;44:1017–1022.

115. Rodier PM, Aschner M, Sager PR. Mitotic arrest in the developing CNS after prenatal exposure to methylmercury. Neurobehav Toxicol Teratol 1987;6:379–385.

116. Rodier PM, Kates B. Histological localization of methylmercury in mouse brain and kidney by emulsion autoradiography 203 Hg. Toxicol Appl Pharmacol 1988;92:224–234.

117. Sager PR. Selectivity of methylmercury effects on cytoskeleton and mitotic progression in cultured cells. Toxicol Appl Pharmacol 1988;94:472–486.

118. Burbacher T, Rodier R, Weiss B. Methylmercury developmental neurotoxicity: a comparison of effects in humans and animals. Neurotoxicol Teratol 1990;12:191–202.

119. Astolfi E, Gotelli C. Monitoreo exotoxicologico del mercurio. Bol Acad Nac Med Buenos Aires 1981;5(Suppl):181–188.

120. Clarkson TW, Friberg L, Hursh JB, Nylander M. The prediction of intake of mercury vapor from amalgams. In: Clarkson TW, Friberg L, Nordberg GF, Sager PR, eds. Biological monitoring of toxic metals. New York: Plenum Press, 1988:247–264.

121. Heidam L. Spontaneous abortions among dental assistants, factory workers, painters and gardening workers. J Epidemiol Commun Health 1984;38:149–55.

122. Ericson A, Kallen B. Pregnancy outcome in women working as dentists, dental assistants or dental technicians. Int Arch Occup Environ Health 1989;61:329–333.

123. Goncharuk G. Problems relating to occupational hygiene of women in production of mercury. Gigiena truda i professional 'nye zabolevaniya 1977;5:17–20 (as reported in Barlow and Sullivan, 1982).

124. Cordier S, Deplan F, Mandereau L, Hemon D. Paternal exposure to mercury and spontaneous abortions. Br J Ind Med 1991;48:375–381.

125. Miller RK, Mattison DR, Plowchalk D. Biological monitoring of the human placenta. In: Clarkson TW, Friberg L, Nordberg GF, Sager PR, eds. Biological monitoring of toxic metals. New York: Plenum Press, 1988:567–602.

126. Vimy M. Maternal-fetal distribution of mercury (203-Hg) released from dental amalgam fillings. Am J Physiol 258:R939–945.

127. Goyer RA. Toxic effects of metals. In: Amdur MO, Doull J, Klaassen CD, eds. Casarett and Doull's toxicology, 4th ed. New York: Pergamon Press, 1991:623–680.

128. Friberg L, Elinder CG, Kjellstrom T, Nordberg G, eds. Cadmium and health, volumes I & II. Boca Raton, FL: CRC Press, 1986.

129. Levin AA, Miller RK, di Sant'Agnese PA. Heavy metal alterations of placental function: a mechanism for the induction of fetal toxicity by cadmium. In: Clarkson TW, Nordberg GF, Sager PR, eds. Developmental and reproductive toxicity of metals. New York: Plenum Press, 1983:663–654.

130. World Health Organization (WHO). Evaluation of certain food additives and contaminants. Technical Report 776. Geneva: WHO, 1989.

131. Thun M, Osorio A, Schober S, Hannon W, Lewis B, Halperin W. Nephrotoxicity in cadmium workers. Br J Ind Med 1989;46:689–696.

132. International Agency for Research on Cancer (IARC). Monograph on evaluations of carcinogenicity, Suppl 7. Geneva: World Health Organization, 1987.

133. Takenaka S, Oldiges H, Konig H, Hockrainer D, Oberdorster G. Carcinogenicity of cadmium chloride aerosols in wistar rats. J Natl Cancer Inst 1983;70:367–373.

134. Kjellstrom T, Friberg L, Rahnster B. Mortality and cancer morbidity among cadmium-exposed workers. Environ Health Perspect 1979;28:199–204.

135. Sorahan T, Waterhouse J. Mortality study of nickel cadmium battery workers by the method of regression models in life tables. Br J Ind Med 1983;40:293–300.

136. Mattison DR, Gates AH, Leonard A, Wide M, Hemminki K, Copius Peereboom-Stegeman, JHJ. Reproductive and developmental toxicity of metals: female reproductive system. In: Clarkson TW, Nordberg GF, Sager PR, eds. Reproductive and developmental toxicity of metals. New York: Plenum Press, 1983:43–91.

137. Parizek J, Zahor Z. Effects of cadmium salts on testicular tissue. Nature 1956;177:1036–1038.

138. Lee IP. Effects of environmental metals on male reproduction. In: Clarkson TW, Nordberg GF, Sager PR, eds. Reproductive and developmental toxicity of metals. New York: Plenum Press, 1983:253–278.

139. Ferm V, Carpenter S. The relationship of cadmium and zinc in experimental teratogenesis. Lab Invest 1968;18:429–432.

140. Mulvihill J, Gamm S, Ferm V. Facial malformation in normal and cadmium treated hamsters. J Embryol Expt Morph 1970;24:393–403.

141. Samawickarama G, Webb M. The acute toxicity and teratogenicity of cadmium in the pregnant rat. Environ Health Perspect 1979;28:345–349.

142. Gabbiani G, Badonnel M, Mathewson S, Ryan G. Acute cadmium intoxication: early selective lesion of endothelial clefts. Lab Invest 1974;30:686–695.

143. Newland MC, Ng WW, Baggs RB, Gentry GD, Weiss B, Miller RK. Operant behavior in transition reflects neonatal exposure to cadmium. Teratology 1986;34:231–241.

144. Dencker L, Danielsson B, Khayat A, Lindgren A. Disposition of metals in the embryo and fetus. In: Clarkson TW, Nordberg GF, Sager PR, eds. Reproductive and developmental toxicity of metals. New York: Plenum Press, 1983:607–632.

145. Ahokas R, Dilts P. Cadmium uptake by the rat embryo as a function of gestational age. Am J Obstet Gynecol 1979;135:219–222.

146. Levin AA, Miller RK. Fetal toxicity of cadmium: maternal vs. fetal injections. Teratology 1980;22:105–110.

147. Levin AA, Plautz JR, di Sant'Agnese PA, Miller RK. Cadmium: placental mechanisms of fetal toxicity. Placenta 1981;3:303–318.

148. Saltzman R, Miller RK. Cadmium exposure on day 12 of gestation in the Wistar rat: distribution, uteroplacental blood flow, and fetal viability. Teratology 1989;39:19–30.

149. White TEC, Baggs RB, Miller RK. Central nervous system lesions in the Wistar rat fetus following direct fetal injections of cadmium. Teratology 1990;42:7–15.

150. Miller RK, Ng WW, Levin AA. The placenta: relevance to toxicology. In: Clarkson TW, Nordberg GF, Sager PR, eds. Developmental and reproductive toxicity of metals. New York: Plenum Press, 1983:569–605.

151. Miller RK, Shaikh Z. Perinatal metabolism: metals and metallothionein. In: Clarkson TW, Nordberg GF, Sager PR, eds. Developmental and reproductive toxicity of metals. New York: Plenum Press, 1983:153–204.

152. Levin A, Miller RK. Fetal toxicity of cadmium in the rat: decreased utero-placental blood flow. Toxicol Appl Pharmacol 1981;58:297–306.

153. di Sant'Agnese PA, Jensen K, Levin AA, Miller RK. Placental toxicity of cadmium: an ultrastructural study. Placenta 1983;4:149–163.

154. Wier PJ, Miller RK, Maulik D, di Sant'Agnese PA. Cadmium toxicity in the perfused human placenta. Toxicol Appl Pharmacol 1990;105:156–171.

155. Wier PJ, Miller RK. The pharmacokinetics of cadmium in the dually perfused human placenta. Trophoblast Res 1987;2: 357–366.

156. Miller RK, Faber W, Asai M, di Sant'Agnese PA, Wier PJ, Shah Y. Placental toxicity of cadmium and retinoids. Trophoblast Res 1992;6:421–435.

157. Daston G. Toxic effects of cadmium on the developing lung. J Toxicol Environ Health 1982;9:51–61.

158. Cox C, Clarkson TW, Marsh DO, Amin-Zaki, Tikriti S, Myers GG. Dose-response analysis of infants prenatally exposed to methylmercury: an application of a single compartment model to single-strand hair analysis. Environ Res 1989;49:318–332.

# 18

Asphyxiants

YORAM SOROKIN

## ASPHYXIA

### Definition

Asphyxia is a condition characterized by inadequate oxygen ($O_2$) and/or increased carbon dioxide ($CO_2$) in the blood and tissues. As shown in Table 18.1, anoxia or hypoxia can result from respiratory compromise, severe anemia, circulatory stagnation, or impaired utilization of $O_2$ by tissues. Perinatal (fetal) asphyxia may be defined as a combination of hypoxia, hypercapnia, and tissue ischemia resulting in anaerobic metabolism and eventually, if not converted, organ death (1). An asphyxiant is an agent (gas) capable of producing asphyxia.

### Fetal Oxygenation

There are several key steps in the journey of oxygen from maternal inspired air to fetal cells (2). Maternal respiratory muscular efforts move air in and out of the lungs. The oxygen pressure in maternal alveoli is regulated by various physiological mechanisms including sensors of $PO_2$, $PCO_2$, and pH. During pregnancy, maternal arterial $PO_2$ is regulated at lower levels than in the nonpregnant state (3), and oxygen diffuses very rapidly from maternal alveoli into the pulmonary capillaries. Oxygen is transported in blood in both free and bounded forms, the sum of which constitutes the oxygen content of the blood.

Oxygen diffusion across the placenta is very complex and follows Fick's equation. Most elements of the equation are constant for short periods of time. However, uterine blood flow (UBF) can vary markedly over brief intervals. UBF cannot increase in response to fetal needs, but many forces tend to decrease it, including normal uterine contractions (4).

Human umbilical venous $PO_2$ is remarkably low. However, the fetal oxygen dissociation curve lies to the left of the adult curve, resulting in a higher affinity of fetal blood for $O_2$ (Fig. 18.1). The basis for the increased oxygen affinity resides in the interaction of fetal hemoglobin (Hgb) with intracellular 2,3-diphosphoglycerate (2,3-DPG). Due to the high affinity of fetal Hgb and the high rate of perfusion of fetal organs in comparison with their oxygen requirements, the fetus is able to transport large amounts of oxygen from the placenta to fetal organs. Fetal blood oxygen capacity is comparable to that of maternal blood. From the point of view of energy metabolism, the fetus normally has access to all of the oxygen that it needs and does not use anaerobic glycolysis as a terminal source of energy (5, 6).

### Fetal Asphyxia

With inadequate oxygenation within the cell, glycolytic metabolism is diverted from the aerobic pathway toward the production of lactic acid. The results are less efficient energy pro-

**Table 18.1.**
**Mechanisms Resulting in Anoxia or Hypoxia[a]**

| Type of Hypoxia | $PaO_2$ | BF | $O_2$Cap | Comments |
|---|---|---|---|---|
| Arterial (anoxic) | ↓ | Nl or ↑ | Nl or ↑ | Pulmonary irritants, respiratory depressants |
| Anemic | Nl or ↑ | Nl or ↑ | ↓ | Decreased Hgb constituents |
| Stagnant (hypokinetic) | Nl | ↓ | Nl | Reduced blood flow |
| Histotoxic | Nl | Nl | Nl | Impaired $O_2$ utilization by tissues, e.g., cyanide poisoning |

[a]$PaO_2$ = arterial partial pressure of $O_2$; BF = rate of blood flow; $O_2$ Cap = $O_2$ capacity; Nl = normal; Hgb = hemoglobin.

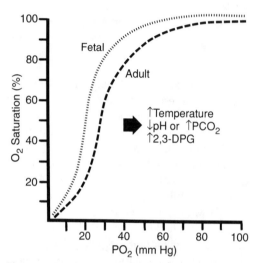

**Figure 18.1.** Oxygen dissociation curves for human adult and fetal blood (pH 7.4, 37°C). Fetal blood has a higher oxygen affinity than adult blood. Note factors that shift the curves to the right.

duction, bicarbonate consumption by lactic acid, and gradual development of metabolic acidosis. When the pH is falling, sensitive enzymes that are necessary for maintenance of vital cellular functions are inoperative. The consequences are cell death, tissue death, and possibly, fetal death.

There are many fetal adaptive mechanisms in response to hypoxemia. During short-term acute reduction in oxygenation, fetal glucose consumption falls and glycogen mobilization increases; fetal lactate concentration rises and may become an important source of substrate. Hypoxemia also results in an increase in fetal hematocrit (7), stimulated erythropoiesis, and decreased fetal blood volume (8).

The fetal environment has oxygen availability that exceeds oxidative needs. When oxygen availability decreases, the fetus can increase fractional oxygen extraction resulting in an increased $PO_2$ difference across the umbilical circulation; ultimately, however, this produces fetal arterial hypoxemia. The degree to which fractional $O_2$ extraction can increase and fetal arterial $PO_2$ can fall before tissue oxygen supplies are inadequate is termed the oxygen margin of safety (9). In ovine studies, fetal oxygen consumption was maintained by increases in $O_2$ extraction until oxygen delivery was reduced by 50% (10). With sustained hypoxemia sufficient to produce lactic acid accumulation, the margin of safety becomes limited and pathological changes may occur.

Cardiac output remains fairly stable at moderate degrees of hypoxia, but decreases as the condition becomes more severe. Blood flow is redistributed by selective vasoconstriction of certain vascular beds and vasodilatation of others: blood flow increases to the brain, heart, and adrenal gland, is maintained in the placenta, and decreases to all other areas of the body (11, 12). Redistribution of blood flow is controlled by the interplay of changes in blood gases, the autonomic nervous system, and hormonal influences (13). With continued $O_2$ deprivation, these compensatory mechanisms are overwhelmed, and the fetus begins to accumulate lactic acid (14).

The fetus can adapt to chronic limitation of oxygen delivery with a decreased rate of oxygen consumption, decreased substrate requirements, and decreased rate of growth, producing intrauterine growth retardation (IUGR) (15, 16).

Fetal body movements decrease with acute short-term hypoxia in the normally grown (17) and IUGR fetus (18), resulting in lower energy expenditure. Reduction in fetal $PO_2$ also abolishes normal rhythmic fetal breathing movements (19). With severe asphyxia, fetal gasping precedes fetal death (20).

When the fetus is subjected to sustained hypoxia or mild graded hypoxia, there is a lower incidence of low voltage electrocortical state, or REM sleep state (21). These findings may reflect a metabolic compensatory response to mild hypoxemia.

When hypoxia is sufficient to result in fetal metabolic acidosis, direct fetal myocardial depression results in late fetal heart rate (FHR) decelerations (22). Most decelerations occur through an autonomic reflex mechanism in nonacidotic early hypoxia (23).

## ASPHYXIANTS

### Carbon Monoxide

PROPERTIES AND OCCURRENCE

Carbon monoxide (CO) is a colorless, odorless, tasteless, nonirritating, combustible toxic gas (24). CO is one of the five most important neurotoxins for humans and is responsible for half of the total poisoning fatalities occurring yearly in the U.S. (25). It is the best known example of an agent that can decrease the oxygen transport capability of the blood and produce anemic hypoxia.

CO is the most abundant pollutant in the lower atmosphere. Natural sources, such as atmospheric oxidation of methane, forest fires, and the ocean (CO produced by microorganisms), are responsible for 90% of the atmospheric CO, while human activity produces 10% (24). Death from fires usually results from CO poisoning rather than from burns. CO is a prominent constituent of flue gas from furnaces and exhaust gas from internal combustion engines. The automobile is the greatest non-natural source of CO. Concentrations as high as 30% have been measured in automobile exhaust gas. Compared to the average atmospheric CO concentration of 0.1 ppm, concentrations in heavy traffic can reach 115 ppm on the freeway, 75 ppm in vehicles on the expressway, and 23 ppm in residential areas (24). The installation of pollution control devices in automobile exhaust systems reduced CO emissions 30-fold, from 90.0 to 3.4 g/mile of automobile travel (26).

CO is a hazard in the steel and mine industries and in many industrial processes. Firefighters, bakers, chauffeurs, garage mechanics, cooks, and furnace repairers have the highest risk of CO exposure among nonindustrial workers. Methylene chloride, a common organic solvent in industrial and commercial products, is metabolized in the body to CO and may cause various degrees of CO poisoning.

In smokers, the carboxyhemoglobin (HbCO) concentration is influenced more by the smoking habit than by air pollution (24). The concentration of CO in tobacco smoke is 4%, and the median HbCO level in heavy smokers (two packs of cigarettes per day) is 5.9% (27). Of the more than 500 different compounds in tobacco smoke, the constituents suspected of exerting harm during pregnancy are CO, cyanide, and nicotine (28, 29).

Endogenous sources of CO result from normal degradation reactions in the body, such as breakdown of heme pigments. In normal women, CO production is doubled during the luteal phase of the cycle and is increased even higher during pregnancy (30). About 15% of this increase results from fetal endogenous CO production.

TOXICOLOGY

Metabolism and Mechanisms of Action

Toxicity from CO is mainly due to its reaction with hemoglobin to form HbCO. In this form, Hgb cannot carry oxygen. Even at very low concentrations, the affinity of Hgb for CO is 220–245 times greater than the affinity of Hgb for oxygen (31). In addition, the shape of the dissociation curve of oxyhemoglobin is altered, so that a smaller portion of blood oxygen is released in tissue capillaries (32). CO also binds to heme-containing proteins in nucleated red cell cytochromes, such as those contained in respiratory enzymes and myoglobin (33). This occurs particularly in severely hypoxic tissues.

CO induces nonischemic hypoxia that initiates cellular injury (34). There is a correlation between HbCO blood levels and the nature and intensity of toxic signs and symptoms. Factors important in the toxicity of CO include CO concentration in the air, duration of exposure, respiratory minute volume, cardiac output, oxygen requirements by the tissues, and Hgb concentration in the blood. At very high inspired CO concentrations (more than 0.5%), dangerous HbCO levels can be reached within minutes. At lower inspired concentrations, blood-gas equilibrium is attained in 1–5 hr in the adult (35). Factors that speed respiration and circulation, such as fever and exercise, accelerate the process of HbCO saturation and shorten the latency period before clinical signs and symptoms appear. Anemia and high altitude also increase the appearance of symptoms.

Carboxyhemoglobin is fully dissociable; once an acute exposure has been terminated, the pigment eventually reverts to oxyhemoglobin, and the CO is excreted via the lungs. A small amount of CO is oxidized to $CO_2$. In a normal resting adult breathing room air, the half-time decrease of CO in the blood is 320 min. However, this half-time is decreased to 45–80 min with 100% oxygen and 20–25 min when 100% oxygen is breathed at hyperbaric pressures (3 atmospheres) (36). This therapeutic effect is achieved by increasing the amount of oxygen dissolved in the plasma.

## Maternal and Fetal Carboxyhemoglobin

Normal maternal HbCO concentration is primarily due to endogenous CO production and is influenced by CO excretion rate, relative affinity of maternal Hgb for CO, concentration of CO in expired air, endogenous CO fetal production, and the rate of CO exchange across the placenta (37, 38). Fetal production of CO accounts for 3% of the total maternal HbCO concentration.

Fetal HbCO concentration varies from 0.7–2.5% as a function of maternal HbCO concentration, fetal CO production rate, placental diffusing capacity for CO, and the relative affinity of fetal Hgb for CO vs. $O_2$. The human fetal/maternal HbCO ratio is 1.1, i.e., fetal HbCO concentration is approximately 10–15% greater than that of the pregnant woman. In the steady state, the ratio depends on the relative $O_2$ and CO affinities of fetal and maternal blood (37).

Longo and Hill (39) exposed chronically instrumented pregnant sheep to CO concentrations of 30–300 ppm. At all levels of CO exposure, the maternal HbCO concentration rose rapidly during the first 2–3 hr, then increased more slowly to a relatively constant level by 7–8 hr; half-time was 2.5 hr. Fetal HbCO concentrations lagged behind maternal levels. Over the first hour, fetal HbCO showed little change, then it rose at a slower rate than in the pregnant woman. Fetal and maternal HbCO concentrations were similar by 5–6 hr, but fetal HbCO levels continued to slowly rise over 24 hr, reaching a steady state by 36–48 hr; fetal half-time was 7 hr.

Using a mathematical model, Hill et al. (40) calculated patterns of human CO uptake and elimination similar to those found in sheep experiments (37, 40). Leonard et al. (41) recently suggested that increased CO elimination during labor may be accompanied by rapid changes in the maternal HbCO concentration, leading to a spuriously high fetal to maternal HbCO ratio at the time of delivery.

## Maternal-Fetal Health Effects

Because of the systemic nature of the hypoxic insult, virtually all body cells are affected by CO. The primary target organs are the tissues with the greatest levels of oxygen consumption: the myocardium, the brain, and, if pregnant, the fetus.

In the rat, pregnancy markedly increases the susceptibility to CO poisoning (42). The mean survival time of pregnant rats exposed to 0.43% CO was 14 min compared to 42 min in nonpregnant female rats with similar exposures. During pregnancy, the 20–30% decrease in blood oxygen capacity (due to decreased Hgb concentration) and the 15–25% increase in oxygen consumption may exacerbate the effects of CO on blood oxygenation. Increased human susceptibility to CO poisoning during pregnancy is logical but remains to be demonstrated.

Injury to the fetus can occur at relatively low levels of fetal HbCO. The fetus has a low arterial oxygen tension and is less able to compensate than the adult by increasing tissue blood flow. Effects noted in rodent studies include decreased fetal weight gain and neurobehavioral deficits after maternal exposures of 125–150 ppm (43–45) and decreased viability at higher exposures (45, 46). Schwetz et al. (47) found no teratogenicity from 250 ppm CO exposure between gestational days 6–15 in mice and days 6–18 in rabbits.

Ginsburg and Myers (48, 49) exposed nine pregnant monkeys near term to air containing concentrations of CO sufficient to produce moderate or severe hypoxia in the fetuses lasting 1 hr. While the mothers tolerated the CO inhalation well, all the fetuses became bradycardic and hypertensive and developed profound metabolic acidosis. The graded hypoxic insults to the fetuses produced three distinct categories of physiological and neuropathological changes. Group 1 fetuses (arterial $O_2$ 21–24 ml/100 ml) recovered after brief ventilation, and no brain injury occurred. A single Group 2 fetus (intermediate level of arterial $O_2$) incurred moderately severe brain damage. Fetuses in Group 3 (arterial $O_2$ 16–18 ml/100 ml) required prolonged mechanical ventilation and showed extensive cerebral hemorrhagic necrosis. Brain edema was the apparent primary cause of death in study animals. The investigators concluded that the fetal monkey brain has a high threshold for the effects of sustained hypoxia, but once a critical level of oxygenation is exceeded, extensive brain damage with early death results.

Sixty human case reports of CO intoxication during pregnancy have been published (50). Only one of these cases occurred in a workplace: a woman 20 weeks pregnant was treated with $O_2$ after exposure to CO from a furnace leak in a restaurant and delivered a normal baby 4 months later. In 42 of the 60 reports, there was sufficient information on maternal toxicity to classify the symptoms as mild, moderate, or severe. Fetal outcome worsened as the severity of maternal symptoms increased. All 11 cases of maternal death were accompanied by fetal death. Of the 27 cases of moderate maternal toxicity (a period of unconsciousness or coma), there were 15 fetal deaths and 10 survivors with anatomical or functional abnormalities. Fetal outcome was generally good when the mother did not experience unconsciousness or coma.

Malformations were reported in six of the 12 cases of CO exposure during the first trimester of pregnancy, and in one of 48 cases of CO exposure later in pregnancy. The malformations included mongoloid-type features, missing and deformed limbs, low-set ears, oral cavity anomalies, hypoplastic organ development, and foot and hip deviations. Functional alterations, such as psychomotor disturbances and subnormal mental development, were not restricted to exposure at any particular stage of pregnancy. In several livebirths, there was evidence of central nervous system (CNS) damage and of poor neurological development. Autopsies of stillbirths showed the CNS to be a target organ for CO-induced damage at any stage of pregnancy.

In a recent multicenter, prospective study, Koren et al. (51) followed 38 women with acute CO poisoning during pregnancy and performed serial developmental assessments on the surviving children up to 3 yr of age. The five pregnancies with severe CO toxicity (depressed sensorium or coma) resulted in two normal births, two stillbirths, and one infant with cerebral palsy and tomographic findings consistent with ischemia. The three cases of adverse outcome had been treated with high flow $O_2$, while the two cases with normal outcome followed hyperbarbic $O_2$ therapy. All of the children born to women with mild or moderate CO poisoning exhibited normal physical and neurobehavioral development. No congenital malformations were reported.

The deleterious effects of maternal smoking on infant birthweight have given rise to the theory that maternal exposure to CO during pregnancy may increase the risk of delivering a low birthweight infant (26, 37). In a case-control study, Alderman et al. (52) used air pollution-monitoring data from the Colorado Department of Health to calculate individual CO exposure for each mother. Low birthweight infants and normal-weight infants were contrasted with respect to ambient levels of CO during the 3 months before delivery in the neighborhoods where their mothers lived at birth. After adjustment for the confounding effects of maternal race and education, there was no association between CO exposure and birthweight.

Wouters et al. (53) examined fetal outcome in 77 uneventful pregnancies and related it to venous cord HbCO levels. Birthweight and birthweight centiles were significantly reduced in children of mothers who smoked. There was a very weak correlation between birthweight centiles and HbCO levels in venous cord blood. In another study of 24 pregnant smokers, changes in maternal heart rate, blood pressure, fetal aortic and umbilical blood flow, and catecholamine levels were related to maternal nicotine levels, but not to CO (54). It seems unlikely that HbCO levels induced in the fetus by maternal smoking can account for the well-known growth retardation associated with tobacco smoke exposure.

## CLINICAL ASSESSMENT

The presenting symptoms of CO poisoning are vague and variable and include headaches (often frontal), lightheadedness, weakness, sleepiness, decreased exercise tolerance, visual disturbances, palpitations, nausea, and vomiting (25, 35). In severe CO poisoning, tissue oxygen tensions are very low, resulting in confusion and syncope.

The presence of HbCO results in a significant decrease in blood $O_2$ content; the ambient CO concentration is rarely high enough to result in a detectable decrease in arterial $PO_2$. The chemoreceptor (carotid body) mechanism may not be triggered, and respiratory parameters may remain within normal limits (55). Peripheral vasodilation occurs in response to a slowly developing hypoxia, and it may exceed the compensatory ability to increase cardiac output. This explains why syncope and fainting are more common than dyspnea in victims of CO poisoning, and why consciousness may be lost for long periods before death.

Carboxyhemoglobin has a cherry red color, and its presence in high concentration in capillary blood may impart an abnormal red color to the skin, mucous membranes, and fingernails. However, in long exposures to low CO concentrations, victims are more apt to exhibit pallor or cyanosis (24). A high index of suspicion is necessary to recognize chronic occult CO poisoning.

There is a syndrome of delayed neuropsychiatric deterioration following severe CO poisoning (25) that is attributable to delayed neuronal death and demyelination. These patients are comatose at the time of poisoning, regain normal neurological function, and then deteriorate at a variable time (2–3 weeks) after the poisoning. The delayed signs include apathy, apraxia, aphasia, disorientation, hallucinations, muscular rigidity, gait disturbances, fecal and urinary incontinence, and coma (25).

Various diagnostic tests are useful in CO poisoning (24, 25, 27). A HbCO level is essential to assess the severity of exposure and to determine the need for hyperbaric oxygen therapy. Other blood tests that may be useful include arterial blood gases, electrolytes, lactic acid, complete blood count (CBC), SGOT, SGPT, glucose, creatine kinase, and lactate dehydrogenase. In addition, an ECG, EEG, and/or CT scan may be indicated. Drug screening may reveal concomitant intoxication with other drugs.

## PREVENTION AND TREATMENT

Cessation of cigarette smoking during pregnancy can have an important impact on maternal and fetal exposure to CO. Reduction of air pollution is another preventive measure. In response to amendments to the Clear Air Act, the U.S. Department of Health Education and Welfare issued the air quality criteria for CO in 1970–1971 (37). Annual maximal permissible exposures are 35 mg/m$^3$ (32 ppm) for 1 hr and 10 mg/m$^3$ (9 ppm) for 8 hr (37).

Most CO poisonings are accidental and are often attributable to leaks from stoves and furnaces. Educational efforts are successful in reducing these CO fatalities. In the mid-1970s, the Allegheny County Health Department in Pittsburgh conducted a program of public education, home inspection, and distribution of CO dosimeters to low-income areas. During the winter following the program, there were no CO fatalities recorded, the first such winter in 8 yr (56).

Death from CO poisoning associated with vehicles are preventable. Production of CO by vehicles can be minimized by regular preventive maintenance, inspection of exhaust systems, and emission testing. Of 68 deaths due to CO poisoning in vehicles in Maryland during 1966–1971, most occurred in parked cars in which the motor was running to provide heat (57).

Since 1968, the average quantity of CO produced by new cars has been reduced by more than 90%. The 1990 amendments to the Clean Air Act mandate oxygenated fuels and more advanced pollution control systems. These measures should result in further reductions of CO emissions (57).

The initial step in treatment of suspected CO poisoning is to remove the victim promptly from the source to fresh air. If respiration has failed, artificial respiration must be instituted. Oxygen is administered to reverse hypoxia and promote CO excretion. In most cases, administration of 100% oxygen with a tight-fitting face mask and a rebreathing reservoir will be adequate. In severe CO poisoning, the patient should be promptly transported to a facility equipped with a hyperbaric chamber (24, 25, 35). The safety of hyperbaric oxygen use during pregnancy has not been established, but it may be beneficial in severe cases (51). If hyperbaric oxygen therapy is not available, 100% $O_2$ should be given for extended periods of time, because the fetus eliminates CO more slowly than the pregnant woman.

Exchange transfusion or transfusions of packed red blood cells has been used in moribund victims. Measures that minimize oxygen consumption by the patient, such as keeping the patient calm, are beneficial. Supplementary care includes correction of hypotension, acidosis, hypoglycemia, electrolyte imbalance, as well as monitoring cardiac function.

## Cyanide

### PROPERTIES AND OCCURRENCE/USES

Hydrogen cyanide (prussic acid, HCN) occurs as a solution or as a gas generated when a cyanide salt reacts with dilute mineral acid. Hydrogen cyanide in aqueous solution is readily absorbed from the skin and from all mucous membranes, e.g., rectum and vagina. The alkali cyanide salts are usually toxic only when ingested (35).

Cyanide is a potent and rapidly active chemical asphyxiant. Cyanide has high affinity for iron in the ferric state (24, 35). When absorbed, it reacts readily with the trivalent cytochrome oxidase in the mitochondria and inhibits cellular respiration (58). The result is lactic acidosis and cytotoxic hypoxia.

Because of its ability to form complexes with metal, cyanide is used in metallurgical and photographic processes, electroplating, and metal cleaning (35). Hydrogen cyanide gas is used to fumigate ships, mills, warehouses, greenhouses, and to sterilize soil. Organically bound cyanides (e.g., acrylonitrile) are also sometimes used as fumigants. In the home, cyanides are found in silver polish, insecticides, rodenticides, and fruit seeds. The salt, cyanogen chloride, can produce cyanide poisoning or induce pulmonary edema with chronic exposures. Amygdalin is a cyanogenic glycoside found in apricot, peach, and other similar fruit pits, as well as in sweet almonds. Amygdalin is the major ingredient of laetrile; this alleged anticancer drug has been responsible for human cyanide poisoning (35).

Hydrogen cyanide gas may be generated during the pyrolysis of wool, polyamides, polyurethanes, polyacrylonitriles, and other substances (24, 35). A recent study (59) suggests that cyanide may be an important cause of poisoning and death in residential fire victims of smoke inhalation.

Sodium nitroprusside is used to treat hypertensive emergencies and in some situations requiring short-term reduction of cardiac preload and/or afterload. This drug is converted to cyanide and thiocyanate and may result in cyanide poisoning if it is infused at a rapid rate or given for prolonged periods (35).

The cytochrome P450-dependent monooxygenases liberate cyanide from organic nitriles (58), as do glutathione S-transferases from organic thiocyanates.

### TOXICOLOGY

#### Metabolism and Mechanisms of Action

Most cyanide poisonings involve accidental or intentional ingestion of hydrocyanic acid or one of its alkali salts (24, 35). The critical toxic lesion induced by HCN is the cell's inability to utilize oxygen. The undissociated acid, hydrogen cyanide, interrupts electron transport by inhibiting the cytochrome a-cytochrome $a_3$ step. As a result, oxidative metabolism and phosphorylation are compromised. Electron transfer from $a_3$ to molecular oxygen is blocked, peripheral tissue oxygen tensions begin to rise, and the unloading gradient for oxyhemoglobin is decreased.

Cyanide directly stimulates the chemoreceptors of the carotid and aortic bodies, resulting in hyperpnea. While cardiac irregularities are often noted, death is due to respiratory arrest of central origin (60).

As with other chemical asphyxiants, the critical organs are those most sensitive to oxygen deficiency: the brain and heart. The demyelinating lesions in the brain obtained in experimental cyanide intoxications are not specific for cyanide, but are similar to those produced by hypoxia (61).

Conversion of cyanide to the relatively harmless thiocyanate ion is the major mechanism of detoxification. This conversion uses an enzymatic reaction mediated by the enzyme, Rhodanese (transsulfurase), which has its greatest activity in the liver, but is widely distributed in tissues (35). The response rate of the Rhodanese system to a cyanide challenge is slow, but it can be accelerated by an exogenous supply of sulfur (thiosulfate). The thiocyanate formed is readily excreted into the urine.

Relatively small amounts of absorbed cyanide are excreted unchanged by the lungs. There are other minor routes of detoxification including trapping the cyanide group on vitamin $B_{12}$ and oxidation to formate and $CO_2$.

## Maternal-Fetal Health Effects

Teratogenic effects of cyanide have been observed in several animal models. Neural tube defects (NTDs), including exencephaly and encephalocele, were the most common anomalies seen after prenatal exposure of explanted chick embryos to sodium cyanide (62) or of hamsters to nitriles (63). Doherty et al. (64) subcutaneously infused sodium cyanide into pregnant golden hamsters between 6 and 9 days of gestation and observed a high incidence of NTDs. Other defects included hydropericardium and crooked tail. Fetal crown rump length was significantly smaller in offspring of cyanide-treated dams than in offspring of control animals. A total dose of 30–40 times the acute subcutaneous $LD_{50}$ dose was administered to the animals before signs of maternal toxicity appeared. The concurrent administration of cyanide and sodium thiosulfate, the

classical cyanide antagonist, protected against both the toxic and the teratogenic effects of cyanide. NTDs have also been found in offspring of hamsters treated with amygdalin, the most common constituent of laetrile (65).

In a two-generation reproduction study in the rat, the oral administration of 25 mg/kg/day of cyanamide produced decreases in dam weight gain, in the number of corpora lutea, in the number of implantations, and in the number of neonates observed in rats of the Fo generation (66). Oral administration of two lower dosages was without effect. No changes were seen in the Fl generation.

Stimulation of the aortic or carotid bodies by sodium cyanide in fetal lambs in utero produces cardiorespiratory responses characterized by bradycardia and respiratory effort, but no significant change in blood pressure (67).

## CLINICAL ASSESSMENT

The initial symptoms of acute cyanide poisoning by ingestion are a bitter taste, numbness in the throat, salivation, nausea, vomiting, hyperpnea, headaches, anxiety, confusion, vertigo, stiffness in the lower jaw, palpitations, and constriction in the chest (24, 35). Respiration is initially stimulated because of the chemoreceptor cells' response to decreased oxygen; as the cyanide level rises, respiration becomes slow, irregular with prolonged expirations, and then stops. Due to initial vasoconstriction, blood pressure rises and the heart rate slows. Thereafter, the pulse becomes rapid and weak, and the skin becomes bright pink in color due to the high oxyhemoglobin concentration of venous blood (35). Hypoxic generalized convulsions occur following unconsciousness, and the victim has bradycardia, paralysis, and undilated pupils. Death is from respiratory arrest.

Inhalation of HCN commonly produces toxic reactions within seconds and death within minutes. Absorption is slower after ingestion of cyanide salts, and death may be delayed as long as hours. Cyanide toxicity from sodium nitroprusside and cyanide preparations used over long periods gives less dramatic symptoms (68). Signs and symptoms include metabolic acidosis, shortness of breath, headaches, nausea, vertigo, flushing, and seizures. The retinal vein and artery are equally red. Patients with reduced renal function who are treated with nitroprusside over long periods (over a week) are at increased risk for cyanide poisoning. The cyanate levels should be checked during therapy.

## PREVENTION AND TREATMENT

Effective treatment of cyanide poisoning must be very rapid. Clinical clues to the diagnosis include the characteristic odor of cyanide (oil of bitter almonds), bright pink color of the skin, or bradycardia in the absence of cyanosis (35). A history from paramedics, police, family members, or co-workers may reveal the presence of pillboxes, photography supplies, peaches, or pesticides. A history of laetrile therapy or employment in jobs using cyanide-containing processes should be noted.

Laboratory tests are seldom useful for prognosis or treatment. Specimens, including gastric contents and plasma, should be saved. Other laboratory tests include CBC, electrolytes, toxicologies, and arterial blood gases (ABGs); ABGs will show a metabolic acidosis with a normal $PO_2$. Whole blood cyanide levels in fatal cases exceed 0.5 mM (more than 3 $\mu g/ml$)(68).

In the apneic victim, intubation and artificial respiration with 100% oxygen are started. Sodium thiosulfate is the best sulfur antidote to cyanide (35). Thiosulfate is nontoxic, has high water solubility, and irreversibly inactivates cyanide. However, sodium thiosulfate has a slow onset of action. Therefore, until the cyanide is detoxified, the usual therapy of cyanide poisoning first includes the conversion of a portion of the circulating hemoglobin into methemoglobin using amyl nitrite by inhalation and sodium nitrite intravenously. (The four ferric heme groups in methemoglobin compete very effectively and rapidly with cytochrome oxidase for cyanide, and cyanomethemoglobin is a dissociable complex.) Aspirols of amyl nitrite are broken in front of the patient's nose or between the patient and the oxygen delivery system one at a time for 30 sec of every minute, while a sodium nitrate 3% solution is being prepared for a 10-ml intravenous administration over 10 min (for adults) (35, 69). Then 50 ml of 25% sodium thiosulfate are administered intravenously in the same site. Repeat doses of sodium nitrite and sodium thiosulfate are usu-

ally half of the original, with the need based on the serum cyanide level and the patient's condition.

In the asymptomatic patient who swallowed cyanide, gastric lavage with saline or a solution of sodium thiosulfate and water 5% and/or administration of syrup of Ipecac may be useful. However, due to the speed of absorption and the rapidity with which symptoms appear, these techniques should be postponed until nitrite and thiosulfate therapy has been given (69).

Patients with cyanide poisoning are transferred to the intensive care unit after the initial acute emergency treatment. Frequent venous oxygen samples are taken to monitor therapy, and the patient is observed for blood pressure instability, cyanosis of the skin or mucous membranes, arrhythmias, and myocardial anoxia. Vasopressors, transfusions, or hemodialysis may be necessary. Treatment of sodium nitroprusside-induced cyanide toxicity includes stopping the nitroprusside infusion, administering antidote therapy, and hemodialysis if necessary to remove thiocyanate (69).

### Hydrogen Sulfide

## PROPERTIES AND OCCURRENCE/USES

Hydrogen sulfide ($H_2S$) is a colorless, highly toxic irritant and asphyxiant gas (35). It is heavier than air and has the odor of rotten eggs. Its smell is detectable at about 0.25 ppm and barely tolerable at 20–30 ppm, but there is no smell at high concentrations because of olfactory fatigue.

An estimated 90–100 million tons of $H_2S$ are produced annually from natural and human-made sources. $H_2S$ is released from decay of organic material, natural gas, volcanic gases, and sulfur springs. It is present in sewers (sewer gas) and cesspools and is a product of putrefaction. $H_2S$ is emitted from a variety of industrial operations including viscose rayon manufacture, paper mills, petrochemical plants, petroleum refineries, natural gas plants, coke oven plants, iron smelters, pesticide and sulfur production, food processing, and tanneries (35, 70). $H_2S$ is used in ton quantities in the preparation of heavy water for nuclear reactors. It is also released in vivo from ingested or injected soluble inorganic sulfides.

In urban areas, the general population is exposed to levels of $H_2S$ below 1 mg/m$^3$ (71). Peak concentrations as high as 2 mg/m$^3$ have been reported in geothermally active areas. Much higher concentrations can occur near industrial sites (up to 200 and even 450 mg/m$^3$). In an episode of severe ambient air contamination by $H_2S$ in Posa Rica, Mexico, caused by malfunction of a sulfur recovery plant, levels of 1500–3000 mg/m$^3$ occurred and resulted in several deaths (72).

Workers are not usually exposed to $H_2S$ concentrations above the occupational exposure limits of 10–15 mg/m$^3$ adopted by many governments. However, there are numerous reports of accidental exposures to much higher concentrations in various industries. Human $H_2S$ poisoning is invariably the result of occupational exposure to the gas.

## TOXICOLOGY

### Metabolism and Mechanisms of Action

$H_2S$ is rapidly absorbed into the body, almost exclusively through inhalation. It is distributed to the brain, kidney, liver, pancreas, and small intestine (70). Half of the absorbed dose is excreted in the urine as sulfate within 24 hr. The major detoxification route of $H_2S$ is by oxidation to sulfate (70); another detoxification route involves methylation. The third metabolic pathway, which is largely responsible for the toxic action of $H_2S$, involves reaction with metal or disulfide-containing proteins (73).

The human body has an inherently large capacity for detoxifying $H_2S$; the toxicity of $H_2S$ gas mixtures is more closely related to concentration than length of exposure. Vapor concentrations of 50 ppm (0.005%) in air cause toxic symptoms, while concentrations of 1000–2000 ppm (0.1%–0.2%) are usually fatal within a few minutes (35). Susceptibility to $H_2S$ varies among individuals, and it has been suggested that previous exposure may increase the sensitivity to $H_2S$.

$H_2S$ has affinity for metals essential to development (copper, magnesium, iron), and the hydrosulfide anion inhibits cytochrome oxidase similarly, but more strongly, than cyanide. In addition, $H_2S$ interferes with protein synthesis in the brain. Neurotoxicity induced by $H_2S$ has been observed in experimental animals and humans. After acute exposure of rabbits, neurotoxicity resulted from inhibition of alkaline phosphatase and adenosine triphosphatase in the cerebral cortex. The CNS effects were due to sulfide binding of metal ions required as enzyme cofactors. Reduced brain protein synthesis was observed in female mice after 2 hr of exposure to 150 mg/m$^3$ $H_2S$. Cumulative effects of $H_2S$ occurred even when exposures were 4 days apart. In Rhesus monkeys, high short-term exposure (750 mg/m$^3$ for 22 min) resulted in necrosis of the cerebral cortex, reduction in Purkinje cells of the cerebellar cortex, and focal gliosis. It is not known whether $H_2S$ exposures can induce transplacental neurotoxicity.

### Maternal-Fetal Health Effects

Franklin et al. (74) exposed gravid rats to low concentrations (20, 50, and 75 ppm) of $H_2S$ for 6 hr daily from day 6 of gestation to term (21 days) and produced a dose-dependent extension of litter delivery time at parturition. In an in vitro study, these researchers showed that low concentrations of sodium disulfide reversibly attenuate the contractile response of the isolated rat uterus to oxytocin without affecting angiotensin II responsiveness (75). Reduction of oxytocin receptors by hydrosulfide ion may be a mechanism by which low levels of $H_2S$ delay parturition in rats (75).

Recently, Hayden et al. (76) studied the effects of low level $H_2S$ on rat growth and development. Gravid rat dams were exposed to $H_2S$ at doses $\geq 75$ ppm from day 6 of gestation until day 21 postpartum. Delivery time was extended in a dose-dependent manner. Maternal liver cholesterol content was elevated significantly on day 21 postpartum. The pups exposed in utero and neonatally exhibited a subtle decrease in time of ear detachment and hair development, but had no other observed changes in growth or development.

In a different study of chronic $H_2S$ exposure (20–50 ppm) during perinatal development, severe alterations in the architecture and growth characteristics of the cerebellar Purkinje cell were found (77). Developing neurons exposed to low concentrations of $H_2S$ may be at risk of severe deficit.

Barilyak (78) described embryotoxicity and a low incidence of retarded ossification, hydrocephalus, and hydronephrosis after simultaneous exposure of rats to carbon disulfide ($CS_2$) and $H_2S$. Saillenfait et al. (79) exposed pregnant rats to various concentrations of $CS_2$ (0, 100, 200, 400, 500 ppm), or $H_2S$ alone (100 ppm) or in combination with $CS_2$ (400 or 800 ppm), during days 6–20 of gestation. Exposure to 400 or 800 ppm $CS_2$ produced maternal toxicity and resulted in a low incidence of club foot and decreased fetal body weight. The latter effect was enhanced by a combination with 100 ppm $H_2S$.

A Finnish study evaluated the frequency of spontaneous abortion occurring over 4 yr in an industrial community of 20,000 inhabitants (80). The rate of spontaneous abortion was related to the occupations of women and their husbands and to the level of air pollution (sulfur dioxide, hydrogen sulfide, $CS_2$) in the family's residential area. Women who were employed in rayon textile jobs and paper product jobs had an increased rate ($p < 0.10$) of spontaneous abortions; the wives of men employed in transport and communication, in rayon textile jobs, and in chemical process jobs also had increased miscarriage rates. After controlling for age, parity, and socioeconomic class, the levels of sulfur dioxide or $CS_2$ were not associated with a risk of spontaneous abortion. In all socioeconomic classes, more miscarriages were noted in areas where the mean annual level of $H_2S$ exceeded 4 mg/m$^3$; however, the difference was not statistically significant.

## CLINICAL ASSESSMENT

The symptoms and signs of poisoning from exposure to $H_2S$ gas or after administration of soluble sulfide salts to animals are similar to those produced by cyanide (35, 70). The only exceptions are due to the irritancy of $H_2S$. Chronic exposure to low concentrations (50–200 ppm) of $H_2S$ causes painful conjunctivitis ("gas eye"), photophobia, lacrimation, and corneal opacity. Low to moderate exposures result in respiratory irritation and pulmonary edema, as well as nausea, vomiting, diarrhea, and profuse salivation. Olfactory nerve paralysis is induced by levels of 225 mg/m$^3$ (70). Direct skin contact with $H_2S$ solution produces pain and

erythema. Tachypnea, palpitations, tachycardia, arrhythmias, sweating, weakness, and muscle cramps may also occur (35, 70).

CNS effects include headaches, vertigo, amnesia, confusion, and loss of consciousness. Exposure to very high concentrations of $H_2S$ vapor (greater than 1400 ppm) causes acute intoxication with sudden collapse and unconsciousness, with or without prior warning (35). Death results from respiratory paralysis after a terminal asphyxial convulsion. The coma disappears promptly after exposure to sublethal dosages, but full recovery is slow. Residual cough, cardiac dilatation, bradycardia, albuminuria, and amnesia or psychic disturbances are common. In most nonfatal cases, eventual recovery is complete.

Laboratory tests that may aid in diagnosis and management include urinalysis (albumin, casts, red blood cells), quantitative blood levels of hydrosulfide ion, and the use of lead-acetate paper to test for the presence of $H_2S$ in air (35).

## PREVENTION AND TREATMENT

Because most cases of acute $H_2S$ poisoning result from occupational exposure, prevention requires stringent control measures in the workplace. A recent report of $H_2S$ poisoning with subendocardial infarction in a factory worker who bent over an open tank (81) and two cases of fatal poisoning during cleaning of a tank that had transported polysulfides (82) illustrate the problem.

The initial step in management of $H_2S$ poisoning is to remove the victim from the exposure area to fresh air (35). If respirations are depressed, artificial respiration is given until normal breathing is restored. Like cyanide, hydrosulfide anion produces its major toxic effects through inhibition of cytochrome oxidase; therefore, induction of methemoglobinemia with sodium nitrite injections can protect against sulfide poisoning. The mechanism involves competition for free sulfide between tissue cytochrome oxidase and circulating methemoglobin, the latter binding sulfide in an inactive form called sulfmethemoglobin.

In severe poisoning, treatment with amyl nitrite and sodium nitrite is given, but the sodium thiosulfate injection is omitted (35). Oxygen is specifically indicated if pulmonary edema occurs. Atropine administered intra-muscularly may provide some symptomatic relief. The conjunctivitis may be treated with olive oil drops in each eye, or 3–4 drops of epinephrine solution (1:1000), given at frequent intervals. Local anesthesia or compresses help relieve the pain.

## REFERENCES

1. Jacobs MM, Phibbs RH. Prevention, recognition, and treatment of perinatal asphyxia. Clin Perinatol 1989; 16:785–807.
2. Meschia G. Placental respiratory gas exchange and fetal oxygenation. In: Creasy R, Resnik R, eds. Maternal fetal medicine: principles and practice. Philadelphia: WB Saunders, 1989:303–313.
3. Gaensler EA. Lung displacement: abdominal enlargement, pleural space disorders, deformities of the thoracic cage. In: Fenn WO, Rahn H, eds. Handbook of physiology, section 3: respiration. Vol. II. Washington, D.C.: American Physiological Society, 1965.
4. Harding R, Sigger NJ, Wickham PD. Fetal and maternal influences on arterial oxygen levels in the sheep fetus. J Dev Physiol 1987;5:267.
5. Hellegers AE, Schruefer JJ. Normograms and empirical equations relating oxygen tension, percentage saturation and pH in maternal and fetal blood. Am J Obstet Gynecol 1961;81:377.
6. Battaglia FC, Meschia G. Principal substrates of fetal metabolism. Physiol Rev 1978;58;499–527.
7. Towell ME. Fetal respiratory physiology. In: Goodwin JW, Godden JO, Chance GW, eds. Perinatal medicine. Toronto: Longman Canada Ltd, 1976:171–186.
8. Brace RA. Fetal blood volume responses to acute fetal hypoxia. Am J Obstet Gynecol 1986;155:889–893.
9. Richardson BS. Fetal adaptive responses to asphyxia. Clin Perinatol 1989;16:595–611.
10. Edelstone DI. Fetal compensatory responses to reduced oxygen delivery. Semin Perinatol 1984;8:184–191.
11. Cohn HE, Sacks EJ, Heymann MA, Rudolph AM. Cardiovascular responses to hypoxemia and acidemia in fetal lambs. Am J Obstet Gynecol 1974;120:817–824.
12. Peeters LLH, Sheldon RE, Jones MD, et al. Blood flow to fetal organs as a function of arterial oxygen content. Am J Obstet Gynecol 1979;135:637–646.
13. Sheldon RE, Peeters LLH, Jones MD Jr, et al. Redistribution of cardiac output and oxygen delivery in the hypoxemic fetal lamb. Am J Obstet Gynecol 1979; 135:1071–1078.
14. Rudolph AM. The fetal circulation and its response to stress. J Dev Physiol 1984;6:11–19.
15. Soothill PW, Nicolaides KH, Campbell S. Prenatal asphyxia, hyperlacticaemia, hypoglycemia and erythroblastosis in growth retarded fetuses. Br Med J 1987;294: 1051–1055.
16. Pardi G, Buscaglia M, Ferrazzi E, et al. Cord sampling for the evaluation of oxygenation and acid-base balance in growth retarded human fetuses. Am J Obstet Gynecol 1987;157:1221–1228.
17. Natale R, Clewlow F, Dawes GS. Measurement of fetal forelimb movements in the lamb in utero. Am J Obstet Gynecol 1981;140:545–551.
18. Bekedam DJ, Visser GHA, de Vries JJ, et al. Motor behavior in the growth retarded fetus. Early Hum Dev 1985;12:155–165.
19. Boddy K, Dawes GS, Fisher R, et al. Foetal respiratory movements, electrocortical and cardiovascular responses to hypoxemia and hypercapnia in sleep. J Physiol (London) 1974;243:599–618.
20. Tchobroutsky C, Monset-Couchard M, Dumez Y, Toubas P. Fetal breathing during moderate asphyxia in sheep and in human related to outcome of pregnancy. Contrib Gynecol Obstet 1979;6:80–87.
21. Patrick J, Richardson B, Rurak D et al. Biophysical variables during sustained hypoxemia in fetal sheep (abstr 8). Soc Gynecol Invest, 1987.
22. Myers RE, Mueller-Heubach E, Adamsons K. Predictability of the state of fetal oxygenation from a quantitative analysis of the components of late decelerations. Am J Obstet Gynecol 1973;115:1083–1094.
23. Martin CB Jr, de Hann J, Van der Wildt B. Mechanisms of late decelerations in the fetal heart rate: a study with autonomic blocking agents in fetal lambs. Eur J Obstet Gynecol Reprod Biol 1979;9:361–373.
24. Goodman LS, Gilman A. The pharmacological basis of therapeutics. 8th ed. New York: Pergamon Press, Inc., 1990.
25. Marzella L, Myers R. Carbon monoxide poisoning. Pract Therap 1986;34:186–194.
26. National Research Council, Committee on Medical and Biologic Effects of Environmental Pollutants. Carbon monoxide. Washington, D.C.: National Academy of Sciences, 1977.
27. Goldsmith JR, Landaw SA. Carbon monoxide and human health. Science 1968;162:1352–1359.
28. Abel EL. Smoking and pregnancy. J Psychoactive Drugs 1984;16:327–338.
29. Pirani BBK. Smoking during pregnancy. Obstet Gynecol Surv 1978;33:1–13.
30. Delivoria Papadopoulos M, Coburn RF, Forster RE. Cyclic variation of rate of carbon monoxide production in normal women. J Appl Physiol 1974;36:49–51.
31. Lilienthal JL Jr, Riley RL, Proemmel DD, Franke RE. The relationships between carbon monoxide, oxygen and hemoglobin in the blood of man at altitude. Am J Physiol 1946;145:351–358.
32. Roughton FJW, Darling RC. The effect of carbon monoxide on the oxyhemoglobin dissociation curve. Am J Physiol 1944;141:17–31.
33. Gutierrez G. Carbon monoxide toxicity. In: Air pollution-physiological effects. In: McGrath JJ, Barnes CD, eds. New York: Academic Press, Inc., 1982:127–147.
34. Siesjo BK. Symposium. Carbon monoxide poisoning: mechanism of damage, late sequelae and therapy. Clin Toxicol 1985;23:247–326.
35. Gosselin RE, Smith RP, Hodge HC, Braddaock JE. Clinical toxicology of commercial products. 5th ed. Baltimore: Williams & Wilkins, 1984.

36. Peterson JE, Stewart RD. Absorption and elimination of carbon monoxide by inactive young men. Arch Environ Health 1970;21:165–171.

37. Longo LD. The biological effects of carbon monoxide on the pregnant woman, fetus, and newborn infant. Am J Obstet Gynecol 1977;129:69–103.

38. Longo LD. Carbon monoxide in the pregnant mothers and fetus and its exchange across the placenta. Ann NY Acad Sci 1970;174:312–341.

39. Longo LD, Hill EP. Carbon monoxide uptake and elimination in fetal and maternal sheep. Am J Physiol 1977;232:H321.

40. Hill EP, Hill JJ, Power GG, Longo LD. Carbon monoxide exchanges between the human fetus and mother: a mathematical model. Am J Physiol 1977;232:H311.

41. Leonard MB, Vreman HJ, Ferguson JE, Smith DW, Stevenson DK. Interpreting the carboxyhemoglobin concentration in fetal cord blood. J Dev Physiol 1989;11: 73–76.

42. Smith E, McMillan E, Mack L. Factors influencing the lethal action of illuminating gas. J Indust Hyg 1935;17:18.

43. Fechter LD, Annau Z. Toxicity of mild prenatal carbon monoxide exposure. Science 1977;197:680–682.

44. Mactutus CF, Fechter LD. Moderate prenatal carbon monoxide exposure produces persistent, and apparently permanent, memory deficits in rats. Teratology 1985;31:1–12.

45. Singh J, Scott LH. Threshold for carbon monoxide induced fetotoxicity. Teratology 1984;30:253–257.

46. Astrup P, Trolle D, Olsen HM, Kjeldsen K. Effect of moderate carbon monoxide exposure on fetal development. Lancet 1972;2:1220–1222.

47. Schwetz BA, Smith FA, Leong BKJ, Staples RE. Teratogenic potential of inhaled carbon monoxide in mice and rabbits. Teratology 1979;19:385–392.

48. Ginsburg MD, Myers RE. Fetal brain injury after maternal carbon monoxide intoxication. Neurology 1976;26: 15–23.

49. Ginsburg MD, Myers RE. Fetal brain damage following maternal carbon monoxide intoxication: an experimental study. Acta Obstet Gynecol Scand 1974;53:309–317.

50. Norman CA, Halton DM. Is carbon monoxide a workplace teratogen? A review and evaluation of the literature. Br Occup Hyg Soc 1990;34:335–347.

51. Koren G, Sharav T, Pastuszak A, et al. A multicenter prospective study of fetal outcome following accidental carbon monoxide poisoning in pregnancy. Reprod Toxicol 1991;5:397–403.

52. Alderman BW, Baron AE, Savitz DA. Maternal exposure to neighborhood carbon monoxide and risk of low infant birth weight. Public Health Rep 1987;102:410–414.

53. Wouters EJM, De Jong PA, Cornelissen PJH, Kurver PHJ, van Oel WC, van Woensel CLM. Smoking and low birth weight: absence of influence by carbon monoxide? Eur J Obstet Gynecol Reprod Biol 1987;25:35–41.

54. Lindblad A, Marsal K, Andersson, KE. Effect of nicotine on human fetal blood flow. Obstet Gynecol 1988;72:371–381.

55. Ayres SN, Giannelli S. Jr, Armstrong RB. Carboxyhemoglobin: hemodynamic and respiratory responses to small concentrations. Science 1965;149:193–194.

56. Centers for Disease Control. Carbon monoxide intoxication—a preventable environmental health hazard. MMWR 1982;31:529–531.

57. Centers for DIsease Control. Fatal carbon monoxide poisoning in a camper-truck—Georgia. MMWR 1991;40: 154–155.

58. Stotz E, Altschuil AM, Hogness TR. The cytochrome c-cytochrome oxidase complex. J Biol Chem 1938; 124:745–754.

59. Baud FJ, Barriot P, Toffis V, et al. Elevated blood cyanide concentrations in victims of smoke inhalation. N Engl J Med 1991;325:1761–1766.

60. Wexler J, Whittenberge JL, Dumke PR. The effect of cyanide on the electrocardiogram of man. Am Heart J 1947;34:163–173.

61. Bass NH. Pathogenesis of myelin lesions in experimental cyanide encephalopathy. Neurology 1968;18:167–177.

62. Spratt NT. Nutritional requirements of the early chick embryo. III. The metabolic basis of morphogenesis and differentiation as revealed by the use of inhibitors. Biol Bull 1950;99:120–135.

63. Willhite CC. Malformations induced by inhalation of acetonitrile vapors in the golden hamster. Teratology 1981;23:698.

64. Doherty PA, Ferm VH, Smith RP. Congenital malformations induced by infusion of sodium cyanide in the golden hamster. Toxicol Appl Pharmacol 1982;64:456–464.

65. Willhite CC. Congenital malformations induced by laetrile. Science 1982;15:1513–1515.

66. Valles J, Obach R, Menargues A, Valles JM, Rives A. Two-generation reproduction-fertility study of cyanide in the rat. Pharmacol Toxicol 1987;61:20–25.

67. Itskovitz J, Rudolph AM. Cardiorespiratory response to cyanide of arterial chemoreceptors in fetal lambs. Am J Physiol 1987;252:H916–H922.

68. Graham DL, Laman D, Theodore J, Robin ED. Acute cyanide poisoning complicated by lactic acidosis and pulmonary edema. Arch Intern Med 1977;137:1051–1055.

69. Cooper K, Albrezzi B. Emergency? It's Cyanide! Am J Nurs 1990;11:42–44.

70. Tabacova A. Maternal exposure to environmental chemicals. Neurotoxicology 1986;7:421–440.

71. World Health Organization Environmental (WHO). Health Criteria 19: hydrogen sulfide. Geneva: WHO, 1981.

72. McCabe LC, Clayton GD. Air pollution by hydrogen sulfide in Posa Rica, Mexico. An evaluation of the incident of Nov. 24, 1950. Am Med Assoc Arch Ind Hyg Occup Med 1952;6:199–213.

73. Beauchamp RO Jr., Bus JS, Popp JA, Boreiko CJ, Jelkovich DA. A critical review of the literature on hydrogen sulfide toxicity. Crit Rev Toxicol 1984;13: 25–97.

74. Franklin KJ, Hayden LJ, Roth SH, Moore GJ. Proc Can Fed Biol Soc 1989;32:11.

75. Hayden LJ, Franklin KJ, Roth SH, Moore GJ. Inhibition of oxytocin-induced but not angiotensin-induced rat uterine contractions following exposure to sodium sulfide. Life Sci 1989;45:2557–2560.

76. Hayden LJ, Goeden H, Roth SH. Growth and development

in the rat during sub-chronic exposure to low levels of hydrogen sulfide. Toxicol Ind Health 1990;6:389–401.

77. Hannah RS, Roth SH. Chronic exposure to low concentrations of hydrogen sulfide produces abnormal growth in developing cerebellar Purkinje cells. Neurosci Lett 1991;122:225–228.

78. Barilyak IR. Effects of small concentrations of carbon disulfide and hydrogen sulfide in the intra-uterine development of rats. Arkh Anat Gistol Embroil 1975;68:77–81.

79. Saillenfait AM, Bonnet P, de Ceaurriz J. Effects of inhalation exposure to carbon disulfide and its combination with hydrogen sulfide on embryonal and fetal development in rats. Toxicol Lett 1989;48:57–66.

80. Hemminki K, Niemi ML. Community study of spontaneous abortions: relation to occupation and air pollution by sulfur dioxide, hydrogen sulfide, and carbon disulfide. Int Arch Occup Environ Health 1982;51:55–63.

81. Vathenen AS, Emberton P, Wales JM. Hydrogen sulphide poisoning in factory worker [Letter]. Lancet 1988;1:305.

82. Campany'a M, Sanz P, Reig R, et al. Fatal hydrogen sulfide poisoning. Medicina Del Lavoro 1989;80:251–253.

# 19

## Organic Solvents

### LAURA S. WELCH

Clinicians are well aware of the fetal alcohol syndrome but may not realize that alcohol belongs to a larger, diverse class of compounds called solvents that may also have adverse developmental or reproductive effects. Exposure to various solvents has been associated with infertility in both experimental animals and men, as well as spontaneous abortion, and birth defects and neurobehavioral deficits in offspring. This chapter reviews the evidence pertaining to the effects of solvents on the reproductive system.

### PROPERTIES AND USES

A solvent is a substance (usually a liquid) that dissolves another substance. Solvents are either water based or hydrocarbon based; the latter group, called organic solvents, is the focus of this chapter. Solvents are used for many purposes including cleaning, degreasing, and thinning of paints and other coatings. Exposures can occur in the workplace or in the community; many household products contain organic solvents, and solvents are often found in community air or water from industrial releases. There are over 30,000 industrial solvents that can be classified by common properties into subclasses. This section reviews some basic principles of solvents, focusing on the properties that may predict risk of adverse reproductive outcome. A broader discussion of the health effects of solvents can be found in several occupational medicine texts (1, 2).

Solvents are classified into groups based on their chemical structures: aliphatic, alicyclic, and aromatic. They can then be classified by the presence of certain functional groups: glycols, ketones, alcohols, esters, ethers, and others. Some examples are provided in Table 19.1. Understanding these basic structures may allow us to extrapolate data on one solvent to another, chemically similar one.

Certain properties of solvents affect exposure of the workers handling them. Solvents vary in lipid and water solubility. Solvents that are both lipid and water soluble pass through intact skin most easily, for skin has both water and lipid compartments. Dermal absorption represents the major route of exposure for many solvents.

The property of a solvent that affects inhalation exposure is its volatility, i.e., its tendency to evaporate into a gas or a vapor. As a general rule, the higher the volatility of a solvent, the more will be present in the breathing zone of a worker, and hence, the higher the exposure. Solvents are readily absorbed across the alveolar capillary membrane of the lung. From 40–80% of the inhaled dose is absorbed at rest, and the total amount absorbed increases with exercise and pregnancy as blood flow to the lung and alveolar ventilation increase. Once absorbed, solvents are distributed throughout the body and, in particular, to lipid-rich tissues. They may be excreted unchanged by exhalation from the lungs or metabolized in the liver and

**Table 19.1.**
**Basic Chemical Structure and Examples of Some Common Organic Solvents**

| Chemical Classification | | Examples |
|---|---|---|
| Aromatic hydrocarbons: characterized by the presence of hydrogen and carbon atoms arranged in a benzene ring structure | Benzene $C_6H_6$ | Benzene Toluene Xylene |
| Halogenated hydrocarbons: hydrogen and carbon atoms with one or more halogen atoms replacing the hydrogens (fluorine, chlorine, bromine, or iodine) | Carbon Tetrachloride $CCl_4$ | Chlorodifluoromethane Trichloroethylene Carbon Tetrachloride Methylene Chloride Perchloroethylene |
| Aldehydes: characterized by a double bonded carbonyl C=O group joined by at least one hydrogen atom | Formaldehyde HCHO | Formaldehyde Acetaldehyde |
| Glycol ethers: one or both of the hydroxyl OH groups of a glycol is replaced by an ether; ethers contain the C—O—C linkage | Ethylene Glycol Monomethyl Ether $C_2H_5OCH_2OH$ | Ethylene Glycol Monomethyl Ether (EGME), Ethylene Glycol Monethyl Ether (EGEE), and their acetates. |
| Ketones: contain a double-bonded carbonyl C=O group and two hydrocarbon groups | Methyl Ethyl Ketone $CH_3C(O)C_2H_5$ | Methyl Ethyl Ketone Acetone |

excreted in the urine. The half-life of a solvent in the body varies greatly from compound to compound, with some as long as several days. A solvent with a half-life longer than 12 hr will accumulate over the work week, resulting in a higher body burden at the end of the week from the same exposure conditions.

As explained in Chapter 10, exposure to some solvents can be determined by biological monitoring, which most commonly involves measuring the solvent or a metabolite in urine or blood. These measurements can be very useful in monitoring exposure to a solvent that is absorbed through the skin, for industrial hygiene monitoring in the workplace only approximates inhalation exposure. In addition, biological monitoring allows the clinician to determine exposure in a particular patient without relying on the employer's ability or willingness to collect exposure data. The usefulness of such monitoring depends on the properties of the solvent. Solvents that are excreted rapidly may not be "captured" by a test performed some time after work and, for solvents with short half-lives, the levels of metabolite may fluctuate so much from hour to hour as to render the tests less than useful measures of overall exposure.

It is important to note that biological monitoring alone cannot determine that an exposure is safe or without reproductive risk. Biological monitoring provides an exposure estimate for an individual, but this estimate must be combined with adequate health data to determine risk. The American Conference of Governmental Industrial Hygienists (ACGIH) has developed a concept called the Biological Exposure Index (BEI), which is the level of a biological indicator that corresponds to ACGIH's air exposure limit (threshold limit value or TLV). The TLVs and BEIs for some common organic solvents are provided in the Appendix at the end of this book. However, since ACGIH does not specifically consider reproductive risk in the development of TLVs or BEIs, these values do not necessarily represent "safe" levels.

Animal studies demonstrate that solvents cross the placental barrier. Many factors are known to affect the rate of transfer of drugs and chemicals from maternal blood to the conceptus including the degree of lipid solubility and protein binding, the pKa of the compound, placental blood flow, placental function, and the degree to which active transport occurs (3). Active transport is not thought to be of major importance. Generally, compounds that have a high affinity for lipid, a low degree of ionization, and a molecular weight less that 1000 are rapidly transferred across the placenta (4). Many solvents fit this description for, by definition, they are lipid soluble and nonpolar.

## REPRODUCTIVE AND DEVELOPMENTAL EFFECTS

### Infertility

Ethylene glycol ethers and their acetates have been shown in animal and human studies to affect sperm count and fertility. Ethylene glycol ethers are widely used in industry in paints, varnishes, and thinners; as solvents in resins; and in textile printing and a variety of coating operations (5).

There are now more than 100 glycol ethers available commercially, and not all carry the same reproductive risk. The National Institute for Occupational Safety and Health (NIOSH) estimates that 850,000 workers in the U.S. are potentially exposed to 2-ethoxyethanol (EGEE), 2-methoxyethanol (EGME), and their acetates, the glycol ethers most clearly associated with reproductive risk. It is likely that the reproductive toxicity of these solvents is due to their metabolites, rather than to the parent compounds. 2-Ethoxyethanol is oxidized by alcohol dehydrogenase and aldehyde dehydrogenase to ethoxyacetic acid; 2-methoxyethanol is similarly metabolized to methoxyacetic acid (6). Inhibition of this metabolism protects against reproductive toxicity, and administration of the metabolites causes the toxicity seen with the parent compounds in vivo (7, 8). Using this hypothesis and set of experiments, glycol ethers that are not biotransformed to alkoxyacetic acid metabolites via this enzyme system are thought not to have reproductive effects (6).

With chronic oral or inhalation exposure, ethylene glycol ethers cause focal testicular atrophy and disruption of the seminiferous tubules in mice, rats, and rabbits (9–15). Two studies of male workers exposed to ethylene glycol monomethyl ether (EGME) or ethylene glycol monoethyl ether (EGEE) found decreased total sperm counts (16, 17), while one found no effect (18). Given the weight of the evidence, clinicians should consider ethylene glycol ethers as reproductive toxicants to male workers. The animal data are strong and reproducible, and an effect is seen near levels achieved in workplaces; in addition, two human studies have found an effect. The National Institute for Occupational Safety and Health has recently completed an updated assessment that reflects the data on the reproductive and developmental effects of these chemicals, and the permissible exposure limits will be reduced in the future.

### Menstrual Disorders

Several studies report that women who work with benzene, toluene, xylene, styrene, carbon disulfide, and formaldehyde have an increased incidence of menstrual disorders. Michon (19) reported prolonged or heavy bleeding in women exposed to benzene, toluene, and xylene in a Polish shoe factory. Mikhailova et al. (20) reported an increase in menstrual disturbances in women exposed to benzene. Zlobina et al. (21) also found an increase in menstrual disorders, including dysmenorrhea or prolonged and heavy bleeding, in women exposed to styrene. Syrovadko (22) noted an increase in menstrual disorders in women exposed to a mixture of toluene and xylene. This group of studies comes from Eastern Europe, and the limited data reported make an assessment ·of exposure and case ascertainment difficult. No information is provided about the doses of solvents or about other potential exposures in the workplace. These results have not been replicated in other studies to date. At this point, it is premature to conclude that these solvents are the cause of menstrual disorders, but future study is warranted.

In a U.S. study of more than 1500 blue collar workers employed in the plastics industry, no association was found between styrene exposure and menstrual disorders in a multiple logistic regression model (23). The authors did find an association between menstrual disorders and smoking, age, chronic disease, and nulliparity. Extensive industrial hygiene data were collected on styrene exposures, and no dose-response relationship was evident. This well-conducted study suggests that there is no association between this one solvent and menstrual disorders. Similarly detailed assessments are not available for the other solvents implicated in the Eastern European studies.

## Maternal Morbidity During Pregnancy

An early report described two cases of pre-eclampsia in women working in a chemical laboratory (24). Exposures to chloroform ranged from 300–1000 ppm, which is 6–20 times the recommended limit, and other laboratory workers had solvent-induced hepatotoxicity. This was the first report to suggest a link between solvents and pre-eclampsia.

More recently, Eskenazi et al. (25) used data from a large cohort of pregnant women to evaluate the relationship between solvent exposure and pre-eclampsia. More than 4000

women completed an interview during pregnancy, on average at 3 months' gestation. An occupational history was included in the interview, and occupation was coded using the system of the U.S. Bureau of the Census. An industrial hygienist selected 98 occupations from the Census lists that could result in exposure to organic solvents. Two industrial hygienists, blinded to case status, then reviewed the questionnaires from the 1059 women so identified to determine if they indeed had solvent exposure; a subset of 90 women with solvent exposure was identified by this method. Analysis of the data revealed that solvent-exposed women were four times more likely to develop pre-eclampsia than women without solvent exposure. A similar result has been reported in studies from Eastern Europe (21, 26); however, the limitations of these studies are similar to those described earlier for menstrual disorders.

The methods used by Eskenazi were rigorous, and the results are biologically plausible. Solvents have been associated with glomerulonephritis in a case series (27) and with proteinuria in some epidemiological studies (28). Given these findings, it would be prudent to monitor women with solvent exposure for hypertension and renal disease during pregnancy.

## Spontaneous Abortion

Increased rates of spontaneous abortion have been reported in women exposed to styrene in the production of reinforced plastics (29) and in women working with glues (26). Hemminki et al. (29) reported an increase in spontaneous abortions in women who were members of the Finnish Union of Chemical Workers; however, no specific exposure data were available to determine if this excess was due to solvents or other agents used in the chemical industry. A recent study investigated spontaneous abortion among all women in Finland who had been biologically monitored for solvents (30). Women exposed to aliphatic solvents had an increased risk for spontaneous abortion.

Several studies have reported an increased rate of spontaneous abortion in women working in laboratories (31, 32), but others have not confirmed this association (33, 34). Laboratory workers are a heterogeneous group with potential exposure to heavy metals, viruses, and other hazards, as well as to solvents. In the study by Lindbohm et al. (31), exposure was determined by job description, and no detailed assessment of solvent exposure was performed; thus, the association with laboratory work is not necessarily related to solvents. Other investigators performed a more detailed exposure assessment as part of a nested case-control analysis among a cohort of female workers in eight Finnish pharmaceutical plants (32). This analysis found an odds ratio of 3.5 (p = 0.05) for exposure to four or more solvents in women with spontaneous abortion, and a similar odds ratio for exposure to methylene chloride as a single agent. Harkonen et al. (35) found no effect of styrene exposure on pregnancy outcome in a study of female lamination workers. However, the sample included only 67 women, and only 230 births were expected; this small sample size limited the study's ability to find an effect.

If we consider the animal equivalent of spontaneous abortion to be fetal resorption, several solvents have caused resorptions when administered at high doses. Chloroform was embryotoxic in several studies (36–38) at doses that produced maternal toxicity. Xylene caused postimplantation losses in exposed rats at doses of 700 ppm (39). Styrene was embryolethal in mice and hamsters (40), but not in rats or rabbits, at doses ranging from 250–1000 ppm. Toluene caused a reduction in birthweight in mice and rats (41, 42).

Most studies have assessed spontaneous abortion as a consequence of exposure to the female. Taskinen et al. (43) conducted a case-control study to determine if paternal exposure to solvents could also cause early fetal loss. Exposure to male workers was ascertained through questionnaires and through biological monitoring data for styrene, toluene, xylene, tetrachloroethylene, trichloroethylene, and 1,1,1-trichloroethane. Paternal exposure to organic solvents, toluene, or "miscellaneous" solvents, in a dose range classified as "high or frequent" (daily use or exposure above established thresholds for biological indices), was associated with an odds ratio of 2.1–2.8, each with confidence intervals excluding one.

Overall, these studies show a fairly consistent association between maternal solvent exposure and spontaneous abortion and suggest that paternal exposure may be important as well. Studies by Taskinen et al. (32) and Lindholm et al. (30) suggest that this effect occurs primarily in the high exposure groups, but further investigation is warranted to characterize the dose-response.

## Birth Defects

Several studies have investigated the link between parental exposure to solvents and birth defects in their offspring. In many of these studies, exposure to specific solvents was not determined, and men or women were simply classified as either exposed or unexposed to solvents. In others, a high rate of birth defects was associated with employment in certain industries; because of solvent use in those industries, solvents were considered a potential cause of the defects.

Some studies have focused specifically on central nervous system (CNS) defects and solvent exposure. The most susceptible period of the CNS to effects of solvents ranges from 10–18 weeks' gestation, a period of rapid growth of the CNS. However, brain development continues until birth and beyond; the effect of solvents on function, rather than structure, is discussed in a subsequent section.

Two case-control studies suggest a link between parental exposure to solvents and CNS defects. A study using occupational titles in Denmark found that malformations of the CNS were higher in children of painters and in men occupationally exposed to solvents (44). A similar study in Finland reported an odds ratio of 5.5 for CNS defects with exposure to organic solvents during the first trimester of pregnancy (45), but an extension of this study did not confirm this finding (46). The authors suggest that the discrepant results might be due to changes in Finnish social policies that substantially decreased chemical exposure to pregnant workers over the latter part of the study period.

McDonald et al. (47) found that exposure to aromatic solvents was more frequent among the mothers of infants with an "important" congenital defect. A case-control analysis was drawn from a comprehensive survey of pregnancies in Montreal; the cases consisted of 301 women who had a child with an important congenital defect, and referents were matched for hospital, age, date of delivery, and education. After a review of job titles for cases and controls, an occupational hygienist visited worksites with potential for chemical exposure to assess in more detail the specific exposures and doses received by study participants during pregnancy. There was a significant excess of solvent exposure among the cases, and most of this excess was due to toluene exposure. The anomalies found were primarily renal-urinary and gastrointestinal.

Holmberg and Nurminen (45) conducted a case-control analysis of the relationship between solvent exposure and the occurrence of cleft palate. Cases were identified through the Finnish Register of Congenital Malformations, and information about exposure was obtained through interviews of the mothers of cases and controls. When necessary to classify exposure better, the industrial hygienists, blinded to case or control status, requested specific information from employers. Exposure to organic solvents was more common among case mothers than referent mothers.

Tikkanen and Heinonen (48) compared the frequency of occupational solvent exposure among mothers of all infants with cardiovascular malformations born in Finland between 1982 and 1984 with exposure among a control group who had normal births. Solvent exposure was determined by structured interviews with the mothers conducted 2–22 weeks after delivery. Using logistical regression, the authors reported an increase in exposure to organic solvents among mothers of infants with ventricular septal defects (OR 1.5, CI 1.0–3.7), but not with all cardiovascular defects (OR 1.3, CI 0.8–2.2). The authors did not attribute these findings to recall bias, for there was no evidence of increased reporting of exposure to anesthesia, glues, or pesticides among the case group. If case mothers recalled solvent exposures "better" than control mothers, one would expect an increase in all exposures thought to be hazardous, not just an increase in solvent exposure.

A series of other studies implicate solvents indirectly. Assuming that solvent exposure occurs in laboratory work, three Swedish studies identified solvents as possible risk factors for congenital malformations. Hansson et al. (49) reported that pregnant women working in laboratories in the pharmaceutical industry had a higher perinatal death rate and a higher rate of major malformations among offspring; however, these results were based on a small number of events. Meirik et al. (50) observed an excess of serious malformations in children born to women working in the laboratories of Uppsala University. In particular, 4 of 245 infants were born with anal or esophageal atresia, when only 1 of 1000 were expected. No specific exposures were identified. Blomqvist et al. (51) reported a high incidence of cleft palate and gut atresia among infants of women working in the laboratories of the pulp and paper industry. Ericson et al. (52) studied birth outcomes in more than 1000 laboratory workers in Sweden and found an excess of serious malformations; this increase was seen in all types of laboratory work, with and without potential exposure to viruses. However, there was no excess of gut atresia or cleft palate in this study. Another case control analysis found no association between laboratory work and malformations of the intestinal tract or oral clefts (44).

Other industries with solvent exposure have also been investigated. Erikson et al. (53) reported an association between gastroschisis and work in the printing industry. Harkonen et al. (54) investigated the occurrence of congenital malformations in children of 1698 male and 511 female workers involved in the production of reinforced plastics. Births were identified for 1963–1979 in the population registry, and birth defects were ascertained from the Finnish Register of Congenital Malformations. No excess of congenital anomalies was found, although the overall numbers of births and birth defects were small, limiting the power of the study.

Some solvents have been tested for teratogenicity in animal systems. Chloroform caused malformations in two rodent studies (37, 38) at doses that did not produce maternal toxicity. Dichloromethane induced some minor skeletal anomalies at exposures of 1250 ppm (55) and caused skeletal abnormalities and retarded kidney development at exposures of 700 ppm in rats (39). The fluorocarbon, chlorodifluoromethane, induced microphthalmia in rats (56). At levels of 3000 ppm, methyl ethyl ketone caused an increase in major malformations in rats (57, 58). Other solvents including benzene, carbon tetrachloride (if given at less than the maternally toxic dose), and dichloroethane were not fetotoxic or teratogenic in well-conducted studies (56, 57).

The ethylene glycol ethers 2-ethoxyethanol, 2-methoxyethanol, and their acetates induce birth defects in exposed animals, including cardiovascular and skeletal malformations. Exposure of rabbits to 160 ppm of EGEE for 7 hr/day from gestational days 1–18 caused a significant increase in cardiovascular abnormalities (59, 60). Rats developed malformations of the heart with exposure to 130 ppm of 2-ethoxyethanol acetate (EGEEA). Dermal exposure to 2-ethoxyethanol, by application of 0.25 ml applied four times a day from gestational days 7–16, resulted in cardiovascular abnormalities (61). The level of exposure to EGEEA that causes no observable fetal effects in animals is 25 ppm (62).

Exposure of pregnant mice to 2-methoxyethanol or its acetate caused a dose-dependent increase in skeletal abnormalities in offspring at doses that were not associated with maternal toxicity (14, 62–66). Toraason et al. (65) studied the effect of EGME on the cardiovascular system and found ventricular septal defects and right ductus arteriosus at 50 mg/kg/day administered orally. At a dose of 25 mg/kg/day, fetuses developed a prolonged QRS complex. Ventricular septal defect, patent ductus arteriosus, and coarctation of the aorta were found after exposure of rabbits to 50 ppm EGME (63). The level at which no effect on fetal development is observed in mice, rats, or rabbits is 10 ppm.

Based on these animal data, NIOSH recommends that workplace exposures not exceed 0.5 ppm and 0.1 ppm for EGEE and EGME (and their acetates), respectively (67).

Considered as a whole, these studies provide data to support an association between solvent exposure during pregnancy and congenital defects. At least two solvents cause birth defects in animal experiments. The human studies suggest a risk for exposure to organic solvents generally, but do not identify a specific solvent responsible for the effect. Most of these studies involved populations occupationally exposed to a mix of solvents, and women were classified as exposed if they had *any* solvent exposure. If the true risk was present only in a subset of women exposed to a particular solvent, many of the women considered exposed would actually not be. This misclassification of exposure makes it very difficult to find a true effect due to only one solvent.

Because the levels of exposure to solvents are not provided in the human studies, we cannot clearly determine which groups might be at risk. The available data suggest that birth defects occurred at whatever level of exposure existed in jobs held by women in Canada and Scandinavia in the early 1980s; exposure in U.S. workplaces in the 1990s is likely to be comparable. Based on this information, it is advisable to reduce exposure to solvents during pregnancy or in women planning to become pregnant. This exposure reduction must occur early in pregnancy to prevent effects during critical periods of organogenesis, and should extend throughout pregnancy to protect the developing CNS.

## Specific Developmental Syndromes: Toluene

A syndrome nearly identical to fetal alcohol syndrome has been reported in the children of women who sniffed toluene during pregnancy for a "high" (68–70). Glue or spray paint sniffing results in significant exposure, and chronic neurological disease (71), renal disease (72), and sudden death (73) have been reported with high levels of exposure to toluene. Case reports of infants born to women who abused toluene during pregnancy describe microcephaly, developmental delay, attentional deficits, and phenotypic defects including small midfaces, narrow bifrontal diameters, short palpebral fissures, deep-set eyes, micrognathia, and limb anomalies. In animal experiments, toluene is fetotoxic, causing reduced fetal growth, but is not teratogenic (41, 42, 74).

A syndrome of mental retardation and spastic quadriparesis has been reported from inhalation of gasoline during pregnancy (75). However, these women inhaled leaded gasoline, so the neurological effects of organic solvents cannot be separated from those of lead.

## Neurodevelopmental Effects

The significant occurrence of mental retardation, learning disabilities, and other neurodevelopmental problems in the population have catalyzed intense efforts to elucidate possible causes. While exposure to high doses of a neurotoxin can cause a structural malformation, lower doses may induce more subtle manifestations of toxicity. Methylmercury, for example, is known to cause a spectrum of neurological defects including mental retardation, a cerebral palsy-like syndrome, and delayed developmental and language milestones. Low-level exposure to lead is associated with decreased cognitive function in children (Chapter 17). As previously described, the toluene-induced syndrome includes an attention deficit and developmental delays.

Solvents are, by nature, lipophilic; they can cross the blood-brain barrier and are known to affect CNS functioning in exposed adults. It would be expected that maternal exposure to solvents would also result in exposure to the developing fetal CNS.

Solvent-induced neurobehavioral effects have been observed in various animal studies. Dichloromethane exposure to rats at 4500 ppm both prepregnancy and during pregnancy caused a decrease in habituation to a new environment in the pups (76, 77). Exposure of female rats to 100 ppm of 2-ethoxyethanol from gestational days 7–13 or days 14–20 resulted in offspring with impaired neuromuscular activity, delayed learning in avoidance conditioning, and decreased activity in a running wheel (78). Exposure of male and female rats to 25 ppm of 2-methoxyethanol caused delayed learning in avoidance conditioning (79). Neurochemical changes were seen in offspring of both paternally and maternally exposed groups, with an increase in acetylcholine and 5-hydroxytryptamine in whole brain and increases in norepinephrine and acetylcholine in the brainstem (79).

In mice, injury to the hippocampus in adults

or in the developing fetus is associated with specific functional deficits. In a model using 5-azacytidine as a developmental toxicant, specific defects were caused by treatment in the first trimester of gestation (80).

Eskenazi et al. (81) compared the neurodevelopment of 41 children whose mothers worked with organic solvents during pregnancy with a group of children matched for maternal age, race, and child's age at testing whose mothers were unexposed. They found no difference between the groups in a range of developmental scales. The investigators were not able to define a precise level of exposure; because all solvent-exposed women were included, some exposure misclassification may have occurred.

At this time, no industrial organic solvent has been shown to exert a neurodevelopmental effect in humans outside of a more severe fetal alcohol-like syndrome induced by very high-dose abuse of toluene. However, identifying more subtle deficits can be difficult. It has, for example, taken skilled researchers years to document the effects of low-level lead exposure on the developing CNS.

## Childhood Cancer

### CENTRAL NERVOUS SYSTEM CANCERS

In adults, there is thought to be a lag of 10 or more years between initial exposure to a carcinogen and the subsequent development of cancer. Nervous system cancer is the most common solid tumor of childhood, and the occurrence of cancer in the first decade suggests that prenatal events or exposures might contribute to development of the disease.

Some studies have noted an excess of brain tumors in children whose parents had exposure to solvents (82, 83), while others have not (84, 85). Hemminki et al. (86) identified 282 cases of brain cancer through the Finnish Cancer Registry and used data from maternity welfare centers to determine maternal and paternal occupations; details of exposure beyond a simple job classification were not available. An increased rate of brain tumors was found among the children of women factory workers and the children of men who worked as painters. Peters and Preston-Martin (83) found that parental work in the printing, chemical, or petroleum industry was associated with an increased risk of brain tumors in children.

One study reported that work in the aircraft industry was associated with a higher incidence of childhood brain cancer (83), while another case-control study of brain cancer cases in Washington State did not find an elevated rate of parental employment in the aerospace industry (87).

A large case-control study in Texas examined the occupations of fathers of 499 children with intracranial and spinal cord tumors (82). Paternal occupational information was obtained from birth certificates, and jobs were categorized as having potential for hydrocarbon exposure or not. Maternal occupation was not known. This study found an increased risk of CNS defects in children of printers, graphic artists, and workers in the chemical and petroleum industries, but not in all workers with exposure to hydrocarbons. It is important to note the potential problem of misclassification in this study, for unexposed fathers could have exposed wives.

A study in New York State (88) examined parental exposures in 338 patients with a primary tumor of the CNS. In this study, occupational information was obtained by telephone interview with the mothers; work history included job title, a description of job duties, and a description of products or services provided by the company. Occupations and industries were assigned U.S. Census codes, and these codes were used to classify individuals as exposed or unexposed to the substances of interest. No consistent relationship between paternal hydrocarbon exposure and CNS defects was found; the number of cases with a mother employed in any exposed job was too small to analyze.

Work in these industries entails exposure to solvents among other substances, although the studies do not describe the specific solvents involved. The limited data available suggest a possible risk of childhood brain tumors from parental (especially paternal) solvent exposure, but more study is needed before any specific action is warranted by a clinician with a patient in these occupations. All of the studies had relatively little exposure information. They could be subject to misclassification bias because job titles were usually used as surrogated markers of exposure. In this case, a worker may be classified as exposed to solvents by his or her job title when, actually, that worker has little exposure, while another worker exposed to solvents may be missed because the job title does not reflect solvent exposure. Random misclassification tends to bias a study toward the null hypothesis, i.e., it makes it more difficult to demonstrate a difference between the groups called "exposed" and "unexposed" (89).

## SUMMARY AND RECOMMENDATIONS

There have been many studies of organic solvent exposure and adverse reproductive and developmental outcomes in both humans and experimental animals. Maternal exposure to organic solvents as a group is consistently associated with a modest increased risk for birth defects and, somewhat less consistently, for spontaneous abortion. Some studies suggest an association with menstrual disorders and preeclampsia, but the data are more limited. Ethylene glycol ethers have been shown to cause testicular dysfunction in exposed male workers. In addition, some data suggest that paternal exposure to organic solvents is associated with spontaneous abortion and childhood cancer.

There is still much more we need to know to make informed clinical decisions. Few of these studies tell us if there is a threshold of exposure below which no adverse outcomes occur or if there is a critical period for exposure, outside of which an exposure might have a reduced effect. In most cases, it is unclear whether the adverse outcome is due to a specific solvent or to a class of solvents. This information is hard to obtain; human studies of adverse reproductive outcome are difficult to perform well, and detailed assessment of exposure may not be possible in industrial settings. More animal research is needed but cannot answer all our questions. Clinicians giving counsel about the risk to a pregnancy or fertility may still be dealing with large areas of uncertainty 10–20 yr from now.

Based on available data, it is prudent to reduce exposure to solvents as much as possible in the industrial setting, particularly if exposure occurs to ethylene glycol ethers or substantial exposure occurs to any solvent. As a working definition, the following criteria to determine substantial exposure to a solvent are proposed:

(a) use in an industrial setting *and*
(b) regular dermal contact *or*
(c) industrial hygiene data showing exposure at or near the TLV *or*
(d) biological monitoring results that reveal exposure near the BEI.

After a determination that substantial exposure may exist, the clinician could ask for more detailed exposure assessment from the employer, while at the same time recommending a job transfer until the level of exposure is clarified. In making recommendations to the employer or discussing job modifications with the employer or worker, some basic principles of exposure reduction are useful.

(a) *Product Substitution.* Replacing a toxic chemical with a safer one is usually the ideal solution but may not be practical when making a determination about a pregnant woman. It can take months or years to determine if an acceptable substitute exists, and a decision about job placement must be made more rapidly during pregnancy.

(b) *Engineering Controls.* Strategies such as improving local exhaust ventilation or enclosing a work process can significantly reduce exposure.

(c) *Administrative Controls.* Instituting work rotations can reduce, but not eliminate, exposure to individual workers. Reassignment for a period of time may be warranted.

(d) *Personal Protective Equipment.* Provision of personal protective equipment such as respirators or gloves can be useful, especially if combined with other, more effective methods of exposure control.

Respirators must be fitted with the proper cartridge for the solvent in use, and there must be an established program for fitting the respirator and determining how frequently to change the cartridge. Some companies allow the worker to determine if the cartridge is spent by reporting a breakthrough in smell. This strategy will not be effective for many solvents, for the smell threshold may exceed the level at which toxic effects occur, or a

worker may develop olfactory fatigue to a solvent in a short period of time and, thus, not detect an odor through the respirator.

Any gloves prescribed must be tested for the particular solvent. Some types of gloves are effective for one solvent but essentially useless for another. The solvent manufacturer can advise the clinician or the employer on appropriate glove material and breakthrough time for specific solvents. Inasmuch as most solvents are dermally absorbed, the individual must pay particular attention to work practices. Does his/her clothing get saturated in the process? Does the solvent get inside the gloves because of splashes or exposure above the glove line?

Finally, significant exposure to organic solvents in pregnancy warrants level II ultrasounds and careful clinical follow-up.

## REFERENCES

1. Rosenberg J. Solvents. In: LaDou J, ed. Occupational medicine. Norwalk: Appleton & Lange, 1990:359–386.
2. Sandmeyer EE. Aromatic hydrocarbons. In: Clayton GD, Clayton FE, eds. Patty's industrial hygiene and toxicology. Volume 2B: Toxicology. New York: John Wiley & Sons, 1981;3253.
3. Nau H. Species differences in pharmacokinetics and drug teratogenesis. Environ Health Perspect 1986;70:113–129.
4. Mirkin BL, Singh S. Placental transfer of pharmacologically active molecules. In: Mirkin BL, ed. Perinatal pharmacology and therapeutics. New York: Academic Press, 1976:1–69.
5. Clapp DE, Zaebst DD, Herrick RF. Measuring exposures to glycol ethers. Environ Health Perspect 1984;57:91–95.
6. Miller RR. Metabolism and disposition of glycol ethers. Drug Metab Rev 1987;18:1–22.
7. Foster PMD, Creasy DM, Foster JR, Thomas LV, Cook MW, Gangolli SD. Testicular toxicity of ethylene glycol monomethyl and monoethyl ethers in the rat. Toxicol Appl Pharmacol 1983;69:385–399.
8. Foster PMD, Creasy DM, Foster JR, Gray TJB. Testicular toxicity produced by ethylene glycol monomethyl and monoethyl ethers in the rat. Environ Health Perspect 1984;57:207–217.
9. Hardin BD. Reproductive toxicity of the glycol ethers. Toxicology 1983;27:91–102.
10. Zenick H, Oudiz D, Niewenhuis RJ. Spermatotoxicity associated with acute and subchronic ethoxyethanol treatment. Environ Health Perspect 1984;57:225–231.
11. Chapin RE, Lamb JC. Effect of ethylene glycol monomethyl ether on various parameters of testicular function in the F344 rat. Environ Health Perspect 1984;57:219–224.
12. Barbee SJ, Terrill JB, DeSousa DJ, Conaway CC. Sub-

chronic inhalation toxicology of ethylene glycol monoethyl ether in the rat and rabbit. Environ Health Perspect 1984;57:157–163.

13. Miller RR, Hermann EA, Young JT, Landry TD, Calhoun LL. Ethylene glycol monomethyl ether and propylene glycol monomethyl ether: metabolism, disposition and subchronic inhalation toxicity studies. Environ Health Perspect 1984;57:233–239.

14. Nagano K, Nakayama E, Oobayshi H, et al. Embryotoxic effects of ethylene glycol monomethyl ether in mice. Toxicology 1981;20:335–343.

15. Hanley TR, Young JT, John JA, Rao KS. Ethylene glycol monomethyl ether (EGME) and propylene glycol monomethyl ether (PGME): inhalation fertility and teratogenicity studies in rats, mice and rabbits. Environ Health Perspect 1984;57:7–12.

16. Ratcliffe JM, Schrader SM, Clapp DE, Halperin WE, Turner TW, Hornung RW. Semen quality in workers exposed to 2-ethoxyethanol. Br J Ind Med 1989;49:399–406.

17. Welch LS, Schrader SM, Turner TW, Cullen MR. Effects of exposure to ethylene glycol ethers on shipyard painters: II. Male reproduction. Am J Ind Med 1988;14:509–526.

18. Cook RR, Bodner KM, Kolesar RC, et al. A cross-sectional study of ethylene glycol monomethyl ether process employees. Arch Environ Health 1982;37:346–351.

19. Michon S. Disturbances of menstruation in women working in an atmosphere polluted with aromatic hydrocarbons [Abstract]. Pol Tyg Lek 1965;20:1648–1649.

20. Mikhailova LM, Kobyets GP, Lyubomudrov VE, Braga GF. The influence of occupational factors on diseases of the female reproductive organs. Pediatriya Akusherstvo Ginekologiya 1971;33:56–58.

21. Zlobina NS, Izyumova AS, Ragule NY. The effect of low concentration of styrene on the specific functions of the female organism [Abstract]. Gig Tr Prof Zabol 1975;12:21–25.

22. Syrovadko ON. Working conditions and health status of women handling organosilicon varnishes containing toluene [Abstract]. Gig Tr Prof Zabol 1977;12:15–19.

23. Lemasters GK, Hagen A, Samuels SJ. Reproductive outcomes in women exposed to solvents in 36 reinforced plastics companies. I. Menstrual dysfunction. J Occup Med 1985;27:490–494.

24. Tylleskar–Jensen J. Chloroform—a cause of pregnancy toxaemia? Nordisk Medicin 1967;77:841–842.

25. Eskenazi B, Bracken MB, Holford TR, Grady J. Exposure to organic solvents and hypertensive disorders of pregnancy. Am J Ind Med 1988;14:177–188.

26. Shumilina AV. Menstrual and reproductive functions of workers with occupational exposure to formaldehyde. Gig Tr Prof Zabol 1975;12:18–21.

27. Churchill SN, Fine A, Gault MH. Association between hydrocarbon exposure and glomerulonephritis: an appraisal of the evidence. Nephron 1983;33:169–172.

28. Brochard P, De Palmas J, Martini M, Blondet M, Lagrue G. Etude de la prevalence des proteinuries depistees chez des sujets exposes professionnellement aux solvents. Presented at the International Congress on Occupational Health, Dublin, Ireland, 1984.

29. Hemminki K, Franssila E, Vainio H. Spontaneous abortions among female chemical workers in Finland. Int Arch Occup Environ Health 1980;45:123–126.

30. Lindbohm M-L, Taskinen H, Sallmen M, Hemminki K. Spontaneous abortions among women exposed to organic solvents. Am J Ind Med 1990;17:449–463.

31. Lindbohm M-L, Hemminki K, Kyyronen P. Parental occupational exposure and spontaneous abortions in Finland. Am J Epidemiol 1984;120:370–378.

32. Taskinen H, Lindbohm M-L, Hemminki K. Spontaneous abortions among women working in the pharmaceutical industry. Br J Ind Med 1986;43:199–205.

33. Axelsson G, Lutz C, Rylander R. Exposure to solvents and outcome of pregnancy in university laboratory employees. Br J Ind Med 1984;41:305–312.

34. Heidam LZ. Spontaneous abortions among laboratory workers: a follow-up study. J Epidemiol Commun Health 1984;38:36–41.

35. Harkonen H, Holmberg PC. Obstetric histories of women occupationally exposed to styrene. Scand J Work Environ Health 1982;8:74–77.

36. Schwetz BA. Teratogenicity of maternally administered volatile anesthetics in mice and rats [Abstract]. Dissertation Abstracts International B 1970;31:3599–B.

37. Schwetz BA, Leong BK, Gehring PJ. Embryo and fetotoxicity of inhaled chloroform in rats. Toxicol Appl Pharmacol 1974;28:442–451.

38. Murray FJ, Schwetz BA, McBride JG, Staples RE. Toxicity of inhaled chloroform in pregnant mice and their offspring. Toxicol Appl Pharmacol 1979;50:515–522.

39. Ungvary G, Tatrai E, Hudak A, Barcza G, Lorincz M. Study on the embryotoxic effect of para-xylene. Egeszsegtudomany 1979;23:152–158.

40. Ragule NY. Embryotropic action of styrene. Gigiena I Sanitariya 1974;11:85–86.

41. Nawrot PS, Staples RE. Embryofetal toxicity and teratogenicity of benzene and toluene in the mouse. Teratology 1979;19:41A.

42. Hudak A, Ungvary G. Embryotoxic effects of benzene and its methyl derivatives: toluene, xylene. Toxicology 1978;11:55–63.

43. Taskinen H, Antilla A, Lindbohm ML, Sallman M, Hemminki K. Spontaneous abortion and congenital malformations among wives of men occupationally exposed to organic solvents. Scand J Work Environ Health 1989; 15:345–352.

44. Olsen J. Risk of exposure to teratogens amongst laboratory staff and painters. Dan Med Bull 1983;30:24–28.

45. Holmberg PC, Nurminen M. Congenital defects of the central nervous system and occupational factors during pregnancy. Case referent study. Am J Ind Med 1980; 1:167–176.

46. Kurppa K, Holmberg PC, Hernberg S, Rantala R, Riala R, Nurminen T. Screening for occupational exposures and congenital malformations. Scand J Work Environ Health 1983;9:89–93.

47. McDonald JC, Lavoie J, Cote R, McDonald AD. Chemical exposures at work in early pregnancy and congenital defects: a case-referent study. Br J Ind Med 1987; 44:527–533.

48. Tikkanen J, Heinonen OP. Cardiovascular malforma-

tions and organic solvent exposure during pregnancy in Finland. Am J Ind Med 1988;14:1–8.

49. Hansson E, Jansa S, Wande H, Kallen B, Ostlund E. Pregnancy outcome for women working in laboratories in some of the pharmaceutical industries in Sweden. Scand J Work Environ Health 1980;6:131–134.

50. Meirik O, Kallen B, Gauffin U, Ericson E. Major malformations in infants born of women who worked in laboratories while pregnant. Lancet 1979;2:91.

51. Blomqvist U, Ericson A, Kallen B, Westerholm P. Delivery outcome for women working in the pulp and paper industry. Scand J Work Environ Health 1981;7:114–118.

52. Ericson A, Kallen B, Zetterstrom R, Eriksson M, Westerholm P. Delivery outcome of women working in laboratories during pregnancy. Arch Environ Health 1984;39:5–10.

53. Erikson JD, Cochran WM, Anderson CD. Birth defects and printing. Lancet 1978;1:385.

54. Harkonen H, Tola S, Korkala ML, Hernberg S. Congenital malformations, mortality and styrene exposure. Ann Acad Med 1984;13:404–407.

55. Schwetz BA, Leong BKJ, Gehring BJ. The effect of maternally inhaled trichloroethylene, perchloroethylene, methyl chloroform, and methylene chloride on embryonal and fetal development in mice and rats. Toxicol Appl Pharmacol 1975;32:84–96.

56. Barlow SM, Sullivan FM. Reproductive hazards of industrial chemicals. New York: Academic Press, 1982.

57. Schwetz BA, Leong BKJ, Gehring PB. Embryo- and fetotoxicity of inhaled carbon tetrachloride, 1, 1-dichloroethane and methyl ethyl ketone in rats. Toxicol Appl Pharmacol 1974;28:452–464.

58. John JA, Pilny MK, Kuna RA, Deacon MM, Yakel HO. Teratogenic evaluation of methyl ethyl ketone in the rat. Teratology 1980;28:452–464.

59. Andrew FD, Buschbom RL, Cannon WC, et al. Teratologic assessment of ethylbenzene and 2-ethoxyethanol. Final report of NIOSH contract 210–79–0037. Richland, WA: Battelle Pacific Laboratories, 1981.

60. Hardin BD, Bond GP, Sikov MR, Andrew FD, Beliles RP, Niemeier RW. Testing of selected workplace chemicals for teratogenic potential. Scand J Work Environ Health 1981;7:66–75.

61. Hardin BD, Niemeier RW, Smith RJ, Kuczuk MH, Mathinos PR, Weaver TF. Teratogenicity of 2-ethoxyethanol by dermal application. Drug Chem Toxicol 1982;5:277–294.

62. Doe JE. Ethylene glycol monoethyl ether and ethylene glycol monoethyl ether acetate teratology studies. Environ Health Perspect 1984;57:33–42.

63. Hanley TR, Yano BL, Nitschke KD, John JA. Comparison of the teratogenic potential of inhaled ethylene glycol monomethyl ether in rats, mice, and rabbits. Toxicol Appl Pharmacol 1984;75:409–422.

64. Horton VL, Sleet RB, John-Greene, Welsch F. Developmental phase-specific and dose-related teratogenic effects of ethylene glycol monomethyl ether in CD-1 mice. Toxicol Appl Pharmacol 1985;80:108–118.

65. Toraason M, Stringer B, Stober P, Hardin BD. Electrocardiographic study of rat fetuses exposed to ethylene

glycol monomethyl ether (EGME). Teratology 1985;32:33–39.

66. Hardin BD, Eisenmann CJ. Relative potency of four ethylene glycol ethers for induction of paw malformations in the CD-1 mouse. Teratology 1987;35:321–328.

67. U.S. Department of Health and Human Services, National Institute for Occupational Safety and Health. Criteria for a recommended standard: occupational exposure to ethylene glycol monomethyl ether, and their acetates. DHHS (NIOSH) publ no. 91–119. Cincinnati: NIOSH, 1991.

68. Toutant C, Lippmann S. Fetal solvents syndrome. Lancet 1979;2:1356.

69. Hersh JH, Podruch PE, Rogers G, Weisskopf B. Toluene embryopathy. J Pediatr 1985;106:922–927.

70. Wilkins-Haug L, Gabow P. Toluene abuse during pregnancy; obstetric complications and perinatal outcomes. Obstet Gynecol 1991;4:504–509.

71. King MD. Neurological sequelae of toluene abuse. Human Toxicol 1982;1:281–283.

72. Goodwin TM. Toluene abuse and renal tubular acidosis in pregnancy. Obstet Gynecol 1988;71:715–718.

73. Winek CL, Collom WD. Benzene and toluene fatalities. J Occup Med 1971;13:259–261.

74. Donald JM, Hooper K, Hopenhayn-Rich C. Reproductive and developmental toxicity of toluene: a review. Environ Health Perspect 1991;94:237–244.

75. Hunter AGW, Thompson D, Evans JA. Is there a fetal gasoline syndrome? Teratology 1979;20:75–80.

76. Hardin BD, Manson JM. Absence of dichloromethane teratogenicity with inhalation exposure in rats. Toxicol Appl Pharmacol 1980;52:22–28.

77. Bornschein RL, Hastings L, Manson JM. Behavioural toxicity in the offspring of rats following maternal exposure to dichloromethane. Toxicol Appl Pharmacol 1980;52:29–37.

78. Nelson BK, Brightwell WS, Setzer JV, Taylor BJ, Hornung RW. Ethoxyethanol behavioral teratology in rats. Neurotoxicology 1981;2:231–249.

79. Nelson BK, Brightwell WS, Burg JR, Massari VJ. Behavioral and neurochemical alterations in the offspring of rats after maternal or paternal inhalation exposure to the industrial solvent 2-methoxyethanol. Pharmacol Biochem Behav 1984;20:269–279.

80. Rodier PM, Reynolds SS, Roberts WN. Behavioral consequences of interference with CNS development in the early fetal period. Teratology 1979;19:327–336.

81. Eskenazi B, Gaylord L, Bracken MB, Brown D. In utero exposure to organic solvents and human neurodevelopment. Dev Med Child Neurol 1988;30:492–501.

82. Johnson CC, Annegers JF, Frankowski R, Spitz M, Buffler PA. Childhood nervous system tumors-an evaluation of the association with paternal occupational exposure to hydrocarbons. Am J Epidemiol 1987;126:605–613.

83. Peters JM, Preston-Martin S. Brain tumors in children and occupational exposure of parents. Science 1981;213:235–237.

84. Sanders BM, White GC, Draper GJ. Occupations of fathers of children dying from neoplasms. J Epidemiol Commun Health 1980;35:245.

85. Gold EB, Diener MD, Szklo M. Parental occupations and cancer in children: a case-control study and review of the methodologic issues. J Occup Med 1982;24:578–584.

86. Hemminki K, Saloniemi I, Salonen T, Partanen T, Vainio H. Childhood cancer and parental occupation in Finland. J Epidemiol Commun Health 1981;35:11–15.

87. Olshan AF, Breslow NE, Daling JR, Weiss NS, Leviton A. Childhood brain tumors and paternal occupation in the aerospace industry. J Natl Cancer Inst 1986;77:17–19.

88. Nasca PC, Baptiste MS, MacCubbin PA, et al. An epidemiologic case-control study of central nervous system tumors in children and parental occupational exposures. Am J Epidemiol 1988;128:1256–1265.

89. Savitz DA, Chen J. Parental occupation and childhood cancer: review of epidemiologic studies. Environ Health Perspect 1990;88:325–337.

# Occupational Exposure to Pharmaceuticals: Antineoplastics, Anesthetic Agents, Sex Steroid Hormones

MELISSA McDIARMID

The reproductive effects of the majority of xenobiotics are not well characterized. However, one group of chemicals for which slightly more is known regarding reproductive toxicity is pharmaceuticals. This knowledge is due largely to more extensive laboratory and animal testing during drug development and to human data derived from treated patients.

Opportunity for occupational exposure to pharmaceuticals occurs primarily in two work sectors, pharmaceutical manufacture and health care delivery, where the majority of workers may be exposed. The National Institute for Occupational Safety and Health (NIOSH) estimates that 1 million workers are at risk of exposure to hazardous pharmaceuticals in health care delivery, including primarily nurses and pharmacists (1).

The three drug classes addressed in this chapter—antineoplastics, hormones, and anes-thetic gases—have all been implicated as reproductive or developmental toxicants in both laboratory and human epidemiological studies of exposed workers. Numerous other pharmaceutical agents are known to exert untoward reproductive effects in patients and are reviewed elsewhere (2).

## ANTINEOPLASTIC DRUGS

The terms "cytotoxic" (meaning "cell killer") and "antineoplastic" are often applied interchangeably to describe the multiple classes of drugs used in cancer therapy. However, not all antineoplastics are cytotoxic, nor are cytotoxics used exclusively for cancer treatment. For example, zidovudine (AZT) is a cytotoxic antiviral agent used in the prophylaxis and treatment of acquired immunodeficiency syndrome (AIDS). Recognizing this discrepancy, the

American Society of Hospital Pharmacists recently described the term "hazardous drug" to include the cytotoxics and other noncytotoxic medications that pose potential genotoxic, oncogenic, mutagenic, teratogenic, or other hazards to exposed workers (3).

## Properties and Occurrence

Antineoplastics can be divided into five structurally unique drug classes: alkylating agents, antibiotics, antimetabolites, mitotic inhibitors, and a miscellaneous class. The majority of these agents are synthetic chemicals, although some of the antibiotics and mitotic inhibitors are derived from natural organic constituents.

Stringent work practices in the manufacturing sector have greatly reduced exposure to pharmaceutical workers. By far, the largest population at risk for potentially significant exposure is health care professionals who mix and administer the drugs (primarily nurses and pharmacists). These activities can generate exposure in a variety of ways. Drug preparation outside of vertical laminar-flow hoods (biological safety cabinets) and improper use or design of personal protective clothing result in significant contamination. Splattering or aerosol generation can occur when drug ampules are opened, during withdrawal or transfer of drugs from vials, and when trapped air is expelled from drug-filled syringes. Leakages in tubing and stopcock connections and spills or accidents represent significant sources of exposure. Finally, contamination can result from improper handling of patient body fluids or careless disposal practices. Environmental exposure can occur when cancer patients are treated with these drugs at home by a visiting nurse or family member.

## Toxicology

### METABOLISM

The primary routes of occupational exposure are inhalation and skin absorption, although ingestion can occur due to workplace and hand contamination.

Most of the antineoplastic drugs are indirect acting, i.e., they require metabolic activation, usually in the liver, to exert their effects. The majority are excreted in their metabolically active form in the urine, creating another potential exposure opportunity for hospital workers handling patient wastes.

Transplacental passage of some antineoplastics is evidenced by documented insult to the developing fetus of treated patients. While fetal malformations and spontaneous abortions are reported in women treated with antineoplastic agents of all classes (4), the alkylating agents and the antimetabolites are most often implicated.

### MECHANISMS OF ACTION

Anticancer agents act by arresting the proliferation of malignant cells. There are three proliferation pathways that can be blocked by anticancer drugs: DNA replication, protein synthesis, and mitosis (5).

Figure 20.1 illustrates the primary mechanisms operative in anticancer therapy. The alkylating agents act by covalently binding to DNA, thus impairing normal DNA replication. The antibiotics work as DNA intercalators, interfering with transcriptional processes in protein synthesis. The antimetabolites interrupt protein synthesis by impeding the production of essential cellular building blocks such as folic acid, purines, and pyrimidines. Antimitotic agents are primarily spindle poisons that arrest mitosis and normal cell division. Antineoplastic drugs in the miscellaneous category exert their effects through a variety of mechanisms.

Carcinogenic risk to exposed hospital workers was the initial occupational health concern expressed for antineoplastic agents. Many of the anticancer drugs are animal carcinogens. Evidence for the human carcinogenicity of these agents accrued through reports of "second malignancy" development in patients treated with antineoplastics for primary neoplasms (6, 7). The International Agency for Research on Cancer (IARC) has evaluated the evidence for carcinogenicity and genotoxicity of common anticancer agents (8). Mutagenicity of most antineoplastic agents across the major drug classes has been reported by IARC to include point mutations and chromosomal effects (Table 20.1).

In his 1989 paper, Vainio (9) postulates potential common mechanisms for carcinogenesis and teratogenesis, including mutation and

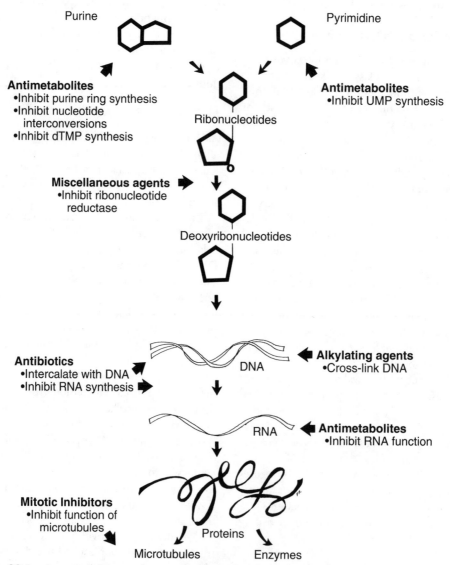

**Figure 20.1.**  Summary of the mechanisms and sites of action of selected classes of antineoplastic agents. Adapted from Gilman GA, Rall TW, Nies AS, Taylor P, eds. The pharmacologic basis of therapeutics.8th ed. New York: Pergamon Press, 1990:1208.

**Table 20.1.**
**Developmental Toxicity and Genotoxicity of Some Common Anticancer Agents[a]**

| Drug Class | Developmental Toxicity | | | Genotoxicity[d] | |
|---|---|---|---|---|---|
| | Animal[b] | | Human[c] | PM | CE |
| | T | E | | | |
| Aklylating Agents | | | | | |
| BCNU | + | + | | + | + |
| Busulfan | + | | + | + | + |
| Chlorambucil | + | + | + | + | + |
| Cyclophosphamide | + | + | + | + | + |
| Nitrogen mustard | + | + | + | + | + |
| Thiotepa | + | | | + | + |
| Cis-diaminedichloroplatinum | | + | | + | + |
| Antibiotics | | | | | |
| Actinomycin | + | + | | + | + |
| Adriamycin | | | | + | + |
| Bleomycin | | | | ± | + |
| Daunomycin | | | + | + | + |
| Antimetabolites | | | | | |
| Cytosine arabinoside | | | + | | |
| 5-Fluorouracil | + | + | + | | + |
| 6-Mercaptopurine | + | + | + | + | + |
| Methotrexate | + | + | + | + | + |
| Mitotic inhibitors | | | | | |
| Vincristine | + | + | + | − | + |
| Vinblastine | + | + | + | − | + |
| Miscellaneous | | | | | |
| DTIC (Dacarbazine) | + | + | | + | |
| Proxarbazine | + | + | + | + | + |

[a] +, positive result; −, negative result; T = teratogenicity; E = embryotoxicity; PM = point mutations; CE = chromosomal effect.
[b] Data judged by the International Agency for Research on Cancer (1975, 1976, 1981). Data summarized from Sorsa M, Hemminki K, Vainio H. Occupational exposure to anticancer drugs: potential and real hazards. Mutat Res 1985;154:135–149.
[c] Data summarized from Gililland J, Weinstein L. The effects of cancer chemotherapeutic agents on the developing fetus. Obstet Gynecol Surv 1983;38:6–13.
[d] Data summarized from Sorsa M, Hemminki K, Vainio H. Occupational exposure to anticancer drugs: potential and real hazards. Mutat Res 1985;154:135–149.

disrupted intercellular communication. The majority of anticancer agents are genotoxic. Several nongenotoxic teratogens such as mirex, ethanol, and some glycol ethers can block cell-cell communication. Likewise, some antineoplastics, although not genotoxic themselves, may act as tumor promotors via a mechanism of disrupted intercellular communication (10).

## REPRODUCTIVE HEALTH EFFECTS

### Gonadal Effects

Evidence for the human reproductive effects of the antineoplastic agents derive primarily from anecdotal case reports of treated patients. To assess effects on spermatogenesis and fertility in males, Richter et al. (11) studied a group of lymphoma patients treated with chlorambucil. They noted oligospermia and azoospermia af-

ter a minimum dose of 400 mg. In a similar investigation, Miller (12) reported aspermia at a minimum dose twice that reported by Richter. Cheviakoff et al. (13) reported reversal of oligospermia 6 weeks after ending chlorambucil treatment in three of five patients tested.

Long-term treatment with cyclophosphamide has also been associated with sterility in males treated with 11.3 g over 4 months (14), azoospermia after 50–100 mg/day for more than 2 months (15), and testicular atrophy at 3 mg/kg/day (16). Males receiving combination chemotherapy with chlorambucil, cyclophosphamide, and other agents experienced altered reproductive capacity (17).

The alkylating agents also exhibit adverse effects in human females. Freckman et al. (18) noted loss of ovarian primordial follicles and cessation of menses after 14–20 mg/day chlorambucil for 2 months. Amenorrhea is a well-documented complication of cyclophosphamide therapy (15, 19) and may, in some cases, be reversible (20). Menstrual irregularities and amenorrhea have also been reported in patients treated with a combination chemotherapy regimen. The alkylating agents may exert their adverse effects on female fertility through action on epithelial cells, direct cytotoxic effects on ova or follicles, or by some combination of these mechanisms (21).

Chapman (22) has reviewed the experience of gonadal injury resulting from chemotherapy. The alkylating agents and vinca alkaloids produce much of the gonadal dysfunction in humans, with additional drugs implicated in male reproductive damage only. Gonadal injury is apparently a function of dose and age at time of exposure, as is reversibility of gonadal insult. Prepubertal children experience less gonadal toxicity than adults. These observations from treated cancer patients have implications for occupational cohorts who may be chronically exposed as adults to antineoplastics over 20 or more years of a working lifetime.

## Developmental Effects

The teratogenicity and embryotoxicity of most antineoplastic agents have been well documented in experimental animal studies and are summarized in Table 20.1. Virtually all of these drugs demonstrate some embryofetal toxicity in animals. While the majority of these studies are performed by dosing female animals and examining outcomes, more recent work investigating male-mediated reproductive effects in animals also deserves discussion.

Trasler and colleagues (23) examined the effect of chronic low dose (1.5–5.0 mg/kg/day × 11 weeks by gavage) cyclophosphamide treatment of adult male rats on pregnancy outcome. Despite minimal effects on the male reproductive system, there were significant effects on the conceptus including a dose-dependent increase in preimplantation loss after 5–6 weeks exposure, postimplantation loss beginning at 2 weeks of exposure, and an increase in malformed and growth-retarded fetuses at 3–4 and 7–9 weeks of exposure. These results document a male-mediated teratogenic

effect from a chronically administered antineoplastic agent.

In another study, Adams et al. (24) reported behavioral deficits in progeny of cyclophosphamide-treated male rats (10 mg/kg/day intraperitoneal × 5 days for 5 weeks). This work may indicate a male-mediated, chemically induced genetic effect manifested by behavioral alterations.

The maternally mediated effects of antineoplastic agents on the fetus have been reviewed by Gililland and Weinstein (4). Adverse outcomes are associated with the majority of drugs, but untoward effects predominate with alkylating agent or antimetabolite treatment. Some abnormalities seen with alkylating agent use include anomalies of the toes with cyclophosphamide (25, 26); eye abnormalities, cleft palate, and streak ovaries (27), and hydronephrosis and absent right kidney (28) after busulfan exposure; absence of kidney and ureter after chlorambucil exposure (29); and foot and toe abnormalities (30) and malpositioned small kidneys (31) after nitrogen mustard treatment. Spontaneous abortions have also been reported in patients treated with some of these agents (23, 32).

The antimetabolites have been associated with multiple fetal abnormalities including cranial anomalies and cleft palate after aminopterin treatment (23), cranial and digital abnormalities after methotrexate therapy (23), and multiple abnormalities of the hands and internal organs after fluorouracil treatment (33).

For all of these cases, trimester of exposure was apparently important in determining fetal outcome, with lesser effects seen if treatment occurred later in pregnancy. Also, there are many reports of apparently normal births following antineoplastic therapy during pregnancy (23, 34), and accumulated data suggest no increase in congenital anomalies in offspring born to women or men formerly treated with mutagenic antineoplastics for childhood cancers (35).

## Occupational Exposure

Evidence for hospital worker exposure began accruing in 1979 when Falck et al. (36) used the *Salmonella* reversion test to demonstrate mutagenic activity in the urine of nurses handling cytostatic agents. As measured by this assay, mutagenicity increased during the work week and decreased over the weekend hiatus from occupational exposure. In 1981, Waksvik et al. (37) found a dose-dependent increase in gaps and breaks in chromosomes of nurses handling cytostatic drugs. One year later, Nguyen et al. (38) reported increases in the mutagenicity of urine of pharmacy personnel preparing antineoplastic drugs. When personnel used recommended safe handling procedures and a biological safety cabinet during drug preparation, urine mutagenicity was decreased or absent. Drug absorption by workers was documented by Hirst et al. (39) in 1984, when they reported measurable amounts of cyclophosphamide in the urine of nurses handling the drug.

Two recent epidemiological studies regarding reproductive outcomes among nurses exposed to antineoplastics are of interest. In a Finnish case-control study, Hemminki et al. (40) noted that first trimester exposure to antineoplastic drugs was significantly more common among nurses who gave birth to malformed infants than among those who delivered normal infants. No association was found between exposure to anticancer agents and fetal loss in this study. However, in another case-control study of nurses employed in Finnish hospitals that ranked high in usage of antineoplastic drugs, Selevan et al. (41) reported a statistically significant association between fetal loss and occupational exposure (at least once per week) to antineoplastics during the first trimester of pregnancy. Because most subjects handled multiple anticancer drugs, separation of the effects of individual agents was not possible.

The discrepancy in fetal loss findings in these two studies may be due to differences in methodology or in the degree of exposure experienced by subjects. In both investigations, frequency of use was employed as a marker of exposure, and no environmental or biological measurements were obtained. Hemminki et al. collected exposure data from the head nurses in individual hospitals; Selevan et al. ascertained exposure through work histories provided by the subjects themselves. This latter method of ascertainment is more prone to recall bias. On the other hand, nurses' exposure levels in the Selevan study may have been higher. The sample was confined to hospitals that reported significant usage of antineoplastics, and only nurses who actually prepared drug doses were considered exposed. Preparation of drugs outside of vertical laminar-flow hoods can result in significant contamination. In the Hemminki study, the data on spontaneous abortions pertained to nurses employed in departments of a general hospital where exposure to antineoplastics was relatively uncommon, and the mode of exposure was not clearly defined. (For the subsequent study of malformations, Hemminki included departments where cancer treatment was extensive).

Although the majority of studies have been performed on oncology nursing and pharmacy personnel, several agents, such as cyclophosphamide, are increasingly employed for nonmalignant illnesses with the potential for exposing workers in other sectors of the medical care setting.

## Clinical Assessment

In the preconception setting or during pregnancy, workers handling antineoplastic drugs may be particularly concerned about potential adverse reproductive or developmental effects. The type, frequency, and degree of exposure should be well documented during history-taking through questions regarding work practices and the availability of control measures at the workplace. It is important to note the occurrence of accidents or spills and to ascertain gestational age at exposure accurately. If a safety officer is available, direct inspection of the patient's work area and environmental monitoring provide more accurate estimates of exposure.

Measuring drug levels in body fluids documents exposure but has little prognostic value. If significant exposure occurs during pregnancy, diagnostic testing, including a level II ultrasound and perhaps amniocentesis, should be considered. It may be prudent for the acutely exposed male or female worker to defer conception for 3 months. This period allows for drug clearance and for regeneration of sperm in the seminiferous epithelium.

## Prevention and Treatment

Since the early 1980s, many organizations and authors have published guidelines for the safe handling of antineoplastic agents. All of these sources recommend the use of a glove-box or vertical laminar air flow hood, protective work apparel, special handling techniques, and specialized waste disposal procedures.

The Occupational Safety and Health Administration (OSHA) published handling guidelines for antineoplastics in 1986 (42). The OSHA Hazard Communication Standard also requires that workers be informed of potential hazards (including reproductive hazards) in their work environment. In addition, OSHA recommends a medical surveillance program for all antineoplastic drug handlers that includes a preplacement physical examination and a complete blood count. This program complements engineering controls and safe handling guidelines in protecting workers from these potentially hazardous agents. A registry of all staff who routinely handle antineoplastics is also suggested; it would tally drug name and total dosage prepared by each worker.

A more detailed medical surveillance protocol for antineoplastic drug handlers has recently been published (43). It focuses on the skin, hematopoietic, hepatic, renal, and urinary systems in the physical examination. These systems should also be emphasized in the medical history, as should a detailed reproductive history. Because of problems with assay sensitivity, cost, and interpretation of results, biological monitoring for specific agents of exposure is not appropriate for routine surveillance of antineoplastic handlers.

According to OSHA recommendations, alternative duties that do not involve handling antineoplastics should be made available on request to male or female workers who are actively trying to conceive or who are pregnant or are breastfeeding (42).

In summary, handling antineoplastic drugs may expose workers to known reproductive or developmental toxicants. Health risks can be prevented by implementing safe handling guidelines, administrative and engineering controls, and a comprehensive medical surveillance program. Taking these steps ensures a safer workplace where these useful therapeutic agents are handled in a way that protects employee health.

## ANESTHETIC AGENTS

The inhalation anesthetics have been in clinical use since the last century. These agents have recently been suspected of causing adverse health effects, including reproductive effects, in exposed workers.

## Properties and Occurrence

At room temperature and pressure, anesthetics are either gases or volatile liquids. Currently, nitrous oxide ($N_2O$) is the only gas in widespread use. Nitrous oxide is a colorless gas that is heavier than air. It has relatively low solubility in blood and is excreted unchanged through the lungs, with a small fraction escaping through the skin due to its rapid diffusion.

The volatile anesthetics are liquids at room temperature and are more soluble in blood and fat than $N_2O$. These agents include halothane (2-bromo-2-chloro-1,1,1-trifluoro-ethane), methoxyflurane (2,2-dichloro-1,1,-difluoroethyl methyl ether), enflurane (2-chloro-1,1,2-trifluoroethyl difluoromethyl ether), and isoflurane (1-chloro-2,2,2-trifluoroethyl difluromethyl ether).

Currently, the most widely used inhalation anesthetic agents in the U.S. are nitrous oxide, enflurane, halothane, and isoflurane (44). The principal source of waste anesthetic gases in the hospital is leakage from anesthetic equipment. NIOSH estimates that 50,000 operating room personnel (excluding surgeons) are exposed to waste anesthetic agents each year (44). These agents are also found in other hospital locations including delivery rooms, dental facilities, emergency rooms, and clinics. Opportunity for exposure also exists for recovery room personnel exposed to waste gases in the expired breath of postoperative patients. Nitrous oxide, halothane, and methoxyflurane have all been measured in the expired breath of patients and operating room personnel for periods ranging from hours to days after anesthetic administration (44).

Measured concentrations of anesthetic agents depend on the method and technique of anesthesia delivery and the scavenger system in place for waste gas. Leakage from anesthetic equipment can be traced to both inadequate work practices of anesthesiologists and nurse anesthetists, as well as faulty installation or poor maintenance of equipment or scavenging systems.

Environmental sampling data published in 1969 and 1970 have documented peak levels of 27 ppm halothane and 428 ppm $N_2O$ in an operating room (45) and average concentrations of 85 ppm halothane and 7000 ppm $N_2O$ in the breathing zone of an anesthesiologist when a nonrebreathing system was used (46). For comparison, current NIOSH recommended exposure limits are 2 ppm for halothane as a 1-hr ceiling limit and 25 ppm nitrous oxide as an 8-hr time weighted average (TWA) (44). In newer facilities with better ventilation systems, appreciably lower levels of these agents have been measured (47). However, occasional peak exposures can still occur during intubation or from face mask leakage.

## Toxicology

### METABOLISM

Inhalation anesthetics rapidly diffuse across the alveolar membrane and achieve various concentrations in blood and other tissues based on solubility of the agent in blood, rate of blood flow to an organ, and fat content of the tissue (5). The concentration effect is reversed after ventilation with anesthetic-free gas washes out the lungs, thus decreasing the blood level of the agent and delivery to tissues. The anesthetic gases are metabolized to a small extent in the body via hepatic microsomal enzyme systems. Production of metabolites may be responsible for some of their toxic effects.

### MECHANISMS OF ACTION

While the anesthetic agents are implicated in animal and human studies as developmental toxicants, their mechanisms of action are poorly understood. Some of these agents, such as halothane and $N_2O$, are mutagenic in various test systems (48, 49). Limited evidence suggests that inhalation anesthetic gas exposure increases cancer risk among exposed populations (50). As previously discussed, carcinogens that function either as genotoxicants or disruptors of cellular

communication may share common mechanisms with developmental toxicants.

An interesting hypothesis proposed by Goldstein et al. (51) regarding nitrous oxide toxicity derives from measures of increased concentrations of nitric oxide (NO) and nitrogen dioxide ($NO_2$) in the operating room. They reasoned that energy-releasing equipment, such as electric cauteries and x-ray machines, may cause oxidation of nitrous oxide. Nitrogen dioxide is reportedly embryolethal, fetotoxic, and teratogenic in rats at levels well below 3 ppm (52). While the concentrations of NO and $NO_2$ were significantly less than recommended threshold limit values, they indicate that the operating environment is not inert and that further investigation is warranted.

## REPRODUCTIVE HEALTH EFFECTS

### Experimental Animal Studies

The majority of laboratory animal studies examining anesthetic gas developmental toxicity have been conducted at relatively high exposure levels, similar to those administered to patients undergoing anesthesia. High-dose $N_2O$ exposure has been reported to cause fetal resorption in the rat (53) and lethality in chick eggs (54). Fink et al. (55), using 50% $N_2O$ for 2, 4, or 6 days of gestation, found rib and vertebral defects in most surviving rat fetuses. These findings have been confirmed by others. Studies of halothane have demonstrated embryolethal and teratogenic effects in the rat, mouse, and hamster (56, 57). A variety of abnormalities were identified including neural groove lesions, such as defects or absence of ribs and vertebrae. In the rabbit, anesthetic concentrations of halothane did not result in embryotoxic or teratogenic effects (58).

Significant findings in experiments conducted at the lower doses experienced by health workers would enhance the plausibility of the developmental toxicity of anesthetic agents. Some animal data suggest low-dose effects. Gofmeckler and co-workers (52) reported $N_2O$-induced embryolethality, fetotoxicity, and teratogenicity in rats at levels below 3 ppm. In addition, Corbett et al. (59) found that trace concentrations of $N_2O$ caused an increased fetal death rate and a reduced average number of offspring in rats. In some studies, exposure of pregnant rats to approximately 10 ppm halothane has been associated with embryolethality, ultrastructurally visible morphological changes in the fetal cerebral cortex, and behavioral disorders in offspring (57).

## Human Studies

Early studies published between 1967 and 1971 from the Soviet Union (60), Denmark (46), and the U.S. (61) first raised the question of an association between occupational anesthetic gas exposure and adverse pregnancy outcomes. However, because of technical limitations and small numbers of subjects, these reports should be regarded as pilot studies only. Numerous other studies have subsequently been published (Table 20.2) and were recently reviewed by Kline (62).

**Table 20.2.**
**Reported Reproductive Effects In Operating Room Personnel[a]**

| Authors (Reference) | Date | Subjects | Referents | Conclusion |
|---|---|---|---|---|
| Cohen et al. (61) | 1971 | 67 F OR nurses<br>50 F anesthetists | 92 F general nurses<br>81 F physicians (other) | +SA |
| Knill-Jones et al. (98) | 1972 | F anesthetists at work | F anesthetists not at work, other F physicians | +CM<br>+INF, +SA |
| Rosenberg and Kirves (99) | 1973 | 124 F OR nurses<br>58 F anesthesia nurses | 75 F ER nurses<br>43 F intensive care nurses | +SA |
| Cohen et al. (63) | 1974 | 1059 anesthesiologists at work<br>7136 F anesthetists<br>12,272 F OR nurses | 639 F pediatricians<br>6560 nurses | +SA, +CM |
| Corbett et al. (64) | 1974 | 268 F nurse-anesthetists with at least one birth and working in pregnancy | 261 F nurse-anesthetists not working in pregnancy | +CM |
| Knill-Jones et al. (65) | 1975 | M and F anesthetists, number not given by sex | Woman exposed vs. neither parent exposed | +SA, −CM |
| Pharoah et al. (100) | 1977 | F anesthetists | Other F physicians working/unexposed or F physicians not working | +CM<br>+SGA |
| Ericson and Kallen (101) | 1979 | 541 women working in pregnancy | All Swedish women medical workers with 19,127 births | −CM, −SA |
| Cohen et al. (66) | 1980 | M dentists exposed<br>F dental assistants exposed | M dentists unexposed<br>F dental assistants unexposed | +CM, +SA |
| Axelsson and Rylander (67) | 1982 | 245 F exposed medical workers | 270 F nonexposed medical workers | +SA[b] |
| Hemminki et al. (68) | 1985 | 217 nurses w/SA<br>46 women w/malformed births | 571 age-matched women with normal births<br>128 age-matched women with normal births | +SA[b]<br><br>+CM[c] |
| Guirguis et al. (69) | 1990 | 8032 M and F exposed operating room and recovery room personnel from 75 Ontario hospitals | 2525 M and F nonexposed hospital workers | +SA<br>+CM |

[a]F = female, M = male, SA = spontaneous abortion, CM = congenital malformation, INF = infertility, SGA = small for gestational age, OR = operating room, ER = emergency room. Adapted from Vainio H. Inhalation anesthetics, anticancer drugs and sterilants as chemical hazards in hospitals. Scand J Work Environ Health 1982;8:94–107; Ericson A, Kallen B. Survey of infants born in 1973 or 1975 to Swedish women working in operating rooms during their pregnancies. Anesth Analg 1979;58:302–305; Kline JK. Maternal occupations: effects on spontaneous abortions and malformations. In: Stein AZ, Hatch MC, eds. Reproductive problems in the workplace. Occupational medicine: state of the art reviews. Philadelphia: Hanely & Belfus, Inc., 1986:381–403.
[b]Not statistically significant.
[c]Too few to give stable estimate of effect.

Three large retrospective studies performed in the mid-1970s compared the obstetric histories of female anesthetists and spouses of male anesthetists with control groups (63–65). An increased risk for spontaneous abortion associated with anesthesia practice of the female, but not the male, was observed in two studies (63, 65). Both male and female anesthetists reported an increase in congenital malformations (63, 64).

A 1980 U.S. study of male dentists and female dental assistants exposed primarily to $N_2O$ revealed a significant increase in spontaneous abortions among the exposed population compared with unexposed controls (66). The rates observed were 8.1/100 pregnancies among the controls and 19.1/100 pregnancies among the heavily exposed. This study is limited, however, by its failure to control for confounding exposure to mercury amalgam.

Despite the generally "positive" findings in studies performed from 1971–1980 (Table 20.2), methodological limitations exist in many of these earlier works including recall and response biases, uncontrolled confounding, and variability of the estimated size of the exposure effect. In most studies, the magnitude of the adverse effect is small, with the largest effect demonstrated in the study by Cohen et al. (61), which reported an odds ratio of 3.7 for spontaneous abortion. More recent work (67, 68) with better methodology does not generally substantiate a significant developmental effect from anesthesia exposure (62). One exception is a recent large, retrospective, questionnaire-based study of Ontario hospital personnel that found increased risks for both spontaneous abortion and congenital malformations among offspring of male and female workers chronically exposed to anesthetic gases compared to unexposed controls (69). In comparison with earlier investigations, this study had higher response rates, improved estimates of exposure, and better control of confounders; however, recall bias remained a significant potential problem.

Inconsistencies in study results may reflect not only differences in study methodologies, but also variations in degree of exposure to anesthetic gases. Findings from earlier studies prompted improved hygiene practices including installation of scavenger systems for waste gases and altered work practices to minimize fugitive gas escape. The positive findings in the recent Ontario study (69) may, in part, be attributable to the long duration of exposure (mean greater than 30 hr/week) and levels of exposure to $N_2O$ (well above the NIOSH TWA of 25 ppm) found for many of the occupational groups in the participating hospitals (70).

In summary, it appears that operating room staff may be at an increased risk of spontaneous abortion in settings without adequate hygiene. Data on congenital malformations are more limited and less consistent. Evidence from the dental study and animal evidence previously cited suggest that high concentrations of $N_2O$ may be the causative factor for adverse outcomes. Failure to demonstrate an increased risk in some recent studies is probably due to newly instituted hygiene practices.

## Clinical Assessment

Workers exposed to excessive amounts of anesthetic gases have symptoms of the anesthetized patient. CNS effects predominate and include drowsiness, irritability, depression, headache, nausea, fatigue, and impairment of judgment and coordination. Workers manifesting these symptoms should be removed from exposure and evaluated in the employee health unit. Assessment includes a basic history and physical examination focusing on the exposure incident and symptoms. Because of reported hepatic and renal toxicity in some exposed workers, blood tests examining the function of these organs should be obtained both immediately after exposure and in a follow-up visit several weeks later. There are no specific treatments or antidotes for overexposure.

If pregnancy is contemplated, it may be advisable to defer conception for 3 months after documented overexposure. There are no grounds for recommending a therapeutic abortion for anesthesia personnel who become pregnant or for the pregnant worker with a one-time overexposure. The overexposed worker, however, should be offered alternative duty away from all hospital reproductive hazards for the remainder of the pregnancy or until appropriate control measures are implemented. The hospital safety department must be informed of the incident so that it can be remedied for the protection of the patient and other workers.

There is currently no OSHA requirement to perform medical surveillance on workers handling anesthetics. Under its Hazard Communication Standard, OSHA does mandate that workers be informed of potential hazards of their work environment. Additionally, NIOSH recommends that workers exposed to anesthetic gases have medical histories that include family, genetic, reproductive, and occupational histories on file and that baseline data be obtained on the hepatic, renal, and hematopoietic systems. Liver and kidney function should be monitored periodically in exposed workers (1).

## Prevention

Prevention of overexposure to anesthetic gases in the operating room is achieved primarily through engineering controls. The International Labour Office suggests three steps to control exposure to anesthetic gases (71): (*a*) install a proper nonrecirculating air conditioning system with a minimum of 20 room air exchanges per hour; (*b*) install a scavenger system for collecting waste gases at the anesthetic breathing level; and (*c*) use low-flow rates of anesthetic gases.

Periodic environmental sampling for specific anesthetic agents should be performed to evaluate engineering controls and work practices. Records of these measures should be kept in workers' medical files. Several excellent reviews of exposure control methods are available (44, 72, 73).

## SEX STEROID HORMONES

The evidence for reproductive or developmental toxicity from occupational sex steroid hormone exposure is relatively sparse. There are, however, a few reports involving the estrogens that deserve review.

## Properties and Occurrence

The estrogens are steroid hormones synthesized by the ovary from cholesterol. The biosynthetic pathway ultimately yields three main estrogenic forms, the most potent being 17-β

estradiol (5). During pregnancy, the placenta also synthesizes estrogen; in men, the testes produce small amounts of estradiol and estrone. The biological actions of estrogens influence the primary and secondary sex characteristics of the female including growth and development of the vagina, uterus, and fallopian tubes; breast enlargement; skeletal growth; growth of axillary and pubic hair; and regional pigmentation of the skin of the nipples and genital region. Estrogens play a vital regulatory role in the menstrual cycle. Estrogens stimulate endometrial proliferation, and the decline in sex steroid hormone concentrations toward the end of the cycle results in menstruation.

Primary concerns about occupational exposure relate to pharmaceutical manufacturing of synthetic estrogens rather than the hospital setting, although nonmanufacturing exposure opportunities are possible. Only two studies have reported occupational exposure to estrogens in detail, and they have involved pharmaceutical production. In one study, estrogen exposure was ascertained by questionnaire (74); in the other, area and personal air samples, as well as blood levels of estrogens in workers, were determined (75). There are no reports of occupational exposure in a hospital or pharmacy setting.

## Toxicology

### METABOLISM

Estrogens are readily absorbed through the skin and mucous membranes. When applied locally, absorption is sufficient to produce systemic effects (5). The estrogens are also well absorbed through the gastrointestinal tract. The natural estrogens are metabolized and inactivated in the liver and excreted in the urine. Several derivatives of the natural estrogens, such as ethinyl estradiol and the nonsteroidal estrogens, are effective orally due to slow inactivation in the body. Ingestion (from contaminated hands) is, therefore, another potential route of exposure for pharmaceutical workers.

### MECHANISMS OF ACTION

Estrogens exert their effects at the nuclear level of the cell in estrogen-responsive tissues (female reproductive tract, breast, pituitary, and hypothalamus). Uptake occurs first through a cytoplasmic and then through a nuclear receptor site. Once inside the nucleus, metabolic processes ensue including synthesis of mRNA and proteins and, ultimately, DNA synthesis.

## REPRODUCTIVE HEALTH EFFECTS

### Experimental Animal Studies

The teratogenic effects of estrogen administration in animals have been confined primarily to intersexual changes. When estrogens are administered, male offspring tend to retain mullerian duct derivatives and female-type genitalia, with suppression of male-type structures. Conversely, androgen administration causes female infants to retain wolffian duct derivatives and male-type genitalia. Numerous studies have documented these effects. For example, Greene et al. (76, 77) reported estrogen-induced feminization of the external genitalia of male fetuses with testes retained in the female position and reduction or absence of the epididymis, vas deferens, seminal vesicles, and prostate. Burns (78) produced ovotestes by treating premature opossum embryos with topical estradiol diproprionate. Yasuda et al. (79) produced ovotestes and intra-abdominal testes with persistent mullerian and wolffian ducts in male fetuses after estradiol administration on days 11–17 of gestation.

There are also a few reports of nonreproductive organ defects from estrogen exposure. In one study, cleft palates occurred in 14% of mouse fetuses after injecting pregnant females with 1 mg estradiol on days 11–16 of gestation and in 12.4% of offspring after maternal estrone injection. The incidence of cleft palate among control fetuses was 0.7% (80).

### Human Studies

There is significant controversy in the literature concerning the teratogenic effects of estrogens in humans. Since the late 1960s, a number of studies have found a positive relationship between exposure to exogenous sex hormones during pregnancy and the birth of malformed infants. Different patterns of anomalies have been reported including neural tube defects (81), cardiovascular malformations (82, 83), and limb reduction defects (84). Numerous other reports have failed to demonstrate an association between exogenous sex hormone exposure and nongenital malformations (85–88). This controversy was extensively reviewed by Wilson and Brent (89) who concluded that a relationship between sex steroid exposure and teratogenic outcomes in nongenital structures is unlikely. Their assertion is based on the epidemiological limitations of many of the studies and the absence of a known mechanism whereby sex hormones could influence development of organs lacking specific hormone-receptor sites. However, because it is impossible to prove that exposure to sex steroids does not cause a malformation in some rare circumstances, they advise prudent use of these agents during pregnancy.

The transplacental carcinogenesis of diethylstilbestrol (DES), a nonsteroidal estrogen, is well established (Chapter 7). This drug causes adenocarcinoma of the vagina in female offspring of treated mothers and disorders of reproductive function in male and female offspring (90, 91). Other suggestions of the carcinogenicity of estrogens have since been raised (92).

Estrogens have also been used as postcoital contraceptives (93, 94). While possible mechanisms for this action are controversial, the result is early pregnancy loss. This additional effect of estrogen is important to the following review of reproductive outcomes in an occupationally exposed population.

### Occupational Studies

Several studies have investigated occupational exposure to estrogens in the pharmaceutical manufacturing setting. A Polish study reported signs of hyperestrogenism in nine women, one man, and seven children following the adults' occupational exposure to DES and other estrogens in a pharmacy plant (95). A U.S. report noted feminizing effects in male workers manufacturing DES (96).

A detailed investigation of a plant in Puerto Rico (75) that formulated oral contraceptives reported gynecomastia or decreased libido in exposed male workers and intermenstrual bleeding in exposed female workers. Personal and area air samples were collected and evaluated for mestranol and norethindrone, and blood was drawn from workers for plasma ethinyl estradiol determinations. All of the affected males (4 of 4) had clinically apparent or a history of gynecomastia and worked in areas with the highest potential exposure to powdered active ingredients. In the highest exposure category, 7 of 28 workers had elevated plasma ethinyl estradiol levels. However, when the data from all 55 workers were stratified into low and high exposure groups, no statistically significant difference in ethinyl estradiol levels was found. The prevalence of intermenstrual bleeding in exposed women was compared with nonexposed controls drawn from local well-women clinics. A matched-pair analysis revealed a relative risk of intermenstrual bleeding for exposed women of 4.26 (95% CI = 1.61–11.26).

In a more recent survey of pregnancy outcomes among women working in the pharmaceutical industry, an increased odds ratio of 4.2 (p = 0.05) was found for spontaneous abortions in women exposed to estrogens during the first trimester of pregnancy (74). While other factors causing spontaneous abortion cannot be excluded, the use of estrogen as a postcoital contraceptive and reports of first trimester fetal losses in women who conceive while using oral contraceptives (97) makes an association between occupational estrogen exposure and spontaneous abortion plausible.

## Clinical Assessment

Clinical assessment includes a history and physical examination focused on symptoms and signs of hyperestrogenism. These markers include loss of libido, gynecomastia, and impotence in males, and intermenstrual bleeding or menorrhagia in females. A careful reproductive history must also be taken from both sexes to identify a history of infertility (possibly due to unrecognized early fetal loss), spontaneous abortion, or malformations or cancer in offspring. Special attention is paid to a history of cancer in estrogen-dependent organs such as the breast, uterus, or prostate. In the absence of adequate environmental sampling data, blood for a specific estrogen level (if agents are known) can be taken for documentation pur-

poses. However, opportunity for exposure and clinical signs and symptoms should take precedence over biological monitoring data that may be limited by technical problems with the assay, half-life of the agent in the circulation, or individual metabolic differences.

## Prevention and Treatment

Primary prevention of overexposure to estrogens in pharmaceutical manufacture depends on engineering controls and good work practices. Exposure to estrogen dust via skin and inhalation can be all but eliminated by enclosing dusty processes, installing efficient local exhaust ventilation, and by having workers use appropriate protective apparel. The OSHA Hazard Communication Standard requires employers to disclose to workers potential health hazards present in the work environment. This standard also applies here and should include information about the potential effects on both workers and their offspring.

While not required by OSHA, many large pharmaceutical plants perform routine pre-employment and periodic medical surveillance on their manufacturing employees to obtain medical history and physical examination data, including comprehensive reproductive histories.

## CONCLUSION

This chapter has reviewed three classes of pharmaceuticals that are potential reproductive health hazards for workers occupationally exposed. Based on their genotoxicity and other mechanisms of action, evidence for the risks caused by antineoplastics is probably the strongest. They are particularly problematic because of difficulties protecting workers during drug handling. There is also epidemiological evidence for a modest reproductive risk from exposure to inhalation anesthetics. It may be, however, that widespread attention to this problem has resulted in better hygiene in operating rooms, with lower resultant waste gas exposure. While evidence for the teratogenicity of estrogens remains controversial, estrogen's postcoital contraceptive effect makes it a possible cause of early fetal loss in exposed workers. Overexposure to estrogens has occurred in pharmaceutical manufacture in the past. Again, however, improved industrial hygiene practices and engineering controls may have greatly reduced exposure-related health risks. Obstetricians and other health practitioners must be aware that workers handling these three types of pharmaceuticals may be at increased risk of adverse reproductive outcomes. Taking an adequate work history may, therefore, sufficiently widen a differential diagnosis to identify an occupationally induced problem correctly.

## REFERENCES

1. National Institute for Occupational Safety and Health. Guidelines for protecting the safety and health of health care workers. DHHS (NIOSH) publ. no. 88–119. Washington, D.C.: U.S. Government Printing Office, 1988.

2. Briggs GG, Freeman RK, Yaffe SJ. Drugs in pregnancy and lactation. 3rd ed. Baltimore: William & Wilkins, 1990.

3. American Society of Hospital Pharmacists. Technical assistance bulletin on handling cytotoxic and hazardous drugs. Am J Hosp Pharm 1990;47:1033–1049.

4. Gililland J, Weinstein L. The effects of cancer chemotherapeutic agents on the developing fetus. Obstet Gynecol Surv 1983;38:6–13.

5. Gilman GA, Rall TW, Nies AS, Taylor P, eds. The pharmacological basis of therapeutics. 8th ed. New York: Pergamon Press, 1990.

6. Davis JL, Prout MN, McDenna PJ, Cole D, Korbity B. Acute leukemia complicating metastatic breast cancer. Cancer 1973;31:543–546.

7. Reimer RR, Hoover R, Fraumeni JF. Acute leukemia after alkylating agent therapy of ovarian cancer. N Engl J Med 1977;297:177–181.

8. International Agency for Research on Cancer (IARC). Chemicals, industrial processes, and industries associated with cancer in humans. Vol. 1–29. IARC Monographs 1982;Suppl 4:292.

9. Vainio H. Carcinogenesis and teratogenesis may have common mechanisms. Scand J Work Environ Health 1989;15:13–17.

10. Trosko JE, Yoffi LP, Warren ST, Tsushimoto G, Chang C. Inhibitors of cell-cell communication by tumor promotors. Carcinog Compr Surv 1987;565–585.

11. Richter P, Calamera JC, Morgenfeld MC, Kierszenbaum AL, Lavieri JC, Mancini RE. Effect of chlorambucil on spermatogenesis in the human with malignant lymphoma. Cancer 1970;25:1026–1030.

12. Miller DG. Alkylating agents and human spermatogenesis. JAMA 1971;217:1662–1665.

13. Cheviakoff S, Calamera JC, Morgenfeld MC, Mancini RE. Recovery of spermatogenesis in patients with lymphoma after treatment with chlorambucil. J Reprod Fertil 1973;33:155–157.

14. Immel L, Schirren C. Azoospermia caused by cytostatic treatment. Z Haut Geschlechtskr 1967;42:643–646.

15. Fairley KF, Barrie JU, Johnson W. Sterility and testicular atrophy related to cyclophosphamide therapy. Lancet 1972;1:568–569.

16. Kumar R, Biggart JD, McEvoy J, McGeown MG. Cyclophosphamide and reproductive function. Lancet 1972;1:1212–1214.

17. Hinkes E, Plotkin D. Reversible drug-induced sterility in a patient with acute leukemia. JAMA 1973;223:1490–1491.

18. Freckman HA, Fry HL, Mendez FL, Maures ER. Chlorambucil-prednisolone therapy for disseminated breast carcinoma. JAMA 1964;189:23–26.

19. Uldall PR, Kerr DN, Tacchi D. Sterility and cyclophosphamide. Lancet 1972;1:693–694.

20. Cameron JS, Ogg CS. Sterility and cyclophosphamide. Lancet 1972;1:1174–1175.

21. Sieber SM, Adamson RH. Toxicity of antineoplastic agents in man: chromosomal aberrations, antifertility effects, congenital malformations and carcinogenic potential. Adv Cancer Res 1975;22:57–155.

22. Chapman R. Gonadal injury resulting from chemotherapy. Am J Ind Med 1983;4:149–162.

23. Trasler JM, Hales BF, Robaire B. Chronic low dose cyclophosphamide treatment of adult male rats: effects on fertility, pregnancy outcome and progeny. Biol Reprod 1986;34:275–283.

24. Adams PM, Fabricant JD, Legator MS. Cyclophosphamide-induced spermatogenic effects detected in the $F_1$ generation by behavioral testing. Science 1981;24:80–82.

25. Greenberg LH, Tanaka KR. Congenital anomalies probably induced by cyclophosphamide. JAMA 1964; 188:423–426.

26. Toledo TM, Harper RC, Moser RH. Fetal effects during cyclophosphamide and irradiation therapy. Ann Intern Med 1971;74:87–91.

27. Diamond I, Anderson MM, McCreadie SR. Transplacental transmission of busulfan (myleran) in a mother with leukemia. Pediatrics 1960;25:85–90.

28. Boros SJ, Reynolds JW. Intrauterine growth retardation following third trimester exposure to busulfan. Am J Obstet Gynecol 1977;129:111–112.

29. Shotton D, Monie IW. Possible teratogenic effect of chlorambucil on a human fetus. JAMA 1963;186:74–75.

30. Garrett MJ. Teratogenic effects of combination chemotherapy. Ann Intern Med 1974;80:667.

31. Mennuti MT, Shepard TH, Mellman WJ. Fetal renal malformation following treatment of Hodgkin's disease during pregnancy. Obstet Gynecol 1975;46:194–196.

32. Stutzman L, Sokal JE. Use of anticancer drugs during pregnancy. Clin Obstet Gynecol 1968;11:416–427.

33. Stephens JD, Golbus MS, Miller TR, Wilber RR, Epstein CJ. Multiple congenital anomalies in a fetus exposed to 5-fluorouracil during the first trimester. Am J Obstet Gynecol 1980;137:747–749.

34. Nicholson HD. Cytotoxic drugs in pregnancy. J Obstet Gynecol Br Commonw 1968;75:307–312.

35. Green DM, Zevon MA, Lowrie G, Seigelstein N, Hall B. Congenital anomalies in children of patients who received chemotherapy for cancer in childhood and adolescence. N Engl J Med 1991;325:141–146.

36. Falck K, Grohn P, Sorsa M, et al. Mutagenicity in urine of nurses handling cytostatic drugs. Lancet 1979;1:1250–1251.

37. Waksvik H, Kleep O, Brogger A. Chromosome analyses of nurses handling cytostatic agents. Cancer Treat Rev 1981;65:607–610.

38. Nguyen TV, Theiss TC, Matney TS. Exposure of pharmacy personnel to mutagenic antineoplastic drugs. Cancer Res 1982;42:4792–4799

39. Hirst M, Mills DG, Tse S, et al. Occupational exposure to cyclophosphamide. Lancet 1984;1:186–188.

40. Hemminki K, Kyyrgronen P, Lindbohm M-L. Spontaneous abortions and malformations in the offspring of nurses exposed to anesthetic gases and other hazards. J Epidemiol Commun Health 1985;39:141–147.

41. Selevan S, Lindbohm M-L, Hornung RW, et al. A study of occupational exposure to antineoplastic drugs and fetal loss in nurses. N Engl J Med 1985;313:1173–1178.

42. Yodaiken RE: OSHA work practice guidelines for personnel dealing with cytotoxic drugs. Am J Hosp Pharm 1986;43:1193–1204.

43. McDiarmid MA. Medical surveillance for antineoplastic drug handlers. Am J Hosp Pharm 1990;47:1061–1066.

44. National Institute for Occupational Safety and Health. Criteria for a recommended standard: occupational exposure to waste anesthetic gases and vapors. DHEW (NIOSH) publication no. 77–140. Cincinnati: U.S. Department of Health, Education and Welfare, 1977.

45. Linde HW, Bruce DL. Occupational exposure of anesthesiologists to halothane, $N_2O$ and radiation. Anesthesiology 1969;30:363–368.

46. Askrog V, Petersen R. Forurening of operationsstuer med lurtformige anaestetika og reontgenbestroaling. Saertryk Nord Med 1970;83:501–504.

47. Vainio H. Inhalation anesthetics, anticancer drugs and sterilants as chemical hazards in hospitals. Scand J Work Environ Health 1982;8:94–107.

48. Garro AJ, Phillips RA. Mutagenicity of the halogenated olefin, 2-bromo-2-chloro-1,1,-difluoroethylene presumed metabolite of the inhalation anesthetic halothane. Mutat Res 1978;54:17–22.

49. Garrett S, Fuerst R. Sex-linked mutations in *Drosophila* after exposure to various mixtures of gas atmospheres. Environ Res 1974;7:286–293.

50. Cohen EN, Brown BW, Bruce DL, et al. Occupational disease among operating room personnel: a national study. Anesthesiology 1974;41:321–340.

51. Goldstein BD, Paz J, Guiffrid JG, Palmes ED, Ferrand EF. Atmospheric derivatives of anesthetic gases as a possible hazard to operating room personnel. Lancet 1976;2:235–237.

52. Gofmeckler VA, Bekhman II, Golotin FG. The embryotropic action of nitrogen dioxide and a complex of atmospheric pollutants. Gigiena I Sanitariya 1977;12:22–27.

53. Shepard TH, Fink BR. Teratogenic activity of nitrous oxide in rats. In: Fink BF, ed. Toxicity of anesthetics: proceedings of a research symposium held in Seattle, May 12–13, 1967. Baltimore: Williams & Wilkins, 1968:308.

54. Smith BE, Gaub ML and Moya F. Teratogenic effects of anesthetic agents: nitrous oxide. Anesth Analg 1965;44:726–732.

55. Fink BR, Shepard TH, Blandau RJ. Teratogenic activity of nitrous oxide. Nature 1967;214:146–148.

56. Bussard DA, Stoelting RK, Peterson C, Sshaq M. Fetal changes in hamsters anesthetized with nitrous oxide and halothane. Anesthesiology 1974;41:275–278.

57. Baeder CH, Albrecht M. Embryotoxic/teratogenic potential of halothane. Int Arch Occup Environ Health 1990;62:263–271.

58. Kennedy GL, Smith SH, Keplinger ML, Calandra JC. Reproductive and teratologic studies with halothane. Toxicol Appl Pharmacol 1976;35:467–474.

59. Corbett TH, Cornell RG, Endres JL, Millard RI. Effects of low concentrations of nitrous oxide on rat pregnancy. Anesthesiology 1973;39:299–301.

60. Vaisman AI. Work in operating theaters and its effect on the health of anesthesiologists. Eksp Khir Anestheziol 1967;12:44–49.

61. Cohen EN, Bellville JW, Brown BW. Anesthesia, pregnancy and miscarriage. A study of operating room nurses and anesthetists. Anesthesiology 1971;35:343–347.

62. Kline JK. Maternal occupation: effects on spontaneous abortions and malformations. In: Stein AZ, Hatch MC, eds. Reproductive problems in the workplace. Occupational medicine: state of the art reviews. Philadelphia: Hanley & Belfus Inc., 1986:381–403.

63. Cohen EN, Brown BW, Bruce DL, Cascorbi HF, Corbett TH, Jones TW, Whitcher CH. Occupational disease among operating room personnel: a national study. Anesthesiology 1974;41:321–340.

64. Corbett TH, Cornell RG, Endres JL, Lieding K. Birth defects among children of nurse-anesthetists. Anesthesiology 1974;41:341–344.

65. Knill-Jones RP, Newman BJ, Spence AA. Anesthetic practice and pregnancy: controlled survey of male anesthetists in the United Kingdom. Lancet 1975;2:807–809.

66. Cohen EN, Brown BW, Wm ML, Whitcher CE, Brodsky JB, Gift HC, Greenfield W, Jones TW, Driscoll EJ. Occupational disease in dentistry and chronic exposure to trace anesthetic gases. J Am Dent Assoc 1980;101:21–31.

67. Axelsson G, Rylander R. Exposure to anesthetic gases and spontaneous abortion: response bias in a postal questionnaire. Int J Epidemiol 1982;11:250–256.

68. Hemminki K, Kyyronen P, Lindbohm MJ. Spontaneous abortions and malformations in the offspring of nurses exposed to anesthetic gases, cytostatic drugs and other potential hazards in hospitals, based on registered information of outcome. J Epidemiol Commun Health 1985;39:141–147.

69. Guirguis SS, Pelmear PL, Roy ML, Wong L. Health effects associated with exposure to anaesthetic gases in Ontario hospital personnel. Br J Ind Med 1990;47:490–497.

70. Rajhans GS, Brown DA, Whaley D, Wong L, Guirguis SS. Hygiene aspects of occupational exposure to waste anaesthetic gases in Ontario hospitals. Ann Occup Hyg 1989;33:27–45.

71. Parmeggiani L, ed. Encyclopedia of occupational health and safety. 3rd (revised) ed. Geneva, Switzerland: International Labour Office, 1983.

72. Whitcher C. Occupational exposure to inhalation anesthetics: an update. Plant technology and safety management series no. 4: hazardous waste management—controlling asbestos and waste anesthetic gases. Chicago: Joint Commission on Accreditation of Healthcare Organizations, 1987:35–45.

73. Guidman LJ, Smith NT. Monitoring occupational exposure to inhalation anesthetics. Stoneham, MA: Butterworth Publishers, 1984:367–403.

74. Taskinen H, Lindbohm ML, Hemminki K. Spontaneous abortions among women working in the pharmaceutical industry. Br J Ind Med 1986;43:199–205.

75. Harrington JM, Stein GF, Rivera RO, de Morales AV. The occupational hazards of formulating oral contraceptives: a survey of plant employees. Arch Environ Health 1978;33:12–15.

76. Greene RR, Burrill MW, Ivy AC. Experimental intersexuality: the paradoxical effects of estrogens on the sexual development of the female rat. Anat Rec 1939;74:429–438.

77. Greene RR, Burrill MW, Ivy AC. Experimental intersexuality: the effects of estrogens on the antenatal sexual development of the rat. Am J Anat 1940;67:305–345.

78. Burns RK. Experimental reversal of sex in the gonads of the opossum Didelphis Virginiana. Proc Nat Acad Sci (USA) 1955;41:669–676.

79. Yasuda Y, Kihara T, Tanimura T, Nishimura H. Gonadal dysgenesis induced by prenatal exposure to ethinyl estradiol in mice. Teratology 1985;32:219–227.

80. Nishihara G. Influence of female sex hormones in experimental teratogenesis. Proc Soc Exp Biol Med 1958;97:809–812.

81. Gal I, Kirman B, Stern J. Hormonal pregnancy tests and congenital malformations. Nature 1967;216:83.

82. Levy EP, Cohen A, Fraser FC: Hormone treatment during pregnancy and congenital heart disease. Lancet 1973;1:611.

83. Janerich DT, Dugan JM, Standfast SF, Strite L. Congenital heart disease and prenatal exposure to exogenous sex hormones. Br Med J 1977;1:1058–1060.

84. Jaffe P, Liberman MM, McFadyen I, Valman HB. Incidence of congenital limb reduction deformities. Lancet 1975;1:526–527.

85. Mulvihill JJ, Mulvihill CG, Neill CA. Prenatal sex-hormone exposure and cardiac defects in man. Teratology 1974;9:A–30.

86. Nishimura H, Uwabe C, Semba R. Examination of teratogenicity of progestogens and or estrogens by observation of the induced abortuses. Teratology 1974;10:93.

87. Yasuda M, Miller JR. Prenatal exposure to oral contraceptives and transposition of the great vessels in man. Teratology 1975;12:239–243.

88. Wiseman RA, Dodda-Smith IC. Cardiovascular birth defects and antenatal exposure to female sex hormones: a re-evaluation of some base data. Teratology 1984; 30: 359–370.

89. Wilson JG, Brent RL. Are female sex hormones teratogenic? Am J Obstet Gynecol 1981;141:567–580.

90. Greenwald P, Barlow JJ, Nasca PC, Burnett WS. Vaginal cancer after maternal treatment with synthetic estrogens. N Engl J Med 1971;285:390–392.

91. Herbst AL, Kurman RJ, Scully RE, Poslanzer DC. Clear-cell adenocarcinoma of the genital tract in young females. N Engl J Med 1972;287:1259–1264.

92. Black MM, Leis HP. Mammary carcinogenesis. Influence of parity and estrogens. NY St J Med 1972;72: 1601–1605.

93. Blye RP. The use of estrogens as postcoital contraceptive agents. Am J Obstet Gynecol 1981;141:567–580.

94. Dixon GW, Schlesselman JJ, Ory HW, Blye RP. Ethinyl estradiol and conjugated estrogens as postcoital contraceptives. JAMA 1980;244:1336–1339.

95. Pacynski A, Budzynska A, Przylecki S. Hiperestrogenizm v pracownikow zakladow farmaceutyczaych i ich dzieci jako choroba zawodowa. Endokrynol Pol (Warsaw) 1971;22:149–154.

96. U.S. Department of Health, Education and Welfare, National Institute for Occupational Safety and Health. Health hazard evaluation report, publ. no. 71–79. Cincinnati: National Institute for Occupational Safety and Health, 1973.

97. Harlap S, Shions PH, Ramcharan S. Spontaneous fetal losses in women using different contraceptives around the time of conception. Int J Epidemiol 1980;9:49–56.

98. Knill-Jones RP, Rodrigues LV, Moir DD. Anesthetic practice and pregnancy: controlled survey of women anesthetists in the United Kingdom. Lancet 1972;1: 1326–1328.

99. Rosenberg P, Kirves A. Miscarriages among operating theater staff. Acta Anesthesiol Scand 1973;53:37–42.

100. Pharoah PO, Alberman E, Doyle P, Chamberlain G. Outcome of pregnancy among women in anesthetic practice. Lancet 1977;1:34–36.

101. Ericson A, Kallen B. Survey of infants born in 1973 or 1975 to Swedish women working in operating rooms during their pregnancies. Anesth Analg 1979;58:302–305.

# 21

.................................................

# Pesticides

## MARION MOSES

Pesticide exposure can be a risk factor for sterility, spontaneous abortion, stillbirth, and birth defects. For certain pesticides, such as the soil fumigant dibromochloropropane (DBCP), the evidence is incontrovertible; for others, such as the herbicide 2,4,5-trichloro-phenoxy acetic acid (2,4,5-T), the evidence is more controversial. Both DBCP and 2,4,5-T are now banned in the United States (Table 21.1).

Most cases of adverse reproductive outcome with putative pesticide exposure do not present to the primary care provider with apparent clinical illness or as a life-threatening poisoning. The client may not know what pesticide is involved or be able to describe the exposures in even a qualitative way. Fear and anxiety may be associated with a strong odor or irritant effects. Often, the exposure occurred several months or more in the past. Parental concerns usually relate to the risk of birth defects in a current pregnancy or whether pesticide exposure could be associated with adverse outcome that has already occurred, such as spontaneous abortion, stillbirth, or birth defects.

Pesticides must be registered with the Environmental Protection Agency (EPA) before they are manufactured or sold in the U.S. There are 729 active ingredient pesticides and 1200 "inert" ingredients formulated into 21,000 different registered pesticide products. Although inert ingredients are not active as

pesticides, they can be more toxic than the pesticide itself or enhance its toxicity. Acute or chronic health effects may be related to the active ingredient pesticide, the inert ingredient, or a combination of the two.

It can be difficult and very time-consuming to obtain information about a specific pesticide's potential for inducing adverse reproductive or other chronic effects; such information is not required to be on the pesticide label. Many pesticides are teratogenic, embryotoxic, or fetotoxic. Other potential effects include impaired fertility, sterility, chromosomal abnormalities, genetic mutations, and adverse effects on DNA synthesis or repair. The state of California requires chronic toxicity data as a condition for continuing registration of pesticides for use in the state. The chapter Appendix summarizes the toxicological data for the pesticides evaluated so far by state toxicologists. Table 21.2 lists some widely used pesticides considered to be teratogens by the EPA.

## USAGE

Agriculture accounts for 80% of the 1 billion pounds of pesticides used annually in the U.S. (1). (Table 21.3). An additional 1 billion pounds are used for wood preservation, including primarily creosote on railroad ties, but also pentachlorophenol, copper, and arsenic compounds for utility poles, dock pilings, and lumber.

**Table 21.1.**
**Pesticides Banned, Suspended, or Severely Restricted in the U.S.**

| Pesticide | Action | Year |
|---|---|---|
| Alar (daminozide) | All food uses canceled | 1990 |
| Aldrin | All uses canceled except termite control | 1974 |
| BHC | All uses canceled | 1978 |
| Chlordane | Cancellation most uses, except termite control | 1978 |
|  | All uses canceled | 1988 |
| Chlordimeform | Registration voluntarily withdrawn | 1989 |
| DBCP | All uses canceled except pineapple in Hawaii | 1979 |
|  | All uses canceled | 1985 |
| DDT | All agricultural use canceled | 1972 |
|  | Used only for public health emergencies |  |
| Diazinon | Use on golf courses, sod farms canceled | 1986 |
| Dieldrin | Cancellation of most uses | 1974 |
| Dinoseb | Emergency suspension, registration canceled | 1986 |
| Ethylene dibromide (EDB) | All uses canceled | 1984 |
| Endrin | Voluntary cancellation | 1985 |
| EPN | Use as mosquito larvacide canceled | 1983 |
| Heptachlor | All uses canceled except seed treatment | 1978 |
|  | Seed treatment use canceled | 1989 |
| Lindane | Indoor smoke fumigation use canceled | 1986 |
| Maleic hydrazide | All uses suspended | 1981 |
| Mirex | All uses canceled except pineapples in Hawaii | 1977 |
| Nitrofen (TOK) | Voluntary cancellation | 1983 |
| 2,4,5-T/Silvex | Emergency suspension | 1979 |
|  | All uses canceled | 1985 |
| Toxaphene | All uses canceled except sheep/cattle dip and bananas/ pineapple in Puerto Rico and Virgin Islands | 1982 |

**Table 21.2.**
**Selected Pesticides Listed As Teratogens by the U.S. Environmental Protection Agency**

| Fungicides | Herbicides | Insecticides |
|---|---|---|
| Benomyl | Acrolein (Aqualin) | Avermectin |
| Captafol | Bentazon (Basagran) | Chlordimeform |
| Folpet | Cyanazine (Bladex) | Endosulfan |
| Hexachlorobenzene | Bromoxynil 24-D | Ethion |
| Mancozeb | Dinocap | Imidan (phosmet) |
| Maneb | Dinoseb | Methyl parathion |
| Tributyltin oxide | Diquat | Mirex |
| Triphenyltin fluoride | Fluazifop-butyl | Trichlorfon |
| Triphenyltin acetate | (Fusilade) |  |
|  | Nitrofen (TOK) |  |
|  | Picloram |  |
|  | Sodium arsenite |  |
|  | 2,4,5-T |  |
|  | Trifulralin |  |

**Table 21.3.**
**Selected Pesticides Widely Used in Agriculture in the U.S.**

| Insecticides | Herbicides | Fungicides |
|---|---|---|
| Aldicarb (Temik) | Alachlor (Lasso) | Benomyl (Benlate)[a] |
| Azinphosmethyl (Guthion) | Atrazine[a] | Captan[a] |
| Carbaryl (Sevin)[a] | 2,4-D[a] | Chlorothalonil (Bravo)[a] |
| Carbofuran (Furadan) | Glyphosate | Maneb (Dithane)[a] |
| Chlorpyrifos (Lorsban, | (Roundup)[a] | Mancozeb (Dithane) |
| Dursban)[a] | Paraquat | Triadimefon (Bayleton) |
| DD (Telone II) | (Gramoxone) | Sulfur |
| Diazinon (Spectracide)[a] | Simazine[a] | |
| Dichlorvos (DDVP)[a] | Trifluralin (Treflan) | |
| Malathion[a] | | |
| Methamidophos (Monitor) | | |
| Methomyl (Lannate) | | |
| Methyl bromide[a] | | |
| Methoxyychlor[a] | | |
| Mevinphos (Phosdrin) | | |

[a]Pesticides with extensive nonagricultural use.

Nonagricultural pesticide uses include the following:

(a) *Structural pest control*. Pesticides are used in the treatment of office buildings, schools, hotels, hospitals, theaters, supermarkets, department stores, restaurants, sports facilities, food storage facilities, aircraft, and homes to control insects and other pests.

(b) *Lawn care and turf management*. Use of insecticides, fungicides, and herbicides is extensive in the treatment of home and commercial lawns, golf courses, park and recreation areas, and for other turf management.

(c) *Maintenance of right-of-way*. Herbicides are widely used for brush and weed management on highways, railroad beds, and power transmission lines.

(d) *Industrial use*. Pesticides are used in paints, glues, pastes, metal-working fluids; in fabrics such as tents, tarpaulins, sails, tennis nets, exercise mats, carpets, upholstery; and in a wide variety of consumer products including cosmetics, shampoos, soaps, household disinfectants, cardboard and other food packaging materials, and many paper products. Water in cooling towers is treated to prevent growth of weeds, algae, fungi, and bacteria, as are canals, ditches, reservoirs, and other water channels.

(e) *Over-the-counter*. Approximately 65 million pounds of pesticides are sold directly to the consumer as aerosols, foggers, pest strips, baits, pet products, lawn and garden chemicals, and insect repellents. With few exceptions, most of the pesticides in home and garden products are different formulations of pesticides used in agriculture.

(f) *Public health*. In the U.S., this use includes primarily mosquito and rodent control and treatment of drinking water. In addition, defoliants and herbicides are used by the federal government for drug eradication programs on federally owned land.

## SOURCES OF EXPOSURE

Exposure to pesticides is ubiquitous because of widespread use in agriculture and the ready availability and use of over-the-counter products and commercial pest control services.

## Occupational Exposures

Workers who handle pesticides or are in contact with crops or commodities sprayed with them have the greatest potential exposures. This category includes workers who mix, load, and apply pesticides in agriculture; structural pest control operators (exterminators); chemical lawn company sprayers; workers employed in maintenance of right-of-way on highways, railroad lines, and parks, golf courses, and other recreation areas; mosquito abatement workers; pet groomers; farm workers; greenhouse and nursery workers; and florists. Janitorial and custodial workers in schools, offices, and other buildings may also be exposed. Exposures may be much lower in pesticide manufacturing workers, since batch processing and closed systems require almost no direct contact.

## Exposure to Community Residents and Bystanders

Rural agricultural community residents surrounded by fruit orchards, citrus groves, or cotton or other fields that are regularly and repeatedly sprayed are potentially exposed to a great variety of pesticides. Suburban residents are increasingly at risk as farm land is purchased and housing developments are built adjacent to agricultural groves, orchards, and fields.

Whether pesticides are applied from the air or on the ground, significant concentrations of pesticides can drift a mile or more from the site of initial application depending on droplet size and wind conditions; lower concentrations can drift many miles (2). Off-gassing from fields, where fumigants such as methyl bromide and metam-sodium are injected or incorporated into the soil, is also a potential source of exposure to community residents.

Populations living near areas where pesticides are manufactured, stored, or disposed have potential exposure from air emissions, water contamination, and other sources. The risk of exposure depends, in part, on toxic control policies at the facility. The transportation of pesticides can result in toxic spills. Recently, for example, derailment of a railroad tank car in California resulted in the release of metam-sodium (a teratogen) into the Sacramento River, killing millions of fish and putting community residents at risk.

## Exposure to the General Public

The general public's exposure to pesticides is ubiquitous because use in agriculture and ani-

mal husbandry results in residues in fresh and processed food and in milk, eggs, meat, fish, and other animal products. The public has expressed a high level of concern about these residues in food. While it is unlikely that typical amounts of pesticide residues in food are sufficient to produce adverse reproductive outcomes, this possibility must be considered in cases of misuse. Among the thousands of consumers poisoned from the illegal application of aldicarb (Temik) to watermelon in California in 1985 were two women who delivered premature, stillborn infants.

Pesticide residues in food are much lower than more direct exposures resulting from use of pesticide services and products for home and garden applications (e.g., insect control, chemical lawn treatment). Recent EPA studies measuring the concentration of pesticides indoors show that residues can persist for long periods of time after application. Another source of direct exposure includes pesticides applied to the skin, such as insect repellents or preparations for the treatment of lice and scabies.

## ABSORPTION AND METABOLIC FATE

Pesticides are readily absorbed through the skin, the respiratory tract, and the gastrointestinal tract. The eye also absorbs pesticides and can be a significant route of exposure with splashes and spills. Most pesticides cross the placenta in humans.

The major route of occupational exposure to pesticides is the skin, and not, as commonly believed, the respiratory system. Fumigants, which are in the form of gases, are a notable exception; however, the skin is a route of absorption for them as well. Pesticides can persist on the skin for many months after the last known exposure (3). The respiratory tract can be an important route of absorption for the general public, because many over-the-counter products are in the form of aerosols, foggers, smoke bombs, and pest strips.

The rate of absorption of pesticides into the body is product-specific and depends on the properties of the active ingredient pesticide and the inert ingredients in a particular formulation.

Dichlorodiphenyltrichloroethane (DDT) and related chlorinated hydrocarbon insecticides were widely used in agriculture from the late 1940s until the early 1970s. Because of environmental persistence, bioaccumulation in the fatty tissue of humans and animals, severe toxic effects on nontarget species (especially birds and fish), potentially devastating ecological effects, and human health concerns, most have been banned or severely restricted in the U.S., including DDT, aldrin, endrin, dieldrin, chlordane, benzene hexachloride (BHC), heptachlor, and toxaphene (Table 21.1).

Chlorinated hydrocarbon pesticides are highly lipophilic and have long half-lives. Their metabolites are persistent and ubiquitous contaminants of human adipose tissues and breast milk (Chapter 6); the most commonly found pesticides or metabolites are DDE, dieldrin, heptachlor epoxide, β-BHC, hexachlorobenzene, and the chlordane metabolites—transnonachlor and oxychlordane.

The banning of the chlorinated hydrocarbons has resulted in an increase in the use of the more acutely toxic organophosphate and N-methyl carbamate insecticides. These chemicals are responsible for most of the occupational and accidental pesticide poisonings and deaths in the U.S. Unlike the chlorinated hydrocarbons, the organophosphates and N-methyl carbamates are readily metabolized and excreted. Widely used organophosphates include parathion, azinphosmethyl (Guthion), chlorpyrifos (Dursban, Lorsban), diazinon, dichlorvos (DDVP, Vapona), methamidophos (Monitor), and malathion. Widely used N-methyl carbamates include aldicarb (Temik), methomyl (Lannate), carbofuran (Furadan), carbaryl (Sevin), and propoxur (Baygon).

## ADVERSE REPRODUCTIVE OUTCOMES

### Birth Defects

#### OCCUPATIONAL STUDIES

Frequently reported birth defects in the offspring of pesticide-exposed populations include neural tube defects, limb reduction defects, and facial clefts. An increased risk for anencephaly has been related to parental occupation of farmer and farm worker (4); neural tube defects, and a combined category of neural tube defects, facial clefts, and renal agenesis have been related to exposure to agricultural chemicals during preconception (5). Increased prevalence of neural tube defects has been observed in areas with heavy use of agricultural chemicals (6, 7).

Limb reduction defects have been associated with occupation as a farm worker and with living in an agricultural area (8, 9). The risk of limb reduction defects was also found to be greater with first trimester pesticide exposure and with repeated exposure.

Maternal pesticide exposure has been found to increase the risk for facial clefts (10, 11) as well as for all congenital malformations. Some studies have shown an increased risk for spina bifida, while others have not (5, 12). In an interview study of crop duster pilots and their sibling controls, there was no difference between the groups in number of birth defects in their offspring (13).

#### COMMUNITY-BASED STUDIES

Birth defect studies have been done in communities with concerns about environmental contamination such as Fresno County, California, where drinking water was contaminated with DBCP; the San Francisco Bay Area, where residential areas were extensively sprayed with malathion; and Oahu, Hawaii, where the island's milk supply was contaminated with heptachlor (14). No adverse developmental effects were found to be related to the exposures. However, all of the studies were ecological in design and did not determine individual exposures of the women who delivered children with birth defects.

#### CASE REPORTS

A couple heavily exposed to 2,4-dichlorophenoxy acetic acid (2,4-D) for 6 months before conception until 5 weeks after the last menstrual period had a chromosomally normal child with severe mental retardation and multiple anomalies who survived. A farm worker woman exposed to the insecticides Metasystox-R (oxydemeton), Phosdrin (mevinphos), and Lannate (methomyl) delivered a chromosomally normal child with multiple severe defects who died 2 weeks later.

## AGENT ORANGE, DIOXIN, AND PHENOXY HERBICIDES

Controversy continues to surround Agent Orange, a 50/50 combination of the phenoxy herbicides 2,4-D and 2,4,5-T used by the U.S. military in Vietnam from 1962–1969. Vietnam veterans have alleged birth defects in their children, among other chronic effects, from their exposure to Agent Orange.

The acute toxicity of 2,4-D and 2,4,5-T is relatively low, and they are readily metabolized and excreted. However, they are contaminated with dioxins, toxic byproducts found in compounds made from chlorinated phenols. There are 75 different dioxin isomers that vary greatly in toxicity. The most toxic dioxin isomer is the one that contaminates 2,4,5-T, known as 2,3,7,8-tetrachlorodibenzo-para-dioxin (2,3,7,8-TCDD). Animal studies show 2,3,7,8-TCDD to be teratogenic when fed to female, but not to male, rats; it is also carcinogenic, but not mutagenic (15). Slowly metabolized, 2,3,7,8-TCDD has been found in human blood and fat many years after the last known exposure (16, 17). It has also been found in breast milk (Chapter 6). The EPA suspended the registration of most uses of 2,4,5-T in 1979 and banned it in 1989. 2,4-D and other phenoxy herbicides can also be contaminated with dioxin, but not with 2,3,7,8-TCDD. There are hundreds of different formulations and mixtures of 2,4-D with other pesticides and fertilizers. Other widely used phenoxy herbicides include 2,4-DP (2,4-dichlorophenoxy propionic acid), 2,4-DB (2,4-dichlorophenoxy butyric acid), MCPA (2-methyl-4-chlorophenoxy acetic acid), MCPP (Mecoprop, 2,4-chloro-2-methylphenoxy propionic acid), and Dicamba (2-methyl-3,6-dichlorobenzoic acid).

Well-conducted studies of Vietnam veterans from the U.S. and Australia and of U.S. Air Force pilots (called Ranch Hands) who flew the planes that sprayed the herbicides found no significant increased risk for them to father children with birth defects (18–20). A Dow Chemical Company survey compared reproductive outcomes among wives of employees potentially exposed to dioxin through the manufacture of trichlorophenol and 2,4,5-T with those among wives of unexposed employees. The number of pregnancies (conceptions) was lower in the exposed group, but no other adverse reproductive outcomes were associated with paternal dioxin exposure (21).

An association between herbicide exposure and facial clefts or neural tube defects has been found in some, but not all, studies in the U.S., Canada, England, Australia, and New Zealand (6, 7, 10, 22–24). The studies were of agricultural sprayers of 2,4,5-T and agricultural populations living in areas of heavy herbicide use. Most were ecological studies in which birth records were reviewed but no attempt was made to document actual exposures.

In northern Italy in 1976, an explosion in a factory manufacturing trichlorophenol released a toxic cloud of 2,3,7,8-TCDD that contaminated Seveso and surrounding towns. Residents living closest to the explosion were evacuated permanently, and those further away were temporarily relocated. No major defects were found in the 26 infants born to women from the most heavily contaminated area who were in the first trimester of pregnancy at the time of the explosion. Only two minor defects were found: one infant had a small flat hemangioma and another had a periurethral cyst (25). A study of the conceptuses of several women who were pregnant at the time of the explosion and had induced abortions because of fear of birth defects found no gross developmental abnormalities and no chromosomal anomalies (26). However, a more recent report noted an increased incidence of chromosomal aberrations in fetal tissue obtained at abortion (27).

In eastern Missouri from 1971–1973, waste oil heavily contaminated with 2,3,7,8-TCDD was used for dust control in horse arenas, commercial truck terminals, church parking lots, and on dirt roads in residential areas. A study using hospital birth records compared birth outcomes among women potentially exposed during pregnancy to more than 1 part per billion (ppb) of dioxin in soil with unexposed births. Increased risks were found for infant, fetal, and perinatal death, for low birthweight, and for some subcategories of birth defects, but none were statistically significant (28).

## Spontaneous Abortion and Stillbirth

Chemical pesticides are toxic substances; many are embryotoxic and fetotoxic. An association with fetal death has been consistently found in several studies of women and men exposed to pesticides. It is possible that birth defects are not more often associated with pesticide exposures because toxicity to the conceptus results in embryofetal death.

Studies of farm worker women in Washington state and female workers in agriculture and horticulture in Finland found increased risks for spontaneous abortion and stillbirth (29, 30). One investigation found substantially increased risk for second trimester, but not first trimester, spontaneous abortion (31). In a large U.S. study of 6386 stillbirths, self-reported pesticide exposure of either parent was weakly related to the risk for stillbirth in their offspring. A study done in India of couples who worked in the vineyards as sprayers and also lived there found a much higher prevalence of spontaneous abortion and stillbirth than in a comparison group (33). The pesticides they were exposed to included DDT, lindane, Dithane M45, Metasystox, parathion, copper sulfate, dichlorvos, and dieldrin.

A study of 314 pilots of crop dusters and 178 of their nonpesticide-exposed siblings showed no difference in the prevalence of spontaneous abortion in their wives (13).

## Sterility/Infertility

Three pesticides for which there is clinical evidence of spermatotoxicity are no longer registered for use in the U.S.: dibromochloropropane (DBCP), ethylene dibromide (EDB), and chlordecone (Kepone).

## DIBROMOCHLOROPROPANE AND ETHYLENE DIBROMIDE

DBCP was widely used as a soil fumigant in agriculture in the U.S. beginning in the early 1950s. In 1977, several men working in the pesticide formulation division of the plant in California where the pesticide was manufactured and formulated reported that they had not recently fathered children. Five of the men initially tested were either azoospermic or oligospermic (sperm count <20 million/ml); all five had been exposed to DBCP.

Further study found that, of those men exposed to DBCP, 13% were azoospermic, 16.8% were oligospermic, and 15.8% had low-normal sperm counts (20–39 million/ml). Corresponding values in unexposed men were 2.9%, 0, and 5.7%. In general, the degree of sperm count suppression was related to the total duration of exposure to DBCP. Two of the sterile workers had not had any exposure to DBCP for 9 and 13 yr, respectively, and both had fathered children before their exposure. The workers in the study were otherwise healthy, and none had symptoms of clinical illness or acute poisoning related to their exposure to DBCP (34, 35).

Testicular biopsy in the most severely affected workers revealed absence of spermatogonia and spermatocytes and atrophy of seminiferous epithelium (36). Elevated serum levels of follicle-stimulating hormone (FSH) and luteinizing hormone (LH) proved to be good indicators of spermatotoxicity.

Workers exposed to DBCP in other parts of the U.S. and in Israel were also found to be azoospermic or oligospermic. Several of the affected men in both countries were followed after cessation of exposure to DBCP. None of the U.S. azoospermics showed any improvement in sperm count 5–8 yr later (37), and 9 of 13 in Israel showed no improvement after 4 yr (38); all had elevated FSH levels. The azoospermics who recovered had lower FSH and LH levels and higher testosterone levels.

Paternal exposure to DBCP sufficient to cause sperm suppression was not found to be associated with any increase in the risk of spontaneous abortion or birth defects in the offspring of men who subsequently recovered testicular function and fathered children. However, a significantly altered sex ratio was found among pregnancies conceived during spermatogenic recovery compared with those conceived before exposure and with the nonexposed (39). A study of 10 children ranging in age from 1–16 yr born to a cohort of workers who recovered from DBCP-induced spermatogenic suppression found normal physical examinations and no abnormalities in chromosomal constitution of peripheral lymphocytes (40).

Ethylene dibromide, which is very similar to DBCP, was used as a grain fumigant and as a substitute for DBCP when it was banned in 1979. Some subsequent studies found decreased fertility among workers at plants where EDB was manufactured (41). A National Institute for Occupational Safety and Health (NIOSH) investigation involving semen analyses of EDB applicators in Hawaii noted reductions in total sperm counts (42). Agricultural use of EDB, which comprises 15% of total EDB use, was banned in the U.S. in 1984. The major current use of EDB is as an additive in lead-containing gasoline.

DBCP was applied by injecting it into the soil, and it is now the most widespread contaminant of groundwater in the state of California. There is no evidence that the levels found in drinking water are sufficient to lead to adverse reproductive outcomes. Ethylene dibromide is a common groundwater contaminant in the state of Florida.

## CHLORDECONE (KEPONE)

One of the most serious outbreaks of poisoning from a chlorinated hydrocarbon pesticide in the U.S. occurred in 1975 in a plant in Virginia that was manufacturing and formulating the insecticide, Kepone, for export. Unlike the DBCP workers, the Kepone-exposed workers were severely poisoned with clinical manifestations of nervousness, tremor, head bobbing, opsoclonus, ataxia, and visual and speech disturbances. In the most severely affected workers, semen samples showed abnormal spermatozoa, oligospermia, and decreased motility; testicular biopsy revealed damage to the germinal epithelium of the testis (43, 44). Kepone was banned in the U.S. in 1975. A very similar pesticide, Mirex, was formerly used extensively for fire ant control; it is a common contaminant in fish from the Great Lakes.

## CLINICAL CONSIDERATIONS

To determine whether or not pesticide exposure may be related to an adverse reproductive outcome, the specific pesticides implicated must be known, as well as the amount and circumstances of the exposure. It is very important to take a thorough occupational and environmental history and to note the patient's symptoms and complaints.

If the name of the pesticide cannot be obtained immediately, all available information should be recorded in the client's record, including what the pesticide was used for, how it was applied, the type of formulation, and any other pertinent information. Often, the client will be able to assist in getting the additional information that is needed. Workers who manufacture or formulate pesticides are covered by the provisions of the Occupational Safety and Health Act. Under the Occupational Safety and Health Administration's (OSHA's) Hazard Communication Standard, these workers have the right to obtain from their employers Material Safety Data Sheets (MSDSs) that list hazardous product ingredients (Chapter 10). Pesticide applicators and agricultural workers are exempt from OSHA regulation, falling instead under the provisions of the Federal Insecticide Fungicide and Rodenticide Act (FIFRA), which is essentially a labeling law administered by the EPA through state working agreements (Chapter 12). In these circumstances, information about product ingredients may be available on product labels or by contacting the pesticide manufacturer or the EPA. However, neither MSDSs nor product labels consistently provide data on reproductive health effects. This information must be obtained through other sources such as computer toxicology databases or government agencies. In addition, national pesticide information hotlines may be helpful (Chapter 10.)

In the case of community exposure, it may be possible to narrow potential exposures if the clinician is familiar with pesticide use patterns and practices in his or her community. Local pest control companies and county and state agencies have this information and are usually willing to share it. If information can be obtained on the specific pesticides involved in the putative exposure, as well as the circumstances, intensity, and duration of exposure, some judgment can often be made regarding the possible role of the pesticide in inducing adverse health effects.

Clinicians may be tempted to dismiss clients' concerns if they are not clinically ill or if they do not have what are considered significant signs and symptoms of exposure. It is instructive to remember that the DBCP-exposed workers were physically and clinically normal except for their azoospermia and oligospermia.

Clinicians may also assume that, unless the putative exposure was maternally toxic, an adverse birth outcome cannot be related to pesticides. This assumption may be unwarranted, especially in regard to fetal death, the most consistently reported finding associated with maternal pesticide exposure.

With few exceptions, such as 2,4,5-T and DBCP, most studies of reproductive toxicity and pesticides pertain to populations occupationally or environmentally exposed to a variety of pesticides in unknown quantities. Many are ecological studies in which the actual exposure of the individuals in the populations being studied is not known. More targeted studies with specification and quantitation of exposures are needed to better characterize pesticides as a risk factor for adverse reproductive outcomes in humans.

## REFERENCES[a]

1. U.S. Environmental Protection Agency (EPA), Office of Pesticide Programs. Pesticide industry sales and usage, 1987 market estimates. Washington, DC: U.S. EPA, 1988.
2. Matthews GA. Pesticide application methods. New York: Longman, Inc., 1982.
3. Kazen D, Bloomer A, Welch R, et al. Persistence of pesticides on the hands of some occupationally exposed people. Arch Environ Health 1974;29:315–318.
4. Polednak AP, Janerick DT. Uses of available record systems in epidemiologic studies of reproductive toxicology. Am J Ind Med 1983;4:329–348.
5. White FMM, Cohen FG, Sherman G, McCurdy R. Chemicals, birth defects and stillbirths in New Brunswick: associations with agricultural activity. Can Med Assoc J 1988;138:117–124.
6. Field B, Kerr C. Herbicide use and incidence of neural tube defects. Lancet 1979;1:1341–1342.
7. Balarajan R, McDowall M. Congenital malformations and agricultural workers. Lancet 1983;1:1112–1113.
8. Schwartz DA, Newsum L, Heifetz RM. Parental occupation and birth outcome in an agricultural community. Scand J Work Environ Health 1986;12:51–54.
9. Schwartz DA, Logerfo JP. Congenital limb reduction defects in the agricultural setting. Am J Public Health 1988;78:654–657.
10. Brogan WF, Brogan CE, Dadd JT. Herbicides and cleft lip and cleft palate. Lancet 1980;2:597–598.
11. Gordon JE, Shy CM. Agricultural chemical use and congenital cleft lip and/or palate. Arch Environ Health 1981;36:213–221.
12. Golding J, Sladden T. Congenital malformations and agricultural workers. Lancet 1983;1:1393.
13. Roan CC, Matanoski GE, McIlnay CQ, et al. Spontaneous abortions, stillbirths, and birth defects in families of agricultural pilots. Arch Environ Health 1984;39:56–60.
14. Marchand LL, Kolonel LN, Siegel BZ, Dendle WH III. Trends in birth defects for a Hawaiian population exposed to heptachlor and for the United States. Arch Environ Health 1986;41:145–148.
15. Silbergeld EK, Mattison DR. Experimental and clinical studies on the reproductive toxicology of 2,3,7,8-tetrachlorodibenzo-p-dioxin. Am J Ind Med 1987; 11:131–144.
16. Patterson DG Jr, Holler JS, Smith SJ, Liddle JA, Sampson EJ, Needham LL. Human adipose data for 2,3,7,8-TCDD in certain U.S. samples. Chemosphere 1986;15:2055–2060.
17. Centers for Disease Control. Serum 2,3,7,8-tetrachlorodibenzo-p-dioxin levels in Air Force health study participants—preliminary report. MMWR 1988;37:309–311.
18. Erickson JD, Mulinaire J, McClain PW, et al. Vietnam veterans' risks for fathering babies with birth defects. JAMA 1984;252:903–912.
19. Donovan JW, MacLennan R, Adena R. Vietnam service and the risk of congenital anomalies: a case-control study. Med J Austral 1984;140:394–397.
20. Lathrop GD, Wolfe WH, Albanese RA, Moynahan PM. An epidemiologic investigation of health effects in Air Force personnel following exposure to herbicides. Brooks Air Force Base, TX: U.S. Air Force, 1984.
21. Townsend JC, Bodner KM, Van Peenan PFD, Olson RD, Cook RR. Survey of reproductive events of wives of employees exposed to chlorinated dioxins. Am J Epidemiol 1982;115:695–713.
22. Nelson CJ, Holson JF, Green HC, Gaylor DW. Retrospective study of the relationship between agricultural use of 2,4,5-T and cleft palate occurrence in Arkansas. Teratology 1979;19:377–383.
23. Hanify JA, Metcalf P, Nobbs CL, Worsley KJ. Aerial spraying of 2,4,5-T and human birth malformation: an epidemiological investigation. Science 1981;212:349–351.
24. Smith AH, Fisher DO, Pearce N, Chapman CJ. Congenital defects and miscarriages among New Zealand 2,4,5-T sprayers. Arch Environ Health 1982;37:197–200.
25. Mastroiacovo P, Spangnolo A, Marni E, Meazza L, Bertollini R, Segni G. Birth defects in the Seveso area after TCDD contamination. JAMA 1988;259:1668–1672.
26. Rehder H, Sanchioni F, Cefes G, Gropp A. Pathological-embryological investigations in cases of abortion related to the Seveso accident. J Swiss Med 1978;108:1817–1825.
27. Tenchini ML, Crimaudo C, Pachetti G, Mottura A, Agosti S, DeCarli L. A comparative cytogenetic study on cases of induced abortions in TCDD exposed and nonexposed women. Environ Mol Mutagen 1983;5:73–85.

---

[a]An extensive bibliography of all the references used for this chapter is available upon request from the author, P.O. Box 420870, San Francisco, CA 94142.

28. Stockbauer JW, Hoffman RE, Schramm WF, Edmonds LD. Reproductive outcomes of mothers with potential exposure to 2,3,7,8-tetrachlorodibenzo-p-dioxin. Am J Epidemiol 1988;128:410–419.
29. Vaughan TL, Daling JR, Starzyk PM. Fetal death and maternal occupation: an analysis of birth records in the state of Washington. J Occup Med 1984;26:676–678.
30. Hemminki K, Saloniemi L, Luoma K, et al. Transplacental carcinogens and mutagens: childhood cancer, malformations and abortions as risk indicators. J Toxicol Environ Health 1980;6:1115–1126.
31. McDonald AD, McDonald JC, Armstrong B, et al. Fetal death and work in pregnancy. Br J Ind Med 1988;45:148–157.
32. Savitz DA, Whelan EA, Kleckner RC. Effect of parents' occupational exposures on risk of stillbirth, preterm delivery, and small-for-gestational-age infants. Am J Epidemiol 1989;129:1201–1218.
33. Rita P, Reddy PP, Venkatram Reddy S. Monitoring of workers occupationally exposed to pesticides in grape gardens of Andhra Pradesh. Environ Res 1987;44:1–5.
34. Whorton D, Krauss RM, Marshall S, Milby TH. Infertility in male pesticide workers. Lancet 1977;2:1259–1261.
35. Milby TH, Whorton D. Epidemiologic assessment of occupationally related, chemically induced sperm count suppression. J Occup Med 1980;22:77–82.
36. Whorton D, Milby TH, Krauss RM, Stubbs HA. Testicular function in DBCP exposed pesticide workers. J Occup Med 1979;21:161–166.
37. Eaton M, Schenker M, Whorton D, Samuels S, Perkins C, Overstreet J. Seven-year follow-up of workers exposed to 1,2-dibromo-3-chloropropane. J Occup Med 1986;28:1145–1150.
38. Potashnik G. A four-year reassessment of workers with dibromochloropropane-induced testicular dysfunction. Andrologia 1983;15:164–170.
39. Goldsmith JR, Potashnik G, Israeli R. Reproductive outcomes in families of DBCP-exposed men. Arch Environ Health 1984;39:85–89.
40. Potashnik G, Abeliovich D. Chromosomal analysis and health status of children conceived to men during or following dibromochloropropane-induced spermatogenic suppression. Andrologia 1985;17:291–296.
41. Dobbins JG. Regulation and the use of "negative" results from human reproductive studies: the case of ethylene dibromide. Am J Ind Med 1987;12:33–45.
42. Ratcliffe JM, Schraeder SM, Steenland K, Clapp DE, Turner T, Hornung RW. Semen quality in papaya workers with long term exposure to ethylene dibromide. Br J Ind Med 1987;44:317–326.
43. Taylor JR, Selhorst JB, Houff SA, Martinez AJ. Chlordecone intoxication in man. Part 1: clinical observations. Neurology 1978;28:626–630.
44. Cohn WJ, Boylan JJ, Blanke RV, Fariss MW, Howell JR, Guzelian PS. Treatment of chlordecone (Kepone) toxicity with cholestyramine. N Engl J Med 1978;298:243–248.

## OTHER GENERAL REFERENCES ON PESTICIDES

1. Farm chemicals handbook. Willoughby, OH: Meister Publishing Co., 1991.
2. Hayes WJ Jr, Laws ERJ, eds. Handbook of pesticide toxicology. Vol. I, General principles. Vol. 2, Classes of pesticides. Vol. 3, Classes of pesticides. San Diego: Academic Press, 1991.
3. Morgan DP. Recognition and management of pesticide poisonings, 4th ed. Washington, DC: United States Environmental Protection Agency, 1989.

....................................................

# Summary of Toxicology Data on Pesticides as of June 1992 Prepared from California Environmental Protection Agency Reports[a]

| Pesticide | OR | OM | RR | BR | BB | GM | CM | DNA |
|---|---|---|---|---|---|---|---|---|
| Acephate (Orthene) | 4 | 1 | 4 | 4 | 4 | 1 | 1 | 1 |
| Acrolein (Aqualin) | 2 | 3 | 3 | 4 | 4 | 1 | 4 | 4 |
| Alachlor (Lasso) | 1 | 1 | 4 | 4 | 4 | 4 | 4 | 1 |
| Aldicarb (Temik) | 4 | 4 | 4 | 4 | 4 | 4 | 4 | 4 |
| Aldrin | 2 | 2 | 2 | 2 | N | N | N | N |
| Allethrin | 4 | 4 | 4 | 4 | 4 | 4 | 4 | 4 |
| Aluminum Phosphide | 0 | 0 | 0 | 0 | 0 | 0 | 0 | 0 |
| Amitraz | 4 | 1 | 1 | 4 | 4 | 1 | 4 | 4 |
| Amitrole | 1 | 1 | 2 | 4 | 1 | 4 | 4 | 1 |
| Anilazine (Dyrene) | 4 | 4 | 4 | 3 | 3 | 1 | 3 | 4 |
| Arsenic (inorganic) | 1 | 1 | N | 1$^m$ | 4 | 1 | 1 | 1 |
| Asulam | 1 | 2 | 2 | 3 | 3 | 3 | 3 | 3 |
| Atrazine | 1 | 4 | 4 | 4 | 4 | 4 | 4 | 4 |
| Azinphos-methyl (Guthion) | 1 | 4 | 4 | 4 | 4 | 4 | 1 | 4 |
| Barban (Carbyne) | N | N | 3 | 3 | N | N | N | N |
| Baythroid (Cyfluthrin) | 3 | 3 | 2 | 2 | 3 | 4 | 4 | 4 |
| Bendiocarb | 3 | 4 | 2 | 2 | 4 | 4 | 1 | 4 |
| Benomyl and MBC (Benlate) | 4 | 1 | 1 | 1 | 1 | 1 | 1 | 1 |
| Bentazon (Basagran) | 4 | 1 | 3 | 1 | 1 | 4 | 4 | 4 |
| Bifenox | 4 | 1 | 3 | 4 | 4 | 4 | 1 | 4 |
| Borax | N | N | 2 | N | N | 2 | N | N |
| Boric acid | N | 1 | 2 | 2 | 1$^m$ | 4 | 4 | 3 |
| Bromacil (Hyvar) | 2 | 1 | 3 | 4 | 4 | 1 | 1 | 4 |
| Bromoxynil | N | N | 3 | 2 | 2 | 4 | 4 | N |
| Calcium hypochlorite | N | 3 | N | 3 | N | N | 3 | N |
| Captafol (Difolatan) | 1 | 1 | 4 | 4 | 4 | 1 | 4 | N |
| Captan | 1 | 1 | 4 | 4$^h$ | 4 | 1 | 1 | 1 |
| Carbaryl (Sevin) | N | 3 | 4 | 4 | 4 | 4 | 1 | 4 |
| Carbofuran (Furadan) | 4 | 4 | 1 | 4 | 4 | 1 | 4 | 4 |
| Carbon tetrachloride | N | N | N | N | N | N | N | N |
| Carboxin | N | 1 | 2 | 4 | 4 | 4 | 1 | 1 |
| Chloramben | 3 | 2 | 3 | 3 | 2 | 2 | 1 | 3 |
| Chlordane | 1 | 1 | 3 | N | 3 | 1 | 3 | 3 |
| Chlorflurenol | 3 | 3 | 2 | N | 3 | 3 | 4 | N |
| Chlorobenzilate | 2 | 2 | 4 | 3 | 3 | 3 | N | 3 |
| Chloroneb | N | N | 3 | 3 | 2 | 4 | 3 | 3 |
| Chloropicrin | 3 | 3 | N | N | N | N | N | N |
| Chlorothalonil (Bravo) | 1 | 1 | 4 | 4 | 4 | 4 | 1 | 4 |
| Chlorpropham | 4 | N | 2 | 3 | 1 | 4 | 1 | 2 |
| Chlorpyrifos (Dursban, Lorsban) | 4 | 4 | 2 | 4 | 4$^m$ | 4 | 4 | 1 |
| Chlorsulfuron | 4 | 4 | 4 | 4 | 4 | 4 | 4 | 4 |
| Coumaphos | 4 | 3 | 2 | 4 | 4 | 4 | 1 | 4 |
| Creosote | N | 2 | N | N | N | 2 | N | N |
| Cryolite | N | N | N | 4 | N | 4 | 4 | 4 |
| Cyanazine | 1 | 4 | 1 | 4 | 4 | 1 | 4 | 1 |

| Pesticide | OR | OM | RR | BR | BB | GM | CM | DNA |
|---|---|---|---|---|---|---|---|---|
| Cycloate | 4 | 3 | 1 | 4 | 4 | 1 | 1 | 1 |
| 2,4-D | 1 | 3 | 1 | 4 | 4 | 4 | 4 | 1 |
| Dacthal (Chlorthal-dimethyl) | 3 | 1 | 2 | 4 | 4 | 4 | 4 | 4 |
| Dalapon | N | 3 | 3 | 2 | N | 3 | 3 | 3 |
| Daminozide (Alar) | 1 | 1 | 4 | 4 | 4 | 4 | 4 | 4 |
| D-D and related compounds | N | N | N | N | N | N | N | N |
| DDVP (Dichlorvos) | 1 | 1 | 3 | 4 | 4 | 1 | 4 | 1 |
| Deet (Off) | N | 3 | 4 | 4 | 3 | 4 | 4 | 4 |
| DEF (Tributylphosphorot-rithiote) | N | 1 | 2 | 4 | 4 | 4 | 4 | 4 |
| Demeton (Systox) | N | N | N | N | N | N | N | N |
| Diazinon (Spectracide) | 4 | 3 | 3 | 3 | 4 | 3 | 1 | 3 |
| Dicamba | 3 | 3 | 3 | 4 | 3 | 4 | 4 | 1 |
| Dichlobenil | 1 | N | 3 | 4 | 4 | 4 | 4 | 4 |
| Dichloro-s-triazinetrione | 4 | 4 | 1 | 3 | 3 | 4 | 3 | 3 |
| Diclofop methyl (Hoelon) | 3 | 2 | 2 | 3 | 3 | 4 | 2 | 4 |
| Diethatyl ethyl | 4 | 4 | 3 | 2 | 4 | 4 | 4 | 4 |
| Diflubenzuron (Dimilin) | 4 | 4 | 2 | 4 | 4 | 4 | 4 | 4 |
| Dimethoate | 4 | 4 | 2 | 4 | 4 | 4 | 4 | 1 |
| 2,4-Dinitrophenol | N | N | N | N | N | N | N | N |
| Dinocap | 3 | 2 | 3 | 3 | 1 | 1 | 4 | 4 |
| Dioxathion | 2 | 3 | 3 | N | N | N | N | N |
| Diphacinone | N | N | N | 3$^m$ | N | 3 | N | N |
| Diphenamid | N | N | 3 | 3 | 3 | 3 | N | 3 |
| Diphenylamine | 3 | N | 3 | 3 | 4 | 4 | 4 | 4 |
| Dipropyl isocinchomeronate | N | N | N | 2 | 4 | 4 | 4 | 4 |
| Diquat | 1 | 3 | 1 | 1 | 1 | 1 | 1 | 1 |
| Diuron | 1 | N | 3 | 4 | 4 | 4 | 1 | 4 |
| Endosulfan (Thiodan) | 3 | 3 | 4 | 4 | 4 | 4 | 4 | 4 |
| Endothall | 1 | 2 | 2 | 4 | 4$^m$ | 4 | 3 | 4 |
| Endrin | 3 | 3 | N | N | N | N | N | N |
| EPTC (Eptam) | 4 | 4 | 4 | 2 | 4 | 1 | 1 | 4 |
| Ethalfluralin | 1 | 4 | 3 | 4 | 4 | 1 | 1 | 4 |
| Ethephon | N | 3 | 3 | 3 | 3 | 2 | 1 | 2 |
| Ethofumesate | 4 | N | 4 | 3 | 1 | 4 | 4 | 4 |
| Ethoprop | 1 | 4 | 1 | 4 | 4 | 4 | 1 | 1 |
| Ethylene dibromide (EDB) | 1 | 1 | N | 2 | N | 1 | 1 | 1 |
| Ethylene dichloride | 2 | 2 | N | N | N | 1 | 3 | N |
| Ethylene oxide (ETO) | 1 | 1 | 2 | 2 | 4 | 1 | 1 | 1 |
| Fenamiphos | 4 | 4 | 3 | 4 | 4 | 4 | 1 | 4 |
| Fenarimol | 1 | 4 | 4 | 4 | 3 | 4 | 4 | 4 |
| Fensulfothion | N | N | N | 4 | 2 | 4 | 4 | 3 |
| Fenthion | 3 | 2 | 1 | 4 | 4 | 1 | 2 | 3 |
| Fenvalerate (Pydrin) | 2 | 2 | 3 | 3$^m$ | 3 | 3 | 3 | 3 |
| Ferbam | N | 3 | N | N | N | N | N | N |
| Fluchloralin | N | 3 | 3 | N | 3 | N | 3 | N |
| Flucythrinate | 2 | 4 | 2 | 3 | 3 | 3 | 3 | N |
| Fluometuron | 4 | 1 | 4 | 4 | 4 | 4 | 4 | 4 |
| Fluvalinate (Mavrik) | 4 | 1 | 1 | 4 | 1 | 1 | 4 | 4 |
| Folpet | 1 | 1 | 4 | 1 | 4 | 1 | 4 | 1 |
| Formaldehyde | 2 | N | N | N | N | 2 | 2 | 2 |
| Fosamine | N | N | 3 | 2 | N | 4 | 1 | 4 |
| Glyphosate (Roundup) | 3 | 1 | 3 | 4 | 4 | 4 | 4 | 4 |
| Heptachlor | 2 | 2 | 2 | N | 3 | 4 | 2 | 2 |
| Imazalil | 4 | 3 | 2 | 1 | 3 | 4 | 4 | 4 |
| Iprodione | 3 | 3 | 3 | 4 | 4 | 4 | 4 | 1 |
| Isoparaffinic hydrocarbon | N | 2 | N | N | N | 4 | 3 | N |
| Kerosene | N | 2 | N | N | N | 4 | 3 | N |
| Lethane | N | N | N | N | N | N | N | N |

| Pesticide | OR | OM | RR | BR | BB | GM | CM | DNA |
|---|---|---|---|---|---|---|---|---|
| Lindane | 2 | 1 | 3 | 4 | 4 | 4 | 2 | 4 |
| Linuron | 1 | 1 | 2 | 4 | 4 | 4 | 4 | 4 |
| Lithium hypochlorite | N | N | 2 | 4 | 3 | 4 | 4 | 4 |
| Magnesium Phosphide | 0 | 0 | 0 | 0 | 0 | 0 | 0 | 0 |
| Malathion | 4 | 4 | 4 | 4 | 4 | 4 | 4 | 4 |
| Maleic hydrazide | 3 | 4 | 4 | 3 | 4 | 3 | 1 | 3 |
| Mancozeb | 1 | 3 | 2 | 4 | 4 | 4 | 1 | 4 |
| Maneb | 4 | 2 | 1 | 2 | 1 | 2 | 1 | 4 |
| Mefluidide | 4 | 4 | 4 | 3 | 4 | 4 | 3 | 3 |
| Metaldehyde | N | N | 2 | N | N | 4 | 4 | N |
| Metam-sodium (Vapam) | N | N | N | 1 | 1 | 1 | 1 | 4 |
| Methidathion (Supracide) | 4 | 1 | 4 | 4 | 4 | 4 | 1 | 4 |
| Methomyl (Lannate) | 4 | 4 | 4 | 4 | 4 | 4 | 4 | 4 |
| Methoxychlor | 3 | 3 | 2 | 2 | N | N | N | N |
| Methyl bromide | 2 | N | 2 | 1 | 1 | 1 | 4 | 1 |
| Methyl parathion | 3 | 3 | 1 | 1 | 3 | 1 | 4 | 4 |
| Methylene chloride | N | N | N | N | N | N | 4 | N |
| Methylenebis (Thiocyanate) | 4 | 4 | 4 | 4 | 4 | 1 | 1 | 4 |
| Methylisothiocyanate (MITC) | 4 | 4 | 2 | 4 | 4 | 1 | 1 | 4 |
| Metolachlor | 1 | 4 | 4 | 4 | 4 | 4 | 4 | 4 |
| Metribuzin (Sencor) | N | 4 | 2 | 4 | 4 | 4 | 1 | 4 |
| Metsulfuron methyl | 2 | 3 | 3 | 4 | 4 | 4 | 1 | 4 |
| Mevinphos (Phosdrin) | N | 4 | 3 | 4 | 3 | 1 | 1 | 1 |
| Molinate (Ordram) | 1 | 1 | 1 | 1 | 4 | 1 | 4 | 4 |
| Monocrotophos (Azodrin) | 4 | 4 | 1 | 4 | 4 | 1 | 1 | 1 |
| Monosodium cyanurate | 1 | 4 | 1 | 3 | 3 | 4 | 3 | 3 |
| MSMA (Monosodium methanearsonate) | P | P | 3 | 3 | 4 | 3 | N | 3 |
| Naled (Dibrom) | 1 | 4 | 1 | 4 | 4 | 4 | 4 | 4 |
| Naphthalene | N | N | N | N | 4 | 4 | 4 | 4 |
| Napropamide | 1 | 3 | 4 | 4 | 4 | 1 | 4 | 4 |
| Naptalam (Alanap) | 3 | 1 | 3 | 3 | 3 | 4 | 1 | 4 |
| Nitrapyrin | 1 | N | 4 | 4 | 4 | 4 | 4 | 4 |
| Norflurazon | 1 | 4 | 4 | 3 | 4 | 4 | 4 | 4 |
| Ortho-benzyl-para-chlorophenol | N | N | N | 4 | 2 | 4 | 3 | 4 |
| Ortho-phenylphenol (OPP) | 1 | 2 | 2 | 4 | 2 | 1 | 1 | 4 |
| Oryzalin | 1 | 4 | 3 | 4 | 4 | 4 | 4 | 4 |
| Oxadiazon | 1 | 1 | 4 | 1 | 1 | 1 | 4 | 1 |
| Oxamyl (Vydate) | 3 | 4 | 2 | 4 | 4 | 4 | 4 | 4 |
| Oxycarboxin | N | N | 3 | 3 | N | 3 | N | N |
| Oxydemeton-methyl (Meta-systox) | 4 | 3 | 1 | 4 | 4 | 1 | 1 | 4 |
| Oxyfluorfen (Goal) | 4 | 1 | 3 | 3 | 4 | 1 | 3 | 4 |
| Oxythioquinox (Morestan) | 3 | 4 | 1 | 1 | 4 | 1 | 1 | 4 |
| Paradichlorobenzene | 3 | 3 | N | 3 | 4 | 4 | 4 | 1 |
| Paraquat (Gramoxone) | 1 | 4 | 4 | 4 | 3[m] | 4 | 1 | 1 |
| Parathion (ethyl) | 1 | 1 | 4 | 4 | 4 | 1 | 4 | 4 |
| Pebulate | 4 | 3 | N | 4 | 4 | 4 | 4 | 4 |
| Pendimethalin | 1 | 4 | 3 | 4 | 4 | 4 | 4 | 4 |
| Pentachloronitrobenzene (PCNB) | 2 | 1 | 3 | 4 | 4 | 4 | 1 | 4 |
| Pentachlorophenol | 3 | 1 | 2 | 1 | 2[h] | 4 | 1 | 2 |
| Permethrin | 4 | 1 | 1 | 4 | 4 | 4 | 4 | 4 |
| Petroleum derivative resin | N | 2 | N | N | N | 4 | 3 | N |
| Petroleum distillate, aromatic | N | 2 | N | N | N | 4 | 3 | N |
| Petroleum distillates | N | N | N | N | N | N | 3 | N |
| Petroleum hydrocarbons | N | 3 | N | N | N | 4 | 3 | N |
| Petroleum naphthlenic oils | N | 2 | N | N | N | 4 | 3 | N |

| Pesticide | OR | OM | RR | BR | BB | GM | CM | DNA |
|---|---|---|---|---|---|---|---|---|
| Petroleum oil, paraffin based | N | 3 | N | N | N | 4 | 3 | N |
| Petroleum distillate refined | N | 2 | N | N | N | 4 | 3 | N |
| Petroleum oil, unclassified | N | 2 | N | N | N | 4 | 3 | N |
| Petroleum, unrefined | N | 2 | N | N | N | 4 | 3 | N |
| Phenothrin | 3 | P | P | 4 | 3 | 4 | 4 | 4 |
| Phenylmercuric acetate | N | N | N | 2 | 2 | 2 | 2 | 3 |
| Phenylmercuric oleate | N | N | N | 2 | 2 | 2 | 2 | 3 |
| Phorate (Thimet) | 4 | 4 | 3 | 2 | 4 | 4 | 4 | 4 |
| Phosalone (Imidan) | N | 4 | 3 | 3 | 1 | 3 | 3 | N |
| Phosmet | N | 4 | 3 | 3 | 3 | 1 | 1 | 4 |
| Phosphamidon | 4 | 3 | 4 | 4 | 4 | 4 | 1 | 4 |
| Picloram | 4 | 3 | 3 | 3 | 2 | 4 | 2 | 2 |
| Pine oil | N | N | N | 4 | N | 4 | 4 | 4 |
| Piperonyl butoxide | 4 | 3 | 4 | 3 | 4 | 4 | 4 | 4 |
| Plictran (Cyhexatin) | 4 | 4 | 3 | 3 | 1 | 4 | 4 | 4 |
| Prometon | 4 | 4 | 4 | 4 | 4 | 4 | 4 | 4 |
| Prometryn | N | 4 | 3 | 4 | 4 | 4 | 4 | 4 |
| Propamocarb | 3 | 3 | 3 | 1 | 4 | 4 | 4 | 4 |
| Propargite (Omite) | 1 | 4 | 1 | 4 | 4 | 1 | 4 | 4 |
| Propetamphos | 4 | 4 | 3 | 4 | 4 | 4 | 3 | 4 |
| Propoxur (Baygon) | 1 | 2 | 4 | 4 | 4 | 4 | 4 | 4 |
| Propyzamide (Kerb) | 3 | 1 | 3 | 4 | 4 | 4 | 4 | 4 |
| Pyrethrins | N | N | N | N | N | N | N | N |
| Resmethrin | 3 | 3 | 2 | 3 | 2 | 4 | 4 | 4 |
| Rotenone | 2 | 2[h] | N | 3 | 3[m] | 3 | 3 | N |
| Simazine (Princep) | 1 | 4 | 3 | 4 | 4 | 4 | 4 | 4 |
| Sodium arsenite | N | N | N | N | N | N | N | N |
| Sodium hypochlorite | N | 3 | N | 3 | N | N | 3 | N |
| Sulfur dioxide | N | N | N | N | N | N | N | N |
| Telone II (1,3-dichloro-propene) | 1 | 1 | 4 | 4 | 4 | 1 | 4 | 1 |
| Terbacil | 3 | 2 | 3 | 4 | 4 | 4 | 4 | 4 |
| Terrazole | 3 | 1 | 3 | 3 | 2 | 4 | 1 | 1 |
| Tetrachlorophenol | N | N | N | N | N | N | N | N |
| Tetrachlorvinphos | 2 | 1 | 3 | 4 | 4 | 4 | 1 | 1 |
| Tetramethrin | 2 | 3 | 1 | 3 | 3 | 4 | 4 | 4 |
| Thiabendazole | 3 | 4 | 4 | 2 | 1 | 4 | 4 | 4 |
| Thiobencarb (Bolero) | 4 | 4 | 4 | 4 | 4 | 4 | 4 | 4 |
| Thiodicarb | 1 | 3 | 3 | 4 | 4 | 1 | 4 | 4 |
| Thiophanate methyl | 3 | 3 | 2 | 3 | 4 | 4 | 3 | 3 |
| Thiram | N | 3 | 2 | 1 | 2 | 4 | 4 | 4 |
| Toxaphene | 2 | 2 | N | N | N | N | CM | N |
| Triadimefon (Bayleton) | 3 | 1 | 1 | 2 | 3 | 4 | 4 | 3 |
| Tributyltin benzoate | N | N | N | N | N | N | N | N |
| Tributyltin oxide | N | N | N | N | N | N | N | N |
| Trichloro-S-triazinetrione | 4 | 4 | 1 | 3 | 3 | 4 | 3 | 3 |
| Trichlorophon (Dipterex) | 4 | 4 | 2 | 4 | 3 | 1 | 1 | 1 |
| Triclopyr (Garlon) | 4 | 4 | 4 | 4 | 4 | 4 | 1 | 4 |
| Trifluralin (Treflan) | 1 | 4 | 4 | 4 | 4 | 4 | 4 | 4 |
| Triforine | N | 3 | 3 | 1 | 3 | 4 | 4 | 4 |
| Vernolate | 4 | 3 | 2 | 1 | 4 | 4 | 1 | 4 |
| Vinclozolin | 3 | 3 | 2 | 1 | 4 | 1 | 4 | 4 |
| Ziram | 1 | 1 | 1 | 3 | 4 | N | N | N |

[a]Abbreviations: N = no study on file; P = study in progress; 1 = possible adverse effect, adequate data (no data gap); 2 = possible adverse effect, inadequate data (data gap); 3 = no adverse effect, inadequate or insufficient data (data gap); 4 = no adverse effect, adequate data (no data gap); [h] = hamster; [m] = mouse; OR = oncogen-rat; OM = oncogen-mouse; RR = reproductive effects-rat; BR = birth defects-rat; BB = birth defects-rabbit; GM = genetic mutation; CM = chromosome damage; DNA = DNA synthesis/repair.

# 22

# Polyhalogenated Biphenyls

MAUREEN PAUL

Polyhalogenated biphenyls represent a diverse class of halogenated aromatic hydrocarbons known for their resistance to degradation and environmental persistence. Two members of this class of compounds—the polychlorinated biphenyls (PCBs) and polybrominated biphenyls (PBBs)—have received significant attention as environmental contaminants. This chapter reviews available data on the reproductive and developmental effects of these toxicants.

## POLYCHLORINATED BIPHENYLS

PCBs were introduced into commerce in the early 1930s. During the ensuing four decades, over 800 million tons of PCBs were produced worldwide (1). Although manufacture and distribution of PCBs were banned in the U.S. in 1977, careless disposal of these persistent chemicals has resulted in widespread environmental contamination.

### Properties and Sources of Exposure

As shown in Figure 22.1, PCBs consist of a biphenyl nucleus with chlorine substituted at various positions. There are 209 possible PCB isomers; widely used commercial preparations were produced as mixtures of chlorinated polycyclic compounds containing 20–60 different PCB isomers. The Monsanto Chemical Company, which marketed their PCB products under the brand name "Aroclor," introduced a

four-digit classification system to describe the predominant components of the mixture (first two digits) as well as the percentage weight of chlorine (last two digits). Thus, Aroclor 1254 describes a PCB mixture containing an average of 54% chlorine by weight. Importantly, commercial preparations were contaminated with small amounts of the chemically similar and highly toxic polychlorinated dibenzofurans (PCDFs) (Fig. 22.1).

The attractive properties of chemical and thermal stability, low volatility, high dielectric constants, and miscibility with organic solvents and polymers resulted in widespread industrial application of PCBs. They were used extensively as dielectric fluids in "closed" system devices, such as transformers and capacitors. They were also incorporated into numerous commercial products including synthetic rubber, plastics and coatings, paints, adhesives, cutting oils, caulking compounds, paper, print inks, flame retardants, and pesticides (2). In the 1970s, the National Institute for Occupational Safety and Health (NIOSH) estimated that 12,000 workers had potential occupational exposure to PCBs (3). Subsequent regulatory restrictions did not affect the use of equipment already containing PCBs in enclosed systems. Therefore, occupational exposure still occurs to workers who service and repair PCB-containing transformers and machinery or who are involved in toxic waste or recycling opera-

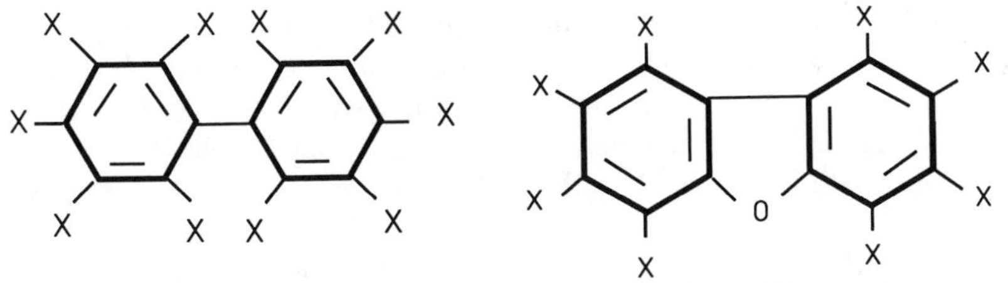

Polychlorinated Biphenyls
(PCBs)

Polychlorinated Dibenzofurans
(PCDFs)

**Figure 22.1.** Basic chemical structures of polychlorinated biphenyls (PCBs) and polychlorinated dibenzofurans (PCDFs). X = chlorine or hydrogen.

tions. Transmission of PCBs to the wives of male workers after laundering contaminated work clothes has also been documented (4).

Unfortunately, the chemical stability that led to the commercial usefulness of PCBs became a serious liability as these chemicals were introduced into the environment, primarily through improper disposal. Resistant to degradation, residues persist in air, soil, water, and sediment. These compounds are highly lipophilic and bioconcentrate in the food chain. Consumption of fish from contaminated waters is a major source of low-level dietary exposure to PCBs (5, 6). Serious poisoning epidemics have also resulted from ingestion of PCB-contaminated cooking oils in Japan and Taiwan (7). The closely related PCDFs have been identified in effluents and wastes from the pulp and paper industry and in municipal incinerator emissions. In addition, PCDFs are released during PCB transformer fires, presenting a potential hazard to firefighters and community residents (8).

Given the widespread pollution of the food chain with PCBs, it is not surprising that detectable tissue levels of PCB residues have been found at high prevalence in unselected populations in the U.S. and other countries (2, 9–11). Fortunately, these levels have gradually declined over the last two decades, reflecting stringent regulation of these chemicals and decreasing environmental exposures (9, 11). Reported serum PCB concentrations in exposed workers are generally higher than those in the general population (12–15).

**Toxicology**

After entering the body through ingestion, inhalation, or dermal absorption, PCBs accumu-

late in adipose tissue. Even low-dose chronic exposures result in detectable body burdens of these chemicals. The liver is the primary site of biotransformation of PCBs via hydroxylation and conjugation with glucuronic acid. Evidence suggests that PCB components in a mixture have widely different metabolic rates and that the highly chlorinated congeners are preferentially retained (16, 17).

Distribution of PCBs to other tissues is related, in part, to their fat content (13). Blood typically has approximately 0.5% fat, and reported human serum to adipose tissue concentrations of PCBs are 1:120 or greater (18). Rogan et al. (19) found higher levels of PCBs in maternal serum than in placenta, which has very little fat. Measurable cord blood PCB concentrations are typically about one-third the levels found in maternal serum, reflecting either the three-fold difference in fat content or the existence of a partial placental barrier (19, 20). Experimental animal studies and reports of congenital PCB poisoning in humans, however, demonstrate that transplacental transmission does occur and may have significant clinical consequences (21, 22).

As discussed in Chapter 6, PCBs are excreted very efficiently into human milk, which is typically comprised of 3–4% fat. Low-level contamination of breast milk with PCBs is ubiquitous worldwide (23). Median concentrations of PCBs in breast milk approach or exceed the Food and Drug Administration's (FDA) tolerance limit of 1.5 ppm (fat weight basis) for PCBs in cow's milk and dairy products in some U.S. studies (19, 24). Rogan et al. (19) found that breast milk levels of PCBs declined substantially with duration of lactation, previous breastfeeding, and serial pregnancies. These data imply that excretion into milk is a major means by which maternal body burden of PCBs is reduced. Other studies provide evidence that infants absorb and accumulate PCBs over the course of lactation (20, 25).

## Reproductive Effects

In experimental animal studies, antispermatogenic effects and impaired fertility are observed in males fed high doses of PCBs. Ovulatory dysfunction, menstrual irregularity, and reduced fertility are noted at lower doses in females (26). In rodents, neonatal exposure to PCBs has been found to impair subsequent reproductive function (26). Male rats exposed to Aroclor 1254 during lactation were less successful in mating and reproducing as adults than were unexposed controls (27).

PCBs induce cytochrome P450- and P448-dependent monooxygenases at rates that are apparently congener-specific. Hepatic induction resulting in alteration of sex steroid hormone levels has been postulated as a mechanism for the reproductive effects of PCBs. Structurally similar to stilbesterol, some PCBs also exhibit weak inherent estrogenic activity (21, 26).

There are no formal studies of fertility impairment among humans exposed to PCBs. Some PCB congeners have been found in human seminal and follicular fluids (28, 29). In an uncontrolled cross-sectional survey, Bush et al. (30) found similarly low concentrations of total PCBs in semen samples from fertile and infertile men. In samples with low sperm counts, however, sperm motility was inversely associated with the presence of three specific PCB congeners. However, the authors expressed skepticism that the low concentrations of PCBs found in this study could produce biological effects and suggested that the measured compounds might signal the presence of other, more potent toxicants. Given animal findings and the potential for PCBs to alter sex steroid hormone concentrations, more research into possible antifertility effects of PCBs is warranted.

## Developmental Effects

The developmental toxicity of PCBs has been studied in a variety of animal species. In general, PCBs do not appear to cause gross structural malformations, but a fairly consistent pattern is seen across species of low birthweight, postnatal growth deficits, and high perinatal mortality following prenatal exposure (26). In most studies, these effects occur at maternally toxic doses. However, low-dose exposure during pregnancy has been associated with neurotoxicity and behavioral deficits in animals (21, 26, 31).

Human data on developmental effects derive from accidental poisoning epidemics and from populations exposed to PCBs through occupation or through low-level dietary sources.

## YUSHO AND YUCHENG OUTBREAKS

In Japan in 1968, contamination of rice bran oil with PCBs, polychlorinated quaterphenyls (PQFs), and PCDFs occurred during the manufacturing process. More than 1000 people who ingested the oil developed "yusho" (oil disease) characterized by chloracne, dermal hyperpigmentation, eye discharge and swelling, headache, respiratory symptoms, limb numbness, along with hematological abnormalities and elevation of liver enzymes. Of 14 children born to exposed women, two were stillborn; all infants were small for gestational age (SGA), and most had deep brown pigmentation of the skin. Other less constant findings included facial edema, eye secretions, gingival hyperplasia, natal teeth, large fontanelles, and spotty calcifications of the skull (7).

A decade later, a similar outbreak occurred in Taiwan where the disease was known as "yucheng." It is estimated that 270 infants were born to poisoned women between 1979 and 1986, although detailed data have been published on relatively few (32). High rates of fetal loss and infant mortality were reported after in utero exposure (32). Although the congenital findings were similar in many ways to those observed in Japan, some variations were noted. For example, blackened noses and acneform rashes were observed in Taiwanese neonates but were not described in Japanese infants. These variations may reflect differences in the composition or concentrations of the oil contaminants (7). In monkeys, treatment with PCDFs produces characteristic ac-neform lesions whereas exposure to purified mixtures of PCBs and PQFs does not, suggesting that PCDFs may be primary etiological agents in the disease (33).

Some follow-up studies in Japan and Taiwan found that low birthweight infants demonstrated catch-up growth if additional exposure to PCBs was limited (32, 34). Harada (35) reported apathy, listlessness, and mild neurological deficits in some 7- to 9-yr-old Japanese children exposed in utero or through breastfeeding. Yu et al. (36) conducted a follow-up study of 128 Taiwanese children exposed prenatally or through breast milk and 115 controls from the same neighborhood at ages ranging from a few months to 7 yr. Developmental delays were found more frequently in the exposed children compared with controls when assessed by interview with the mothers, neurological examinations, and cognitive testing. Delays were greater in children who were smaller in size and in those who had exhibited neonatal symptoms of intoxication.

## OCCUPATIONAL STUDIES

High serum concentrations of PCBs have been found among occupationally exposed cohorts in the U.S. and elsewhere. A study of Japanese capacitor manufacturing workers revealed PCB levels in whole blood of workers and in breast milk of exposed lactating women to be 10–100 times those of nonexposed Japanese and far in excess of levels found in typical yusho patients (14). In a NIOSH study of U.S. workers occupationally exposed to PCBs, mean serum concentrations of electrical equipment manufacturing workers exceeded background community levels by 8–50 times for the lower chlorinated biphenyls (LPCBs) and two to four times for the higher chlorinated biphenyls (HPCBs) (37). Evidence from occupational studies suggests that the decline of blood PCB levels is rapid for the easily metabolized congeners and much slower for the long-lived components (16, 17); recent exposure is associated with more of the biodegradable PCB congeners that account for the highest serum PCB concentrations found in the occupational cohorts studied (38).

Chloracne and subclinical alterations of liver enzymes have been reported in some workers exposed to PCBs (14, 15, 37, 39, 40). In general, however, biological effects in workers are mild compared to yusho and yucheng patients despite higher serum levels of PCBs. These findings again suggest that adverse effects depend on the particular PCB components and contaminants present in the commercial mixtures to which various populations are exposed (33). Japanese investigators demonstrated that the blood PCB composition in occupationally exposed cohorts clearly differed from yusho patients and that the former were not exposed to PCQs or PCDFs (14, 40).

Very few studies have evaluated developmental effects resulting from occupational exposure to PCBs. In an uncontrolled study, Hara (14) reported nail decay, gingival pigmentation, and dental abnormalities among some children of workers exposed to high levels of PCBs through lactation. However, the findings were mild compared to those observed in yusho patients and showed no correlation with the children's blood PCB levels.

In a study involving female workers employed at two capacitor manufacturing plants in upstate New York, Taylor et al. (41) examined the association between occupational exposure to highly chlorinated (high homolog) PCBs and birthweight and gestational age of offspring. Based on personnel records and industrial hygiene data, workers were categorized into a high exposure group comprised of jobs with direct contact with PCBs and a low exposure group with no direct contact. Interviews were conducted with study participants, and birthweights and gestational ages were verified through medical or vital records. Infants born to highly exposed women had slightly reduced birthweights, due primarily to a modest decrease in gestational age. However, tobacco and alcohol consumption were not controlled in this study. The authors noted that the magnitude of the observed effects was quite small compared to other known determinants of gestational age and birthweight.

## U.S. GENERAL POPULATION COHORT STUDIES

Developmental outcomes have been studied in two U.S. cohorts with low-level dietary intake of PCBs. The North Carolina Breast Milk and Formula Project (19) is a prospective birth cohort study of over 800 children who were born between 1978 and 1982 to a self-selected sample of female volunteers. The project involved measurement of PCBs in maternal serum, cord blood, placenta, and serial samples of breast milk; administration of questionnaires to mothers; and collection of data on infants from medical records, clinical examinations, and serial developmental testing. Maternal body burden of PCBs at birth, estimated by combining the results of all samples collected from each woman into a summary concentration of PCBs in milk fat at birth, was used as an index of transplacental exposure to the embryofetus. Cumulative postnatal breast milk exposure, expressed as total milligrams of PCBs consumed by an infant, was estimated from the concentration of the chemical in milk and the duration of lactation. Multiple regression analyses were employed to examine the association between transplacental or breast milk PCB exposures and postnatal outcomes while adjusting for relevant confounders. Higher transplacental exposure to PCBs was associated with hypotonicity and hyporeflexia in newborns and with lower psychomotor scores on serial testing up to 2 yr of age; however, developmental deficits were no longer apparent on testing at 3, 4, or 5 yr of age (42, 43). Breast milk exposure was unrelated to developmental test scores at any age (43). Transplacental PCB exposure was not related to birthweight (42), and subsequent breast milk exposure had no effect on infant growth or occurrence of illnesses in the first year of life (44).

The second U.S. cohort followed for developmental outcomes includes infants born in 1981–1982 to women who consumed PCB-contaminated fish from Lake Michigan before and during pregnancy. Data on fish consumption and other important variables were collected by interview with mothers shortly after delivery. PCBs were measured in cord blood, maternal serum, and breast milk. Postnatal outcomes were ascertained through review of medical records, physical examinations, and serial developmental testing. The exposed group was comprised of 242 infants whose mothers recalled eating more than 11.8 kg of

contaminated fish over a 6-yr period; mothers of 71 control infants reported no Lake Michigan fish consumption.

Fish consumption predicted breast milk and maternal serum PCB levels which, in turn, predicted cord concentrations (5, 45). After adjustment for confounders, exposed newborns weighed 160–190 g less than controls (45). Head circumference was disproportionately small in relation to both birthweight and gestational age, a finding in keeping with experimental studies in monkeys and data collected from the Japanese poisoning epidemics (7). Prenatal exposure was associated with persistent growth deficits at 5 months and 4 yr of age (46). Developmental testing revealed an association between maternal fish consumption and motor impairment and hyporeflexia in newborns (47). Prenatal PCB exposure (but not breast milk exposure) was also related to impaired visual recognition memory at 7 months (48) and subtle verbal and memory deficits at 4 yr (49). Children's 4-yr serum PCB levels, an index of lactation exposure, were associated with reduced activity in a dose-dependent fashion (46).

## Summary and Clinical Recommendations

Developmental effects resulting from high-dose exposure to commercial PCB mixtures are well documented in experimental animal studies and in reports from Japanese and Taiwanese poisoning epidemics. The most consistent findings include low birthweight, abnormal skin pigmentation, prenatal and postnatal mortality, and developmental delays. Low-dose prenatal exposure through dietary sources has also been associated in some studies with decreased fetal growth and nonpersistent neurobehavioral deficits in children. PCBs are effectively transferred to infants through breast milk and accumulate in the infant over the course of lactation. With the exception of one recent study suggesting reduced activity in children exposed to PCBs through lactation (46), there are no reports of adverse health effects in breastfed infants attributed to PCBs at population levels. Limited data suggest that PCBs may result in adverse reproductive effects through hepatic enzyme induction and alteration of sex steroid hormone levels.

The toxicity of PCB mixtures depends, in part, on the composition of congeners and contaminants in the mixture. There is evidence that the severe clinical manifestations found in yusho and yucheng patients were due to the concentration of PCDFs in the oil, contaminants not generally found in other occupationally or environmentally exposed populations. Because most studies to date rely on indirect indices of exposure or on biological measures of total PCB concentrations, little is known about the relative contribution of various PCB congeners to reproductive or developmental effects.

Given the ubiquitous contamination of food sources with PCBs, virtually everyone is exposed to low levels of these chemicals. Mean serum PCB levels range from 4–7 ppb in various U.S. population studies, and levels in adipose tissue and milk fat are much higher (15, 50). There is no established dose-response relationship between PCB exposure and adverse reproductive or developmental outcomes. For these reasons, routine biological screening for PCBs is not recommended.

Measurement of PCBs in serum or breast milk should be obtained only when excessive exposure is suspected through the history or clinical findings. While no standards for breast milk PCB concentrations have been set, one author suggests limiting the duration of breastfeeding if PCB levels exceed 2.3 ppm (milk fat basis) (24). Patients should be advised to minimize consumption of fish from contaminated waters and to avoid excessive weight reduction, which may mobilize chemicals stored in adipose tissue. Because PCBs are also potential carcinogens, occupational exposures should be kept to the lowest feasible limit through engineering controls, provision of personal protective equipment, and safe work practices.

## POLYBROMINATED BIPHENYLS

PBBs are similar in chemical structure to PCBs, with bromine substituted for chlorine on the biphenyl nucleus. Like PCBs, PBBs are lipophilic and bioaccumulate in fatty tissue.

Commercial mixtures of PBBs consist of a number of different congeners with varying metabolic rates. Some PBB components are resistant to degradation, resulting in long biological half-lives and persistence in the environment.

Manufacture of PBBs in the U.S. was discontinued in 1974. Production was largely limited to a Michigan firm that marketed PBB-based products as flame retardants under the brand name Firemaster. This company also produced a nontoxic cattle feed supplement known as Nutrimaster. In the summer of 1973, bags containing PBBs were inadvertently sold as Nutrimaster, resulting in significant contamination of animal feed. Several months passed before the source of the contamination was identified. Affected farms (primarily in Michigan's Lower Peninsula) were quarantined and thousands of animals destroyed. By that time, however, a large proportion of Michigan residents had been exposed to contaminated meat and dairy products. Significant occupational exposure most likely also occurred during manufacture of the PBB products and during and after the contamination incident (51).

Field observations of contaminated herds in Michigan revealed decreased milk production and pregnancy wastage. In laboratory animal experiments, developmental effects of PBBs are generally similar to PCBs and include growth deficits, decreased survival, and neurobehavioral abnormalities. Teratogenicity has also been noted in rodents exposed to high doses. Like PCBs, these chemicals induce hepatic enzymes and may alter sex steroid hormone levels. Ovulatory dysfunction, altered spermatogenesis, and decreased fertility have been noted in various toxicological studies (26, 52).

Despite the high prevalence of detectable PBB levels in tissue samples from a large cohort of persons residing in Michigan in 1973–1974, no adverse health effects have yet been causally linked to PBBs in this population (53–55). Like PCBs, the highest concentrations of PBBs have been found in adipose tissue and human milk fat (22, 56, 57). Cord blood levels are approximately one-tenth those found in maternal sera (22, 57). Blood PBB levels in children at 4 yr of age correlate with concentrations in maternal milk and duration of breastfeeding (58).

In an ecological study, Humble and Speizer (59) found similar fetal death rates in Michigan counties with high proportions of quarantined farms vs. those with no quarantined farms during an 8-yr period after the PBB contamination incident. Weil et al. (60) examined 33 Michigan farm children exposed to PBBs in utero or in early infancy and 20 unexposed controls at a mean age of 37–38 months. Although exposed children were reported by their parents to have had more minor illnesses and increased clumsiness, objective examination revealed no differences between the groups in physical or neurological parameters. Exposed and unexposed children performed similarly on developmental tests selected to measure a range of perceptual-motor, attentional, and verbal abilities. However, within the exposed group, a significant inverse relationship was observed between PBB fat level and cognitive test performance (61). This association was not confirmed by other investigators who administered more extensive developmental tests to the same exposed cohort at approximately 5 yr of age (62). Whether these discrepant findings reflect methodological differences in the two studies or true early deficits that improved over time is unclear (63).

Human data on the reproductive effects of PBBs are limited. Rosenman et al. (64) performed semen analyses 4 yr after the contamination incident on 41 exposed farmers, 11 former workers from the PBB production facility, and 52 unexposed graduate students. No significant differences were observed among the groups in sperm count, motility, or morphology, and there was no correlation between serum PBB level and sperm concentration.

In summary, unlike the ubiquitous contamination of the environment with PCBs, exposure to PBBs is much more limited. Available health effects data on Michigan residents exposed to low levels of PBBs are reassuring, and no significant adverse reproductive or developmental effects have been confirmed.

## REFERENCES

1. Brinkman UAT, DeKok A. Production, properties, and usage. In: Kimbrough RD, ed. Halogenated biphenyls, terphenyls, napthalenes, dibenzodioxins and related products. New York: Elsevier/North-Holland 1980: 1–40.

2. Finkles J, Priester LE, Creason JP, Hauser T, Hinners T, Hammer DI. Polychlorinated biphenyl residues in human plasma expose a major urban pollution problem. Am J Public Health 1972;62:645–651.

3. National Institute for Occupational Safety and Health. Criteria for a recommended standard. Occupational exposure to polycyclic biphenyls. NIOSH publication 77–225. Cincinnati: National Institute for Occupational Safety and Health, 1977.

4. Fischbein A, Wolff MS. Conjugal exposure to polychlorinated biphenyls (PCBs). Br J Ind Med 1987;44:284–286.

5. Schwartz PM, Jacobson SW, Fein G, Jacobson JL, Price HA. Lake Michigan fish consumption as a source of polychlorinated biphenyls in human cord serum, maternal serum, and milk. Am J Public Health 1983;73:293–296.

6. Fiore BJ, Anderson HA, Hanrahan LP, Olson LJ, Sonzogni WC. Sport fish consumption and body burden levels of chlorinated hydrocarbons: a study of Wisconsin anglers. Arch Environ Health 1989;44:82–88.

7. Miller RW. Congenital PCB poisoning: a reevaluation. Environ Health Perspect 1985;60:211–214.

8. Tiernan TO, Taylor ML, Garrett JH, et al. Sources and fate of polycyclic dibenzodioxins, dibenzofurans and related compounds in human environments. Environ Health Perspect 1985;59:145–158.

9. Kutz FW, Wood PH, Bottimire DP. Organochlorine pesticides and polychlorinated biphenyls in human adipose tissue. Rev Environ Contam Toxicol 1991;120:1–82.

10. Phillips LJ, Birchard GF. Regional variations in human toxics exposure in the USA: an analysis based on the National Human Adipose Tissue Survey. Arch Environ Contam Toxicol 1991;21:159–168.

11. Robinson PE, Mack GA, Remmers J, Levy R, Mohadjer L. Trends of PCB, hexachlorobenzene, and beta-benzene hexachloride in levels in the adipose tissue of the U.S. population. Environ Res 1990;53:175–192.

12. Smith AB, Schloemer J, Lowry LK, et al. Metabolic and health consequences of occupational exposure to polychlorinated biphenyls. Br J Ind Med 1982;39:361–369.

13. Rogan WJ, Gladen BC, Wilcox AJ. Potential reproductive and postnatal morbidity from exposure to polychlorinated biphenyls: epidemiologic considerations. Environ Health Perspect 1985;60:233–239.

14. Hara I. Health status and PCBs in blood of workers exposed to PCBs and of their children. Environ Health Perspect 1985;59:85–90.

15. Wolff MS. Occupational exposure to polychlorinated biphenyls (PCBs). Environ Health Perspect 1985;60: 133–138.

16. Yakushiji T, Watanabe I, Kuwabara K, et al. Rate of decrease and half lives of polychlorinated biphenyls in the blood of mothers and their children occupationally exposed to PCBs. Arch Environ Contam Toxicol 1984;13:341–345.

17. Phillips DL, Smith AB, Burse VW, Steele GK, Needham LL, Hannon WH. Half-life of polychlorinated biphenyls

in occupationally exposed workers. Arch Environ Health 1989;44:351–354.

18. Wolff MS, Fischbein A, Thorton J, Rice C, Lilis R, Selikoff IJ. Body burden of polychlorinated biphenyls among persons employed in capacitor manufacturing. Arch Environ Health 1982;49:199–208.

19. Rogan WJ, Gladen BC, McKinney JD, et al. Polychlorinated biphenyls (PCBs) and dichlorodiphenyl dichloroethene (DDE) in human milk: effects of maternal factors and previous lactation. Am J Public Health 1986;76:172–177.

20. Kodama H, Ota H. Transfer of polychlorinated biphenyls to infants from their mothers. Arch Environ Health 1980;35:95–100.

21. Lione A. Polychlorinated biphenyls and reproduction. Reprod Toxicol 1988;2:83–89.

22. Jacobson JL, Fein GG, Jacobson SW, Schwartz PM, Dowler JK. The transfer of polychlorinated biphenyls (PCBs) and polybrominated biphenyls (PBBs) across the human placenta and into maternal milk. Am J Public Health 1984;74:378–379.

23. Jensen AA. Chemical contaminants in human milk. Residue Rev 1983;89:1–128.

24. Wickizer TM, Brilliant LB, Copeland R, Tilden R. Polychlorinated biphenyl contamination of nursing mothers' milk in Michigan. Am J Public Health 1981;71:132–137.

25. Kuwabara K, Yakushiji T, Watanabe I, et al. Relationship between breast feeding and PCB residues in blood of the children whose mothers were occupationally exposed to PCBs. Int Arch Occup Environ Health 1978;41:189–197.

26. Barlow SM, Sullivan FM. Reproductive hazards of industrial chemicals. London: Academic Press, 1982.

27. Sager DB. Effect of postnatal exposure to polychlorinated biphenyls on adult male reproductive function. Environ Res 1983;31:76–94.

28. Trapp M, Baukloh V, Bohnet HG, Heeschen W. Pollutants in human follicular fluid. Fertil Steril 1984;42:146–148.

29. Schlebusch H, Wagner U, van der Ven H, Al-Hasani S, Diedrich K, Krebs D. Polychlorinated biphenyls: the occurrence of the main congeners in follicular and sperm fluids. J Clin Chem Clin Biochem 1989;27:663–667.

30. Bush B, Bennett AH, Snow JT. Polychlorobiphenyl congeners, p,p'-DDE, and sperm function in humans. Arch Environ Contam Toxicol 1986;15:333–341.

31. Pantaleoni GC, Fanini D, Sponta AM, Palumbo G, Giorgi R, Adams PM. Effects of maternal exposure to polychlorobiphenyls (PCBs) on F1 generation behavior in the rat. Fundam Appl Toxicol 1988;11:440–449.

32. Yen YY, Lan SJ, Ko YC, Chen CJ. Follow-up study of reproductive hazards of multiparous women consuming PCBs-contaminated rice oil in Taiwan. Bull Environ Contam Toxicol 1989;43:647–655.

33. Kunita N, Hori IS, Obana H, et al. Biological effects of PCBs, PCQs and PCDFs present in the oil causing yusho and yu-cheng. Environ Health Perspect 1985;59:79–84.

34. Yamashita F, Hayashi M. Fetal PCB syndrome: clinical features, intrauterine growth retardation and possible alteration in calcium metabolism. Environ Health Perspect 1985;59:41–45.

35. Harada M. Intrauterine poisoning. Bull Institute Constitutional Medicine Kumamoto University 1976;25(suppl):1–60.

36. Yu M-L, Hsu C-C, Gladen BC, Rogan WJ. In utero PCB/PCDF exposure: relation of developmental delay to dysmorphology and dose. Neurotoxicol Teratol 1991;13:195–202.

37. Smith AB, Schloemer J, Lowry LK, et al. Metabolic and health consequences of occupational exposure to polychlorinated biphenyls. Br J Ind Med 1982;39:361–369.

38. Wolff MS, Schecter A. Accidental exposure of children to polychlorinated biphenyls. Arch Environ Contam Toxicol 1991;20:449–453.

39. Chase KH, Wong O, Thomas D, Berney BW, Simon RK. Clinical and metabolic abnormalities associated with occupational exposure to polychlorinated biphenyls (PCBs). Occup Med 1982;24:109–114.

40. Takamatsu Makoto, Oki M, Maeda K, Inoue Y, Hirayama H, Yoshizuka K. Surveys of workers occupationally exposed to PCBs and of yusho patients. Environ Health Perspect 1985;59:91–97.

41. Taylor PR, Stelma JM, Lawrence CE. The relation of polychlorinated biphenyls to birthweight and gestational age in the offspring of occupationally exposed mothers. Am J Epidemiol 1989;129:395–406.

42. Rogan WJ, Gladen BC, McKinney JD, et al. Neonatal effects of transplacental exposure to PCBs and DDE. J Pediatr 1986;109:335–341.

43. Gladen BC, Rogan WJ. Effects of perinatal polychlorinated biphenyls and dichlorodiphenyl dichloroethene on later development. J Pediatr 1991;119:58–63.

44. Rogan WJ, Gladen BC, McKinney JD, et al. Polychlorinated biphenyls (PCBs) and dichlorodiphenyl dichloroethene (DDE) in human milk: effects on growth, morbidity, and duration of lactation. Am J Public Health 1987; 77:1294–1297.

45. Fein GG, Jacobson JL, Jacobson SW, Schwartz PM, Dowler JK. Prenatal exposure to polychlorinated biphenyls: effects on birth size and gestational age. J Pediatr 1984; 105:315–320.

46. Jacobson JL, Jacobson SW, Humphrey HEB. Effects of exposure to PCBs and related compounds on growth and activity in children. Neurotoxicol Teratol 1990;12:319–326.

47. Jacobson JL, Schwartz PM, Fein GG, Dowler JK. Prenatal exposure to an environmental toxin: a test of the multiple effects model. Develop Psychol 1984;20:523–532.

48. Jacobson SW, Fein GG, Jacobson JL, Schwartz PM, Dowler JK. The effect of intrauterine PCB exposure on visual recognition memory. Child Develop 1985;56:853–860.

49. Jacobson JL, Jacobson SW, Humphrey HEB. Effects of in utero exposure to polychlorinated biphenyls and related contaminants on cognitive functioning in young children. J Pediatr 1990;116:38–45.

50. Kimbrough RD. Laboratory and human studies on polychlorinated biphenyls (PCBs) and related compounds. Environ Health Perspect 1985;59:99–106.

51. Kingsley K. Polybrominated biphenyls (PBB) environmental contamination in Michigan, 1973–76. Environ Res 1977;13:74–93.

52. Fries G. The PBB episode in Michigan: an overall appraisal. CRC Crit Rev Toxicol 1985;16:105–156.

53. Wolff MS, Anderson HA, Selikoff IF. Human tissue burdens of halogenated aromatic chemicals in Michigan. JAMA 1982;247:2112–2116.

54. Landrigan PJ, Wilcox KR Jr, Silva J Jr, Humphrey HEB, Kauffman C, Health CR Jr. Cohort study of Michigan residents exposed to polybrominated biphenyls: epidemiologic and immunologic findings. Ann NY Acad Sci 1979; 320:284–94.

55. Kreiss K, Roberts C, Humphrey HEB. Serial PBB levels, PCB levels, and clinical chemistries in Michigan's PBB cohort. Arch Environ Health 1982;37:141–147.

56. Miller FD, Brilliant LB, Copeland R. Polybrominated biphenyls in lactating Michigan women: persistence in the population. Bull Environ Contam Toxicol 1984;32:125–133.

57. Eyster JT, Humphrey HEB, Kimbrough RD. Partitioning of polybrominated biphenyls (PBB) in serum, adipose tissue, breast milk, placenta, cord blood, biliary fluid and feces. Arch Environ Health 1983;38:47–53.

58. Jacobson JL, Humphrey HEB, Jacobson SW, Schantz SL, Mullin MD, Welch R. Determinants of polychlorinated biphenyls (PCBs), polybrominated biphenyls (PBBs), and dichlordiphenyltrichloroethane (DDT) levels in sera of young children. Am J Public Health 1989;79:1401–1404.

59. Humble CG, Speizer FE. Polybrominated biphenyls and fetal mortality in Michigan. Am J Public Health 1984;74:1130–1132.

60. Weil WB, Spencer M, Benjamin D, Seagull E. The effect of polybrominated biphenyl on infants and young children. J Pediatr 1981;98:47–51.

61. Seagull EAW. Developmental abilities of children exposed to polybrominated biphenyls (PBB). Am J Public Health 1983;73:281–285.

62. Schwartz EM, Rae WA. Effect of polybrominated biphenyls (PBB) on developmental abilities in young children. Am J Public Health 1983;73:277–281.

63. Nebert DW, Elashoff JD, Wilcox KR. Possible effect of neonatal polybrominated biphenyl exposure on the developmental abilities of children. Am J Public Health 1983;73:286–289.

64. Rosenman KD, Anderson HA, Selikoff IJ, Wolff MS, Holstein E. Spermatogenesis in men exposed to polybrominated biphenyl (PBB). Fertil Steril 1979;32:209–213.

# 23

· · · · · · · · · · · · · · · · · · · · · · · · · · · · · · · · · · · · · · · · · · · ·

# Viral Infections

BARBARA JANTAUSCH, JOHN L. SEVER

Viral infections can represent significant hazards to pregnant women in the workplace. Some agents cause maternal morbidity, which also indirectly affects fetal outcome. Others exert direct toxic effects on the fetus that can result in spontaneous abortion, intrauterine fetal death, and birth defects.

This chapter reviews potential risks to the woman and fetus of rubella, human *Parvovirus* B19, cytomegalovirus, varicella, and hepatitis B virus. The chapter describes how these viruses can be acquired in the workplace and outlines prophylactic and postexposure recommendations to minimize complications to pregnancy. Human immunodeficiency virus is covered separately in Chapter 24.

## RUBELLA

Rubella is an RNA virus and member of the Togavirus family, genus *Rubivirus*. Rubella infection during pregnancy can result in spontaneous abortion, stillbirth, and congenital defects. Although no major rubella epidemics have occurred in the U.S. since introduction of a vaccine in 1969, sporadic outbreaks do occur.

## Epidemiology

Approximately 10–20% of women of childbearing age remain susceptible to the rubella virus (1, 2). During 1978 in England and Wales, the attack rate for rubella was noted to be 1.7/1000 pregnant women (3).

Populations at risk include unimmunized individuals and those with no natural history of rubella infection who lack a protective titer to the virus. School and day care personnel, health care providers, and those within a confined population, such as college students, have increased risk of exposure. Reinfection may also occur (4).

The number of cases of congenital rubella syndrome (CRS) reported to the Centers for Disease Control (CDC) dropped from 67 in 1970 (1.8/100,000 livebirths/yr) to three cases in 1987 (0.08/100,000 livebirths/yr) (5). However, one group estimates that as many as 100 cases of CRS may have occurred in the U.S. during 1982–1985 (2). It is projected that CRS will continue to be a problem for the next 10–30 yr until the childbearing population is immune.

## Modes of Transmission

The human is the only host for the rubella virus. Disease is present during winter and spring with peak periods in March, April, and May. The organism is transmitted through droplet contact. The incubation period is 12–21 days, with an average of 18 days. Virus can be isolated from nasopharyngeal secretions from 7 days before to 14 days after appearance of the rash.

Infants with CRS can shed the virus for 1 yr or longer in nasopharyngeal secretions or urine. There have been isolated case reports of viral shedding in older children and in a 29-yr-old adult with CRS (6, 7).

## Maternal and Fetal Health Consequences

Rubella infection is asymptomatic in 25–50% of adult cases. When symptomatic, the pregnant woman may experience a transient febrile illness with rash and arthralgias (3). Women have delivered infected infants with clinical manifestations of rubella syndrome after an asymptomatic pregnancy with no known history of rubella exposure. Rubella-specific IgM or a four-fold rise in acute and convalescent sera are usually used to establish the diagnosis.

CRS is characterized by intrauterine growth retardation, hearing loss, congenital heart defects, eye defects, and central nervous system (CNS) abnormalities (8). In some infants, growth retardation or deafness is the only sign of rubella infection (3). Others present with thrombocytopenia, encephalitis, and hepatitis at birth (8). A blueberry muffin-like rash, hepatosplenomegaly, and radiolucent bone lesions may also be present. Late sequelae including neurological deficits, developmental delay, hearing defects, and endocrinopathies may be apparent only on follow-up examination (9).

Whether transmission of rubella virus to the fetus results in spontaneous abortion, stillbirth, congenital defects, or asymptomatic infection depends on the gestational age at the time of infection. Maternal infection during the preimplantation period usually results in embryolethality, although CRS has been described (10). The majority of defects attributable to CRS occur after maternal infection during the first 16 weeks of pregnancy (11). In one study, all infants who were infected before the 11th week were born with congenital defects (3). In another study, no defects were noted in 20 children with maternal infection after the 17th week; however, one case of deafness occurred after maternal infection at 17 weeks (11). A hearing deficit was noted in one patient following transmission of infection to 117 infants during gestational weeks 17–24 (12).

Maternal reinfection with rubella can occur during pregnancy; infection is usually asymptomatic, can generate maternal rubella-specific

IgM, and is generally considered to be of low risk to the fetus (13, 14). However, fetal damage after maternal reinfection has been reported (15).

Diagnosis in the infant can be made by isolation of the virus from the nasopharynx, urine, or cerebrospinal fluid; by detection of rubella-specific IgM; or by persistence of rubella-specific IgG for greater than 1 yr. At present, the detection of rubella-specific IgM antibody in the first 6 months of life is usually used to confirm the diagnosis of congenital rubella.

## Prevention and Patient Management

### IMMUNIZATION

RA 27/3 is the live attenuated rubella vaccine currently available for immunization in the U.S. The Advisory Committee for Immunization Practices (ACIP) recommends that susceptible women of childbearing age who are not immunocompromised and not pregnant, including women in the postpartum period and those who are postabortion, receive rubella vaccine. Because the vaccine can cross the placenta, women should be counseled to avoid conception for 3 months after immunization. However, no cases have been reported of infant defects secondary to maternal rubella immunization during pregnancy. The maximum theoretical risk of CRS related to the vaccine is less than 2% (16).

Vaccine virus is transmitted in breast milk but is not a contraindication to breastfeeding (17). Administration of blood products or anti-Rho (D) immune globulin (human) is not a contraindication to vaccination. However, if vaccination follows administration of these products, blood should be drawn 6–8 weeks after immunization to document seroconversion. Susceptible children and household contacts of pregnant women should also be immunized (17).

### OTHER CONTROL STRATEGIES

Patients with CRS who are secreting virus should be placed in strict isolation and be cared for only by rubella-immune personnel. In the event of an outbreak in the workplace, susceptible pregnant women should be transferred from the high-risk environment for the duration of the outbreak and undergo clinical and serological monitoring and counseling by their health care providers (18).

## COUNSELING FOR WOMEN INFECTED DURING PREGNANCY

For women infected during pregnancy, gestational age at the time of infection should be well documented. These individuals are appropriately counseled regarding occurrence of defects at various gestational ages. The decision to continue or to terminate pregnancy is made by the individual with her health care provider. Women with asymptomatic rubella infection during pregnancy should be treated in the same manner as those who experience clinical disease. Women reinfected with rubella virus during pregnancy are advised of the very low risk to the fetus. Women who incidentally receive vaccine during pregnancy should be counseled that the risk for fetal damage due to rubella is less than 2%.

## HUMAN *PARVOVIRUS* B19

Human *Parvovirus* (HPV) B19 is a DNA virus belonging to the family Parvoviridae. The virus causes erythema infectiosum (EI) or so-called fifth disease, which most commonly occurs in school-aged children. Symptoms of EI usually include a prodrome of fever and flu-like illness followed by the onset of a characteristic "slapped cheek" facial rash and a generalized maculopapular exanthem on the trunk and extremities (19). Infection also produces transient aplastic crisis (TAC) in patients with hemolytic anemias and conditions requiring increased erythrocyte production, and chronic anemia in immunodeficient individuals (20). Infection during pregnancy has resulted in fetal loss and nonimmune hydrops fetalis.

## Epidemiology

Human *Parvovirus* B19 infection occurs worldwide. Clinical infection is most common among school-aged children 5–15 yr of age. Antibody is present in 5–10% of preschool children and 50% of the adult population (21).

Populations at increased risk of infection include teachers, school nurses, day care workers, health care personnel, and household contacts of susceptible individuals. Presence of IgG is usually protective; however, infection has been reported in one volunteer with low-titer antibody (22).

The attack rate for susceptible household contacts exposed to persons with EI or TAC is approximately 50% (20). During school epidemics, seroconversion among susceptible staff can reach 20–30% (23). Attack rates of 36–38% have occurred among susceptible health care workers during nosocomial outbreaks (24).

In a woman whose serological status is unknown, the risk of fetal death secondary to HPV B19 infection is calculated to be less than 2.5% following exposure to an infected household contact and less than 1.5% after significant exposure at a school where EI is prevalent (23). The only prospective study published to date found a fetal loss rate of 5% among 39 pregnant women with serological evidence of recent infection (25).

## Modes of Transmission

The human is the only host for HPV B19. Although infection occurs throughout the year, epidemics of EI among school children occur most commonly in the late winter and spring. The virus is present in the respiratory secretions and blood of infected individuals. Disease is transmitted through aerosol droplet spread, through contact with blood, and through transfusion of infected blood and blood products (26). The incubation period for EI is 4–14 days extending to 20 days; for TAC, 6–12 days extending to 20 days or longer. Shortly after appearance of the rash, patients with EI are no longer infectious. Individuals with TAC, however, are infectious throughout their clinical course.

## Maternal and Fetal Health Consequences

Human *Parvovirus* B19 infection during pregnancy can be asymptomatic or present with arthralgias and, less frequently, with a maculopapular rash. Arthritis, fever, headache, malaise, and photophobia may also be present (27–29). In some cases, infection is suspected only by a history of exposure during an outbreak of EI or to an individual with clinical disease.

Recent maternal infection can be documented by a positive serum B19 IgM test; however, only 80% of women with recent infection will have detectable IgM levels. A simultaneous positive IgG and negative IgM denotes previous infection; these women are presumed to be immune to subsequent infection (28).

*Parvovirus* B19 can cause asymptomatic fetal infection (29), spontaneous abortion, nonimmune fetal hydrops, or intrauterine fetal death (25–30). It is believed that viral infection of fetal erythroid precursor cells generates a fetal aplastic crisis with anemia, cardiovascular failure, and eventual development of nonimmune hydrops (30). Myocarditis has been diagnosed with viral particles detected by electron microscopy in the myocardial cells (31). An anencephalic fetus was delivered to a B19-positive mother; however, this was believed to represent coincidental infection (28). Two other reports have described abortuses with eye defects, including one with abnormal bronchial and cardiac tissue (32, 33).

Intrauterine *Parvovirus* infection should be suspected when there is clinical disease or a history of exposure in the pregnant woman. Positive maternal B19 IgM serology makes fetal infection a possibility, and detection of hydrops by ultrasound strengthens the diagnosis. Confirmation of fetal infection requires identification of B19 IgM in fetal blood samples or in the newborn, or persistence of B19 IgG in the infant. *Parvovirus* DNA has been detected in fetal tissues by in situ hybridization studies; electron microscopy can detect virus particles in serum and amniotic fluid. As yet, it is not possible to grow the virus routinely.

## Prevention and Patient Management

### CONTROL STRATEGIES

There is no human *Parvovirus* B19 vaccine currently available.

Patients with hereditary hemolytic anemias in aplastic crisis and immunodeficient patients with chronic B19 infection are most contagious. The former have high concentrations of virus in their serum and nasopharyngeal secretions. Nosocomial transmission of B19 infection after contact with these patients has occurred primarily in nurses, but also in one play therapist who had no direct patient contact (24).

Both groups of patients should be admitted to private rooms with gown and glove isolation for the duration of the illness. Masks are recommended for close contact (21, 34) and may be advisable whenever entering the rooms of these patients.

Pregnant women should be excluded from caring for individuals with aplastic crisis because these patients can be very infectious (21). However, policies to exclude pregnant women routinely from the workplace during outbreaks of EI have generally not been recommended due to the ubiquity of the virus. Removal from child care or teaching may lessen the risk of infection, but does not eliminate it (21). Decisions about work transfer or removal during an outbreak of EI should be made by the pregnant worker in consultation with her health care provider and public health officials (23).

To minimize risk of infection during an outbreak of fifth disease, pregnant school and day care workers should avoid close contact with children and refrain from using water fountains or sharing glasses and utensils (28). In addition, pregnant women should avoid household contacts of patients with EI or contacts of viremic patients (35).

Universal precautions are advisable when handling the products of conception from women infected with HPV B19. Infected mothers should be isolated for the duration of their postpartum hospital stay. Newborns surviving B19 infection may secrete virus, and isolation is also warranted. Universal precautions and good handwashing are recommended for personnel caring for these infants.

### COUNSELING FOR WOMEN INFECTED DURING PREGNANCY

Pregnant women who are symptomatic or suspect exposure to HPV B19 infection should be counseled regarding potential risks and serology drawn for B19 IgM and IgG (Fig. 23.1). Serological testing is available through some

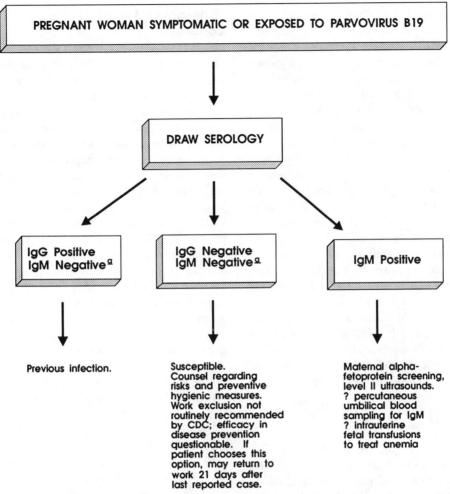

**PREGNANT WOMAN SYMPTOMATIC OR EXPOSED TO PARVOVIRUS B19**

**DRAW SEROLOGY**

**IgG Positive
IgM Negative[a]**

**IgG Negative
IgM Negative[a]**

**IgM Positive**

Previous infection.

Susceptible.
Counsel regarding
risks and preventive
hygienic measures.
Work exclusion not
routinely recommended
by CDC; efficacy in
disease prevention
questionable.  If
patient chooses this
option, may return to
work 21 days after
last reported case.

Maternal alpha-
fetoprotein screening,
level II ultrasounds.
? percutaneous
umbilical blood
sampling for IgM
? intrauterine
fetal transfusions
to treat anemia

**Figure 23.1.**   Proposed management protocol for pregnant women exposed to human *Parvovirus* B19.
[a]Only 80% of women with recent *Parvovirus* infection will have detectable IgM levels.

state health departments, some commercial laboratories, and the CDC. Women who are IgM positive should be followed with serial maternal serum α-fetoproteins because elevated levels have been associated with fetal infection (30). Serial level II ultrasounds are performed weekly for at least 8 weeks to look for development of hydrops fetalis (25). If hydrops is present, percutaneous umbilical blood sampling and intrauterine blood transfusion (IBT) have been considered to correct fetal anemia (25, 28, 36). However, the efficacy of IBT has not been established for the treatment of B19-induced hydrops fetalis and is not routinely recommended. Some cases of hydrops fetalis have been found to recover spontaneously.

## CYTOMEGALOVIRUS

Cytomegalovirus (CMV) is a DNA virus and member of the herpesvirus group. It is the virus with the highest incidence of in utero transmission (37). Congenital CMV infection can occur with primary maternal infection or in infants of seropositive ("immune") mothers (38) through reactivation of latent virus or reinfection. However, recurrent infection is much less likely to produce clinical sequelae in the infant.

### Epidemiology

Most women are infected with CMV at some point in their lives. While seropositivity among adults in developed nations averages about

40%, it approaches 100% in developing countries (39). Prospective studies have shown seropositive rates of 35–55% among pregnant women from middle and higher income groups and 77–82% among pregnant women from lower income groups (40, 41). Personnel who have contact with children, who deliver patient care, or who work in clinical laboratories are at increased risk of exposure to CMV disease (42).

The annual rate of acquisition of primary CMV infection among women of childbearing age is approximately 2.5% for women in middle to high income populations and 6.8% for those from low income groups. The occurrence of in utero transmission of primary CMV infection is 30–40%, with no significant difference in frequency noted between high and low income populations (40). The rate of in utero transmission of recurrent CMV infection is 1–2% (43).

Congenital CMV infection occurs in 0.2–2.0% of all livebirths, with an average annual infection rate of approximately 1%. In the U.S., approximately 30,000 infants are born with congenital CMV infection each year (37).

## Modes of Transmission

The human is the only reservoir for CMV. The virus is found worldwide and has no seasonal variation. Virus may be present in urine, saliva, tears, cervical secretions, breast milk, blood, semen, and feces. Infection is transmitted from person to person through sexual or other direct contact with infected body fluids, organ transplantation, and through contact with contaminated fomites such as diapers and toys (43, 44).

CMV may be transmitted to the fetus after maternal viremia. Infants can also acquire the virus perinatally from contact with infected genital secretions or by ingestion of contaminated breast milk (45). The incubation period for acquired CMV infection is 28–60 days, with an average of 40 days (46). Infants can also acquire CMV infection through multiple blood transfusions or nosocomial spread.

Individuals are infectious while shedding virus. Congenitally infected infants can shed virus in the urine for as long as 4–8 yr. Virus shedding from the throat is less persistent (47, 48).

## Maternal and Fetal Health Consequences

The majority of CMV infections during pregnancy are asymptomatic but can present with a self-limited mononucleosis-like illness. Signs of infection include fever, lymphadenopathy, splenomegaly, and elevation of peripheral lymphocyte count and liver enzymes (46, 49).

Seroconversion during pregnancy can be documented by comparison of paired acute and convalescent sera using ELISA tests. While the presence of positive CMV IgM by ELISA or radioimmunoassay helps confirm primary infection (50, 51), the test is positive in only 80% of women with primary infection and it is also positive in some recurrent infections. Recovery of CMV from urine or genital secretions is not a sensitive indicator of primary infection inasmuch as it can also occur with reactivation of virus. Attempts to recover virus from amniotic fluid have proven unreliable (50).

The majority of infants (90–95%) with congenital CMV infection are asymptomatic at birth. However, asymptomatic infants are at risk for developmental impairment, especially lowered IQ and hearing deficits. In one study, 16% of infants with positive CMV IgM antibody from cord blood had an IQ of 79 or lower, and 11% had bilateral hearing deficits (52).

Symptomatic newborns have a fatality rate of approximately 20% (37) and may present with thrombocytopenia, petechiae, hepatosplenomegaly, hyperbilirubinemia, microcephaly, small size for gestational age, prematurity, and chorioretinitis. Follow-up examination of survivors has noted microcephaly, mental retardation, cerebral palsy, hearing loss, and eye defects (53, 54). The majority of survivors of symptomatic infection have CNS or perceptual deficits.

The effect of gestational age at the time of infection on transmission of CMV or clinical outcome is as yet undetermined (40). Congenital infection resulting from primary maternal CMV infection is more commonly associated with clinical sequelae, while in utero transmission secondary to recurrent infection is less commonly of clinical consequence to the child (41). In one study of infants congenitally infected with CMV, 25% of infants born to mothers with primary CMV infection during pregnancy developed sequelae, whereas 8% of infants born to mothers with immunity to CMV (recurrent infection) did (55). In another study, all infants who were symptomatic at birth (5/33 or 15%) were born to mothers with primary infection; none of 27 infected infants born to mothers with recurrent infection was symptomatic (41). However, one case report of a child born to a mother with recurrent CMV infection during pregnancy describes hepatosplenomegaly and thrombocytopenia at birth and subsequent bilateral sensorineural deafness (56). Overall, congenital infection occurs more commonly in lower income populations. Congenital infection after primary maternal CMV, however, is more prevalent in upper socioeconomic groups (41).

Perinatal acquisition of CMV infection by healthy term infants does not usually result in major morbidity or mortality. However, significant sequelae can occur in premature infants including neutropenia, thrombocytopenia, hepatosplenomegaly, and respiratory compromise (57).

The most sensitive and specific method of identification of congenital infection is isolation of virus from the infant's urine within the first week of life (58). This method is well correlated with detection of CMV IgM in cord blood (51).

## Prevention and Patient Management

### CONTROL STRATEGIES

There is currently no licensed vaccine for CMV. Although studies are in progress on a CMV vaccine, it is likely to be restricted to nonpregnant women.

To prevent transmission of CMV infection, pregnant women should practice good personal hygiene, especially handwashing. Universal precautions are indicated for hospital and laboratory workers potentially exposed to CMV. Sound educational programs should inform pregnant workers about the risks of CMV infection, potential effects on the fetus, and appropriate infection control practices to minimize seroconversion. Routine serological testing is not indicated (51).

The literature suggests that pediatric health care workers may be at increased risk of CMV infection (59). However, several studies have shown that, when adequate hygiene is practiced, there is no increased risk of CMV infection for pediatric nurses compared with young women in the community (60–62). Reported annual attack rates of CMV are 2.5% for young, middle class women in the community, 3.3% for pediatric nurses, and 5.5% for young, middle class women between pregnancies (60).

Preschool-aged children, especially those attending day care, represent a significant source of CMV for parents, child care workers, and the community (42, 43). A 15% seroconversion rate among parents of children in day care centers has been reported (42). Day care workers have been noted to have an increased annual rate of acquisition of CMV infection (11–20% seroconversion per year) (63, 64). A study from Alabama revealed a yearly seroconversion rate of 20% among day care personnel (63). In this investigation, workers having 20 or more contact hours per week with children younger than 3 yr of age had a markedly increased annual seroconversion rate of 31.4%, compared with 13.2% among workers with lesser contact.

Day care workers who are pregnant or who are considering pregnancy should be appropriately counseled and offered serological testing to determine their CMV status (63). Adequate hygiene practices may help minimize acquisition of infection. Suggested measures include frequent handwashing, use of gloves when changing diapers, and precautions against secretions (including respiratory secretions). Assignment of these women to the care of older children may also reduce the risk of seroconversion (64).

Any woman who develops clinical symptoms resembling mononucleosis and is heterophile negative should be tested for primary CMV infection. If positive, appropriate counseling is offered (50). For the purpose of comparison of acute and convalescent sera for CMV as well as for other infectious agents, it may be prudent to collect and to store a serum sample at the beginning of pregnancy for all women (43).

## COUNSELING FOR WOMEN INFECTED DURING PREGNANCY

Women with documented primary or recurrent CMV infection during pregnancy should be counseled about the potential risks of infection to the infant. No correlation can be made between gestational age and outcome for the infant, nor is there any standard reliable means available to document in utero transmission of infection.

There are currently no indications for recommending termination of pregnancy after early primary CMV infection (51). Of 100 women with primary CMV infection during pregnancy, approximately 30% will transmit infection to the infant in utero. Of these 30 congenitally infected infants, approximately 18% will have clinical symptoms at birth and be at risk for major sequelae and an additional 7% may develop sequelae after birth (55). Of all asymptomatic newborns, 10–15% will have intellectual or perceptual (primarily hearing) deficits. Recurrent CMV infection rarely produces congenital defects in the infant; however, 8% of infected infants born to mothers with recurrent infection can have sequelae (55). Some authorities recommend culturing amniotic fluid or fetal blood for the virus, but data are not available correlating culture results with outcome of the infant.

## VARICELLA

Varicella-zoster virus (VZV) is a DNA virus and member of the herpesvirus family. The virus causes chickenpox in children and adults and can result in latent infection; reactivation of infection results in herpes zoster or "shingles." Transmission of the virus in utero can cause varicella embryopathy (VE) and varicella of the newborn (VON) (65).

### Epidemiology

At least 3 million cases of chickenpox occur in the U.S. each year (65), with the majority in individuals below 15 yr of age. Individuals over 20 yr old account for only 1.8% of cases (66). Varicella is uncommon during pregnancy; its incidence is estimated at 1/7500 based on eight cases occurring in 60,000 pregnancies prospectively studied (67). The annual incidence of herpes zoster in the U.S. is 0.3–0.5%, with the majority of cases occurring in adults over 50 yr of age. Among U.S. women of childbearing age, the mean incidence is 2.16/1000/yr (68).

After household exposure, approximately 90% of susceptible contacts will develop varicella. Most individuals living in temperate regions are immune to varicella by adulthood, while those from tropical areas are more likely to be susceptible. Among adults having a negative or uncertain history of varicella, approximately 85–95% will be immune; thus, the attack rates for adults after household or hospital exposure is 5–15% (69). McGregor et al. (70) noted that 71% of pregnant women with negative histories of VZV infection, and 90% of those with uncertain histories, were seropositive. With the exception of bone marrow transplant recipients, adults with a positive history of varicella are considered immune, usually for life (69).

Susceptible individuals include those who have not had VZV and immunocompromised patients. The latter may develop a fulminant course with dissemination and fatality.

### Modes of Transmission

The human represents the only reservoir of infection. The infection is most common in late winter and early spring. The organism is transmitted from person to person via vesicular skin lesions, by aerosol, and possibly through respiratory droplet spread (71). Susceptible individuals can develop chickenpox after exposure to patients with zoster.

Individuals with chickenpox are contagious 1–2 days before and 5–6 days after the onset of rash. Immunocompromised persons are contagious while new lesions are appearing. The incubation period for chickenpox is 10–21 days, with an average of 14–16 days. The use of varicella-zoster immune globulin (VZIG) prolongs the incubation period; individuals who have received VZIG are considered contagious for 28 days (72).

### Maternal and Fetal Health Consequences

Varicella-zoster lesions typically begin on the scalp or trunk and spread centrifugally. They appear first as erythematous macules, then vesicles, and finally crust and form scabs. The patient may be febrile to 101–102° F through the first few days of rash. Dissemination to other organs causing encephalitis, pneumonia, or hepatitis is rare and occurs more commonly in adolescents and adults than in children. Herpes zoster, occurring as a reactivation of latent infection, presents as a vesicular skin rash along sensory dermatomes (73).

Diagnosis can be made by isolation of virus from vesicular lesions or by immunofluorescent staining of cells from the floor of vesicles. Serological diagnosis is possible through detection of varicella IgM or comparison of acute and convalescent titers using Fluorescent Antibody against Membrane Antigen (FAMA), ELISA, immune adherence, hemagglutination, or neutralization titers. Complement fixation is more readily available than these methods but is less sensitive.

Pregnant women are subject to the same complications of VZV infection as are other adults. There are a number of reports of maternal fatality, intrauterine fetal death, and prematurity after maternal varicella pneumonia (74–77). Of 43 pregnant women studied by Paryani, four of them (9%) developed varicella pneumonia; two patients required ventilatory support, and one patient died (74). In another review, seven of 17 (41%) mothers with varicella pneumonia died (75). Acyclovir and adenine arabinoside have been used in a limited number of cases of maternal varicella pneumonia, with resultant clinical resolution in the mother and delivery of a live infant (78, 79). Routine use of acyclovir cannot be recommended during pregnancy; however, acyclovir should be considered in cases where the possible risks to the fetus are outweighed by the potential therapeutic benefits of treating life-threatening disease in the pregnant woman (78, 79).

Infants of women with VZV infection during pregnancy may develop an embryopathy characterized by low birthweight, cortical atrophy, seizures, chorioretinitis, cataracts, microophthalmia, hypotrophic limbs, hemiatrophy, and skin lesions (74, 80, 81). These defects usually occur after maternal infection in the first half of pregnancy. However, one report describes an infant with significant skin and soft tissue scarring of an extremity after maternal varicella infection at 28 weeks' gestation (82).

Infants who are born to mothers who had been infected with VZV up to 3 weeks before delivery are usually asymptomatic but they may develop herpes zoster at an early age (83). Infants who develop varicella following maternal infection 6–21 days before delivery usually have a benign course; however, if maternal varicella develops within 5 days of delivery or during the first 2 postpartum days, the newborn is at risk for serious disseminated varicella infection and should receive VZIG (69).

Congenital varicella infection can be diagnosed in a number of ways. Symptomatic varicella or characteristic anomalies may be noted at birth, or herpes zoster may develop in infancy. The presence of VZV IgM during the neonatal period and the persistence of VZV IgG at 1 yr of age or older without prior history of varicella infection confirms the diagnosis (74).

The role of zoster during pregnancy is controversial. No birth defects were noted in 14 infants after maternal herpes zoster infections, the majority of which (64%) occurred during the third trimester (74). However, limb atrophy and dermal scarring were noted in one infant born to a mother with herpes zoster during the 12th week of pregnancy with positive serological studies for VZV in mother and infant (84).

## Prevention and Patient Management

### CONTROL STRATEGIES

Live varicella vaccine is not currently licensed in the U.S.

Susceptible individuals should avoid exposure to patients with chickenpox or herpes zoster or those in the incubation period for chickenpox. In the occupational setting (e.g., health care facilities, day care centers, schools), it is advisable that pregnant women without a history of varicella infection or serological evidence of immunity avoid contact with infected individuals. The administration of VZIG to susceptible pregnant women has been recommended (74) after a significant varicella exposure (69) to prevent maternal complications of

VZV infection. For maximum efficacy, it should be given as soon as possible and within 96 hr of exposure (69). Whether the administration of VZIG mitigates fetal complications is unknown.

Individuals exposed to varicella are considered infectious from days 10–21 postexposure and days 10–28 if VZIG was administered. Persons who contract varicella should be placed in strict isolation until all skin lesions are crusted over (usually 6 days). If a woman develops varicella after delivery, the infant is isolated from the mother until all vesicles have crusted over. It is not known whether VZV is excreted in the breast milk of mothers with chickenpox (65).

## COUNSELING FOR WOMEN INFECTED DURING PREGNANCY

Women with chickenpox during pregnancy should be counseled regarding the potential risks of VZV to the fetus based on gestational age. The occurrence of birth defects after maternal varicella infection during the first trimester is low (4.9%), as determined by combined data from 61 infants in prospective studies (68, 74, 81). In one report, the frequency was as low as 2.3% (85). Defects do occur after maternal varicella infection during the second and third trimesters, but they are very uncommon (80, 82). Birth defects after zoster infection are rare. If varicella develops within 5 days before or 2 days postdelivery, the infant can develop severe disease and should receive VZIG as soon as possible.

## HEPATITIS B

Hepatitis B is a DNA virus. It has the potential to cause chronic liver infection leading to cirrhosis and to predispose to hepatocellular carcinoma. Maternal infection can be transmitted to the fetus in utero, at the time of birth, or during the postnatal period.

### Epidemiology

The presence of hepatitis B virus (HBV) antibody in the U.S. ranges from 5% in the general population to 100% within certain high-risk groups. In the U.S., 200,000–300,000 new cases of hepatitis B occur each year. The carrier rate among young adults is 6–10%. Chronic active hepatitis occurs in one-fourth of carriers and predisposes to cirrhosis of the liver (86).

The prevalence of hepatitis B surface antigen (HBsAg) among pregnant women varies according to the population studied: it is lowest among women from the U.S. and northern Europe and highest among Chinese women (87). In screening of pregnant women from France, the U.S., and China, the proportion of women positive for HBsAg was 0.63% (28/4452), 0.88% (136/15,399) and 15% (204/1343), respectively (88–90).

Populations at higher risk for acquiring or having HBV include intravenous drug users, homosexuals, residents of endemic areas, recipients of multiple blood transfusions, persons with multiple episodes of sexually transmitted diseases, household contacts of HBV carriers, personnel or residents of institutions for the mentally retarded, prisoners, hemodialysis patients, health care workers (especially those exposed to blood from potentially infectious patients), and sexual contacts of these groups. After needlestick exposure with blood positive for both HBsAg and hepatitis B e antigen (HBeAg), 19% of recipients developed hepatitis B (91, 92).

In the U.S., it is estimated that 16,500 infants are born to HBsAg-positive women each year; 3500 infants become chronic HBV carriers (93). Among infants born to mothers who are both HBsAg and HBeAg positive, 95% become infected by 3 months of age. Of these infants, 85–93% become chronic carriers, as compared with 31% of infants born to HBeAg-negative mothers (94, 95).

### Modes of Transmission

Hepatitis B virus is found in humans and some nonhuman primates. It has a worldwide distribution with a high prevalence in Africa and Asia. Virus can be found in blood, urine, saliva, feces, semen, vaginal secretions, bile, amniotic fluid, gastric aspirates of newborn infants, and breast milk (91, 96). The most common routes of transmission are through percutaneous inoculation of blood, mucous membrane contact with blood and body fluids, and through sexual contact (97). Individuals are infectious while they are HBsAg positive. The incubation period for acquired infection is 50–180 days, with an average of 120 days (98).

Maternal-fetal transmission usually occurs at the time of birth; in utero transmission accounts for only 5–10% of infants who become carriers (94).

## Maternal and Infant Health Consequences

Most pregnant women who are positive for HBsAg are asymptomatic chronic carriers. Some patients develop acute hepatitis, and a minority have fulminant disease characterized by hepatic failure, encephalopathy, and a high mortality rate. Hepatitis B infection can also cause chronic persistent and chronic active hepatitis, the latter leading to cirrhosis and death in some patients (97). In general, the course of the disease is not altered during pregnancy.

Maternal HBV infection can result in preterm delivery, especially if symptomatic (99), but is not associated with teratogenic effects. Women positive for HBeAg are more likely to be infectious (92, 95), and risk of fetal infection is enhanced in these cases (94, 95).

The majority of infants infected with HBV become asymptomatic carriers, including 90% of unvaccinated infants born to HBsAg-positive and HBeAg-positive mothers. Like adults, infants may develop acute hepatitis, chronic persistent hepatitis, chronic active hepatitis, and fulminant disease (87, 88, 100).

The presence of HBsAg in the blood of neonates confirms infection. Cord blood samples positive for HBsAg cannot be used for this purpose (101).

## Prevention and Patient Management

### IMMUNIZATION

Plasma-derived hepatitis B vaccine (Heptavax) is no longer produced in the U.S. The currently available vaccines are manufactured by recombinant DNA technology (Recombivax HB, Engerix-B). When given in appropriate doses, protective levels of antibody are produced in over 90% of healthy recipients. For adults and children with normal immune status, protection lasts for at least 5 yr. Declining antibody levels in at-risk individuals may warrant administration of booster doses of vaccine (102).

There is no contraindication to vaccination for pregnant women in whom it is otherwise indicated. Guidelines from the CDC (102) and the Occupational Safety and Health Administration (OSHA) (103) recommend Hepatitis B vaccine for susceptible workers at significant risk for HBV infection. This group includes health care workers (medical, dental, and laboratory personnel), public safety workers, and others who work in high-risk areas or who have potential contact with blood, blood products, body fluids, or tissues from infected patients. Other vaccine candidates are personnel and residents of institutions for the mentally retarded, hemodialysis patients, intravenous drug users, prison inmates, household and sexual contacts of HBV carriers, and other members of high-risk groups (86). Table 23.1 delineates the recommended immunization dosages and schedules for high-risk groups and postexposure prophylaxis.

Recently, the CDC has recommended routine hepatitis B vaccination of all infants (102). It is particularly important to report positive HBsAg serology in the mother to pediatric personnel so that the infant receives hepatitis B immune globulin (HBIG) and appropriate doses of hepatitis B vaccine (Table 23.1). Use of combined active-passive immunization protocols has reduced carrier rates of infants born to HBsAg-positive mothers by 85–90% (94, 104).

### OTHER CONTROL STRATEGIES

All pregnant women should be tested for HBsAg as part of initial prenatal screening. Testing based solely on the identification of risk categories will exclude a significant percentage of antigen-positive women (89, 93). Follow-up testing is not recommended unless there is a history of exposure, acute hepatitis is suspected, or high-risk behavior, such as intravenous drug use, is identified.

More than 90% of women positive for HBsAg on routine screening are chronic carriers. Infected women should be thoroughly evaluated; household members and sexual con-

**Table 23.1.**
**Recommendations for Hepatitis B Prophylaxis (Centers for Disease Control, 1991)[a]**

| Population | Recommendations |
|---|---|
| Pre-exposure | |
| High-risk populations | Recombivax HB 10 μg or Engerix-B 20 μg IM (deltoid muscle) at 0, 1, 6 months; booster dose is 10 μg Recombivax or 20 μg Engerix-B; doses are usually halved for children <11 yr old, except Recombivax dose is 2.5 μg; Recombivax dose for children 11–19 yr old is 5 μg; use 40-μg doses in hemodialysis patients and immunocompromised patients (Engerix-B is a four-dose regimen at 0, 1, 2, 6 months in these patients); test for HBsAb levels annually in hemodialysis patients and give a booster dose when HBsAb level falls below 10 mIU/ml; dialysis staff and HIV-positive individuals should be tested for seroconversion to HBsAb 1–6 months after vaccine completion; testing those at risk for occupational exposure for seroconversion after vaccination should also be considered |
| Neonates born to HBV-negative mothers | Give Recombivax 2.5 μg or Engerix-B 10 μg IM within 12 hr of birth, and at 1 and 6 months of age (Engerix-B is also licensed for four doses given at 0, 1, 2, and 12 months of age); alternative dosing regimen for infants born to HBsAg-negative mothers is 1–2 months, 4 months, 6–18 months of age |
| Postexposure | |
| Personnel with needlestick/body fluid exposure | At time of exposure, draw hepatitis B serology on exposed person and potential source; if exposed susceptible and source HBsAg positive, administer HBIG (0.06 ml/kg IM) as soon as possible (best within 24 hr) and commence vaccine series described above |
| Neonates born to HBV-positive mothers | Give HBIG 0.5 ml IM within 12 hr after birth *and* Recombivax 5 μg or Engerix-B 10 μg IM within 12 hr of birth, and at 1 and 6 months of age; infants should be tested for HBsAb and HBsAg when 9–15 months old, or 3–9 months after vaccination is complete |
| Neonates born to mothers of unknown HBV status | Test the mother for HBsAg and, while results are pending, give the neonate Hepatitis B vaccine within 12 hr of birth at a dose for infants born to HBsAg-positive mothers; if the mother is found to be positive, give the infant HBIG as soon as possible within 7 days of birth; continue vaccination of the infant at the appropriate dose and schedule as directed by maternal serology |

[a]Centers for Disease Control. Hepatitis B virus: a comprehensive strategy for eliminating transmission in the United States through universal childhood vaccination: recommendations of the Immunization Practices Advisory Committee (ACIP). MMWR 1991;40:1–25. HBIG = Hepatitis B Immune Globulin; IM = intramuscular.

tacts are tested and, if susceptible, offered vaccination. Use of the fetal scalp electrode during labor may represent a portal of inoculation for the fetus.

Women should be rescreened during each pregnancy. Although highly reliable, positive HBsAg tests should be confirmed (93). Women who were not screened prenatally should be tested on admission for delivery, so that results are available within 24 hr postpartum.

In addition to vaccination, individuals at risk for HBV infection in the workplace should practice universal precautions in accordance with CDC and OSHA guidelines (103, 105).

Avoidance of needlestick injury is particularly important. Pregnant women exposed to hepatitis B should follow CDC guidelines for postexposure prophylaxis and be retested for HBsAg later in pregnancy.

## COUNSELING FOR WOMEN INFECTED DURING PREGNANCY

Mothers positive for HBsAg should be counseled regarding risks of transmission to the infant and the recommendation for active and passive immunization of the infant at birth.

## REFERENCES

1. Centers for Disease Control. Elimination of rubella and congenital rubella syndrome—United States. MMWR 1985;34:65–66.
2. Bart KJ, Orenstein WA, Preblud SR, Hinman AR. Universal immunization to interrupt rubella. Rev Infect Dis 1985;7S:S177–S184.
3. Miller E, Cradock-Watson JE, Pollock TM. Consequences of confirmed maternal rubella at successive stages of pregnancy. Lancet 1982;2:781–784.
4. Evans AS, Niederman JC, Sawyer RN, et al. Prospective studies of a group of Yale university freshmen. II. Occurrence of acute respiratory infections and rubella. J Infect Dis 1971;123:271–278.
5. Centers for Disease Control. Rubella and congenital rubella syndrome United States, 1985–1988. MMWR 1989;38:173–178.
6. Shewmon DA, Cherry JD, Kirby SE. Shedding of rubella virus in a 4 1/2-year-old boy with congenital rubella. Pediatr Infect Dis J 1982;1:342–343.
7. Menser MA, Forrest JM, Slinn RF, Nowak MJ, Dorman DC. Rubella viruria in a 29-year-old woman with congenital rubella. Lancet 1971;2:797–798.
8. Cherry JD. Rubella. In: Feigin RD, Cherry JD, eds. Textbook of pediatric infectious diseases. Philadelphia: WB Saunders, 1987:1810–1831.
9. Sever JL, South MA, Shaver KA. Delayed manifestations of congenital rubella. Rev Infect Dis 1985;7:S164–S169.
10. Ueda K, Nishida Y, Oshima K, Shepard TH. Congenital rubella syndrome: correlation of gestational age at time of maternal rubella with type of defect. J Pediatr 1979; 94:763–765.
11. Munro ND, Sheppard S, Smithells RW, Holzel H, Jones G. Temporal relations between maternal rubella and congenital defects. Lancet 1987;2:201–204.
12. Grillner L, Forsgren M, Barr B, Bottiger M, Danielsson L, De Verdies C. Outcome of rubella during pregnancy with special reference to the 17th-24th weeks of gestation. Scand J Infect Dis 1983;15:321–325.
13. Morgan-Capner P, Hodgson J, Hambling MH, et al. Detection of rubella-specific IgM in subclinical rubella reinfection in pregnancy. Lancet 1985;1:244–246.
14. Grangeot-Keros L, Nicolas JC, Bricout F, Pillot J. Rubella reinfection and the fetus. N Engl J Med 1985; 313:1547.
15. Eilard T and Strannegard O. Rubella reinfection in pregnancy followed by transmission to the fetus. J Infect Dis 1974; 129:594–596.
16. Advisory Committee on Immunization Practices. Rubella vaccination during pregnancy—United States 1971–1986. MMWR 1987;36:457–461.
17. Centers for Disease Control. Rubella prevention. MMWR 1984; 33:301–317.
18. Greaves WL, Orenstein WA, Stetler HC, Preblud SR, Hinman AR, Bart KJ. Prevention of rubella transmission in medical facilities. JAMA 1982;248:861–864.
19. Plummer FA, Hammond GW, Forward K, et al. An erythema infectiosum-like illness caused by human parvovirus infection. N Engl J Med 1985;313:74–79.
20. Chorba T, Coccia P, Holman RC, et al. The role of parvovirus B19 in aplastic crisis and erythema infectiosum (fifth disease). J Infect Dis 1986;154:383–393.
21. American Academy of Pediatrics, Committee on Infectious Diseases 1989–1990. Parvovirus, erythema infectiosum and pregnancy. Pediatrics 1990;85:131–133.
22. Anderson MJ, Higgins PG, Davis LR, et al. Experimental parvoviral infection in humans. J Infect Dis 1985;152:257–265.
23. Centers for Disease Control. Risks associated with human parvovirus B19 infection. MMWR 1989;138:81–97.
24. Bell LM, Naides SJ, Stoffman P, Hodinka RL, Plotkin SA. Human parvovirus B19 infection among hospital staff members after contact with infected patients. N Engl J Med 1989;321:485–491.
25. Rodis JF, Quinn DL, Gary W, et al. Management and outcome of pregnancies complicated by human B19 parvovirus infection: a prospective study. Am J Obstet Gynecol 1990;163:1168–1171.
26. Mortimer PP, Luban NL, Kelleher JF, Cohen BJ. Transmission of serum parvovirus-like virus by clotting-factor concentrates. Lancet 1983;2:482–484.
27. Anand A, Gray E, Brown T, Clewley JP, Cohen BJ. Human parvovirus infection in pregnancy and hydrops fetalis. N Engl J Med 1987;316:183–186.
28. Rodis JF, Hovick TJ, Quinn DL, Rosengren SS, Tattersall P. Human parvovirus infection in pregnancy. Obstet Gynecol 1988;72:733–738.
29. Woernle CH, Anderson LJ, Tattersoll P, Davison JM. Human parvovirus B19 infection during pregnancy. J Infect Dis 1987;156:17–20.
30. Carrington D, Gilmore DH, Whittle MJ, et al. Maternal serum alpha-fetoprotein—a marker of fetal aplastic crisis during intrauterine human parvovirus infection. Lancet 1987;1:433–435.
31. Naides SJ, Weiner CP. Antenatal diagnosis and palliative treatment of non-immune hydrops fetalis secondary to fetal parvovirus B19 infection. Prenat Diagn 1989;9:105–114.
32. Weiland HT, Vermey-Keers C, Salimans MM, Fleuren GJ, Verwey RA, Anderson MJ. Parvovirus B19 associated with fetal abnormality [Letter]. Lancet 1987;1:682–683.
33. Hartwig NG, Vermeij-Keers C, Van Elsacker-Niele AM, Fleuren GJ. Embryonic malformations in a case of intrauterine parvovirus B19 infection. Teratology 1989;39: 295–302.
34. Leads from the MMWR. Risks associated with human parvovirus B19 infection. JAMA 1989;261:1555–1563.

35. Naides SJ. Infection control measures for human parvovirus B19 in the hospital setting. Infect Control Hosp Epidemiol 1989;10:326–329.

36. Schwarz TF, Roggendorf M, Hottentrager B, et al. Human parvovirus B19 infection in pregnancy. Lancet 1988;2:566–567.

37. Stagno S, Pass RF, Dworsky ME, Alford CA. Congenital and perinatal CMV infections. Semin Perinatol 1983; 7:31–42.

38. Stagno S, Reynolds DW, Huang E, Thames SD, Smith RJ, Alford CA. Congenital cytomegalovirus infection: occurrence in an immune population. N Engl J Med 1977;296:1254–1258.

39. Krech U. Complement-fixing antibodies against cytomegalovirus in different parts of the world. Bull WHO 1973;49:103–106.

40. Stagno S, Pass RF, Cloud G, et al. Primary cytomegalovirus infection in pregnancy: incidence, transmission to fetus and clinical outcome. JAMA 1986;256:1904–1908.

41. Stagno S, Pass RF, Dworsky ME, et al. Congenital cytomegalovirus infection. The relative importance of primary and recurrent maternal infection. N Engl J Med 1982;306:945–949.

42. Pass RF, Hutto C, Ricks R, Cloud G. Increased rate of cytomegalovirus infection among parents of children attending day-care centers. N Engl J Med 1986;314:1414–1418.

43. Adler SP. Cytomegalovirus transmission among children in day care, their mothers and caretakers. Pediatr Infect Dis J 1988;7:279–285.

44. Hanshaw JB. Cytomegalovirus. In: Feigin RD, Cherry JD, eds. Textbook of pediatric infectious diseases. Philadelphia: WB Saunders, 1987:1558–1566.

45. Stagno S, Reynolds DW, Pass RF, Alford CA. Breast milk and the risk of cytomegalovirus infection. N Engl J Med 1980; 302:1073–1076.

46. Betts RF. Cytomegalovirus infection epidemiology and biology in adults. Semin Perinatol 1983;7:22–30.

47. Reynolds DW, Stagno S, Stubbs KG et al. Inapparent congenital cytomegalovirus infection with elevated cord IgM levels. N Engl J Med 1974;290:291–296.

48. Hanshaw JB. Congenital cytomegalovirus infection: a fifteen year perspective. J Infect Dis 1971;123:555–561.

49. Ho M. Cytomegalovirus. In: Mandell GL, RG Douglas, JE Bennett, eds. Principles and practice of infectious diseases. New York: Churchill Livingstone, 1990:1159–1172.

50. Onorato IM, Morens DM, Martone WJ, Stansfield SK. Epidemiology of cytomegaloviral infections: recommendations for prevention and control. Rev Infect Dis 1985;7:479–496.

51. Griffiths PD, Baboonian C. A prospective study of primary cytomegalovirus infection during pregnancy: final report. Br J Obstet Gynaecol 1984;91:307–315.

52. Hanshaw JB, Scheiner AP, Moxley AW, Gaer L, Abel V, Scheiner B. School failure and deafness after "silent" congenital cytomegalovirus infection. N Engl J Med 1976;295:468–470.

53. Williamson WD, Desmond MM, La Fevers N, Taber LH, Catlin FI, Weaver TG. Symptomatic congenital cytomegalovirus. Disorders of language, learning and hearing. Am J Dis Child 1982;136:902–905.

54. Pass RF, Stagno S, Myers GJ, Alford CA. Outcome of symptomatic congenital cytomegalovirus infection: results of long-term longitudinal follow-up. Pediatrics 1980;66:758–762.

55. Fowler KB, Stagno S, Pass RF, Britt WJ, Boll TJ, Alford CA. The outcome of congenital cytomegalovirus infection in relation to maternal antibody status. N Engl J Med 1992;326:663–667.

56. Ahlfors K, Harris S, Ivarsson S, Svanberg L. Secondary maternal cytomegalovirus infection causing symptomatic congenital infection. N Engl J Med 1981;305:284.

57. Yeager AS, Palumbo PE, Malachowski N, Ariagno RL, Stevenson DK. Sequelae of maternally derived cytomegalovirus infections in premature infants. J Pediatr 1983;102:918–922.

58. Stagno S, Pass RF, Reynolds DW, Moore MA, Nahmias AJ, Alford CA. Comparative study of diagnostic procedures for congenital cytomegalovirus infection. Pediatrics 1980;65:251–257.

59. Friedman HM, Lewis MR, Nemerofsky D, Plotkin SA. Acquisition of cytomegalovirus infection among female employees at a pediatric hospital. Pediatr Infect Dis J 1984;3:233–235.

60. Dworsky ME, Welch K, Cassady G, Stagno S. Occupational risk for primary cytomegalovirus infection among pediatric health care workers. N Engl J Med 1983;309:950–953.

61. Ahlfors K, Ivarsson S-A, Johnsson T, Renmarker K. Risk of cytomegalovirus infection in nurses and congenital infection in their offspring. Acta Paediatr Scand 1981;70:819–823.

62. Balcarek KB, Bagley R, Cloud G, Pass RF. Cytomegalovirus infection among employees of a children's hospital. No evidence for increased risk associated with patient care. JAMA 1990;263:840–844.

63. Adler SP. Cytomegalovirus and child day care. Evidence for an increased infection rate among day-care workers. N Engl J Med 1989;321:1290–1296.

64. Pass RF, Hutto C, Lyon MD, Cloud G. Increased rate of cytomegalovirus infection among day care center workers. Pediatr Infect Dis J 1990;9:465–470.

65. Brunell PA. Fetal and neonatal varicella-zoster infections. Semin Perinatol 1983;7:47–56.

66. Preblud SR, D'Angelo LJ. Chickenpox in the United States, 1972–1977. J Infect Dis 1979;140:257–260.

67. Sever J, White LR. Intrauterine viral infections. Annu Rev Med 1968;19:471–486.

68. Enders G. Varicella-zoster virus infection in pregnancy. Prog Med Virol 1984;29:166–196.

69. Advisory Committee on Immunization Practices. Varicella-zoster immune globulin for the prevention of chickenpox. MMWR 1984;33:84–100.

70. McGregor JA, Mark S, Crawford GP, Levin MJ. Varicella zoster antibody testing in the care of pregnant women exposed to varicella. Am J Obstet Gynecol 1987;157:281–284.

71. Leclair JM, Zaia JA, Levin MJ, Congdon RG, Goldman DA. Airborne transmission of chickenpox in a hospital. N Engl J Med 1980;302:450–453.

72. American Academy of Pediatrics, Committee on Infectious Diseases. Varicella-zoster infections. In: Report of the Committee on Infectious Diseases. Elk Grove Village, IL: American Academy of Pediatrics, 1988:456–462.

73. Brunell PA. Varicella-zoster infections. In: Feigin RD, Cherry JD, eds. Textbook of pediatric infectious diseases. Philadelphia: WB Saunders, 1987:1602–1607.

74. Paryani SG, Arvin AM. Intrauterine infection with varicella-zoster virus after maternal varicella. N Engl J Med 1986;314:1542–1546.

75. Harris RE, Rhoades ER. Varicella pneumonia complicating pregnancy. Report of a case and review of literature. Obstet Gynecol 1965;25:734–740.

76. Fish SA. Maternal death due to disseminated varicella. JAMA 1960;173:978–981.

77. Purtilo DT, Bhawan J, Liao S, Brutus A, Yang JP, Balogh K. Fatal varicella in a pregnant woman and a baby. Am J Obstet Gynecol 1977;127:208–209.

78. Glaser JB, Loftus T, Ferrangamo V, Mootabar H, Castellano M. Varicella-zoster infection in pregnancy [Letter]. N Engl J Med 1986;315:1416.

79. Landsberger EJ, Hager WD, Grossman JH. Successful management of varicella pneumonia complicating pregnancy: a report of three cases. J Reprod Med 1986;31:311–314.

80. Brice JE. Congenital varicella resulting from infection during second trimester of pregnancy. Arch Dis Child 1976;51:474–476.

81. Siegel M. Congenital malformations following chickenpox, measles, mumps and hepatitis. Results of a cohort study. JAMA 1973;226:1521–1524.

82. Bai PV, John TJ. Congenital skin ulcers following varicella in late pregnancy. J Pediatr 1979;94:65–67.

83. Higa K, Dan K, Manabe H. Varicella-zoster virus infections during pregnancy: hypothesis concerning the mechanisms of congenital malformations. Obstet Gynecol 1987;69:214–222.

84. Broomhead I, Dudgeon JA. Viral diseases of the fetus and newborn. In: Hanshaw JB, Dudgeon JA, eds. Major problems in clinical pediatrics. Vol 17. Philadelphia: WB Saunders, 1978:192–208.

85. Preblud SR, Cochi SL, Orenstein WA. Varicella-zoster infection in pregnancy [Letter]. N Engl J Med 1986;315:1416–1417.

86. Centers for Disease Control. Protection against viral hepatitis: recommendations of the Immunization Practices Advisory Committee (ACIP). MMWR 1990;39:5–22.

87. Overall JC. Viral infections of the fetus and neonate. In: Feigin RD, Cherry JD, eds. Textbook of pediatric infectious diseases. Philadelphia: WB Saunders, 1987:985–988.

88. Dupuy JM, Giraud P, Dupuy C, Drouet J, Hoofnagle J. Hepatitis B in children. II. Study of children born to chronic HBsAg carrier mothers. J Pediatr 1978;92:200–204.

89. Summers PR, Biswas MK, Pastorek JG, Pernoll ML, Smith LG, Bean BE. The pregnant hepatitis B carrier: evidence favoring comprehensive antepartum screening. Obstet Gynecol 1987;69:701–704.

90. Stevens CE, Beasley RP, Tsui J, Lee W. Vertical transmission of hepatitis B antigen in Taiwan. N Engl J Med 1975;292:771–774.

91. Gerberding JL. Risks to health care workers from occupational exposure to hepatitis B virus, human immunodeficiency virus, and cytomegalovirus. Infect Dis Clin North Am 1989;3:735–745.

92. Werner BG, Grady GF. Accidental hepatitis-B-surface-antigen-positive inoculations. Use of e antigen to estimate infectivity. Ann Intern Med 1982;97:367–369.

93. Advisory Committee on Immunization Practices. Prevention of perinatal transmission of hepatitis B virus: prenatal screening of all pregnant women for Hepatitis B surface antigen. MMWR 1988;37:341–351.

94. Beasley RP, Hwang L-Y, Lee GC, et al. Prevention of perinatally transmitted hepatitis B virus infections with hepatitis B immune globulin and hepatitis B vaccine. Lancet 1983;2:1099–1102.

95. Beasley RP, Trepo C, Stevens CE, Szmuness W. The e antigen and vertical transmission of hepatitis B surface antigen. Am J Epidemiol 1977;105:94–98.

96. Lee AK, Ip HM, Wong VC. Mechanisms of maternal-fetal transmission of hepatitis B virus. J Infect Dis 1978;138:668–671.

97. Robinson WS. Hepatitis B virus and hepatitis delta virus. In: Mandell GL, Douglas RG, Bennett JE, eds. Principles and practice of infectious diseases. New York: Churchill Livingstone, 1990:1204–1231.

98. American Academy of Pediatrics, Committee on Infectious Diseases. Hepatitis B. In: Report of the Committee on Infectious Diseases. Elk Grove, IL: American Academy of Pediatrics, 1988:217–227.

99. Smithwick EM, Pascual E, Go SC. Hepatitis-associated antigen: a possible relationship to premature delivery. J Pediatr 1972;81:537–540.

100. Delaplane D, Yogev R, Crussi F, Shulman S. Fatal hepatitis B in early infancy: the importance of identifying HBsAg-positive pregnant women and providing immunoprophylaxis to their newborns. Pediatrics 1983;72:176–180.

101. Gerety RJ, Schweitzer IL. Viral hepatitis type B during pregnancy, the neonatal period, and infancy. J Pediatr 1977;90:368–374.

102. Centers for Disease Control. Hepatitis B virus: a comprehensive strategy for eliminating transmission in the United States through universal childhood vaccination: recommendations of the Immunization Practices Advisory Committee (ACIP). MMWR 1991;40:1–25.

103. U.S. Department of Labor, Occupational Safety and Health Administration. Occupational exposure to bloodborne pathogens; final rule. 29 CFR Part 1910.1030, 1991.

104. Stevens CE, Toy PT, Tong MJ, et al. Perinatal hepatitis B virus transmission in the United States. Prevention by passive-active immunization. JAMA 1985;253:1740–1745.

105. Centers for Disease Control. Update: universal precautions for prevention of transmission of human immunodeficiency virus, hepatitis B virus, and other bloodborne pathogens in health-care settings. MMWR 1988;37:377–382,387–388.

## 24

....................................................

# Human Immunodeficiency Virus (HIV) and the Workplace

ELIZABETH AVERILL

Both in terms of magnitude of the epidemic and severity of the disease, acquired immunodeficiency syndrome (AIDS) represents a major public health crisis today. The World Health Organization (WHO) estimates that 8–10 million adults and 1 million children worldwide are infected with human immunodeficiency virus (HIV), the etiological agent of AIDS (1). In the U.S., the initial cases of the disease were reported in June of 1981. In the subsequent 10 yr, nearly 200,000 AIDS cases were registered by the Centers for Disease Control (CDC) (2); one-fourth of these cases were reported in 1990 alone. By 1992, AIDS will be the second leading cause of death among men 25–44 yr of age in the U.S. and is likely to be one of the five leading causes of death among women (3).

The dramatic increase in the incidence of AIDS cases has been accompanied by shifts in recognized modes of transmission and populations at risk for the disease. In 1981, 97% of the 189 cases recorded by the CDC were among men, the majority of whom were homosexual or bisexual; no cases were reported among children. In 1990, women accounted for more than 11% of the 43,339 reported cases, and nearly 800 cases occurred among children who were less than 13 yr old (1). While homosexual and bisexual men and intravenous drug users still account for the largest number of adults with AIDS, cases associated with heterosexual and perinatal transmission of HIV have been steadily increasing (Fig. 24.1).

Much has been learned about this enigmatic disease since its initial description over a decade ago. We have identified the causative agent of AIDS and characterized many clinical and epidemiological aspects of the disease. We have mobilized educational resources to reduce transmission, discovered drugs that can extend life, and found promise in preliminary vaccine research. At the same time, justifiable and sometimes bitter battles continue to be fought over the very shape and scope of our society's response to this crisis. Basic assumptions about research, drug testing and distribution, social policy, and our health care delivery system have been called into question. Among the many significant challenges that still confront us is the necessity to achieve a balance between irrational fear and risky behavior.

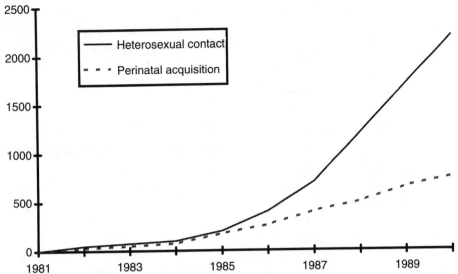

**Figure 24.1.** AIDS cases among women reporting heterosexual contact with HIV-infected or at-risk individuals and perinatally acquired pediatric AIDS cases, United States, 1981–1990. Reproduced from Centers for Disease Control. The HIV/AIDS epidemic: the first 10 years. MMWR 1991;40:360–361.

Meeting this challenge is critical both to the well-being of the uninfected and to the compassionate, nondiscriminatory, and effective treatment of the infected. This chapter explores HIV-related risks to reproduction particularly within the context of the work environment, where achieving such a balance is of critical import.

## HIV AS AN OCCUPATIONAL RISK FACTOR

In exploring HIV as an occupational risk factor, it is universally recognized that the virus is not casually contracted. Transmission of HIV requires direct contact with infected blood or bodily secretions as typically occurs during unprotected anal and vaginal sexual intercourse or sharing of contaminated needles among intravenous drug users. Only workers who come into direct contact with infected biological fluids at their jobs risk exposure to HIV.

### At-risk Occupations

According to the Occupational Safety and Health Administration (OSHA), there are more than 5 million U.S. workers at risk of exposure to HIV (4). Health care workers (HCWs) are the most commonly recognized risk group. This occupational category includes nurses, physicians, health aides, laboratory technicians, dentists and hygienists, emergency medical technicians, housekeeping and custodial staff, and central supply personnel (5). The reported frequency of HCWs with AIDS (approximately 5%) is consistent with the relative proportion of HCWs in the labor force (6). Less obvious but potentially at-risk occupations include police and firefighters, correction officers and mental health attendants, sewage workers, hazardous medical waste incinerator operators, plumbers, mortuary attendants, and others (5).

Only a very small proportion of all AIDS cases reported to the CDC are attributed to occupational exposure (7). As of June 1990, 24 HCWs in the U.S. had documented seroconversion after occupational exposure to HIV (8). Most HCWs with AIDS report other known nonoccupational risk factors for the disease. However, when compared with non-HCWs with AIDS, nearly twice as many HCWs with AIDS (2.8% vs. 5.3%) have no other identified risk factors (6, 8). Whether this difference reflects occupational risk or reporting bias is unknown.

### Sources and Risks of Transmission

Potential sources of HIV transmission in the occupational setting include needlestick or sharp instrument injuries and mucous membrane or open skin lesion contact with infected body fluids (4, 6, 9). In specific cases followed by the CDC, presumed sources of exposure included puncture wounds from syringes in phlebotomists, nurses, and other health professionals (several involving resheathing episodes); exposure through a large-gauge biopsy needle; skin contact through an open wound; blood spilled over arms and forearms while manipulating an apheresis machine; exposure when glass vials of blood broke; eye, hand, and mouth splashes; hand contact with infant feces and blood; cuts from medical instruments and from cleaning contaminated instruments; and exposure during a pressure bandage intervention.

As of July 1988, the CDC Cooperative Needlestick Surveillance Group (10) had prospectively followed 1201 HCWs (including physicians, nurses, laboratory workers or technicians, respiratory technicians, and housekeeping staff) exposed to blood from HIV-infected patients. Of the HCWs in the study, 80% were exposed through needlestick injuries, 8% were cut with sharp objects, 7% were exposed via contaminated open wounds, and 5% had mucous membrane exposures. Three documented seroconversions occurred among the 860 HCWs parenterally exposed to HIV-infected blood through needlesticks or sharp instrument cuts, for a seroconversion rate of 0.35%. As of June 1991, the number of percutaneously exposed HCWs enrolled in the CDC surveillance study increased to 1366 with four documented seroconversions, for an infection rate of 0.29% (CDC, unpublished data). In another prospective cohort study of at-risk HCWs, Gerberding et al. (11) found a slightly higher seroconversion rate of 0.47%. In contrast, the risk of developing hepatitis B virus (HBV) infection after needlestick exposures to HBV-infected patients ranges from 6–30% (9). Among laboratory personnel who handle concentrated HIV virus, the risk of seroconversion is estimated to be 0.48/100 person-years of exposure (12). Risk estimates are not available for non-HCW occupational sectors with potential for exposure to blood or bodily secretions.

The precise magnitude of occupational risk is not known with certainty because many workplace exposures have not been identified or tracked for outcome. Available data indicate that parenteral exposure to infected blood presents a higher risk of seroconversion than other sources of exposure; even then, the risk is apparently low.

## HIV AND REPRODUCTION

### HIV Infection in Women and Children

Through December 1990, 15,493 cases of AIDS in women were reported to the CDC, representing approximately 10% of all reported adult cases (7). A disproportionate number of AIDS cases occurs among women of color, and the vast majority involve women of childbearing age. While the greatest proportion of cases among women are attributable to intravenous drug use, nearly one-third are associated with heterosexual contact with a person with AIDS or at risk for AIDS (13).

Reported HIV seroprevalence rates among women vary according to survey methods, to the geographic locations and types of settings studied, and to population risk factors. Studies from family planning and obstetrical settings that do not specifically target high-risk populations reveal seroprevalence rates ranging from 0–4.3%. Higher rates have been found in urban areas such as Newark, Baltimore, Manhattan, and Washington, DC. Among female intravenous drug users, seroprevalence rates up to 25% have been reported at delivery and greater than 50% at some inner city drug treatment centers (14).

Of the cumulative 2525 pediatric AIDS cases reported to the CDC as of August 1990, 83% presumably acquired the virus perinatally (7). Transplacental passage of HIV has been documented (15, 16), even as early as 8 weeks' gestation (17). Data suggest that the cells responsible for in utero infection may be the CD4 lymphocytes and mononuclear phagocytes (18). Although not yet directly substantiated, it is assumed that perinatal transmission can also occur through contact with infected maternal blood and secretions during delivery. Finally, HIV has been recovered from breast milk (19), and transmission via lactation has been demonstrated (20). Most prospective studies indicate that 25–50% of infants born to

HIV-positive mothers will contract the infection (21), with clinical disease developing in 80% of infected infants within the first 2 yr of life (22, 23). Symptomatic maternal infection and the severity of CD4 cell depletion may be risk factors for perinatal transmission (21).

## Reproductive and Developmental Risks

There is no conclusive evidence that pregnant women are at increased risk for HIV seroconversion or that pregnancy accelerates the interval to symptomatic disease. These concerns have been raised primarily because pregnancy alters certain markers of cellular immunity (24), and some other viral diseases can be more virulent during gestation. In early studies, reported rates of disease progression were enhanced among asymptomatic pregnant women followed for 28–30 months postpartum compared with other HIV-infected cohorts (25, 26). However, these uncontrolled studies were confined to women who delivered infected infants, a factor that may reflect longer duration of disease or more compromised immune function. More recent controlled investigations have failed to demonstrate an adverse effect of pregnancy on disease progression (21, 27).

Children with congenital HIV infection have high rates of morbidity and mortality. In a prospective study of 172 infants diagnosed with perinatally acquired infection, 50% had died by 36 months of age (23). Neurological complications are common among infants with congenital HIV infection. These effects are believed to be directly due to HIV infection because secondary CNS infections are uncommon among children with AIDS (28).

Determining the contribution of maternal HIV infection to adverse developmental outcomes requires adequate control of other risk factors commonly found among HIV-positive populations. For example, individuals infected with HIV are predisposed to opportunistic and secondary teratogenic infections such as cytomegalovirus (CMV) and toxoplasmosis. Potential developmental effects of AIDS-related treatment drugs are unknown. Low socioeconomic status, limited access to medical care, substance abuse, and the high prevalence of other sexually transmitted diseases among HIV-infected women may also affect pregnancy outcome.

Recent prospective, controlled studies have not corroborated earlier reported associations between HIV infection and spontaneous abortion, low birthweight, preterm delivery, or premature rupture of the membranes, at least in asymptomatic women (21, 29–31). In addition, the AIDS virus has not been established as a teratogen (21, 27).

There are no published reports regarding the effects of HIV on male reproductive capacity. However, it is reasonable to conjecture that the neurological dysfunction and debilitating symptoms experienced by many people with AIDS, along with the treatments they undergo, could impair male sexual functioning.

## HIV-Related Reproductive Risks in the Workplace

There are a number of potential reproductive risk considerations that are not specific to HIV but nonetheless confront workers, particularly in the health care setting. These issues derive from the care of immunocompromised patients with opportunistic infections or with cancer requiring treatment with potentially hazardous chemotherapeutic agents.

Individuals with AIDS are susceptible to some infections that are known to affect pregnancy outcome adversely, such as toxoplasmosis and CMV. Toxoplasmosis encephalitis occurs in approximately 5–10% of all AIDS patients (32). However, because the organism is principally found in the cerebrospinal fluid and brain in AIDS patients and there is no evidence for direct human-to-human transmission, it should not pose a significant risk to caregivers.

Reactivation of CMV is common among AIDS patients, and rates of CMV shedding increase with worsening immune dysfunction (33). As explained in Chapter 23, primary infection with CMV during gestation accounts for most cases of serious congenital disease. Over half of women of childbearing age are seroimmune to CMV, and transmission of the virus requires close contact with infected body fluids. When adequate personal hygiene is practiced, the risk of spread of CMV to health care workers appears to be no greater than in nonmedical populations (34). In one prospective study of HCWs with intensive exposure to HIV-infected patients, rates of CMV seroconversion were similar to reported rates in other HCWs and community-based populations (11).

Some hospitals may restrict pregnant women from caring for patients at high risk of CMV shedding or assign only seroimmune women to work with these patients (34). However, most patients shedding CMV are not identified, and there are no data to suggest that reassigning seronegative workers actually lowers the risk of transmission (35). Pregnant personnel who care for HIV-infected patients are not known to be at greater risk of acquiring HIV or related opportunistic infections than are their nonpregnant co-workers (36). While voluntary transfer options may be considered under some circumstances, quality worker education and adherence to stringent hygiene practices are generally effective means of preventing transmission of CMV in the occupational setting (33–35).

There are no specific data regarding occupational reproductive risks to HCWs from administration of chemotherapeutic agents to combat AIDS. Many of the drugs are experimental in nature and have not been fully tested for toxicity. In one study unrelated to AIDS, fetal loss among nurses was associated with frequent mixing and administration of antineoplastic agents such as cyclosporin, doxorubicin, and vincristine during the first trimester (37). Many of the conditions that historically allowed for exposure to these agents among HCWs have now been rectified through provision of hoods and protective clothing to workers or through centralized drug preparation under better-controlled conditions. Nonetheless, the clinician should assess drugs that the HCW administers for their mechanisms of action and modes of administration. For example, is the drug aerosolized, thereby presenting a possible inhalation hazard? Does the HCW come into direct contact with the agent during its administration? If not involved in direct patient care, is the worker otherwise exposed in the manufacture or disposal of the agent? In all cases,

hospitals should adhere to OSHA guidelines pertaining to use of antineoplastics (38), and employees should be trained in safer work practices.

At present, no data are available regarding potential reproductive effects of antiviral agents used in AIDS research protocols. A study assessing the risks and benefits of azidothymidine (AZT) therapy in pregnant women is currently underway.

## WORKPLACE CONTROLS

It is infeasible to identify all patients infected with HIV. Routine serological testing of patients and staff is not recommended as a means of reducing transmission of the virus. Moreover, screening tests may be falsely negative in recently infected individuals who have not yet developed detectable levels of antibodies to HIV. Therefore, stringent workplace controls are required to minimize exposure of workers to potentially infected blood and body fluids. In general, measures to prevent transmission of the virus to all workers would also be expected to reduce potential reproductive risks.

The CDC has developed guidelines to prevent the transmission of HIV to health care and public safety workers (39). In addition, OSHA recently issued a standard to reduce occupational risks from blood-borne pathogens, including HIV and HBV (4). The standard delineates employer responsibilities regarding worker training, labeling, decontamination and disposal procedures, provision of safety equipment and engineering controls, medical surveillance, reporting requirements, and emergency response procedures. Special provisions apply to research laboratories that produce or use concentrated HBV or HIV. The scope of the standard is based on the potential for occupational exposure to blood and other potentially infectious materials, whether or not the individual is employed in the health care industry. It applies to 24 Standard Industrial Classification (SIC) codes representing over 500,000 establishments and more than 5 million at-risk workers. While the standard addresses potential hazards confronting law enforcement officials, corrections officers, and firefighters, many of these workers are employed within the public sector and are, therefore, exempt from OSHA regulation.

## Universal Precautions

The CDC (36, 40) and OSHA (4) have adopted the strategy of universal blood and body fluid precautions to prevent transmission of HIV in occupational settings.

Universal Precautions is an approach to infection control. According to the concept of Universal Precautions, all human blood and certain human body fluids are treated as if known to be infectious for HIV, HBV, and other blood-borne pathogens (4).

While blood is the single most important source of HIV exposure in the occupational setting, universal precautions also apply to amniotic, peritoneal, pericardial, pleural, synovial, and cerebrospinal fluids as well as to semen and vaginal secretions. Because occupational transmission has not been documented for breast milk, nasal secretions, sputum, tears, or sweat, universal precautions do not extend to these fluids unless they contain visible blood. Saliva is also excluded, except in the dental setting where it is typically contaminated by blood (4, 40). However, when emergency medical personnel encounter body fluids under uncontrolled circumstances where differentiation is difficult, all fluids should be treated as hazardous (4, 39). Most hospitals do not specifically modify these guidances for pregnant women, except by reinforcing the importance of strict infection control practices.

## Personal Protective Equipment

Personal protective equipment should be made available to all at-risk workers and should be donned before administering patient care. Under the OSHA standard, employers must provide appropriate and well-fitting personal protective equipment at no cost to workers and ensure compliance with its use (4). Gloves are key protective barriers. The vinyl or latex gloves manufactured for medical use provide comparable barrier effectiveness (40). Double gloving for surgery procedures has been found to decrease the risk of inner glove perforation and cutaneous hand exposure to blood (41). For situations where sharp edges are likely to be encountered and thin gloves are not required by the nature of the task, OSHA-approved structural firefighting gloves are advised. In all cases, contaminated gloves should be disposed of in leakage-resistant bags, or if reusable, be properly disinfected. Extra gloves should be readily available. Masks, eyewear, and gowns should be used in accordance with the anticipated risk of exposure. They should also be available on all emergency vehicles where unknown levels of hazards are likely (39).

## Engineering Controls

For the HCW, the most common source of potential HIV exposure involves percutaneous needlestick injuries (4, 10). These incidents typically occur during disassembly of equipment and resheathing. Recently, safer devices have been developed, such as self-sheathing syringes, to protect HCWs from inadvertent injury. Other engineered solutions include the provision and use of puncture-resistant containers for disposal of needles and other sharp devices, mechanical pipetting devices, centrifuge safety equipment, and disposable airway equipment and resuscitation bags. Mechanical resuscitation assist devices should be available on all emergency vehicles.

## Other Interventions

In mental health and correctional facilities, where workers risk exposure to physical assault, implementation of universal precautions may not be feasible. Increased staffing patterns can help reduce violent behavior. Although controversial, the CDC has advocated isolation of violent HIV-infected individuals who attempt to attack correctional facility staff if other methods of control prove inadequate (5). These situations are clearly difficult, and establishing the parameters for control strategies raises major ethical questions.

Under the OSHA standard (4), employers must provide comprehensive training to all at-risk workers regarding the risks of blood-borne infectious diseases and measures to minimize exposure. In addition, copies of the OSHA standard and the employer's exposure control plan must be readily accessible to workers.

## CLINICAL MANAGEMENT

Given the scope and severity of the AIDS epidemic, all primary care providers must be prepared to address the complex needs of HIV-exposed or infected patients. Table 24.1 provides a selected list of helpful resources for clinicians and patients.

## Patient Screening

As part of the preconception or prenatal history, the clinician should explore with the pa-

**Table 24.1.**
**AIDS Resources**

| | |
|---|---|
| Information lines | |
| National AIDS Hotline (CDC) | (800) 342–2437 |
| | (800) 344–7432 (Spanish Access) |
| | (800) 243–7889 (Deaf Access) |
| National AIDS Information Clearinghouse (CDC) | (800) 458–5231 |
| AIDS Clinical Trials Information Service (U.S. Public Health Service collaborative) | (800) 874–2572 |
| Project Inform | (800) 822–7422 |
| Resource and referral organizations | |
| American Foundation for AIDS Research | (212) 719–0033 |
| National Association of People with AIDS | (202) 429–2856 |
| National Coalition of Hispanic Health and Human Services Organizations | (800) 243–7123 |
| National Minority AIDS Council | (202) 544–1076 |
| Women's AIDS Network | (415) 864–4376 |
| American Civil Liberties Union | (212) 382–0557 |

Patient education resources
  Service Employees International Union (SEIU). *The AIDS Book: Information for Workers,* 3rd ed. Washington, DC: SEIU, 1988.
  Lingle VA, Wood S. *How to Find Information About AIDS.* New York: Harrington Press, 1988.
  World Health Organization, International Labour Office. *AIDS and the Workplace: What You Need to Know about AIDS.* Geneva: World Health Organization, 1989.
  *AIDS Treatment News.* Call (415) 255–0588 to subscribe.

tient and partner all work-related and nonoccupational risk factors for HIV transmission. It is critical to ascertain job title and function, reviewing in depth job duties that might entail contact with blood or other body fluids. Discuss details of specific work practices, availability of appropriate protective equipment, and employer infection control practices and policies. It is also important to evaluate the patient's knowledge about HIV transmission and to assess the quality of employer- or union-sponsored education provided to the worker.

The Centers for Disease Control (42) and the American College of Obstetricians and Gynecologists (ACOG) (43) recommend that women at risk for AIDS who are pregnant or who are considering pregnancy be offered confidential HIV testing. According to the CDC, risk factors that warrant testing include illicit intravenous drug use after 1977, a history of blood transfusions, prostitution, at-risk sexual partners (bisexual, intravenous drug users, hemophiliacs), and prior or current residence in high-risk geographic areas (44). While not included on this list, it is reasonable also to offer testing to patients and partners employed in high-risk occupational settings. Hepatitis B virus screening is also warranted during pregnancy or employment in jobs where exposure may occur. Serological testing for CMV is not routinely recommended during pregnancy; however, concerned health care or day care workers may desire screening. All patients who consent to HIV testing should be assured confidentiality and be appropriately counseled about the meaning of test results, measures to prevent transmission, and perinatal issues.

## Post-HIV Exposure Management

Under CDC guidelines (39) and the recent OSHA standard (4), the employer has a responsibility to provide a program of medical management for workers with possible exposure to HIV. Any worker exposed to a source positive for HIV or with unknown status should be counseled regarding the risk of viral transmission. The source individual should be tested for serological status if it is unknown and consent is provided (4). Confidential clinical and serological evaluations should be offered to the worker as soon as possible after the exposure incident to serve as a baseline, and subsequently at 6 weeks, 12 weeks, and 6 months. The individual should be counseled to watch for signs of febrile illness, with particular attention to development of rash and lymphadenopathy. In addition, symptoms commonly attributed to pregnancy, such as emesis and fatigue, may be clinical manifestations of HIV infection. During the postexposure follow-up period, the worker should be advised to refrain from blood donation and to take appropriate precautions to protect personal contacts (40). Circumstances surrounding the exposure incident should be documented in the medical record. Patient confidentiality is critical to prevent unnecessary stigma or discrimination.

Many hospitals now offer postexposure protocols involving administration of prophylactic AZT to reduce the risk of seroconversion. However, given the relatively low rate of seroconversion and the potential adverse reactions of the drug, the merits of this course of action are debated. Prophylactic AZT is not currently recommended during pregnancy because the effects of the drug on the developing fetus are unknown.

## Counseling the HIV-Exposed and HIV-Infected Pregnant Woman

Workers with documented exposures to HIV typically feel varying degrees of emotional trauma and distress. In one study of 20 HIV-exposed workers (45), 55% reported severe acute distress and 35% reported persistent moderate distress; one-fourth reported a significant impact upon their sexual relations, and 30% quit their jobs. While the number of workers interviewed is small, this study suggests that occupational HIV exposure evokes considerable anxiety, despite evidence of a low seroconversion risk. Pregnant workers were not considered in this report; however, it is reasonable to conjecture that the stress experienced by pregnant women in the postexposure period might be compounded by fears of possible fetal transmission. Without denigrating the concern, it is important to explain that, among the thousands of cases of documented worksite exposures, very few people have contracted HIV infection.

In the unlikely event of seroconversion, the pregnant woman should be counseled about the nature of the disease, risk of fetal transmission, and ways to prevent spread of the virus. In addition, she should be informed that therapeutic trials of antiviral agents that may influence the course of the disease currently exclude pregnant women. Options regarding continuation or termination of the pregnancy should be explored. The specter of pediatric AIDS may prompt prejudicial attitudes toward infected pregnant women that contradict their basic rights to reproductive freedom and informed choice. Specifically, some providers may feel that prevention of perinatal transmission warrants efforts to discourage or terminate pregnancy among HIV-positive women. This attitude runs counter to the basic tenets of nondirective counseling, which is a critical component of rational and nondiscriminatory treatment of HIV-infected pregnant women.

A clear multidisciplinary management plan should be formulated with the patient that addresses her medical, psychosocial, financial, nutritional, and other identified needs. At the initial prenatal visit, the HIV-positive patient should be screened for common sexually transmitted diseases (gonorrhea, syphilis, chlamydia, HBV) and tuberculosis. Baseline antibody titers to CMV and toxoplasmosis can be helpful in diagnosis should symptoms occur. Because CMV and herpes simplex virus can be reactivated during pregnancy, careful surveillance during pregnancy is important (46). Fetal surveillance may include serial ultrasound evaluations and antepartum testing. There is no evidence that the mode of delivery modifies perinatal transmission rates, and Cesarean section is not routinely recommended. Fetal scalp electrodes and scalp sampling should be avoided (21). Breastfeeding is not advised for women in industrialized nations where contamination of infant formulas is generally not a problem (Chapter 6).

The ACOG Committee on Ethics holds that physician responsibility to care for HIV-infected patients does not differ from the responsibility to care for other patients (47). The American Medical Association reiterates this position, emphasizing the ethical obligations of physicians to provide competent, compassionate, and nondiscriminatory care to HIV-infected patients and to respect their rights to privacy and confidentiality (48).

## SUMMARY

As the AIDS epidemic enters its second decade, obstetricians and other primary health care providers will be increasingly involved in preventive education and in the care of HIV-exposed or infected patients. While the contributions of sexual practices and intravenous drug use to transmission of HIV disease cannot be underestimated, potential occupational risks are also important. In particular, clinicians must address the concerns of patients planning or experiencing pregnancy who work in jobs with potential exposure to HIV and related infections. Most occupational exposures to HIV and other blood-borne infections are avoidable if workers are properly educated and adhere to strict infection control practices. If seroconversion does occur, care of the infected patient requires a compassionate, multidisciplinary approach that addresses a complexity of needs while respecting the patient's rights to confidentiality, freedom from discrimination, and informed choice.

## ACKNOWLEDGMENTS

The author gratefully acknowledges the insightful comments on this chapter made by Drs. Maureen Paul, David Christiani, and Sheldon Samuels.

## REFERENCES

1. Centers for Disease Control. The HIV/AIDS epidemic: the first 10 years. MMWR 1991;40:357–363, 369.
2. Centers for Disease Control. HIV/AIDS surveillance report. Atlanta: U.S. Department of Health and Human Services, Centers for Disease Control, November 1991.
3. Centers for Disease Control. Mortality attributable to HIV infection/AIDS—United States, 1981–1990. MMWR 1991;40:41–44.
4. U.S. Department of Labor. Occupational Safety and Health Administration. Occupational exposure to bloodborne pathogens; final rule. 20 CFR Part 1910.1031, 1991;64004–64182.
5. Service Employees International Union. The AIDS book: information for workers. U.S.A.: Service Employees International Union, AFL-CIO, CLC, 1988.
6. Centers for Disease Control. Update: acquired immunodeficiency syndrome and human immunodeficiency virus infection among health-care workers. MMWR 1988;37:229–239.
7. Centers for Disease Control. HIV/AIDS surveillance: U.S. AIDS cases reported through August 1990. Atlanta: U.S. Department of Health and Human Services, Centers for Disease Control, 1990.
8. Chamberland ME, Conley LJ, Bush TJ, Ciesielski CA, Hammett TA, Jaffe HW. Health care workers with AIDS: national surveillance update. JAMA 1991;266:3459–3462.
9. American Hospital Association, Technical Panel on Infections within Hospitals. Management of HIV infection in the hospital. Am J Infect Control 1989;17:24A–44A.
10. Marcus R, The Cooperative Needlestick Surveillance Group. Surveillance of health care workers exposed to blood from patients infected with the human immunodeficiency virus. N Engl J Med 1988;319:118–123.
11. Gerberding JL, Bryant-LeBlanc CE, Nelson K, et al. Risk of transmitting the human immunodeficiency virus, cytomegalovirus, and hepatitis B virus to health care workers exposed to patients with AIDS and AIDS-related conditions. J Infect Dis 1987;156:1–8.
12. Weiss SH, Goedert JJ, Gartner S, et al. Risk of human immunodeficiency virus (HIV-1) infection among laboratory workers. Science 1988;239:68–71.
13. Ellerbrock TV, Bush TJ, Chamberland ME, Oxtoby MJ. Epidemiology of women with AIDS in the United States, 1981 through 1990. JAMA 1991;265:2971–2975.
14. Shapiro CN, Schulz SL, Lee NC, Dondero TJ. Review of human immunodeficiency virus infection in women in the United States. Obstet Gynecol 1989;74:800–808.
15. Lapointe N, Michand J, Pekovic C, et al. Transplacental transmission of HTLV-III virus. N Engl J Med 1985;312:1325–1326.
16. Hill WC, Bolton V, Carlson JR. Isolation of acquired immunodeficiency syndrome virus from the placenta. Am J Obstet Gynecol 1987;157:10.
17. Lewis SH, Reynolds-Kohler C, Fox HE, et al. HIV-1 in trophoblastic and villous Hofbauer cells, and haematological precursors in eight-week fetuses. Lancet 1990;335:565.
18. Mano H, Chermann JC. Fetal immunodeficiency virus type 1 infection of different organs in the second trimester. AIDS Res Hum Retroviruses 1991;7:83–88.
19. Thiry L, Sprecher-Goldberger S, Jonckheer T, et al. Isolation of AIDS virus from cell-free breast milk of three healthy virus carriers. Lancet 1985;2:891–892.
20. Zeigler JB, Cooper DA, Johnson RO, Gold J. Postnatal transmission of AIDS-associated retrovirus from mother to infant. Lancet 1985;1:896–898.
21. MacGregor SN. Human immunodeficiency virus infection in pregnancy. Clin Perinatol 1991;18:33–50.
22. Hutto C, Parks WP, Lai SH, et al. A hospital-based prospective study of perinatal infection with human immunodeficiency virus type 1. J Pediatr 3;118:347–353.
23. Scott GB, Hutto C, Makuch RW, et al. Survival in children with perinatally acquired human immunodeficiency virus type 1 infection. N Engl J Med 1989;321:1791–1796.

24. Coyne BA, Landers DV. The immunology of HIV disease and pregnancy and possible interactions. Obstet Gynecol Clin North Am 1990;17:595–606.

25. Scott GB, Fischl MA, Klimas N, et al. Mothers of infants with the acquired immunodeficiency syndrome: evidence for both symptomatic and asymptomatic carriers. JAMA 1985;253:363–366.

26. Minkoff H, Nanda D, Menez R, et al. Pregnancies resulting in infants with acquired immunodeficiency syndrome or AIDS-related complex. Follow-up of mothers, children, and subsequently born siblings. Obstet Gynecol 1987;69:288–291.

27. Sweet RL, Gibbs RS. Infectious diseases of the female genital tract. 2nd ed. Baltimore: Williams & Wilkins, 1990:170–199.

28. Curless RG. Congenital AIDS: review of neurologic problems. Childs Nerv Syst 1989;5:9–11.

29. Selwyn PA, Schoenbaum EE, Davenny K, et al. Prospective study of human immunodeficiency virus infection and pregnancy outcomes in intravenous drug users. JAMA 1989;261:1289–1294.

30. Minkoff HL, Henderson C, Mendez H, et al. Pregnancy outcomes among mothers infected with human immunodeficiency virus and uninfected control subjects. Am J Obstet Gynecol 1990;163:1598–1604.

31. Butz A, Hutton N, Larson E. Immunoglobulins and growth parameters at birth of infants born to HIV seropositive and seronegative women. Am J Public Health 1991; 81:1323–1326.

32. McCabe R, Remington JS. Toxoplasmosis: the time has come. N Engl J Med 1988;318:313–315.

33. Schooley RT. Cytomegalovirus in the setting of infection with human immunodeficiency virus. Rev Infect Dis 1990;12 (Suppl)7:S811–S818.

34. Valenti WM. Infection control and the pregnant health care worker. Am J Infect Control 1986;14:20–27.

35. Brady MT. Cytomegalovirus infections: occupational risk for health professionals. Am J Infect Control 1986;14:197–203.

36. Centers for Disease Control. Recommendations for prevention of HIV transmission in health care settings. MMWR 1987;36(Suppl):16–16S.

37. Selevan SG, Lindbohm ML, Hornung RW, Hemminki K. A study of occupational exposure to antineoplastic drugs and fetal loss in nurses. N Engl J Med 1985;313:1173–1178.

38. Yodaiken RE, Bennett D. OSHA work-practices guidelines for personnel dealing with cytotoxic (antineoplastic) drugs. Am J Hosp Pharm 1986;43:1193–1204.

39. Centers for Disease Control. Guidelines for prevention of transmission of human immunodeficiency virus and hepatitis B virus to health-care and public-safety workers. MMWR 1989;38:1–37.

40. Centers for Disease Control. Update: universal precautions for prevention of transmission of human immunodeficiency virus, hepatitis B virus, and other bloodborne pathogens in health-care settings. MMWR 1988;37:377–388.

41. Gerberding JL, Littell C, Tarkington A, Brown A, Schecter WP. Risk of exposure of surgical personnel to patients' blood during surgery at San Francisco General Hospital. N Engl J Med 1990;322:1788–1793.

42. Centers for Disease Control. Recommendations for assisting in the prevention of perinatal transmission of human T lymphotrophic virus type III/lymphadenopathy-associated virus and acquired immunodeficiency syndrome. MMWR 1985;34:721.

43. American College of Obstetricians and Gynecologists. ACOG committee statement: prevention of human immunodeficiency virus infection and acquired immunodeficiency syndrome. Washington, DC: American College of Obstetricians and Gynecologists, 1987.

44. Centers for Disease Control. Public health service guidelines for counseling and antibody testing to prevent HIV infection and AIDS. MMWR 1987;36:833.

45. Henry K, Campbell S, Jackson B, et al. Long-term follow-up of health care workers with work-site exposure to human immunodeficiency virus. JAMA 1990;263:1765–1766.

46. Hauer LB, Dattel BJ. Management of the pregnant woman infected with the human immunodeficiency virus. J Perinatol 1988;8:258–262.

47. American College of Obstetricians and Gynecologists, Committee on Ethics. Human immunodeficiency virus infections: physicians' responsibilities. Obstet Gynecol 1990;75:1043–1045.

48. American Medical Association, Council on Ethics and Judicial Affairs. Ethical issues involved in the growing AIDS crisis. JAMA 1988;259:1360–1361.

# 25

........................................................

# Chemical Dependency

## H. WESTLEY CLARK, MERYLE WEINSTEIN[a]

Society has long tolerated and even encouraged the use of mind-altering substances such as alcohol and tobacco products. Although efforts are often made to separate legal from illegal drug use, this distinction has little relevance in the clinical setting and may, in fact, detract from health-promoting objectives.

Dependence on psychoactive substances is linked to a number of social and economic factors that influence patients' behaviors and options. Alcoholics and other drug abusers may experience dysfunctional family relationships, low educational status, poor self-esteem, compromised income, psychiatric problems, and vulnerability (1). Yet, unprecedented efforts are underway to "solve" the problem of substance abuse in the U.S. through criminalization. Pregnant women, in particular, are subject to routine toxicology testing, with positive results prompting criminal prosecution for child abuse. Unparalleled media attention is lavished on the babies of mothers who smoke alkaloidal ("crack") cocaine. In some cases, prosecutors and child protective services have encouraged obstetricians to exploit their proximity to the patient to collect incriminating information. Rather than ameliorating the problem, these initiatives serve as a disincentive to substance abusers to seek greatly needed health care and social services.

[a]The writing of this chapter was supported by NIDA Grant R18-DA06097.

In this chapter, we promote an ecological model of care that is based on an informed public health approach to the patient, rather than one that is punitive and legalistic. The former approach recognizes the need for prevention and treatment based on science, discouraging the use of harmful substances through education and support. The latter perspective emphasizes punishment as a possible deterrence and all but ignores the untoward health effects of licit substances and adverse socioeconomic conditions. Importantly, an ecological model recognizes that substance abuse is inextricably linked to multiple factors that must be comprehensively addressed for successful intervention to occur.

## EPIDEMIOLOGY

### Prevalence of Drug Use in the United States

The prevalence of psychoactive drug use varies with the substance, as well as with gender, race, and social class. According to 1990 estimates by the National Institute on Drug Abuse (NIDA), over 13% of the noninstitutionalized U.S. population uses illicit drugs (2). In addition, 27% are smokers and 66% drink alcohol (one-third on a regular basis). Of the 34.5 million women in the 18- to 34-yr-old age group, more than 7 million use illicit drugs, 13 million are current smokers, and 26 million drink alcohol to some extent. Prevalence of use rates are generally higher among men than among women.

## Bias in Conducting Drug Studies

Results of studies on substance abuse and pregnancy must be viewed with caution. The political, academic, and social climate concerning substance abuse influences the orientation and publishability of results. Koren et al. (3) found that negative studies regarding the effects of cocaine use during pregnancy were less likely to be accepted for presentation at a scientific meeting than those extolling the harm of cocaine, even when the negative studies had better methodology.

Numerous factors can distort the interpretation of studies assessing the impact of substance abuse on perinatal outcome. First, the majority of U.S. studies use data collected from low-income women of color recruited and delivered in public hospitals. This method of data collection focuses attention on women who are already at high risk for poor obstetrical outcomes due to social factors such as poverty, malnutrition, and lack of prenatal care. Few studies are concerned with white, middle class women who are cared for by private physicians. Therefore, the results are not generalizable, and analysis of drug-induced effects requires careful control of the multiple health and socioeconomic factors that affect the course and outcome of pregnancy.

Second, polydrug use is extremely common among subjects, especially among heavy users. It is difficult to single out the effects of one drug when it is used in combination with other harmful substances. Assessing the relative contribution of specific drugs to pregnancy outcome is further complicated by the differing methods of exposure ascertainment used for licit and illicit substances. Most recent studies employ urine toxicology screens to identify users of cocaine, amphetamines, and narcotics, whereas data on smoking and alcohol consumption are collected by patient interview. Results of laboratory testing for drug metabolites may be confounded by medications administered during labor or by use of common over-the-counter drugs that produce similar urinary derivatives. One-time testing reflects only recent use for many common substances of abuse. Data collected by interview is well known to result in under-reporting of substance use. In these circumstances, misclassification of drug use may result.

Third, few studies distinguish "recreational" drug users from addicted populations. Any woman who admits to the use of illicit substances or who tests positive for a metabolite of an illicit substance may be regarded as an addict. Little information is available on the effects of occasional drug use during pregnancy.

Other studies have small numbers of subjects and do not use control groups of comparable nondrug-using women. In addition, the potential influence of passive smoke exposure or paternal drug use on pregnancy outcome is virtually ignored in studies to date.

Finally, it is common to find reviews of published research on perinatal maternal drug abuse that exaggerate the findings of the original research. Hyperbole sells.

## SELECTED DRUGS OF ABUSE

In this section, we discuss a select number of psychoactive substances that may constitute hazards to reproduction. These drugs include alcohol, cigarettes, marijuana, cocaine, heroin/methadone, and amphetamines. Space limitations preclude a review of caffeine, phencyclidine (PCP), the benzodiazepines, or hallucinogens. Toluene abuse is addressed in Chapter 19.

## Alcohol

Excessive alcohol consumption remains a major public health problem in the U.S. In the words of one author (4): "Excluding cigarette smoking, alcoholism is probably the most serious drug problem in the United States and other countries."

It is difficult to obtain estimates on the rate of alcohol use among pregnant women. Underreporting of alcohol and other drug use is common, and testing for alcohol use during pregnancy is rare. Alcohol consumption exceeding 45 drinks per month during pregnancy is reported in 2.9–14.0% of various prenatal populations (5).

While heavy alcohol consumption has long been recognized as a major factor in poor pregnancy outcomes, the effects of smaller amounts of alcohol remain unclear. Methods used to estimate alcohol consumption are not uniform among studies, and women classified as "heavy" drinkers in one study may be grouped with "moderate" or "social" drinkers in another. Some studies average consumption over a specified time period, making it impossible to separate effects of binge drinking from low-level, daily ingestion. In many studies, "heavy" alcohol consumption is defined as two *or more* drinks daily, raising the distinct possibility that observed effects are attributable primarily to the subset of very heavy drinkers embedded in this category. In addition, failure to control for the many factors that may influence perinatal outcome will overestimate the risk caused by alcohol. Recent reviews by notable experts have considered these shortcomings and concluded that scientific data are lacking to substantiate an adverse effect of light drinking on pregnancy outcome (6, 7).

Fetal alcohol syndrome (FAS) is the most well-established effect of excessive prenatal exposure to alcohol. According to most studies, the syndrome occurs in approximately 2–8% of infants born to alcoholic women (8). It is characterized by pre- and postnatal growth deficiency; congenital malformations including facial anomalies, minor joint and limb abnormalities, and cardiac defects; and central nervous system (CNS) dysfunction, including mental retardation and neurological deficits (9). Affected infants exhibit a range of clinical manifestations associated with the syndrome, from the most severe to very mild ones. Bingol et al. (10) found that full or partial manifestations of FAS were much more common among children of low socioeconomic status than among children in higher social classes, despite a similar degree of heavy alcohol consumption by the mothers. These data suggest that poverty, malnutrition, and other socioeconomic factors may play significant roles in the occurrence of the syndrome.

In one cohort study, daily drinkers were found to have more second trimester spontaneous abortions than either occasional drinkers or nondrinkers. The highest risk occurred among women who reported an average of three or more drinks per day (11). Women who con-

sumed less than one drink per day had the same risk as nondrinkers. In a large Canadian study, the risk of self-reported spontaneous abortion increased with increasing alcohol consumption during pregnancy, with an abrupt rise between zero and one to two drinks per week (12). Kline et al (13) found that consumption of 1 oz of absolute alcohol twice a week was the minimum threshold for increased risk of aborting. Differential recall of exposure was a potential problem in these latter studies because controls were interviewed during pregnancy or after delivery of livebirths, and cases were interviewed after miscarriage. In addition, the excess risk found by Kline et al. was confined to patients receiving public health care; no association between alcohol consumption and fetal loss was detected in women receiving private care (14). Marbury et al. (15) found that self- reported consumption of 14 or more drinks per week increased the risk of abruptio placentae.

Less severe effects of alcohol consumption, designated as fetal alcohol effects (FAE), are reported to include lower birthweight (16–20); smaller length and head circumference (16, 18), congenital malformations (18–22), impaired neurobehavioral development (23–25) and alcohol-related withdrawal symptoms (26, 27). Most studies have found FAE to occur more frequently among infants born to heavy drinkers. Some studies suggest effects at moderate levels of alcohol consumption; however, due to methodological shortcomings, these findings should be viewed with caution (6, 7).

Two studies are frequently cited to support the contention that moderate drinking influences birthweight. Little (17) found a 160-g decrement in birthweight among infants born to women who drank *at least* 1 oz of absolute alcohol (approximately two drinks) daily during the latter half of pregnancy. Mills et al. (20) reported that infants of women who *averaged* one to two or three to five drinks daily were lighter by 83 g and 165 g, respectively, compared to infants of nondrinkers. These studies leave open the possibility that the effects were concentrated among heavier or binge drinkers. In addition, some important confounders such as pregnancy weight gain and marijuana use were not controlled (7). Other studies with better control of confounders found no association between moderate alcohol consumption and birthweight (15, 28, 29). Rosett et al. (19) did not observe growth retardation in infants born to heavy drinkers who stopped or decreased consumption before the third trimester. Whether the benefits derived solely from alcohol cessation or also from accompanying changes in other health behaviors is unclear.

Reported congenital malformations associated with alcohol use apart from FAS include genitourinary, craniofacial, and limb malformations (21, 22, 28). Ernhart et al. (22) found that drinking less than three drinks per day during pregnancy was unlikely to affect fetal development. Similarly, Mills and Graubard (30) did not find these malformations to be significantly higher among women who had one to two drinks daily. Other studies support the contention that moderate drinking is not associated with an increased risk of teratogenesis (15, 28).

A withdrawal syndrome has been observed in infants exposed to excessive alcohol prenatally. Pierog et al. (26) reported symptoms among FAS infants including tremors, irritability, increased muscle tone, repeated yawning and sneezing, convulsions, startles, abdominal distention, and vomiting. Among non-FAS newborns, those whose mothers stopped drinking during pregnancy showed no withdrawal symptoms; infants of mothers who continued to drink experienced tremors, sleeplessness, hypertonia, abnormal reflexes, excessive mouthing, and inconsolable crying (27).

Streissguth et al. (31) reported developmental problems, including poor attention span and longer reaction times, in middle class children tested at 4 yr of age whose mothers reported consumption of more than 1.5 oz of absolute alcohol (approximately three drinks) daily during early pregnancy; at 7 1/2 yr of age, children from this same cohort had lower IQ scores and persistent attention deficits compared to nonexposed children (25). Maternal binge drinking (five or more drinks on one occasion during the first trimester) was also associated with increased learning problems.

Certain limitations of this study deserve consideration. First, prenatal alcohol consumption was ascertained by maternal interview, raising the likelihood of under-reporting. Second, important confounders such as parental IQ were not controlled. Third, it is extremely difficult to isolate potential effects from prenatal exposure to alcohol from those attributable to other environmental influences in postnatal life. Finally, the clinical significance of subtle deficits found on neurobehavioral testing is unclear. In fact, the IQ and other test scores of children born to moderate drinkers in this study were well within the normal range. In another longitudinal study of a socioeconomically disadvantaged cohort of children assessed repeatedly between 6 months and 5 yr of age, Greene et al. (32) found that the home environment significantly predicted children's cognitive function, but prenatal alcohol exposure did not.

As explained in more detail in Chapter 5, exposure of male animals to alcohol has been variably reported to decrease litter size and to affect the growth and survivability of offspring. Recent animal experiments have also demonstrated a paternally mediated effect on offspring behavior (33, 34). Little and Sing (35) found a 137-g reduction in birthweight among infants whose fathers drank regularly (average of two or more drinks daily or binge drinking) in the month before conception; the effect was independent of maternal alcohol or drug use. While this study suffers from many of the same methodological problems previously discussed, it emphasizes the importance of including paternal drinking habits in all research related to alcohol and pregnancy outcomes.

Alcohol reduces fertility in laboratory animals; its effects on humans have been studied primarily in male subjects. Acute and chronic alcohol consumption has been associated with impotence, abnormal spermatozoa, and decreases in gonadotropic hormones and plasma testosterone levels (36, 37). In women, chronic alcohol consumption has been related to infertility and menstrual disorders (38), but information on specific hormonal effects is limited (39).

## Cigarettes

While the number of people who smoke in the U.S. has decreased, cigarette smoking continues to be a major contributor to poor reproductive outcomes. Estimates of the prevalence of smoking among women vary, and there is evidence that pregnancy motivates women to quit (40). A recent national survey determined that the median prevalence of current smoking was 26.5% among women of reproductive age and 17.7% among pregnant women (41).

Although animal data indicate a relationship between impaired fertility and cigarette smoking, human studies are limited. Delayed conception and infertility were associated with smoking in three studies (42–44), but not in a recent study from France (45). Among men, cigarette smoking has been associated with lower sperm penetration (46), lower sperm density and motility (47, 48), and greater morphological abnormalities (49); one study, however, found no association between smoking and impaired sperm motility (50).

Obstetrical complications associated with cigarette smoking include an increased risk of fetal loss (51–53) and abruptio placentae (54, 55). A dose-response relationship has also been found between ectopic pregnancy and smoking, with risk increasing at more than 10 cigarettes per day (56, 57).

A wide range of neonatal problems has been associated with maternal cigarette smoking. These include lower birthweight (15, 54, 56–63), smaller infant length (58, 60, 63), smaller head circumference (16, 60), premature delivery (52, 54, 64), neonatal mortality (52, 54, 64–66), neurobehavioral deficits (16, 31, 67, 68), and infantile apnea (61). An association between parental smoking and childhood cancer has also been suggested (69).

After controlling for factors such as maternal weight gain, socioeconomic status, educational attainment, and nutritional intake, birthweights of infants born to smokers differ from nonsmokers by as much as 234 g (58, 66). Several investigators have observed a dose-response relationship between maternal smoking and infant birthweight (16, 56, 57, 62, 66). In some studies, reducing the number of cigarettes to less than five per day (56, 57, 66) or stopping smoking before the third trimester (16, 62) modified the risk.

Second-hand smoke inhalation by pregnant women may also affect infant birthweight. In a study of 3891 pregnant patients, 24% did not smoke cigarettes during gestation but were exposed to second-hand tobacco smoke for at least 2 hr daily. When compared to nonexposed infants, maternal smoking reduced infant birthweight by 137 g, and passive inhalation by 30 g (70).

Late fetal/neonatal mortality due to maternal cigarette smoking has also been related to number of cigarettes smoked. Butler et al. (66) found the highest risk among women who smoked over four cigarettes daily. Kleinman and colleagues (65) noted a 25% increase in infant mortality among women smoking less than one pack per day and a 56% increase among those smoking one or more packs daily. Causes of mortality related to maternal cigarette smoking are Sudden Infant Death Syndrome (SIDS) (71, 72) and abruption (54).

Some studies have found a relationship between maternal cigarette smoking and neurobehavioral deficits in children including lower psychomotor development (67), decreased auditory responsiveness (67), and poorer orientation and attention spans (31). Effects were most pronounced among infants of mothers who smoked at least 10 cigarettes per day throughout pregnancy. On the other hand, one investigation found no differences between children of smokers and nonsmokers in regard to growth measures, intelligence, academic achievement, visual-motor perception, or language ability (63).

## Marijuana

The main psychoactive ingredient of marijuana is δ-9-tetrahydrocannabinol (THC). Reported use of marijuana among pregnant women ranges from 5–30% (29, 73). The use of marijuana is highly correlated with consumption of alcohol and cigarettes, making the independent effects of marijuana on pregnancy difficult to decipher.

Some studies suggest that regular use of marijuana shortens the length of gestation (74, 75), while others do not (29, 76). A prospective Australian investigation revealed a significantly higher incidence of preterm births among 36 women reporting marijuana use two or more times per week compared to lesser or nonusers, after adjustment for maternal age, parity, and alcohol and tobacco use (74). Fried et al. (75) noted a 0.8-week decrease in gestational age at birth among heavy marijuana users (more than six times/week) when compared with nonusers.

In these studies, marijuana use did not affect birthweight independent of gestational age. Zuckerman et al. (29) also found no association between self-reported marijuana use and infant birthweight; however, women identified as users by positive urine assays delivered significantly lighter infants than nonusers (mean difference 79 g). Hatch and Bracken (73) found an increased incidence of low-birthweight infants among white women who used marijuana two to three times a month during pregnancy (8.2%) compared to nonusers (2.7%); the effect was not observed in infants born to women of color. In a well-controlled prospective study based on self-reported marijuana use during pregnancy, Day et al. (76) found a significant association with decreased birth length, but only heavy users (average one joint per day) delivered lighter infants than abstainers.

Marijuana is not established as a human teratogen. Neurobehavioral symptoms attributed to prenatal marijuana exposure include altered visual responses, decreased habituation, increased tremors, and neonatal jitteriness (77, 78). After appropriate control of other prenatal and postnatal risk factors, no lasting effects on cognitive or motor function have been documented (79).

While marijuana affects pituitary gonadotropins and inhibits ovulation in experimental animals, human data are limited. In one double-blinded study of 16 women, marijuana smoking significantly depressed luteinizing hormone (LH) levels for up to 120 minutes when compared with a placebo (80). In men, chronic heavy use was associated with a significant decline in sperm concentration, total sperm count, and sperm motility in one study (81), but not in another (46). Kolodny et al. (82) found a decrease in plasma testosterone levels with chronic marijuana use, while Mendelson et al. (83) did not.

## Opioids

### HEROIN

A significant proportion of female heroin addicts experience menstrual aberrations and in-

fertility, although the effects of the drug itself are difficult to separate from other risk factors such as poor nutrition, pelvic infections, and emotional stress. Pregnant heroin addicts typically have little prenatal care. They are at high risk for medical complications ranging from anemia to bacterial endocarditis, hepatitis, and other infections transmitted through contaminated needles or sexual contact. In addition, polydrug use is common among addicts, and heroin may be cut with other toxic substances.

Reported complications in pregnant heroin addicts include premature rupture of membranes, abruptio placentae, preeclampsia, and increased meconium staining (84, 85). Labor in women addicted to heroin is reportedly shorter than in nonusers, although it is unclear whether this is due to the drug or to delay in seeking medical care until labor is well advanced out of fear of withdrawal.

Heroin exposure during gestation is associated with growth retardation (84, 86–89), although catch-up growth has been observed by 1 yr of age (87). Lifschitz et al. (88) found that mean birth length did not differ among heroin-exposed and nonexposed infants after adjustment for other perinatal, biological, and environmental risk factors; furthermore, the postnatal growth of children exposed to narcotics during pregnancy was comparable to that of a high-risk comparison group born to nondrug users. Other reported effects include prematurity (84–87); fetal/infant mortality (84, 89), including increased incidence of SIDS (72); and impaired neurobehavioral development (87, 89–91). A longitudinal study by Wilson et al. (91) found that preschool children born to untreated heroin addicts performed less well on tests of psycholinguistic ability and visual, tactile, and auditory perception than nonexposed controls, but no differences were noted in later school performances or attention span. Most studies show normal cognitive development as measured by the Bayley Scales of Infant Development (90, 91).

### METHADONE

Medical professionals agree that it is better for women to be maintained on methadone during pregnancy than to continue using street heroin. In addition to decreasing medical complications from illicit heroin use, enrollment in a methadone maintenance program increases the availability and use of prenatal care and allows for identification and treatment of other substance use.

Many studies comparing the effects of heroin and methadone have found little differences between the drugs in terms of obstetrical and postnatal complications (92, 93). Two investigations, however, found a relative advantage to methadone over heroin. One study found that heroin exposure was associated with more fetal distress than methadone exposure; methadone-exposed infants also weighed more than heroin-exposed infants, although both groups weighed significantly less than drug-free controls (94). Another study also found that methadone-exposed infants weighed more and that the longer the mother was on methadone, the higher the infant birthweight (95). In contrast, Wilson et al. (87) reported that prenatal methadone exposure was associated with poorer motor development at 1 yr of age than heroin exposure.

An important difference between the two drugs is the number and severity of neonatal withdrawal symptoms. Methadone produces more severe withdrawal than heroin (94, 95). Symptoms include tremors, irritability, difficulties in feeding and sleeping, hyperactivity, poor habituation to light and sound stimulation, inconsolability, abnormal crying, hypertonia, excessive sneezing, vomiting, and diarrhea. Withdrawal symptoms appear early in heroin-exposed infants, while some methadone-exposed infants may take as long as 4 days to develop symptoms (95).

There are no consistent findings regarding the long-term effects of in utero exposure to methadone. Some studies have found differences in mental and/or psychomotor development at 12–18 months of age (90, 92, 94), while others have found no long-term behavioral deficits (96).

## Cocaine

Cocaine use increased dramatically in the U.S. in the mid-1980s, but has been recently declining. According to NIDA, reported annual use rates among 18- to 25-yr-olds declined from approximately 12% in 1988 to 7.5% in 1990 (2);

however, the estimated number of Americans using the drug on a daily basis remained at approximately 300,000. Reported prevalence of use rates among pregnant women in large urban teaching hospitals range from 8–18% (29, 97–99), although frequency of use during pregnancy varies considerably. In one large obstetrical population, approximately one-third of cocaine users reported use less than once per month, while approximately 50% used more than once per week. The majority reported use only during a single trimester, with first trimester use significantly more common than later use (98).

Studies conducted in the U.S. focus on low-income women of color who receive little prenatal care and have multiple risk factors for adverse pregnancy outcomes (98). Few studies have been large enough to control adequately for these important variables. In addition, studies of cocaine use and pregnancy outcome are invariably subject to exposure misclassification and confounding by polydrug use. Despite the plethora of articles assessing the perinatal risks of cocaine, the magnitude of the independent contribution of cocaine use to poor pregnancy outcome remains unclear (100).

The most consistent finding in studies to date is an association between cocaine use and intrauterine growth retardation including lower birthweight, shorter infant length, and smaller head circumference (29, 97, 101–112). In a large prospective study of a low socioeconomic prenatal population, Zuckerman et al. (29) found that infants born to women who had positive urine assays for cocaine were 500 g lighter, 2 cm shorter, and had 1.3 cm smaller head circumferences than infants of nonusers. After control for multiple confounders including cigarette smoking, pregnancy weight gain, and marijuana use in a multivariate model, these differences remained significant but decreased to 93 g, 0.7 cm, and 0.43 cm, respectively. Another well-controlled study recently found that duration of prenatal cocaine exposure accounted for 18% of the observed variance in birthweight, while maternal health and obstetrical factors (including access to prenatal care) contributed 22% (112).

Data on length of gestation are conflicting.

Most studies involve polydrug users or have very small subsets of women who use cocaine only (97, 101, 104, 107, 109, 110). In these investigations, the mean length of gestation is similar among all drug-using groups and is decreased by up to 2 weeks compared to non-drug-using controls. Cherukuri et al. (106) found a three-fold increased risk of preterm delivery among 55 women who reported only crack use during pregnancy compared with an equal number of nondrug-using women matched for age, parity, socioeconomic status, alcohol use, and degree of prenatal care. In contrast, the prospective investigation by Zuckerman et al. (29) found no effect of cocaine use on length of gestation.

Studies showing a high incidence of abruptio placentae have involved small numbers of cocaine users (101–104, 113). In contrast, larger studies have failed to confirm this association (107, 114, 115). While increased rates of spontaneous abortion have been noted in previous pregnancies of cocaine and polydrug users (103), studies assessing current pregnancies have found no effect (102, 105, 107). Other complications reported in case studies that have not been confirmed by larger-scale investigations include pregnancy-induced hypertension (97), maternal intracerebral hemorrhage (116), acute rupture of ectopic pregnancies (117), and uterine rupture (118).

In an analysis of data from the population-based Atlanta Birth Defects Case-Control Study, Chavez et al. (119) found a significant association between reported cocaine use during early pregnancy and an increased risk for urinary tract anomalies. Although the number of these malformations among cocaine exposed infants was small, these findings are consistent with previous reports (101, 103, 120). Other reported abnormalities include intestinal atresia and enterocolitis, cardiac anomalies, skull defects, and limb reduction defects (97, 102, 121). However, not all studies have found a significantly increased risk of malformation (29, 112); the suspected teratogenicity of cocaine requires confirmation through large-scale epidemiological investigations.

Neonates exposed to cocaine in utero may be at risk for cerebral infarctions and seizures (104, 122, 123), possibly due to higher mean arterial blood pressure and cerebral blood flow velocity (124). Echoencephalographic examinations demonstrate a significantly higher incidence of CNS hemorrhage among stimulant-exposed (cocaine and methamphetamines) asymptomatic infants than among other infants, including those exposed to narcotics (123).

Early, small studies reported a high incidence of SIDS among neonates born to cocaine abusers (103, 105, 113). In a larger study that assessed exposure to cocaine and marijuana through interview and urine screening, only 1 of 175 cocaine-exposed infants died of SIDS; this risk of approximately 5/1000 births was not significantly different from the non-exposed group (125). The mother of the infant who died of SIDS was African-American, poor, and smoked cigarettes, all of which are possible risk factors for SIDS. The rate of SIDS in this study is about the same as that associated with abuse of nicotine (72) and that found in indigent populations (125), and is lower than rates reported with opiate abuse (72).

Studies of infants born to polydrug/cocaine abusers have noted withdrawal symptoms including tremors, irritability, hypertonia, abnormal sleep patterns, and poor feeding (102, 104, 105, 108). One study of infants whose mothers smoked crack during pregnancy reported similar findings (106). However, other investigations that included groups exposed only to cocaine noted mild withdrawal symptoms compared to other drug-exposed infants (102, 108); one study found no difference between cocaine-exposed infants and drug-free controls (126).

Singer et al. (127) recently reviewed studies that used the Brazelton scale to assess neonatal neurobehavioral sequelae of in utero cocaine exposure. Early investigations found that cocaine-exposed newborns had depressed interactive behavior and impaired responses to environmental stimuli compared with infants of nondrug-using controls (101, 103). However, these studies were small and failed to control for alcohol consumption and other risk factors. Three larger recent studies used similar scoring systems to assess the neurobehavioral status of term infants exposed prenatally to cocaine, while controlling for important confounders through multivariate analysis (110–112). Results were inconsistent. Eisen et al. (110) found impaired habituation to adverse or repetitive stimuli among cocaine-exposed infants, while other investigators did not (111). Two of the studies followed infants during the first postnatal month. While one study noted small decrements in motor function among infants of cocaine users, this association became nonsignificant after controlling for examiner variables, other substance use, and perinatal risk factors (111). The second study found increased abnormal reflexes and autonomic depression in the exposed group, but these effects were also independently associated with other risk factors and were not thought to have clinical significance (112).

These scoring systems are designed to detect subtle neurobehavioral deficits and may be poor predictors of future performance (127). Long-term developmental data are as yet lacking. However, as the newer studies poignantly illustrate, future research in this area must control for the many socioenvironmental variables that influence child development to avoid attributing to prenatal drug exposure what may belong elsewhere. In addressing the role of parenting as one potentially important factor, Singer et al. (127) remind us of an often neglected point, i.e., that fathers count too.

Prenatal care can reduce pregnancy complications in drug-abusing populations. In a study from the Perinatal Center for Chemical Dependence in Chicago, cocaine abusers who received comprehensive prenatal care had better obstetrical and perinatal outcomes than cocaine-using women not enrolled in a prenatal care program (109). Women participating in the program had longer durations of pregnancy and delivered significantly heavier infants than women not enrolled.

Limited data are available on social users. A Canadian study found that social users who discontinued cocaine use during the first trimester had no increased risk of adverse pregnancy outcomes (128). Chasnoff et al. (101) compared two groups of women enrolled in a prenatal program for substance abusers with a general obstetrical population; one group stopped using cocaine during the first trimester and the other used throughout pregnancy.

Women who discontinued cocaine during the first trimester had infants similar to nondrug-using controls as measured by birthweight, head circumference, and length. Richardson and Day (129) also found no differences in obstetrical outcomes between moderate cocaine users, most of whom decreased use as pregnancy progressed, and drug-free controls.

## Amphetamines and Methamphetamines

Amphetamines are used both legally and illegally. It is common for polydrug users to include amphetamines among their substances of abuse. Few studies are available on the effects of amphetamine consumption during pregnancy. This class of drugs is pharmacologically similar to cocaine, and similar obstetric and neonatal effects have been reported (108, 123). However, one study noted that users of cocaine and methamphetamine differed by race, socioeconomic status, and access to health care (108). While cocaine users were predominately inner city blacks, users of methamphetamines were predominately whites residing in both urban and rural areas. Surprisingly, methamphetamine users were less likely to be involved in a system of health care.

In case reports or small studies, amphetamine use has been associated with pregnancy complications such as eclampsia (130), placental hemorrhage and abruption (108), anemia (108), cardiac arrest during cesarean section (131), and pulmonary edema after cesarean section (132). The latter complications may be due to the combined effects of amphetamines and anesthesia.

Studies assessing neonatal effects from amphetamine and methamphetamine use during pregnancy are inconclusive. While some studies support an association with low birthweight, decreased length and head circumference, increased prematurity, and altered neonatal behavioral patterns (132, 133), others do not (134, 135). Likewise, an increased risk of congenital malformations is noted in some studies (136, 137), but not in others (133). Dixon et al. (108, 123) report similar rates of occurrence of brain lesions and hemorrhages in cocaine and methamphetamine-exposed infants. While the methamphetamine-exposed infants appeared less impaired during the first year than those exposed to cocaine, the authors postulate that abnormalities may manifest at school age, when more complex visual-motor and social cognition tasks are required.

The most complete assessment of the effects of amphetamine use during pregnancy comes from the Karolinska Institute in Sweden (135, 138–141). This study followed 69 amphetamine-addicted women during pregnancy and their children for 4 yr after birth. Postpartum hemorrhage and retained placenta were the most common obstetrical complications. Among the infants born to mothers using amphetamines throughout pregnancy, higher rates of preterm delivery and perinatal mortality were found than among infants born to mothers who stopped during the first trimester. Withdrawal symptoms were noted in 10 of the infants. At 1 and 4 yr of age, growth and general health were similar to nondrug-exposed children. Behavioral adjustment problems observed among the drug-exposed children were attributed by the authors to the home environment rather than to the drug exposure.

## SPECIAL CLINICAL CONSIDERATIONS

### Human Immunodeficiency Virus and Sexually Transmitted Diseases

The dramatic increase in the incidence of human immunodeficiency virus (HIV) infection among women has been attributed largely to substance abuse. Among women with AIDS whose cases were reported to the Centers for Disease Control through December of 1990, 51% were infected through IV drug use and another 21% through sexual contact with IV drug users (142). This disease is now among the 10 leading causes of death in women of reproductive age. The age-adjusted death rate for women 15–44 yr old has increased steadily since 1985. For black women, this rate rose from 4.4/100,000 in 1986 to 10.3/100,000 in 1988; in contrast, the rate for white women increased from 0.6/100,000 to 1.2/100,000. The prevalence of HIV infection among women who delivered infants in 1988 was 140/100,000,

a rate 60 times higher than the HIV/AIDS mortality rate for women 15–44 yr of age. Of the children with AIDS, 80% acquired the infection from their mothers who were drug abusers or sexual partners of drug abusers.

Drug-related behavior such as prostitution or trading sex for drugs places the substance abuser at high risk for sexually transmitted diseases (STDs). In addition, HIV infection itself has been associated with an increased risk of STDs. Minkoff et al. (143) found that seropositive women were twice as likely to become infected with STDs than seronegative women. The use of crack has been associated with higher rates of unprotected sex and syphilis among sexually active black teenage girls, placing them at high risk for HIV infection and pregnancy (144). Adverse pregnancy outcomes among HIV-infected women have been attributed to drugs and adverse socioeconomic factors, but not to the infection itself (143, 145). However, increased numbers of cases of antepartum pneumonia due to HIV seropositivity and immune system compromise have been reported (146).

It is clear that the issue of perinatal substance abuse is a matter of life or death not only for the neonate, but also for the pregnant woman. Uninfected drug abusers who are denied substance abuse treatment risk continued exposure to HIV. Women who fear legal retribution or loss of their children as a result of engaging the health care delivery system are also at a greater risk.

### Perinatal Drug Testing

A growing number of experts are advocating routine testing for illicit drugs during prenatal care or at delivery (3, 147). Table 25.1 lists specific criteria that have been developed to identify possible drug addicts. Recently, the State of Minnesota passed a law requiring physicians to drug screen all women who used cocaine, heroin, phencyclidine (PCP), or amphetamines (but not alcohol or cigarettes) at any time during pregnancy and to report results to the Department of Health. Similar laws have been enacted in other states (148).

Using a laboratory test to identify drug users is problematic for several reasons. This instru-

**Table 25.1.**
**Maternal Risk Factors For Drug Screens**[a]

No or poor prenatal care (less than three or erratic visits)
Suspicion of placental abruption
History/physical signs of substance abuse
Bizarre behavior or psychiatric history
History of prostitution
Family substance abuse or incarceration

[a]Reproduced by permission from Dattel J. San Francisco General Hospital, Department of Obstetrics, Gynecology and Reproductive Science.

mental approach, especially when linked to reporting requirements, subverts the traditional patient-provider relationship based on open and confidential communication. The rationale for drug testing is based on the fact that some women misrepresent their use of psychoactive substances. This is as true for legal substances such as alcohol as it is for illicit drugs. However, drug screens are not always reliable indicators of drug use due to the short half-lives of many substances and the possibility of false positive results. For example, ingestion of nonsteroidal anti-inflammatory agents has produced false-positive assays for THC (149). Passive exposure to marijuana smoke can result in positive urine screens (150). On the other hand, cocaine metabolites are detectable in urine for only 8–48 hr postexposure (149). While drug tests give a "snapshot" view of recent use, they provide little insight into frequency, dosage, or patterns of drug use. We agree with Jessup who states (151): "Though toxicologic screening is a valuable part of the assessment of a patient and invaluable indeed for the neonatologist, it cannot measure a patient's motivation for treatment, the chronicity of her disease, nor her willingness to seek recovery."

It is not unusual for drug screens to be obtained on pregnant women without informed consent. This approach violates standards established for other medical procedures and robs pregnant women of the rights afforded other population sectors subject to drug screening. For example, Department of Transportation regulations that govern the screening of applicants for jobs provide for specific due process protections, including notice before being tested or before disclosing medical infor-

mation to a physician. Patients admitted to alcohol and drug abuse programs receive written warning that confidentiality will be breached if information suggesting child abuse is disclosed (152). Clearly, pregnant women who present for health care should be afforded similar rights.

The judicious use of toxicological screening should occur in the context of a therapeutic and confidential provider-patient relationship. Once a clinician chooses to employ drug screening, great procedural care must be exercised. Patients should be given advanced notice and an opportunity for informed consent before testing. Urine or blood specimens must be collected with forensic care, including chain of custody signatures that track the passage of the specimen from the point of collection to the point of analysis. If the clinic or hospital uses a screening methodology such as immunoassay (e.g., EMIT), a positive urine specimen must be confirmed by a more reliable analytic procedure, such as gas chromatography-mass spectrometry (GC/MS). Finally, drug testing should be linked to an effective program of intervention based on advocacy and treatment, rather than social control and legal retribution.

## Treatment of Addiction in Women

From 1986–1991, more than 300 articles were published on various aspects of psychoactive substance abuse by pregnant women. During the same time period, not more than 25 articles focused on drug and alcohol treatment processes for women. While many have been quick to highlight the horrors of the drug epidemic, inadequate resources have been committed to understanding and addressing the needs of women substance abusers.

As Chavkin (153) points out, the availability of drug treatment programs for women in general, and pregnant women in particular, is severely limited. Yet Jessup (151) contends that comprehensive treatment programs for addicted pregnant women do work and suggests that physicians are ideal case managers for the network of services that are required for pregnant addicted women. Hoegerman et al. (154) describe a multidisciplinary perinatal team that is focused on the complex needs of the mother-child dyad; this team is composed of representatives from obstetrics, pediatrics, developmental psychology, nursing, social work, occupational therapy, psychiatry, substance abuse, and child care. While it will be some time before adequate data are available on treatment effectiveness, it is clear that the notion of comprehensiveness is crucial to addressing the needs of pregnant addicts.

## CONCLUSION: TOWARD AN ECOLOGICAL MODEL OF CARE

Abuse of psychoactive substances is a complex phenomenon reflective of deep-rooted individual and societal problems. Yet many authorities advocate a punitive or control model of intervention rather than one based on education, treatment, and allocation of social goods and services. While substance abuse is not restricted to any given race or class, poor and ethnic minority populations have borne the burden of the hostile reaction of the medical and legal communities (155).

Under the control model, evidence of substance use during pregnancy has become synonymous with child abuse. Women are held individually to blame, while social service agencies are called upon to "rescue" the child from the negligent mother. This attitude creates a false dichotomy, as it presumes that the pregnant woman and the child-to-be have interests that are at loggerheads; it presumes that the substance-using pregnant woman either wants to be a drug addict or alcoholic or wants to harm the child-to-be. An element of the underlying moral basis for this presumption is that the pregnant substance abuser has the option to abort if she does not want to be pregnant, and that failing to exercise this option subordinates her moral position. Another presumption is that the social services system best serves the interests of the child, while the pregnant substance user cannot. In other words, using illicit substances precludes proper parenting.

These presumptions and their underlying moral arguments are in general specious. First, mere use of psychoactive substances does not produce addiction and is not equivalent with addiction. Second, few addicts want to be addicts; pregnant women addicts are no different.

Third, addicted pregnant women do not want to harm their children-to-be. The supposition of maternal-fetal conflict only serves to subvert assistance that could be provided to the substance-using mother. As a result of state assumption of custody, large numbers of drug-exposed children are brought into an already overburdened and ill-equipped foster care system. Furthermore, state assumption of custody removes an important incentive for the drug dependent woman's participation in clinical services, if they are available. Therefore, the woman is punished and the child is punished.

An ecological model of care operates with the clinician functioning as both advocate and treatment provider. The traditional ethical basis of beneficence exercised by the clinician toward the pregnant woman is respected. This model promotes the notion that all women have a right to substance abuse education and treatment, in addition to prenatal and postnatal care. It recognizes that the use of psychoactive substances is part of a dynamic in human behavior that must be altered through intervention in multiple spheres of a woman's life—environment, housing, jobs, family relationships, and psychological make-up. An ecological model embraces advocacy as a critical role for clinicians. The position statement of the California Advocates for Pregnant Women found in Table 25.2 embodies this advocacy-centered approach.

Major medical organizations have begun to respond to the problem of drug abuse in important ways. In November of 1990, the Board of Trustees of the American Medical Association published a report on legal interventions during pregnancy (156). The report holds that criminal sanctions or civil liability for harmful behavior by a pregnant woman toward her fetus are inappropriate. It recommends that pregnant substance abusers be provided appropriate treatment.

While drug and alcohol abuse during pregnancy are certainly not desirable, the response of responsible clinicians should be to work with the pregnant woman in a joint effort to address the problem of addiction. Referral to agencies such as child welfare services should not occur until every effort has been exhausted to foster compliance with rational treatment protocols.

**Table 25.2.**
**Advocacy and Treatment**[a]

In the context of prenatal care and drug and alcohol recovery services, the offer of advocacy by the helping professional to the pregnant or postpartum woman is therapeutic and appropriate. With advocacy and trust as the basis of the relationship, there is the potential for the woman who uses alcohol and other drugs to remain in treatment for the duration of the pregnancy and beyond. The advocacy model includes the following:

1. that treatment is a right and is available and offered to each woman who needs it;
2. that emotional support, social services and a positive treatment alliance with staff knowledgeable about chemical dependency are essential and available and offered to each woman who needs it;
3. that the health care provider/advocate actively and strongly encourages full participation and compliance by the woman in prenatal care and drug and alcohol recovery services;
4. that the institution, agency, clinic, or private practice has the responsibility to educate the pregnant woman about the specific risks to the developing fetus and to her own health with continued drug or alcohol use and that information be provided in educational and culturally appropriate written and verbal formats;
5. that the institution, agency, clinic, or private practice has the responsibility to conduct the advocacy-oriented intervention as described herein;
6. that the health care provider/advocate will continue to advocate for the woman who uses alcohol and other drugs by providing input to the obstetric-pediatric team and by providing information as to her participation in prenatal care and drug and alcohol recovery services and her appropriateness as a parent;
7. that the institution, agency, clinic, or private practice has the responsibility to inform the woman who uses alcohol or other drugs of the potential for evaluation and action by child protective services in the course of the delivery or postpartum period; that it is not the intent of this health care provider/advocate to report her to child protective services during the pregnancy and that this health care provider will continue to advocate for the woman as needed.

[a]Reproduced with permission from California Advocates for Pregnant Women, San Diego, CA.

## REFERENCES

1. Jarvik M. The drug dilemma: manipulating the demand. Science 1990;250:387–392.
2. National Institute on Drug Abuse (NIDA). NIDA national household survey on drug abuse: population estimates 1990. Washington, DC: U.S. Government Printing Office, 1991.
3. Koren G, Shear H, Graham K, et al. Bias against the null hypothesis: the reproductive hazards of cocaine. Lancet 1989;2:1440–1442.
4. Dattel BJ. Substance abuse in pregnancy. Semin Perinatol 1990;14:179–187.
5. Weiner L, Rosett HL, Edelin KC, et al. Alcohol consumption by pregnant women. Obstet Gynecol 1983;61:6–12.
6. Knupfer G. Abstaining for foetal health: the fiction that even light drinking is dangerous. Br J Addict 1991; 86:1063–1073.
7. Alpert JJ, Zuckerman B. Alcohol use during pregnancy: what is the risk? Pediatr Rev 1991;12:375–379.
8. Abel EL, Sokol RJ. Incidence of fetal alcohol syndrome and economic impact of FAS-related anomalies. Drug Alcohol Depend 1987;19:51–70.
9. Clarren SK, Smith DW. The fetal alcohol syndrome. N Engl J Med 1978;298:1063–1067.
10. Bingol N, Schuster C, Fuchs M, et al. The influence of socioeconomic factors on the occurrence of fetal alcohol syndrome. Adv Alcohol Subst Abuse 1987;6:105–118.
11. Harlap S, Shiono PH. Alcohol, smoking, and incidence of spontaneous abortions in the first and second trimester. Lancet 1980;2:173–176.
12. Armstrong BG, McDonald AD, Sloan M. Cigarette, alcohol, and coffee consumption and spontaneous abortion. Am J Public Health 1992;82:85–87.
13. Kline J, Shrout P, Stein Z, et al. Drinking during pregnancy and spontaneous abortion. Lancet 1980;2:176–180.
14. Kline J, Levin B, Stein Z, Warburton D. Epidemiologic detection of low dose effects on the developing fetus. Environ Health Perspect 1981;42:119–126.
15. Marbury MC, Linn S, Monson R, et al. The association of alcohol consumption with outcome of pregnancy. Am J Public Health 1983;73:1165–1168.
16. Fried PA, O'Connell CM. A comparison of the effects of prenatal exposure to tobacco, alcohol, cannabis and caffeine on birth size and subsequent growth. Neurotoxicol Teratol 1987;9:79–85.
17. Little RE. Moderate alcohol use during pregnancy and decreased infant birth weight. Am J Public Health 1977;67:1154–1156.
18. Day NL, Jasperse D, Richardson G, et al. Prenatal exposure to alcohol: effect on infant growth and morphologic characteristics. Pediatrics 1989;84:536–541.
19. Rosett H, Weiner L, Lee A, et al. Patterns of alcohol consumption and fetal development. Obstet Gynecol 1983;61:539–546.
20. Mills JL, Graubard BI, Harley EE, et al. Maternal alcohol consumption and birth weight: how much drinking during pregnancy is safe? JAMA 1984;252:1875–1879.
21. Aro T. Maternal diseases, alcohol consumption and smoking during pregnancy associated with reduction limb defects. Early Hum Dev 1983;9:49–57.
22. Ernhart CB, Sokol RJ, Ager JW, Morrow-Tlucak M, Martier S. Alcohol related birth defects: assessing the risk. Ann NY Acad Sci 1989;562:159–172.

23. O'Connor MJ, Brill NJ, Sigman M. Alcohol use in primiparous women older than 30 years of age: relation to infant development. Pediatrics 1986;78:444–450.

24. Coles CD, Smith I, Fernoff PM, et al. Neonatal neurobehavioral characteristics as correlates of maternal alcohol use during gestation. Alcohol Clin Exp Res 1985;9:454–460.

25. Streissguth AP, Barr HM, Sampson PD: Moderate prenatal alcohol exposure: effects on child IQ and learning problems at 7-1/2 years. Alcohol Clin Exp Res 1990;14:662–669.

26. Pierog S, Chandavasu O, Wexler I. Withdrawal symptoms in infants with the fetal alcohol syndrome. J Pediatr 1977;90:630–633.

27. Coles CD, Smith IE, Fernhoff PM, et al. Neonatal ethanol withdrawal: characteristics in clinically normal, nondysmorphic neonates. J Pediatr 1984;105:445–451.

28. Kaminski M, Franc M, Lebouvier M, duMazaubrun D, Rumeau-Rouquette C. Moderate alcohol use and pregnancy outcome. Neurobehav Toxicol Teratol 1981;3:173–181.

29. Zuckerman B, Frank D, Hingson R, et al. Effects of maternal marijuana and cocaine use on fetal growth. N Engl J Med 1989;320:762–768.

30. Mills JL, Graubard BI. Is moderate drinking during pregnancy associated with increased risk for malformations? Pediatrics 1987;80:309–314.

31. Streissguth AP, Martin DC, Barr HM, et al. Intrauterine alcohol and nicotine exposure: attention and reaction time in 4 year old children. Dev Psychobiol 1984;20:533–541.

32. Greene T, Ernhart CB, Ager J, Sokol R, Martier S, Boyd T. Prenatal alcohol exposure and cognitive development in the preschool years. Neurotoxicol Teratol 1991;13:57–68.

33. Tan SE, Zajac CS, Moore C, Rudel D, Zajac C, Abel EL. Effects of paternal alcohol consumption on behavior of offspring in rats. Alcohol Clin Exp Res 1987;11:3.

34. Abel EL, Lee JA. Paternal alcohol exposure affects offspring behavior but not body or organ weights in mice. Alcohol Clin Exp Res 1988;12:349–355.

35. Little RE, Sing CF. Father's drinking and infant birth weight: report of an association. Teratology 1987;36:59–65.

36. Smith GC, Asch RH. Drug abuse and reproduction. Fertil Steril 1987;48:355–373.

37. Irwin M, Dreyfus E, Baird S, Smith TL, Schuckit M. Testosterone in chronic alcoholic men. Br J Addiction 1988;83:949–953.

38. Wilsnack SC, Klassen AD, Wilsnack RW. Drinking and reproductive dysfunction among women in a 1981 national survey. Alcohol Clin Exp Res 1984;8:451–458.

39. Mendelson JH, Mello NK, Ellingboe J. Acute alcohol intake and pituitary gonadal hormones in normal human females. J Pharmacol Exp Ther 1981;218:23–26.

40. Williamson DF, Serdula MK, Kendrick JS, et al. Comparing the prevalence of smoking in pregnant and nonpregnant women, 1985 to 1986. JAMA 1989;261:70–74.

41. Centers for Disease Control. Cigarette smoking among reproductive-aged women: behavioral risk factor surveillance system, 1989. MMWR 1991;40:719–723.

42. Olsen J, Rachootin P, Schiodt AV, et al. Tobacco use, alcohol consumption and infertility. Int J Epidemiol 1983;122:179–184.

43. Baird DD, Wilcox AJ. Cigarette smoking associated with delayed conception. JAMA 1985;253:2979–2983.

44. Howe G, Westhoff C, Martin Vessey, et al. Effects of age, cigarette smoking, and other factors on fertility: findings in a large prospective study. Br Med J 1985;290:1697–1700.

45. De Mouzon J, Spira A, Schwartz D. A prospective study of the relation between smoking and infertility. Int J Epidemiol 1988;17:378–384.

46. Close CE, Roberts PL, Berger RE. Cigarettes, alcohol and marijuana are related to pyospermia in infertile men. J Urol 1990;144:900–903.

47. Kulikauskas V, Blaustein D, Ablin RJ. Cigarette smoking and its possible effects on sperm. Fertil Steril 1985;44:526–528.

48. Campbell JM, Harrison KL. Smoking and infertility. Med J Austral 1979;1:342–343.

49. Evan HJ, Fletcher J, Torrance M, et al. Sperm abnormalities and cigarette smoking. Lancet 1981;1:627–629.

50. Oldereid NB, Rui H, Clausen OPF, et al. Cigarette smoking and human sperm quality assessed by laser-Doppler spectroscopy and DNA flow cytometry. J Reprod Fertil 1989;86:731–736.

51. Kline J, Stein Z, Susser M, et al. Smoking: a risk factor for spontaneous abortion. New Engl J Med 1977;297:793–796.

52. Johnston C. Cigarette smoking and the outcome of human pregnancies: a status report on the consequences. Clin Toxicol 1981;18:189–209.

53. Kline J, Levin B, Shrout P, et al. Maternal smoking and trisomy among spontaneously aborted conceptions. Am J Hum Genet 1983;35:421–431.

54. Meyer MB, Jonas BS, Tonascia JA. Perinatal events associated with maternal smoking during pregnancy. Am J Epidemiol 1976;103:464–476.

55. Naeye RL. The duration of maternal cigarette smoking, fetal and placental disorders. Early Hum Dev 1979;3:229–237.

56. Hebel JR, Fox NL, Sexton M. Dose response of birth weight to various measures of maternal smoking during pregnancy. J Clin Epidemiol 1988;41:483–489.

57. Kleinman JC, Madans JH. The effects of maternal smoking, physical stature, and educational attainment on the incidence of low birth weight. Am J Epidemiol 1985;121:843–845.

58. Sexton M, Hebel JR. A clinical trial of change in maternal smoking and its effect on birth weight. JAMA 1984;251:911–915.

59. Ericson A, Kallen B, Westerholm. Cigarette smoking as an etiologic factor in cleft lip and palate. Am J Obstet Gynecol 1979;135:348–351.

60. Beaulac-Baillargeon L, Desrosiers C. Caffeine-cigarette interaction on fetal growth. Am J Obstet Gynecol 1987;157:1236–1240.

61. Toubas PL, Duke JC, McCaffree MA, et al. Effects of maternal smoking and caffeine habits on infantile apnea: a retrospective study. Pediatrics 1986;78:159–163.

62. MacArthur C, Knox EG. Smoking in pregnancy: effects of

stopping at different stages. Br J Obstet Gynaecol 1988;95:551–555.

63. Hardy JB, Mellits ED. Does maternal smoking during pregnancy have a long-term effect on the child? Lancet 1972;2:1332–1336.

64. Shiono PH, Klebanoff MA, Rhoades GG. Smoking and drinking during pregnancy: their effects on preterm birth. JAMA 1986;255:82–84.

65. Kleinman JC, Pierre MB, Madans JH, et al. The effects of maternal smoking on fetal and infant mortality. Am J Epidemiol 1988;127:274–282.

66. Butler NR, Goldstein H, Ross EM. Cigarette smoking in pregnancy: its influence on birth weight and perinatal mortality. Br Med J 1972;2:127–130.

67. Fried PA. Cigarettes and marijuana: are there measurable long-term neurobehavioral teratogenic effects? Neurotoxicology 1989;10:577–584.

68. Saxton DW. The behavior of infants whose mothers smoke in pregnancy. Early Hum Dev 1978;2/4:363–369.

69. John EM, Savitz DA, Sandler DP. Prenatal exposure to parents' smoking and childhood cancer. Am J Epidemiol 1991;133:123–132.

70. Martin TR, Bracken MB. The association between low birthweight and caffeine consumption during pregnancy. Am J Epidemiol 1986;124:633–642.

71. Haglund B, Cnattingius S. Cigarette smoking as a risk factor for Sudden Infant Death Syndrome: a population-based study. Am J Public Health 1990;80;1:29–32.

72. Kandall SR, Gaines J. Maternal substance use and subsequent Sudden Infant Death Syndrome (SIDS) in offspring. Neurotoxicol Teratol 1991;13:235–240.

73. Hatch E, Bracken M. Effect of marijuana use in pregnancy on fetal growth. Am J Epidemiol 1986;124: 986–993.

74. Gibson GT, Baghurst PA, Colley DP. Maternal alcohol, tobacco and cannabis consumption and the outcome of pregnancy. Aust NZ J Obstet Gynaecol 1983;23:15–19.

75. Fried PA, Watkinson B, Willan A. Marijuana use during pregnancy and decreased length of gestation. Am J Obstet Gynecol 1984;150:23–27.

76. Day N, Sambamoorthi U, Taylor P, et al. Prenatal marijuana use and neonatal outcome. Neurotoxicol Teratol 1991;13:329–334.

77. Parker S, Zuckerman B, Bauchner H. Jitteriness in full-term neonates: prevalence and correlates. Pediatrics 1990;85:17–23.

78. Fried PA, Watkinson B. 36- and 48-month neurobehavioral follow-up of children prenatally exposed to marijuana, cigarettes, and alcohol. J Dev Behav Pediatr 1990;11:49–58.

79. O'Connell CM, Fried PA. Prenatal exposure to cannabis: a preliminary report of postnatal consequences in school-age children. Neurotoxicol Teratol 1991;13:631–639.

80. Mendelson JH, Mello NK, Ellingboe J. Marijuana smoking suppresses luteinizing hormone in women. J Pharmacol Exp Ther 1986;237:862–866.

81. Hembree WC, Nahas GG, Zeidenberg P, et al. Changes in human spermatozoa associated with high dose marijuana smoking. In: Nahas GG, ed. Marijuana, biological effects. Oxford: Pergamon Press, 1979:429–439.

82. Kolodny RC, Masters WH, Kolodner, Toro G. Depres-

sion of plasma testosterone levels after chronic intensive marijuana use. N Engl J Med 1974;290:872–874.

83. Mendelson JH, Kuehnle J, Ellingboe J, Babor T. Plasma testosterone levels before, during and after chronic marijuana smoking. N Engl J Med 1974;291:1051–1055.

84. Ostrea EM, Chavez CJ. Perinatal problems (excluding neonatal withdrawal) in maternal drug addiction: a study of 830 cases. J Pediatr 1979;74:292–295.

85. Stone ML, Salerno LJ, Green M, et al. Narcotic addiction in pregnancy. Am J Obstet Gynecol 1971;109:716–723.

86. Little BB, Snell LM, Klein VR, et al. Maternal and fetal effects of heroin addiction during pregnancy. J Reprod Med 1990;35:159–262.

87. Wilson GS, Desmond MM, Wait RB. Follow-up of methadone-treated and untreated narcotic-dependent women and their infants: health, developmental, and social implications. J Pediatr 1981;98:716–722.

88. Lifschitz MH, Wilson GS, Smith EO, Desmond MM. Fetal and postnatal growth of children born to narcotic-dependent women. J Pediatr 1983;102:686–691.

89. Vargas GC, Pildes RS, Vidyasagar D, et al. Effect of maternal heroin addiction on 67 liveborn neonates. Clin Pediatr 1975;14:751–757.

90. Strauss ME, Starr RH, Ostrea EM, et al. Behavioral concomitants of prenatal addiction to narcotics. J Pediatr 1976;89:842–846.

91. Wilson GS. Clinical studies of infants and children exposed prenatally to heroin. Ann NY Acad Sci 1989; 562:183–194.

92. Hans SL. Developmental consequences of prenatal exposure to methadone. Ann NY Acad Sci 1989;562: 195–207.

93. Rosner MA, Keith L, Chasnoff IJ. The Northwestern University drug dependence program: the impact of intensive prenatal care on labor and delivery outcomes. Am J Obstet Gynecol 1982;144:23–27.

94. Stimmel B, Adamsons K. Narcotic dependency in pregnancy: methadone maintenance compared to use of street drugs. JAMA 1976;235:1121–1124.

95. Zelson C, Lee SJ, Casalino M. Neonatal narcotic addiction: comparative effects of maternal intake of heroin and methadone. N Engl J Med 1973;289:1216–1220.

96. Kaltenbach K, Finnegan LP: Perinatal and developmental outcome of infants exposed to methadone in-utero. Neurotoxicol Teratol 1987;9:311– 313.

97. Little BB, Snell LM, Klewin VR, et al. Cocaine abuse during pregnancy: maternal and fetal implications. Obstet Gynecol 1989;73:157– 160.

98. Frank DA, Zuckerman BS, Amaro H, et al. Cocaine use during pregnancy: prevalence and correlates. Pediatrics 1988;82:888–895.

99. McCalla S, Minkoff HL, Feldman J, et al. The biological and social consequences of perinatal cocaine use in an inner-city population: results of an anonymous cross-sectional study. Am J Obstet Gynecol 1991;164:625–630.

100. Mayes LC, Granger RH, Bornstein MH, Zuckerman B. The problem of prenatal cocaine exposure. A rush to judgment. JAMA 1992;267:406–408.

101. Chasnoff IJ, Griffith DR, MacGregor S, et al. Temporal

patterns of cocaine use in pregnancy: perinatal outcome. JAMA 1989;261:1741–1744.

102. Bingol N, Fuchs M, Diaz V, et al. Teratogenicity of cocaine in humans. J Pediatr 1987;110:93–96.

103. Chasnoff IJ, Burns WJ, Schnoll SH, et al. Cocaine use in pregnancy. N Engl J Med 1985;313:666–669.

104. Oro AS, Dixon SD. Perinatal cocaine and methamphetamine exposure: maternal and neonatal correlates. J Pediatr 1987;111:571–578.

105. Ryan L, Ehrlich S, Finnegan L. Cocaine abuse in pregnancy: effects on the fetus and newborn. Neurotoxicol Teratol 1987;9:295–299.

106. Cherukuri R, Minkoff H, Feldman, et al. A cohort study of alkaloidal cocaine ("crack") in pregnancy. Obstet Gynecol 1988;72:147–151.

107. Chouteau M, Namerow PB, Leppert P. The effect of cocaine abuse on birth weight and gestational age. Obstet Gynecol 1988;72:351–354.

108. Dixon SD. Effects of transplacental exposure to cocaine and methamphetamine on the neonate. West J Med 1989;150:436–442.

109. MacGregor SN, Keith LG, Bachicha JA, et al. Cocaine abuse during pregnancy: correlation between prenatal care and perinatal outcome. Obstet Gynecol 1989; 74:882–885.

110. Eisen LN, Field TM, Bandstra ES, et al. Perinatal cocaine effects on neonatal stress behavior and performance on the Brazelton scale. Pediatrics 1991;88: 477–480.

111. Neuspiel DR, Hamel SC, Hochberg E, Greene J, Campbell D. Maternal cocaine use and infant behavior. Neurotoxicol Teratol 1991;13:229–233.

112. Coles C, Platzman K, Smith I, James M, Falek A. Effects of cocaine and alcohol use in pregnancy on neonatal growth and neurobehavioral status. Neurotoxicol Teratol 1992;14:23–33.

113. Chasnoff IJ, Burns KA, Burns WJ. Cocaine use in pregnancy: perinatal morbidity and mortality. Neurotoxicol Teratol 1987;9:291–295.

114. Neerhof MG, MacGregor SN, Retsky SS, et al. Cocaine abuse during pregnancy: peripartum prevalence and perinatal outcome. Am J Obstet Gynecol 1989;161: 633–638.

115. Gillogley KM, Evans AT, Hansen RL, Samuels SJ, Batra KK. The perinatal impact of cocaine, amphetamine, and opiate use detected by universal intrapartum screening. Am J Obstet Gynecol 1990;163:1535–1542.

116. Mercado A, Johnson G, Galver D, et al. Cocaine, pregnancy, and postpartum intracerebral hemorrhage. Obstet Gynecol 1989;73:467–468.

117. Thatcher S, Corfman R, Grosso J, et al. Cocaine use and acute rupture of ectopic pregnancies. Obstet Gynecol 1989;74:478–479.

118. Gonsoulin W, Borge D, Moise KJ. Rupture of unscarred uterus in primigravid women in association with cocaine abuse. Am J Obstet Gynecol 1990;163:526–527.

119. Chavez GF, Mulinare J, Cordero JF. Maternal cocaine use during early pregnancy as a risk factor for congenital urogenital anomalies. JAMA 1989;262:795–798.

120. Chasnoff IJ, Chisum GM, Kaplan WE. Maternal cocaine use and genitourinary tract malformations. Teratology 1988;37:201–204.

121. Hoyme HE, Jones KL, Dixon SD, et al. Prenatal cocaine exposure and fetal vascular disruption. Pediatrics 1990;85:743–747.

122. MacGregor SN, Keith LG, Chasnoff IJ, et al. Cocaine use during pregnancy: adverse perinatal outcome. Am J Obstet Gynecol 1987;157:686–690.

123. Dixon SD, Bejar R. Echoencephalographic findings in neonates associated with maternal cocaine and methamphetamine use: incidence and clinical correlates. J Pediatr 1989;115:770–778.

124. van de Bor M, Walther FJ, Sims ME. Increased cerebral blood flow velocity in infants of mothers who abuse cocaine. Pediatrics 1990;85:733–736.

125. Bauchner H, Zuckerman B, McClain M, et al. Risk of Sudden Infant Death Syndrome among infants with in utero exposure to cocaine. J Pediatr 1988;113:831–834.

126. Hadeed AJ, Siegel SR. Maternal cocaine use during pregnancy: effect on the newborn infant. Pediatrics 1989;84:2:205–210.

127. Singer LT, Garber R, Kliegman R. Neurobehavioral sequelae of fetal cocaine exposure. J Pediatr 1991; 119:667–672.

128. Graham K, Dimitrakoudis D, Pellegrini E, et al. Pregnancy outcome following first trimester exposure to cocaine in social users in Toronto, Canada. Vet Hum Toxicol 1989;31:143–148.

129. Richardson GA, Day NL. Maternal and neonatal effects of moderate cocaine use in pregnancy. Neurotoxicol Teratol 1991;13:455–460.

130. Elliott RH, Rees GB. Amphetamine ingestion presenting as eclampsia. Can J Anaesth 1990;37:130–133.

131. Samuels SI, Maze A, Albright G. Cardiac arrest during cesarean section in a chronic amphetamine abuser. Anesth Analg 1979;58:528–530.

132. Smith DS, Gutsche BB. Amphetamine abuse and obstetric anesthesia. Anesth Analg 1980;59:710–711.

133. Little BB, Snell LM, Gilstrap LC. Methamphetamine abuse during pregnancy: outcome and fetal effects. Obstet Gynecol 1988;72:541–544.

134. Briggs GC, Samson JH, Crawford DJ. Lack of abnormalities in a newborn exposed to amphetamine during gestation. Am J Dis Child 1975;129:249–250.

135. Eriksson M, Larsson G, Winbladh B, et al. The influence of amphetamine addiction on pregnancy and the newborn infant. Acta Paediatr Scand 1978;67:95–99.

136. Nora JL, Vargo TA, Nora AH, et al. Dexamphetamine: A possible environmental trigger in cardiovascular malformation. Lancet 1970;1:1290–1291.

137. Gilbert EF, Khoury GH. Dextroamphetamine and congenital cardiac malformation. J Pediatr 1970:638.

138. Billing L, Eriksson M, Steneroth G, et al. Pre-school children of amphetamine-addicted mothers. I. Somatic and psychomotor development. Acta Paediatr Scand 1985;74:179–184.

139. Larsson G, Eriksson M, Zetterstrom R. Amphetamine addiction and pregnancy: psycho-social and medical aspects. Acta Psychiatr Scand 1979;60:334–346.

140. Eriksson M, Larsson G, Zetterstrom R. Amphetamine addiction and pregnancy. II. Pregnancy, delivery and the neonatal period. Sociomedical aspects. Acta Obstet Gynecol Scand 1981;60:253–259.

141. Billing L, Eriksson M, Larsson G, et al. Amphetamine addiction and pregnancy. III. One year follow-up of the children. Psychosocial and pediatric aspects. Acta Paediatr Scand 1980;69:675–680.

142. Ellerbrock TV, Bush TJ, Chamberland MD, Oxtoby MJ. Epidemiology of women with AIDS in the United States, 1981 through 1990: a comparison with heterosexual men with AIDS. JAMA 1991;265:2971–2975.

143. Minkoff HL, Henderson C, Mendez H, et al. Pregnancy outcomes among mothers infected with human immunodeficiency virus and uninfected control subjects. Am J Obstet Gynecol 1990;163:521–526.

144. Fullilove RE, Fullilove MT, Bowser BP, et al. Risk of sexually transmitted disease among black adolescent crack users in Oakland and San Francisco, California. JAMA 1990;263:851–855.

145. Selwyn PA, Schoenbaum EE, Davenny K, et al. Prospective study of human immunodeficiency virus infection and pregnancy outcomes in intravenous drug users. JAMA 1989;261:1289–1294.

146. Berkowitz K, LaSala A. Risk factors associated with the increasing prevalence of pneumonia during pregnancy. Am J Obstet Gynecol 1990;163:981–985.

147. Bays J. Substance abuse and child abuse. Pediatr Clin North Am 1990;37:881–904.

148. Moss K. Substance abuse during pregnancy. Harvard Women's Law Journal 1990;13:278–299.

149. Warner A, Hassan M, Fant WK. Drug abuse testing: pharmacokinetic and technical aspects. Am Assoc Clin Chem 1986;8:1–9.

150. Cone EJ, Johnson RE. Contact highs and urinary cannabinoid excretion after passive exposure to marijuana smoke. Clin Pharmacol Ther 1986;40:247–256.

151. Jessup M. The treatment of perinatal addiction—identification, intervention, and advocacy. West J Med 1990;152:553–558.

152. Clark HW. The role of physicians as medical review officers in workplace drug testing programs: in pursuit of the last nanogram. West J Med 1990;152:514–524.

153. Chavkin W. Drug addiction and pregnancy: policy crossroads. Am J Public Health 1990;80:483–487.

154. Hoegerman G, Wilson CA, Thurmond E, et al. Drug exposed neonates. West J Med 1990;152:559–564.

155. Chasnoff IJ, Landress JH, Barrett ME. The prevalence of illicit drug or alcohol use during pregnancy and discrepancies in mandatory reporting in Pinellas County, Florida. N Engl J Med 1990;322:1202–1220.

156. Board of Trustees, American Medical Association. Legal interventions during pregnancy-court ordered medical treatments and legal penalties for potentially harmful behavior by pregnant women. JAMA 1990;264:2662–2670.

# 26

Common Household
Exposures

MAUREEN PAUL

The average family in the U.S. uses approximately 55 gallons of hazardous household products each year. Products that may contain toxic chemicals include household cleaners, lawn and garden supplies, paint supplies, automotive products, craft and hobby supplies, personal care products, and others. Measures to improve home energy efficiency have resulted in increased concentrations of chemical contaminants and radon in indoor air. Household water is an important source of exposure to toxicants, either by ingestion or through inhalation of volatized chemicals during showering or laundering (Chapter 27).

People in the U.S. typically spend 90% of their time indoors, about two-thirds of which is spent in the home. In the 1980s, the Environmental Protection Agency (EPA) conducted the Total Exposure Assessment Methodology (TEAM) Study to estimate environmental and personal exposures to toxic volatile organic compounds (VOCs) among populations residing in various U.S. cities (1–3). In all locations and for virtually all measured chemicals, mean indoor (residential) air concentrations exceeded those in outdoor air by at least a factor of two, and sometimes, by more than 10-fold. Personal exposures were significantly increased by common practices such as use of

room air fresheners and toilet deodorizers (*p*-dichlorobenzene), automatic washing of clothes and dishes (chloroform), visiting a dry cleaners (1,1,1-trichloroethane, tetrachloroethylene), smoking (benzene, styrene), painting or removing paint (n-decane, n-undecone), cleaning a car engine with solvents (xylene, ethylbenzene, tetrachloroethylene), or visiting a service station (benzene) (1, 3).

Many consumers remain unaware of the potential hazards associated with household products and the activities of daily living. Some of these exposures may contribute to adverse reproductive or developmental outcomes. In addition, anticipation of pregnancy or birth may prompt home renovations that increase exposure to lead, solvents, and other toxicants. It is, therefore, essential that clinicians evaluate home exposures and educate patients about ways to minimize risk. This chapter provides information on household exposures of common concern to pregnant patients or those with reproductive problems. Home use of pesticides is covered in Chapter 21 and drinking water contamination is discussed in Chapter 27.

## ELECTRIC BLANKETS

Electric blankets expose users to power-frequency (60 Hz) electric and magnetic fields.

While this low-frequency electromagnetic energy emanates from all electrical household appliances, electric blankets are of particular concern because they are in close proximity to the body for long periods of time. In fact, electric blankets probably represent the most intense prolonged exposure to electromagnetic fields (EMF) commonly encountered in the home environment.

## How Electric Blankets Work

As shown in Figure 26.1, an electric blanket consists of heating elements that run in longitudinal channels through the blanket and a thermostatic controller that regulates blanket temperature. The most common controller contains a bimetal strip thermally coupled to a small, resistive heater. When the switch is closed, the bimetal strip makes contact with a stationary metal element, initiating warming of the small heater and blanket heating coils. As the bimetal strip heats, it curves away from its contact until the electrical circuit is eventually broken. The setting on the controller determines the temperature at which this occurs by regulating the pressure of the bimetal strip against its fixed contact. The room temperature determines the length of time required for the bimetal strip to cool sufficiently to reclose the switch. In conventional electric blankets, thermoswitches located along the blanket heating elements protect against overheating; some newer types of blankets are thermally self-limiting and require no thermoswitches (4). The duty cycle is the proportion of time that current is being drawn to operate the blanket and depends on the controller dial setting and room temperature. The average population-based duty cycle is approximately 40–50% (4, 5), i.e., heat is being generated about half the time the blanket is in use.

The degree of exposure to electromagnetic fields from electric blanket use varies according to blanket design features and individual factors affecting duty cycle, body size and posture, degree of blanket coverage, body-blanket separation, and duration of use. Reported blanket-induced electric field exposures range from approximately 40 to over 100 volts/meter (V/m), compared with typical household back-

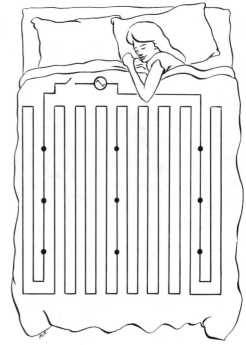

**Figure 26.1.** A conventional electric blanket consists of longitudinal heating elements that run through the blanket and a thermostatic controller (single or dual, depending on blanket size). Thermoswitches (indicated by *black dots*) protect against overheating.

ground exposures of ≤15 V/m (5, 6). Wertheimer and Leeper (7) measured 60-Hz magnetic field exposures of approximately 15 milligauss (mG) from electric blankets; background residential levels are usually less than 2 mG. Using a three-dimensional computer model to estimate magnetic field exposures within human forms as a function of blanket type and varying conditions of use, Florig and Hoburg (4) estimated body average magnetic fields of 15–33 mG across the U.S. blanket-using population. Recently, low-emission electric blankets have been marketed that reduce magnetic field exposures. In recent EMF measurements by the U.S. Food and Drug Administration (FDA), magnetic fields at 5 cm from the surface of low-emission blankets ranged from less than 1–3 mG, compared with 30–40 mG for standard electric blankets. At the same distance, electric fields measured approximately 200 V/m for both the standard and new blanket types (FDA, personal communication).

## Potential Reproductive and Developmental Effects

The properties and potential biological actions of low-frequency electromagnetic fields are discussed in Chapters 13 and 14 and elsewhere (6, 8). Briefly, in vitro studies suggest effects of low-frequency fields on a variety of cell-physiological endpoints including synthesis of DNA, RNA, and proteins; cell proliferation; membrane calcium fluxes; immune responses; and membrane signals involving hormones, enzymes, and neurotransmitters. While most whole animal experiments have not shown teratogenic effects as a result of low-frequency EMF exposure, some have been positive (9). These latter investigations have primarily involved exposure of chick embryos to magnetic fields, and effects differ as a function of field frequency, intensity, and other exposure parameters. Of potential relevance to the reproductive endocrine system, experimental animal and human data reveal alterations in pineal gland function as a result of EMF exposure (6, 10); effects on catecholamines and other central nervous system (CNS) hormones are less consistent.

To date, only one research group has examined the association between electric blanket use and pregnancy outcome. Wertheimer and Leeper (11, 12) collected data on births and prior fetal losses from Denver-area birth records and conducted telephone interviews to ascertain retrospectively use of electric blankets or heated waterbeds. They observed a statistically significant seasonal variation in fetal loss rates among users of electrically heated beds, with the highest concentration of miscarriages occurring in the months of September-January, when cold weather was increasing. No seasonal pattern of spontaneous abortion was noted among nonusers.

Unfortunately, the precise timing of EMF exposure in relation to conception or the period of pregnancy preceding fetal loss is not well established in these reports. In addition, the observed pattern of fetal loss does not provide altogether consistent support for an association with electrically heated beds. For example, the excess of fetal loss observed in September would require heated bed use during midsummer, which seems unlikely. Moreover, exposures during January and February would result in excess loss in the spring season, which was not observed. The researchers explain this latter discrepancy by asserting that intense exposure during the coldest winter months results in early, preclinical loss, while lower but increasing exposure during late summer/early fall allows for longer survival of the conceptus before (clinically recognized) loss occurs. While interesting, this hypothesis remains unsubstantiated.

As explained in Chapter 7, several studies suggest an association between residential or occupational EMF exposure and the development of cancer. In a recent case-control study, Savitz et al. (13) examined the relationship between childhood cancer and exposure to magnetic fields from household electrical appliances, including electric blankets. Parents of cases and controls were interviewed in detail about the use of electric appliances by the woman during pregnancy and by the child postnatally. After adjustment for income, prenatal electric blanket exposure was associated with a statistically significant increase in the incidence of childhood brain cancer (OR 2.5, CI 1.1–5.6). Cancer risk was enhanced with first trimester blanket use and nightly duration of use exceeding 8 hr, but was not related to blanket setting. In another case-control study, electric blanket use did not increase the risk of germ cell testicular cancer in adult white males (14).

To date, no human study has been large enough to examine the association between electric blanket use and the risk of congenital anomalies. Experimental animal data regarding teratogenic effects of electromagnetic fields remain inconsistent, and it is unlikely that the heat generated by electric blankets is sufficient to induce malformations (Chapter 16). In addition, low-frequency EMF exposures do not appear to be mutagenic (15, 16). Fertility impairment among electric blanket users has not been investigated; however, the possibility remains intriguing given the exquisite sensitivity of the male germ cell to heat and the data suggesting EMF-induced alterations in neuroendocrine parameters and pineal gland function.

## Recommendations

There are very few human studies that examine the effects of electric blanket use on pregnancy outcome and none that assess other reproductive parameters. At present, evidence of an association between prenatal electric blanket use and fetal loss or childhood cancer remains inconclusive. After a review of the available data, an FDA Scientific Advisory panel recently recommended further research with improved methodology and continued collaboration between the FDA and blanket manufacturers to reduce EMF emissions (17).

Because risk has not been ruled out and thermal comfort is easily achievable through other means, it is prudent to avoid exposure to electric blankets in the periconception period and during pregnancy. There is little harm in preheating beds electrically and turning off the power just before retiring. This recommendation may change as new data accumulate and as low-emission blankets are improved and tested.

## RADON

Few environmental issues have generated as much attention in recent years as radon. According to the National Council on Radiation Protection and Measurements (NCRP), radon contributes over half of the average annual dose equivalent of ionizing radiation received by U.S. residents from all sources (18). While radon primarily targets the respiratory tract and is unlikely to pose a reproductive risk, pregnancy often prompts questions that clinicians should be prepared to answer.

## Definition and Properties

Radon is a naturally occurring inert gas formed from spontaneous radioactive decay of uranium-238, which is found in most rocks and soil. As shown in Figure 26.2, radon itself undergoes radioactive decay to produce so called radon "daughters" (isotopes of polonium, bismuth, and lead). The short-lived progeny are responsible for the known adverse health effects associated with radon.

As explained in Chapter 13, decay of radioactive elements releases energy either in the

| Uranium-238 | $4.47 \times 10^9$ yr |
| Radium-226 | 1600 yr |
| Radon-222 | 3.82 day |
| Polonium-218 | 3.05 min |
| Lead-214 | 26.8 min |
| Bismuth-214 | 19.7 min |
| Polonium-214 | $1.64 \times 10^{-4}$ sec |
| Lead-210 | 21 yr |
| Bismuth-210 | 5 day |
| Polonium-210 | 138 day |
| Lead-206 | stable |

**Figure 26.2.** Uranium-238 decay series generating radon-222 and its progeny. Half-life of each isotope indicated on the right. $\alpha$ = Alpha particle emission; $\beta$ = beta particle emission; $\gamma$ = gamma radiation. Data from U.S. Department of Health and Human Services, Agency for Toxic Substances and Disease Registry. Toxicological profile for radon. Bethesda, MD: Agency for Toxic Substances and Disease Registry, 1990:62.

form of particles (e.g., $\alpha$ or $\beta$ particles) or photons (e.g., $\gamma$ or x-rays). The $\alpha$ radiation emitted by external radon does not penetrate through the skin. Moreover, with a half-life of nearly 4 days, most inhaled radon gas is exhaled before it decays and deposits a significant radiation dose to lung tissue. Radon daughters, on the other hand, are not gases but tiny solid particles. These progeny attach to the surface of ambient aerosol particles and, when inhaled, deposit in the lining of the respiratory tract. The $\alpha$ radiation emitted by the short-lived polonium isotopes can cause significant localized damage to the bronchial epithelium (19).

Radon and its progeny reach the gastrointestinal tract by ingestion of radon-contaminated water or after swallowing daughter particles cleared from the lungs by the mucociliary blanket. Apparently, most ingested radon is absorbed by the stomach and small intestines (20), and more than 90% of the absorbed dose is rapidly eliminated by exhalation (21). Because radon is highly lipid soluble, chronic exposure can result in storage of radon and its long-lived daughter products (e.g., polonium-210, lead-210) in body fat. Lead-210 has also been found in bone and teeth after prolonged human exposure to radon (22–24). In experimental animal studies, smaller fractions of radon and its progeny have been found in blood, brain, liver, kidney, heart, muscle tissues, and testes (25).

Because most radon in water is rapidly released into the air, the relative contributions of dermal and inhalation routes to radon body burden are difficult to determine. In one study of subjects bathing in radon-contaminated water while breathing compressed air, blood concentrations of radon reached approximately 1% of the concentration in the bath water (26).

The activity of radioactive elements is measured in Curies (Ci) or Becquerels (Bq), the latter being equal to 1 disintegration per second. The activity concentration of radon in air is commonly expressed in pCi/liter of air (1 pCi $= 1 \times 10^{-12}$ Ci).

Because routine measurement of radon progeny is infeasible, the "working level" (WL) is used to describe the amount of $\alpha$ radiation emitted from the short-lived radon daughters. The WL represents any combination of these progeny in 1 liter of air that emits $1.3 \times 10^5$ million electron volts of $\alpha$ energy from complete decay. When radon is in equilibrium with its daughters, 1 WL equals 100 pCi radon-222/liter of air. In a typical house, where ventilation and other factors affect the equilibrium, 1 WL is usually associated with approximately 200 pCi/liter.

## Sources of Radon Exposure

Sources of radon exposure in the home are depicted in Figure 26.3. Uranium-238 and its long-lived decay product, radium-226, are found in abundance in the earth's crust. Radon gas is continually being formed from radium-226 and is released into air pockets between soil and rock particles. Radon gas flows into the home through cracks and pores in the foundation as a result of indoor/outdoor pressure differences. Indoor air concentrations of radon are usually higher in basement areas and in energy-efficient homes where ventilation is de-

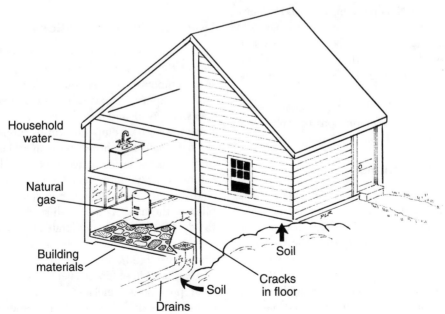

**Figure 26.3.** Sources of indoor radon include soil under homes, household water, natural gas supplies, and building materials.

creased. Studies of indoor radon levels in the U.S. reveal average concentrations of 1.5–4.2 pCi/liter of air, compared to mean atmospheric levels of approximately 0.25 pCi/liter (27, 28). Some building materials also release very small amounts of radon.

Radon in rock and soil can also contaminate groundwater, which is a major source of household water in the U.S. Radon-contaminated water can be directly ingested, or radon can be released into indoor air when water is used for laundering, bathing, and other purposes. Average levels of radon in groundwater are approximately 350 pCi/liter of water (29).

## Potential Health Effects

The primary target organ of radon is the respiratory tract. Several epidemiological studies of miners chronically exposed to high doses of radon (approximately 50–150 pCi/liter air) reveal increased rates of lung cancer and non-neoplastic respiratory diseases, particularly in smokers (24). A few Scandinavian studies also suggest that residential exposure to radon is associated with an increased risk of lung cancer (30, 31).

Due to its low solubility in body fluids, only very small amounts of radon reach the tissues of the reproductive tract. The NCRP estimates that, for the U.S. population, whole body ionizing radiation doses from radon average 200 mrem per year, with the upper limit of exposure to the gonads averaging 10 mrem (18). While no studies have directly evaluated the developmental toxicity of radon and its progeny, this estimated dose is 1/1000th of the radiation dose at which observable malformations or embryotoxicity is expected (Chapter 13).

## Recommendations

While reproductive or developmental effects from residential radon exposure are unlikely, the data on radon-induced lung disease warrant measures to minimize risk. The EPA recommends that indoor radon levels be <4 pCi/liter of air or approximately 0.02 WL (32).

A number of resources are available for home radon testing. In some areas, state or local government agencies are providing homeowners with detectors. Names of reputable firms that have completed the EPA's Radon and Radon Progeny Measurement Proficiency Program are available from regional EPA offices. The EPA suggests that citizens initially utilize a short-term, inexpensive screening method to detect a potential radon problem. More sophisticated testing is recommended if screening results are ≥0.02 WL or 4 pCi/liter, and immediate remedial action should be taken if levels exceed 1 WL or 200 pCi/liter (32).

Remediation generally involves blocking points of radon entry and diverting or removing radon through ventilation mechanisms. Cessation of smoking is also important, since smoke provides a nidus for radon daughter attachment and increases lung cancer risk.

Several educational publications are available to providers and the public through the EPA, including *A Citizen's Guide to Radon* and *Radon Reduction Methods: A Homeowner's Guide*.

## HAIR CARE PRODUCTS

One question that arises repeatedly in clinical practice concerns the safety of using hair dyes and permanent wave solutions during pregnancy. This section briefly reviews the data on this subject.

### Hair Coloring Preparations

Hair colorants fall into three categories that reflect the longevity of the color imparted to hair: temporary (washes out with first shampoo), semipermanent (washes out after successive shampoos), and permanent (lasts until the hair grows out). Temporary rinses simply coat the hair shaft. In contrast, permanent hair coloring involves an oxidative process. Alkaline solutions of dye intermediates mixed with an oxidizing agent (hydrogen peroxide) are applied to the hair. As the alkali swells the hair, the dye intermediates penetrate and oxidize to form insoluble pigments irreversibly bound to the hair itself (33).

Dyes used in semipermanent and permanent color preparations include aromatic nitro and amino compounds (33, 34). Common examples include nitrophenylenediamine, nitroaminophenol, and benzenediamines such as *p*-phenylenediamine, $p$-aminodiphenylamine, or 2,5-diaminotoluene. Other constituents of permanent color products include soaps or detergents, conditioners, solubilizing agents (alcohols, glycols), and antioxidants (e.g., polyhydroxyphenols, sodium sulfite, thioglycolic acid). Metallic hair dyes containing lead and other toxic metals are no longer in common usage.

The hair dye ingredients that have generated the most concern are the aromatic amines. While these compounds bind to hair and skin, some percutaneous absorption can occur (35). Many aromatic amines in hair dyes demonstrate mutagenic activity in bacterial assays and mammalian cell culture (36–38). Teratogenicity testing is limited; studies of hair dyes containing various phenylenediamines and 2,5-toluenediamine are negative in rats and demonstrate embryotoxicity or malformations in mice only at very high (usually maternally toxic) doses (39–41). Some oxidative hair dyes are carcinogenic in laboratory animals, but human studies do not indicate an increased cancer risk from nonoccupational use of hair dyes (42, 43).

## Permanent Wave Preparations

Permanent waving of hair is a two-step process. First, wave solution containing a reducing agent (ammonium thioglycate or glyceryl monothioglycolate) is applied to rolled hair and left on for 15–20 minutes. The reducing agent disrupts the disulfide bonds in the hair keratin. In the second step, an oxidizing agent is applied to "neutralize" the wave solution and stimulate reformation of the disulfide bonds into a new permanent wave set. While the most common neutralizer is hydrogen peroxide, some solutions contain bromate salts (34, 44).

The primary known health effect of permanent wave products is dermatitis. These products do not contain reported animal teratogens, and no human studies have been performed. Because hydrogen peroxide solutions degrade to oxygen and water at the site of application, systemic toxicity is not expected (45).

## Recommendations

There is no direct evidence that the personal use of hair dyes or permanent wave solutions is harmful during pregnancy. However, patients should be informed about the paucity of human data and the potential mutagenicity of semipermanent and permanent hair dyes. In all cases, gloves should be worn while dyeing or perming at home, and solutions should not be left on for excessive periods of time.

Henna is a natural, semipermanent vegetable dye available to patients who prefer to avoid exposure to synthetic chemical products. It consists of the dried powdered leaves of a tree native to parts of Asia and Africa, and the active dye ingredient is 2-hydroxy-1,4-naphthaquinone (33). Homemade hair rinses can also be made from nontoxic plant materials (46).

## HOME HOBBIES

Millions of people in the U.S. enjoy a variety of home hobbies, ranging from arts and crafts to furniture restoration to auto mechanics. It is estimated, for example, that some 50 million adults are engaged in pottery-making, woodworking, and other crafts, and another 22 million enjoy painting, drawing, or sculpture (47).

One person's home hobby may very well be another's occupation. In a survey of over 300 artists in New York City, more than half had home studios that were often in common living spaces such as bedrooms or kitchens. Forty-seven percent of the female artists and 20% of the wives of the male artists were exposed to potentially hazardous art materials during pregnancy (48).

Because hobbies are undertaken for recreational purposes, patients may be unaware of potential health hazards associated with these activities. Hobbyists often use products containing the same toxicants found in the workplace, but few have the technical knowledge or resources necessary to control exposures in the home adequately.

This section briefly discusses potential reproductive or developmental toxicants used in some common arts and crafts hobbies. Table 26.1 summarizes this information and provides recommendations to prevent untoward outcomes. Most of the materials of concern are toxic metals and organic solvents that are discussed in other chapters of this book. Excellent and comprehensive publications on health hazards in the arts and crafts are also available (49–51).

**Table 26.1.**
**Selected Arts and Crafts Hobbies: Reproductive Hazards and Recommendations**

| Hobby | Product(s) | Hazardous Exposures | Recommendations |
|---|---|---|---|
| Ceramics | Glazes and fluxes | Heavy metals, e.g., lead, antimony, cadmium, chromium, lithium, copper, manganese, nickel, cobalt, zinc, barium | Use prepared glazes, but avoid skin contact; do not use lead glazes or eat or drink from lead-glazed containers; do not spray glazes |
| | Kiln | Toxic gases, e.g., carbon monoxide; metallic fumes | Kilns must have efficient exhaust ventilation |
| Painting | Pigments | Heavy metals (see ceramic glazes), solvents | Use premixed paints; avoid leaded paints; use acrylics or watercolors instead of oil paints |
| | Lacquers, thinners, cleaners/strippers | Solvents, e.g., alcohols, acetone, methyl ethyl ketone, toluene, xylene, mineral spirits, turpentine, methylene chloride | Cautious use of shellac, mineral spirits, or acetone probably safer than aromatic or chlorinated hydrocarbon solvents; minimize spraying of solvent-based products, and use adequate ventilation |
| Photography | Developers, dye-couplers (color) | Aminophenol derivatives or substituted $p$-phenylenediamine compounds | Simple black and white photographic processing safe if basic precautions used; avoid color processing and after-treatments such as intensification and toning, or use stringent control measures (see text); do not mix dry chemicals; avoid exposure of cyanide salts to acid, heat, or ultraviolet light (hydrogen cyanide gas released); darkrooms should be well ventilated ($\geq$10 air changes/hr or $\geq$170 cfm); use local exhaust for processing tanks and solvents |
| | Intensifiers | Dichromate salts | |
| | Reducers | Ferrocyanide salts, iodine | |
| | Toners | Heavy metals, e.g., gold, selenium, uranium, platinum, iron | |
| | Restrainers | Bromide salts, hydroxylamine hydrochloride (color) | |
| | Bleaching agents (color) | Bromide salts | |
| | Hardeners, stabilizers | Formalin (40% formaldehyde) | |
| | Film Cleaners | Solvents, e.g., methylene chloride, 1,1,1,trichloroethane, freons | |
| Screen printing | Inks | Solvents | Use prepared water-based inks without solvent additives |
| | Screen cleaners | Solvents | Clean screens in well-ventilated area and immediately dispose of soaked rags or newspapers |
| | Photoemulsions | Dichromates | Use diazo photoemulsions instead of dichromate |
| Stained glass | Came | Lead | Avoid during preconception period, pregnancy, and nursing or use lead-free materials with adequate precautions (see text) |
| | Solder | Lead-tin alloy | |

## Painting

Paint consists of powdered pigment particles evenly dispersed in a liquid medium (vehicle). The vehicle in which the pigment is suspended differs according to the type of paint used by the art hobbyist (52): linseed and other oils are used in oil paints; an aqueous solution of gum in watercolors and pastels; acrylic polymer mixed with water or organic solvents in acrylic paints; egg, gum, oils, or wax emulsions in tempera paints; and epoxy (plastic) resin combined with solvents and hardeners in epoxy paints. Common additives to art paints include metal-based driers and stabilizers and preservatives such as formalin or phenol.

There are two general types of pigments used in art paints: organic and inorganic. Pigments of each type can derive from either natural or synthetic materials. Inorganic pigments contain a variety of toxic metals including lead, chromium, cadmium, cobalt, mercury, nickel, and manganese. (While these pigments have been largely eliminated from architectural coatings, they are still allowed in artists' materials). Of utmost concern are the two lead-containing pigments used in oil paints known as flake white (or white lead) and Naples yellow (or antimony yellow). Large quantities of white lead in oil may also be used for priming canvases. The raw materials for synthetic organic pigments are coal tar or petroleum derivatives (52).

Art hobbyists commonly use spray paints and ancillary paint products that contain a variety of organic solvents. For example, varnishes are employed as finishes or protective coatings on paintings. They typically consist of oil and resins dissolved in turpentine, alcohols, or aromatic hydrocarbon solvents such as toluene or xylene. In pastel painting, fixatives containing similar materials may be sprayed onto pictures to prevent the colors from dusting off. Thinners used to reduce the viscosity of paints and varnishes include turpentine (distilled sap of coniferous trees), petroleum distillates (e.g., mineral spirits), alcohols, and products containing aromatic hydrocarbons. Paint and varnish removers may contain methylene chloride, a solvent that is metabolized in the body to carbon monoxide.

Occupational exposure to organic solvents has been associated with fetal loss and congenital malformations in some studies (Chapter 19). While these studies have methodological limitations and exposure scenarios differ in the workplace and home settings, they still sound a cautionary note for art hobbyists who use solvent-based products.

One solvent commonly found in paint-related products that has received particular attention in recent years is toluene. A few human case reports suggest that recreational abuse of toluene through chronic sniffing of spray paint is associated with maternal renal tubular acidosis, preterm delivery, and an embryopathic "fetal solvent syndrome" (53–55). Noted abnormalities include growth retardation, microcephaly, facial anomalies, minor limb defects, and developmental delay.

Toluene has also been implicated as a teratogen in a limited number of occupational epidemiological investigations. One large Canadian case-control study found a significant excess of major birth defects among infants whose mothers were occupationally exposed to aromatic solvents in the first trimester; most of the excess was associated with toluene exposure, although the severity of exposure was not considered in this analysis (56). Recently, Taskinen et al. (57) conducted a case-control study to evaluate the risk of fetal loss among the wives of men occupationally exposed to organic solvents. Finnish registry data were used to identify pregnancy outcomes, and organic solvent exposures were assessed through personal biological monitoring and questionnaires. After controlling for maternal age and alcohol consumption and smoking by either spouse, the risk of spontaneous abortion was significantly increased with paternal "high or frequent" exposure to organic solvents in general (OR 2.8, CI 1.2–5.9) and to toluene in particular (OR 2.3, CI 1.1–4.7).

It is important that art hobbyists take precautions to avoid excessive exposure to the toxic ingredients in paint-related products. Because significant exposure to toxic pigment powders can occur if artists mix their own paints, use of premixed paint formulations is safer. In addition, hobbyists should avoid use of paints containing lead, cadmium, chromium, or other toxic metals. Brush painting is preferable to spray or air-brush techniques that generate hazardous mists. Products containing toxic organic solvents should be avoided or used only with adequate ventilation and personal protective clothing. In general, painting with watercolors or acrylic or tempera paints is safer than oil painting or use of epoxy paints.

## Screen Printing

Screen printing is a modern stencil-based printmaking technique used to produce multicolored textile or poster designs. The process involves squeezing ink through a framed piece of fine-meshed fabric that contains a stenciled design and that is in contact with the material being printed. Stencils are made by cutting designs into stencil films; by blocking out designs with glues, waxes, shellac, or solvent-based lacquers; or by using photochemical techniques. The inks used in screen printing contain many of the same pigments found in oil paints. Aromatic and aliphatic hydrocarbon solvents are commonly used as ink media, thinners, or modifiers. In addition, various organic solvents may be used to clean blockout materials or inks from the screens.

Exposure to pigment dust is usually not of concern with screen printing because most hobbyists use preprepared inks. Water-based inks are generally preferable to those containing organic solvents. (Ingredients should be carefully checked because some water-based inks also contain organic solvents.) Cleaning ink from the screens with solvent-soaked newspapers and rags is probably the most hazardous step in screen printing, and stringent control measures are necessary to minimize exposure (49).

## Ceramics

Ceramics is a form of pottery-making that typically involves the application of glazes. The fundamental building block of ceramic art is clay that is composed of silica, alumina, oxygen, and lesser amounts of other elements (58).

A ceramic piece is usually finished by applying a glaze that, when fired, creates a durable surface tightly bonded to the clay body. Glazes are composed of clay, colorants, color modifi-

ers, and fluxes that alter the melting properties of silica. Colorants added to glazes include titanium, chromium, cadmium, copper, cobalt, lead, manganese, and other toxic metals. Traditionally used by ceramists, lead fluxes are still present in many commercial glazes. Other fluxes include bone ash (calcium, phosphorus); boron; tin or zinc oxide; and barium, lithium, or magnesium carbonates (58). Fluxes are generally present in glazes in much higher concentrations than colorants.

In the past, ceramists prepared their own glazes by grinding the raw materials; this process produced toxic dusts, and lead poisoning was common among potters. Today, glaze materials can be purchased preground, although exposure by inhalation or ingestion can still occur when handling and weighing the dry glaze powders. In most commercial leaded glazes, lead frits (lead compounded with other materials into a type of ground glass) have replaced raw lead compounds. However, significant lead exposure can still occur during glaze preparation and application. Lead-glazed pottery should never be used as containers for food or drinking liquids; lead may be released from the glazes, especially by acidic substances (49).

Firing clay can result in release of carbon monoxide or sulfur dioxide gas. Depending on the temperatures required for firing and the glazes used, glaze firing can produce toxic chlorine, flourine, and nitrogen gases. In addition, glaze metals may volatilize during firing, creating toxic metal fumes. Lead is not used in stoneware glazes, since the high firing temperatures required volatilize lead oxide (49).

Ceramic hobbyists must take stringent precautions to avoid the potential hazards of their art. Glazes free of lead, chromium, and other toxic metals should be used whenever possible. In all cases, the ceramist should handle dry glaze powders in a fume hood or wear a NIOSH-approved respirator designed to protect against toxic dusts and mists. Dust particles that contaminate floors or work surfaces should be wet-mopped rather than swept. Glaze spraying is most safely performed in an efficiently ventilated spray booth. Finally, inside kilns must be exhaust ventilated to prevent exposure to toxic fumes and gases (49, 58).

## Stained Glass

The colored glass used in this craft is manufactured in the factory. Silica sand is mixed with pigments (metallic oxides), heated, and formed into sheets. In the hands of the craftsperson, the glass is cut into various pieces that are connected by lead came (channeled lead strips) or copper foil and soldered. Techniques to decorate the glass include painting, enameling, or etching with hydrofluoric acid (59).

In terms of reproductive effects, the most hazardous steps in stained glass work involve manipulation of the lead came and soldering. Cutting or sanding the came produces fine lead dust that can be inhaled or ingested. During soldering, strips of lead came or copper foil are joined, not directly, but through the use of a solder material that melts at a lower temperature than the metals to be connected. The solder traditionally used in stained glass work is an alloy composed of 60% tin and 40% lead. Toxic lead fumes may be generated by soldering, and contamination of work surfaces with solder residues creates an ingestion hazard.

Paints or enamels may be applied to the glass and fired in a kiln. Like ceramic glazes, these materials often contain metallic oxides (commonly lead) that impart color upon heating, and their preparation and firing present similar hazards. Exposure to solvents can occur when cleaning stained glass or when using epoxy adhesives to glue slab glass into decorative or architectural pieces (49).

Stained glass work involving lead came or lead-containing solder should not be performed in the preconception period or during pregnancy or nursing. In place of lead came, zinc and other metals are used by some hobbyists. Lead-free solders are also available, although they are not as easy to use as the traditional lead-tin alloy (51).

## Photography

Photography is one of the most popular hobbies in the U.S., and many hobbyists process their film in home darkrooms. While the techniques involved in black and white and color photographic processing differ somewhat, they both employ a wide variety of chemicals. In addition, many photographic processes have been adapted for printmaking uses including photolithography, photoetching, and photo silkscreening (51).

Black and white film is coated with an emulsion consisting of a suspension of silver halide in gelatin. Exposure to light creates a latent image in the emulsion that is converted into a visible image during the development process. In the darkroom, the film is first immersed in a chemical developing bath that reduces the exposed silver halide to metallic silver. Common developers include hydroquinone ($p$-dihydroxybenzene), $p$-aminophenol compounds, and phenidone. The bath also contains preservatives (sodium bisulfite or potassium metabisulfite) to prevent the combination of the developer with oxygen, accelerators to maintain proper pH, and restrainers or antifogging agents (e.g., bromide salts) that prevent the developer from reducing unexposed silver grains. The film is next immersed in a stop bath of acetic acid solution that halts the silver halide reduction, followed by a fixer (hypo or sodium thiosulfate) that forms a soluble complex with the unexposed silver halide grains. After washing with a hypo eliminator to remove the fixing chemicals, the negative is hung to dry (60).

Aftertreatment of negatives includes intensification to increase the density of the image or reduction to lighten the image by selective removal of silver. Dichromate salt solutions are commonly used in intensification. Reduction is usually accomplished with a solution of hypo and potassium ferricyanide (49).

In the making of a print or positive, the image on the negative is transferred to sensitized paper by exposure to a printing light. The prints are then developed in a manner similar to the processing of negatives. Toning is an aftertreatment process that alters the image color by replacing silver with brown silver sulfide or other metals such as gold, selenium, uranium, or iron. Negatives and prints may be cleaned with products containing 1,1,1,trichloroethane, freons, or other organic solvents (49).

While similar in some ways to black and white developing, color processing is more complex and involves potential exposure to a wider range of toxic chemicals. Instead of one silver halide layer, color film consists of three superimposed layers of emulsion sensitive to blue, green, and red, respectively. On contact with color developing agents, the exposed silver halide is reduced, and the oxidized developer reacts with the specific coupler in each layer to form the dye image. Color developing solutions may contain phenylenediamine derivatives and a number of organic solvents. (Ethylene glycol ethers were removed from film developing solutions in the early 1980s but may still be found in products used for photoetching.) Color processing also requires use of a "bleach" or strong oxidizing agent (e.g., ferric EDTA, cyanide or bromide salts) to remove the black silver image and render the color image visible. Other important steps involve hardeners and stabilizers (e.g., formalin) to reduce the fading of the dye image (60).

No studies have specifically examined reproductive or pregnancy outcomes among workers or hobbyists engaged in photoprocessing. However, some of the chemicals involved are of concern and warrant measures to mitigate exposure. In one case report, excessive maternal exposure to bromide salts in a photographic laboratory caused neonatal bromism, characterized by hypotonia and general central nervous system (CNS) depression (61). As explained in Chapter 19, significant occupational exposure to a combination of organic solvents has been associated in some epidemiological studies with adverse pregnancy outcomes. Aftertreatment techniques can expose photographers to toxic metals such as mercury or uranium. Asphyxiant gases are released if cyanide, sulfide, or selenium salts are mixed with acid, and chronic exposure to the color restrainer, hydroxylamine hydrochloride, can cause methemoglobinemia. Finally, some photoprocessing chemicals are suspected mutagens, such as the substituted $p$-phenylenediamine compounds used as color developers and formaldehyde used as a hardener or stabilizer in fixing baths.

In the preconception period and during pregnancy, hobbyists should either refrain from color photoprocessing and aftertreatments such as intensification and toning or use stringent control measures to minimize exposures. Simple black and white photographs can be processed safely if basic precautions are taken. Premixed solutions should be used whenever possible; if it is necessary to weigh and mix photoprocessing chemicals, a NIOSH-certified dust respirator, rubber gloves, and goggles are recommended. Direct skin contact can be avoided through the use of tongs to immerse and remove film from chemical baths. Adequate ventilation is extremely important. Kodak recommends 10 room-air changes per hour for simple black and white processing, or a minimum of 170 cubic feet per minute (cfm) (49). Local exhaust systems are advisable for mixing photochemicals and for color processing and aftertreatments. Finally, the chemical baths should be covered when not in use, and housekeeping should be maintained to avoid accidents and spills.

## Summary

This review of selected arts and crafts hobbies illustrates the importance of including questions about home hobbies in the exposure history of each patient. Information about specific product ingredients can be obtained by calling the manufacturer or a poison control center or by obtaining Material Safety Data Sheets (MSDSs) from manufacturers or retail stores. In addition, the recent Labeling of Hazardous Art Materials Act specifically requires that labels for arts and crafts materials identify ingredients causing chronic hazards, including reproductive effects (62). More information about hazards in the arts and ways to minimize exposures can be obtained from the Center for Safety in the Arts (212–227–6220) or Arts, Crafts, and Theater Safety (212–777–0062).

## HOME RENOVATIONS

Clinicians who care for pregnant patients know that anticipation of childbirth often prompts home renovations, the most common of which is painting the nursery. Potentially hazardous exposures can occur both with removal of existing household paint and with repainting.

### Removal of Old Paint

In the 1970s, efforts to address the problem of childhood lead poisoning included major federal legislation to reduce lead paint exposure in the home (63). The Lead-Based Paint Poisoning Prevention Act of 1971 prohibited the use of leaded paint in residential structures built or rehabilitated by the federal government or with federal assistance and mandated procedures for lead paint abatement in existing public or federally assisted housing stock. In 1977, a regulation by the Consumer Product Safety Commission (CPSC) established a maximum permissible lead content in household paints of 0.06% (600 parts per million lead by dry weight).

Despite these initiatives, toxicity from residential lead paint exposure remains a significant public health problem. An estimated 42 million dwellings in the U.S. still contain lead-based paint (64). While housing built before 1977 is, by far, the dominant source of lead paint exposure, newer residences are not completely exempt. With rare exception, all patients considering home renovations should assume a lead paint problem until proven otherwise.

As explained in Chapter 17, federal authorities have recently reduced the blood lead level of concern to 10 μg/dl (65). Removal of lead-based paint by scraping, sanding, or heating can result in dramatic increases in lead body burden through absorption of dust or fumes. Both deleaders and home occupants are at risk. There are a number of case reports of lead poisoning in adults involved in home lead paint removal (66, 67). Rabinowitz et al. (68, 69) found that recent home refinishing activity was a significant predictor of children's blood lead levels. Other investigators report significant increases in children's blood lead concentrations following residential lead paint abatement, even if children were removed from the home during the deleading process (70, 71). Modified abatement practices, including improved clean-up and repeated dust removal, are more effective than traditional methods (72, 73).

Before initiating home renovations, residential paint should be tested for lead. While home test kits are available, they have not been evaluated by the CPSC and are not as accurate as other methods. Alternatives include in-home testing by trained professionals using x-ray fluorescence or sending paint samples to a qualified laboratory for analysis. Clinicians and patients can contact their local departments of public health for more information on testing and abatement.

Abatement may involve replacing items such as leaded doors; paint removal; or covering leaded surfaces with sealants, wallboard, fiberglass cloth barriers, or durable wallpaper. Lead paint removal should be performed only by licensed deleaders, and home occupants should relocate until certified inspectors designate the removal and clean-up as adequate. Simply repainting leaded surfaces is not sufficient (74). If the history identifies recent home refinishing or lead abatement, clinicians should monitor blood lead levels in all family members.

## Repainting

### ARCHITECTURAL PAINT CONSTITUENTS

Paints used for architectural coatings are broadly classified as interior or exterior paints, each of which includes latex (water-thinned) and solvent-based formulations. The majority of paints marketed for household use are latex paints (75). These products are commonly based on emulsions of polyvinyl acetate or acrylic resins; the polymerization reactions that form these synthetic resins occur within water droplets, creating water-soluble polymers that become insoluble after drying (76). Organic solvents are added in limited quantity to latex paints to improve the performance properties of the paint film. The most common organic solvents found in latex paints are glycol ethers. Fortunately, most manufacturers have substituted the toxic ethylene glycol ethers with the less hazardous propylene series. Oil-based wall paints, as well as enamels used on floors and trim, contain an alkyd resin or oil varnish and are commonly thinned with mineral spirits (34).

The pigments used in architectural paints are almost exclusively metal-based inorganic pigments. White or pale pastel paints typically contain titanium compounds that are replaced by a variety of other metals such as zinc, aluminum, or iron to create deeper colors (34). As discussed above, household paints manufactured after 1977 cannot lawfully contain significant amounts of lead; in addition, the use of other toxic metals, such as cadmium or chrome, has been significantly curtailed. Mineral fillers and extenders, often made from crystalline quartz, are used to modify the color, body, and luster of paints (76).

Biocides, including formaldehyde releasers and other antimicrobial agents, are added to paints for in-can preservation. For years, mercury compounds were also used for this purpose. However, in 1989, a case of childhood mercury poisoning was reported following in-home application of 17 gallons of latex paint. Release of mercury vapors from phenylmercuric acetate in the paint was identified as the probable source of exposure (77). Subsequently, the EPA prohibited the addition of mercury to interior latex paints manufactured after August 20, 1990.

## POTENTIAL REPRODUCTIVE AND DEVELOPMENTAL EFFECTS

Many of the hazardous ingredients found in industrial and art paints have been removed from products intended for household use. In addition, methods of preparation and application differ. For example, unlike paint production workers and some artists, users of architectural paints do not handle and mix dry pigments. Spray painting is a common mode of application in the workplace but is unusual among home renovators. The pigments and other fillers in contemporary household paints probably do not pose a health hazard to the home renovator when brushed or rolled onto surfaces (78).

No studies have specifically assessed reproductive or developmental health risks associated with painting during home renovations. Inferences must, therefore, be made from data on specific constituents of architectural paints and on occupational cohorts exposed to paint products.

The additives of greatest concern in household paints include organic solvents and biocides. Although inorganic mercury was removed from latex paints manufactured after August 1990, use of older paints may still provide a source of exposure to this toxicant.

While organic methyl mercury is a known human teratogen, the developmental effects of

the elemental or inorganic forms have not been extensively investigated. Experimental animal studies indicate that mercury vapor crosses the placenta, especially during the latter part of gestation, and is oxidized in fetal tissues to inorganic mercury. On the other hand, mercuric ions and phenylmercury (rapidly converted to mercuric ions in maternal tissues) accumulate in the placenta, but only small amounts enter the fetal circulation (79). Mercury selectively concentrates in the ovary and testis and has been associated with ovulatory dysfunction, with lengthening of the estrus cycle, and with altered spermatogenesis in animals (80, 81).

A few epidemiological studies have reported menstrual disturbances in women occupationally exposed to mercury vapor (82, 83). While loss of libido has been reported in male workers acutely poisoned by exposure to metallic mercury vapor, most epidemiological studies reveal no effects on fertility or birth outcomes (84–86). In one recent study of male workers at a chloralkali plant, a dose-response relationship was found between the average concentrations of mercury in the workers' urine before conception and rates of self-reported spontaneous abortion among their wives ($p = 0.07$)(87).

While organic solvents can be found in all paints, their concentration is considerably less in latex products than in oil-based formulations. Exposure to a variety of organic solvents can also occur with use of varnishes, lacquers, thinners, and cleaners.

A few of the epidemiological studies of solvent exposure and pregnancy outcome have specifically considered painting as an occupation. In a historical cohort study from the Danish county of Funen (88), reproductive life histories were collected by questionnaire from women in selected occupations, including 76 trade union painters. Shop assistants and vegetable warehouse workers comprised the "less exposed" comparison group. After controlling for gravidity, pregnancy order, and age, the job of painter was associated with an increased risk for self-reported spontaneous abortion (OR 2.9, CI 1.0–8.8). When only hospital-registered miscarriages were considered, the risk estimate decreased and was nonsignificant (OR 1.4, CI 0.4–2.5).

Another study from the same Danish county

evaluated the relationship between parental occupational organic solvent exposure and birth defects in offspring (89). Computerized registry data were used to identify cases of infants with malformations of the (CNS), intestinal canal, or extremities and a control group of infants with other nonteratogenic congenital conditions. Parental occupational titles from birth certificates were categorized into occupational codes, one of which included "painter, decorator, or automobile paint shop worker." None of the mothers in the study was employed in this category. Paternal occupation as painter was associated with a significantly increased risk of fathering a child with a CNS malformation (OR 4.9, CI 1.4–17.1). However, multiple comparisons were made in this study, making it likely that some associations occurred by chance.

In a U.S. retrospective cohort study, Daniell and Vaughan (90) examined Washington State birth certificates for associations between pregnancy outcomes (low birthweight, preterm birth, infant sex ratio, Apgar scores, and fetal loss in last pregnancy) and paternal employment in solvent-related occupations. After adjusting for several important confounders, a significant association was found between low birthweight in infants delivered after 37 weeks' gestation and paternal employment as autobody painter relative to a general control group (RR 1.6, CI 1.1–2.4). No excess risks were found among the solvent-exposed cohorts for any other pregnancy outcome. Again, multiple comparisons were made in this study.

In 1974, Fabia and Thuy (91) reported a two-fold excess risk of cancer death among preschool-aged children whose fathers were employed in hydrocarbon-related occupations at the time of birth. Most of the excess risk was attributed to painters, automobile mechanics, machinists, and miners. Since then, over 20 epidemiological studies have explored the association between parental employment in jobs involving exposure to hydrocarbon solvents and the risk of total or specific childhood cancers. These studies have important methodological limitations that are reviewed in Chapter 7 and elsewhere (92–95).

Many of the childhood cancer studies have considered parental painting occupations, usually as part of a broader job category involving potential hydrocarbon exposure. Because few women are employed as architectural or industrial painters, the majority of studies have focused on paternal occupation. Even in these investigations, the number of subjects employed as painters is small. In general, studies of total childhood cancer risk among offspring of fathers employed in broad occupational categories have yielded little conclusive information. Evidence suggesting that paternal exposure to hydrocarbons increases the risk of specific cancers in children (leukemia, brain cancer, Wilms tumor) is stronger, but still contradictory. Certainly, however, the findings warrant reasonable caution and continued research.

## Summary and Recommendations

Home refinishing activities frequently involve removal of old, potentially lead-based paint and the use of paint-related products containing organic solvents and biocides. While the hazards of lead paint removal are well established, data regarding in-home use of paint and paint products are extremely limited. Some epidemiological studies indicate that chronic high-dose recreational or occupational exposure to organic solvents can increase the risk of adverse pregnancy outcomes, including birth defects. Preliminary evidence also suggests an association between parental exposure to hydrocarbons on the job and the occurrence of specific types of childhood cancer. However, compared to home refinishing, painting as an occupation is more likely to involve exposure to solvent-based product formulations at doses that are higher and occur more frequently. The implications of occupational studies for the home renovator are, therefore, uncertain.

Optimally, home renovations should be completed before conception occurs. If this is not feasible, it is preferable that the pregnant woman refrain from the more hazardous refinishing activities (93). In all cases, the following recommendations are important to follow. First, old paint should not be removed until it is tested and determined to be lead-free. Leaded paint in the home warrants contact with public health officials to determine appropriate abatement measures and biological testing of family members for lead. Under no circumstances should removal of lead-based paint be undertaken by household members! Second, renovators should obtain MSDSs from retailers or manufacturers for all products they intend to use. Latex paints containing ethylene glycol ethers, mercury, or formaldehyde-releasing biocides should be avoided. Finally, use of ancillary paint products containing ethylene glycol ethers or hydrocarbon solvents should be minimized or used with extreme caution. Protective measures include effective ventilation (use outside if possible) and wearing of personal protective equipment, including gloves and NIOSH-approved organic vapor respirators for prolonged or high-dose exposures. Respirators should be fit-tested by occupational medicine specialists. With a well-functioning and fitted respirator, the wearer should not be able to smell solvent odors. If odors are detectable, either the respirator does not fit properly or the organic vapor cartridge needs replacement.

## ACKNOWLEDGMENTS

My sincere appreciation to Drs. David Savitz, Anthony Scialli, and Michael McCann for their thoughtful commentaries on this chapter.

## REFERENCES

1. Wallace LA, Pellizzari ED, Hartwell TD, et al. The TEAM Study: personal exposure to toxic substances in air, drinking water, and breath of 400 residents of New Jersey, North Carolina, and North Dakota. Environ Res 1987;43:290–307.
2. Wallace LA, Pellizzari E, Hartwell T, et al. The California TEAM study: concentrations and personal exposures to 26 volatile organic compounds in air and drinking water of 188 residents of Los Angeles, Antioch, and Pittsburg, CA. Atmos Environ 1988;22:2141–2163.
3. Wallace LA, Pellizzari ED, Hartwell TD, Davis V, Michael LC, Whitmore RW. The influence of personal activities on exposure to volatile organic compounds. Environ Res 1989;50:37–55.
4. Florig HK, Hoburg JF. Power frequency magnetic fields from electric blankets. Health Phys 1990;4:493–502.
5. Preston-Martin S, Peters JM, Yu MC, Garabrant DH, Bowman JD. Myelogenous leukemia and electric blanket use. Bioelectromagnetics 1988;9:207–213.
6. U.S. Congress, Office of Technology Assessment. Biological effects of power frequency electric and magnetic fields—background paper, OTA-BP-E-52. Washington, DC: U.S. Government Printing Office, 1989.
7. Wertheimer N, Leeper E. Adult cancer related to electrical wires near the home. Int J Epidemiol 1982;11:345–355.
8. Tenforde TS, Kaune WT. Interaction of extremely low frequency electric and magnetic fields with humans. Health Phys 1987;53:585–606.
9. Juutilainen J. Effects of low frequency magnetic fields on embryonic development and pregnancy. Scand J Work Environ Health 1991;17:149–158.
10. Wilson BW, Chess EK, Anderson LE. 60-Hz electric field effects on pineal melatonin rhythms: time course for onset and recovery. Bioelectromagnetics 1986;7:239–242.
11. Wertheimer N, Leeper E. Possible effects of electric blankets and heated waterbeds on fetal development. Bioelectromagnetics 1986;7:13–22.
12. Wertheimer N, Leeper E. Fetal loss associated with two seasonal sources of electromagnetic field exposure. Am J Epidemiol 1989;129:220–224.
13. Savitz DA, John EM, Kleckner RC. Magnetic field exposure from electric appliances and childhood cancer. Am J Epidemiol 1990;131:763–773.
14. Verreault R, Weiss NS, Hollenbach KA, Strader CH, Daling JR. Use of electric blankets and risk of testicular cancer. Am J Epidemiol 1990;131:759–762.
15. Cohen MM, Kunska A, Astemborski JA, McCulloch D, Paskewitz DA. Effects of low-level 60-Hz electromagnetic fields on human lymphoid cells. I. Mitotic rate and chromosomal breakage in human peripheral lymphocytes. Bioelectromagnetics 1986;7:415–423.
16. Reese JA, Jostes RF, Frazier ME. Exposure of mammalian cells to 60-Hz magnetic or electric fields: analysis for DNA single-strand breaks. Bioelectromagnetics 1988;9:237–247.
17. U.S. Food and Drug Administration (FDA), Center for Devices and Radiological Health. TEPRSSC discusses fluoroscopy, mercury vapor lamps, and ELF fields and electric blankets. In: FDA. Radiol Health Bull 1990;24(12):24:1–3.
18. National Council on Radiation Protection and Measurements. Ionizing radiation exposures of the population of the United States, report no. 93. Washington, DC: National Council on Radiation Protection and Measurements, 1987.
19. Hart BL, Mettler FA, Harley NH. Radon: is it a problem? Radiology 1989;172:593–599.
20. Dundulis W, Bell W, Kenne B, Dostie P. Radon-222 in the gastrointestinal tract: a proposed modification of the ICRP publication 30 model. Health Phys 1984;47:243–252.
21. Hursh J, Morken D, Davis T, Lovaas A. The fate of radon ingested by man. Health Phys 1965;11:465–476.
22. Fry F, Smith-Briggs J, O'Riordan M. Skeletal lead-210 as an index of exposure to radon decay products in mining. Br J Ind Med 1983;40:58–60.
23. Clemente G, Renzetti A, Santori G, et al. Relationship between the 210 Pb content of teeth and exposure to Rn and Rn daughters. Health Phys 1984;47:253–262.
24. U.S. Department of Health and Human Services, Agency for Toxic Substances and Disease Registry. Toxicological profile for radon. Bethesda, MD: Agency for Toxic Substances and Disease Registry, 1990.

25. Nussbaum E, Hursh J. Radon solubility in rat tissue. Science 1957;125:552–553.

26. Pohl E. Dose distribution received on inhalation of Ra 222 and its decay products. In: International Atomic Energy Agency (IAEA). Radiological health and safety in mining and milling of nuclear materials, vol 1. Vienna: IAEA, 1964:221–236.

27. Alter H, Oswald R. Nationwide distribution of indoor radon measurements: a preliminary database. J Air Pollut Control Assoc 1987;37:227–231.

28. Nero A, Schwehr M, Nazaroff W, et al. Distribution of airborne radon-222 concentrations in U.S. homes. Science 1986;234:922–997.

29. Cothern C, Lappenbusch W, Michel J. Drinking-water contribution to natural background radiation. Health Phys 1986;50:33–47.

30. Axelsson O, Edling C, Kling H. Lung cancer and residency—a case-referent study on the possible impact of exposure to radon and its daughters in dwellings. Scand J Work Environ Health 1979;5:10–15.

31. Svensson C, Pershagen C, Klominek J. Lung cancer in women and type of dwelling in relation to radon exposure. Cancer Res 1989;49:1861–1965.

32. U.S. Environmental Protection Agency. A citizen's guide to radon: what it is and what to do about it. Washington, DC: U.S. Government Printing Office, 1986.

33. Marks JG Jr. Occupational skin disease in hairdressers. In Adams RM, ed. Occupational medicine, state of the art reviews: occupational skin diseases. Philadelphia: Hanley and Belfus, 1986:273–284.

34. Gosselin RE, Smith RP, Hodge HC. Clinical toxicology of commercial products. 5th edition. Baltimore: Williams & Wilkins, 1984.

35. Bronaugh RL, Congdon ER. Percutaneous absorption of hair dyes: correlation with partition coefficients. J Invest Dermatol 1984;83:124–127.

36. Ames BN, Kammen HO, Yamasaki E. Hair dyes are mutagenic: identification of a variety of mutagenic ingredients. Proc Natl Acad Sci 1975;72:2423–2427.

37. Ferguson LR, Robertson AM, Berriman J. Direct-acting mutagenic properties of some hair dyes used in New Zealand. Mutat Res 1990;245:41–46.

38. Kirkland DJ, Venitt S. Cytotoxicity of hair colorant constituents: chromosomal damage induced by two nitrophenylenediamines in cultured chinese hamster cells. Mutat Res 1976,40:47–56.

39. DiNardo JC, Picciano JC, Schnetzinger RW, Morris WE, Wolf BA. Teratological assessment of five oxidative hair dyes in the rat. Toxicol Appl Pharmacol 1985;78:163–166.

40. Indouye M, Murakami U. Teratogenicity of 2,5-diaminotoluene, a hair dye component, in mice. Teratology 1976;14:241–242.

41. Marks TA, Gupta BN, Ledoux TA, Staples RE. Teratogenic evaluation of 2-nitro-p-phenylenediamine, 4-nitro-o-phenylenediamine, and 2,5-toluenediamine sulfate in the mouse. Teratology 1981;24:253–265.

42. Green A, Willett WC, Colditz GA, et al. Use of permanent hair dyes and risk of breast cancer. J Natl Cancer Inst 1987;79:253–257.

43. Hartge P, Hoover R, Altman R, et al. Use of hair dyes and risk of bladder cancer. Cancer Res 1982;4784–4787.

44. Wickett RR, Wisconsin R. Permanent waving and straightening of hair. Cutis 1987;39:496–497.

45. Koren G, Bologa M. Teratogenic risk of hair care products. JAMA 1989;262:2925.

46. Dadd DL. Nontoxic, natural, and earthwise: how to protect yourself and your family from harmful products and live in harmony with the earth. Los Angeles: Jeremy P Tarcher, Inc, 1990.

47. Associated Councils on the Arts. Americans and the arts: a survey of public opinion. New York: Associated Councils on the Arts, 1975:23.

48. McCann M, Hall N, Klarnett R, Plotz P. Reproductive hazards in the arts and crafts. Presented at the Annual Meeting of Society for Occupational and Environmental Health, Bethesda, MD, April 29, 1986.

49. McCann M. Artists beware. New York: Watson-Guptill, 1979.

50. McCann M. Health hazards manual for artists. 3rd edition. New York: Nick Lyons Books, 1985.

51. Rossol M. The artist's complete health and safety guide. New York: Allworth Press, 1990.

52. Mayer R. The artist's handbook of materials and techniques. 5th edition. New York: Viking Penguin, 1991.

53. Hersh JH, Podruch PE, Rogers G, Weisskopf B. Toluene embryopathy. J Pediatr 1985;106:922–927.

54. Goodwin TM. Toluene abuse and renal tubular acidosis in pregnancy. Obstet Gynecol 1988;71:715–718.

55. Wilkins-Haug L, Gabow PA. Toluene abuse during pregnancy: obstetric complications and perinatal outcomes. Obstet Gynecol 1991;77:504–509.

56. McDonald JC, Lavoie J, Cote R, McDonald AD. Chemical exposures at work in early pregnancy and congenital defect: a case-referent study. Br J Ind Med 1987;44:527–533.

57. Taskinen H, Anttila A, Lindhohm ML, Sallmen M, Hemminki K. Spontaneous abortions and congenital malformations among the wives of men occupationally exposed to organic solvents. Scand J Work Environ Health 1989;15:345–352.

58. Zakin R. Ceramics: mastering the craft. Radnor, PA: Chilton Book Co., 1990.

59. Isenberg A, Isenberg S. How to work in stained glass. 2nd edition. Radnor, PA: Chilton Book Co., 1983.

60. U.S. Environmental Protection Agency (EPA), Office of Research and Development. Guides to pollution prevention: the photoprocessing industry. EPA/625/7–91/012. Cincinnati: U.S. EPA, 1991.

61. Mangurten HH, Kaye CI. Neonatal bromism secondary to maternal exposure in a photographic laboratory. J Pediatr 1982;100:596–598.

62. U.S. Consumer Product Safety Commission. Consumer product safety alert: CPSC promotes safety labeling for art and craft materials. Washington, DC: Consumer Product Safety Commission, 1990.

63. Mushak P, Crocetti AF. Methods for reducing lead exposure in young children and other risk groups: an integrated summary of a report to the U.S. Congress on childhood lead poisoning. Environ Health Perspect 1990;89:125–135.

64. Agency for Toxic Substances and Disease Registry (ATSDR). The nature and extent of lead poisoning in the United States: a report to Congress. Atlanta: U.S. Public Health Service, ATSDR, 1988.

65. Clean Air Scientific Advisory Committee/Science Advisory Board, U.S. Environmental Protection Agency. Report of the Clean Air Scientific Advisory Committee (CASAC): review of the OAQPS lead staff paper and the ECAO air quality criteria document supplement, report no. EPA-SAB-CASAC-90-002. Washington, DC: U.S. Environmental Protection Agency, 1990.

66. Fischbein A, Anderson KE, Sassa S, et al. Lead poisoning from "do-it-yourself" heat guns for removing lead based paint: report of two cases. Environ Res 1981;24:425–431.

67. Schneitzer L, Osborn H, Bierman A, Mezey A, Kaul B. Lead poisoning in adults from renovation of an older home. Ann Emerg Med 1990;19:415–420.

68. Rabinowitz M, Leviton A, Bellinger D. Home refinishing activity, lead paint, and infant blood levels. Am J Public Health 1985;75:403–404.

69. Bellinger D, Leviton A, Rabinowitz M, Needleman H, Waternaux C. Correlates of low-level lead exposure in urban children at two years of age. Pediatrics 1986;77:826–833.

70. Amitar Y, Graef JW, Brown MJ, Gerstle RS, Kahn N, Cochrane PE. Hazards of deleading homes of children with lead poisoning. Am J Dis Child 1987;141:758–760.

71. Chisolm JJ Jr, Mellits ED, Quaskey SA. The relationship between the level of lead absorption in children and the age, type, and condition of housing. Environ Res 1985;38:31–45.

72. Charney E, Kessler B, Farfel M, Jackson D. Childhood lead poisoning. A controlled trial of the effect of dust-control measures in blood lead levels. N Engl J Med 1983;309:1089–1093.

73. Farfel MR, Chisolm JJ Jr. Health and environmental outcomes of traditional and modified practices for abatement of residential lead-based paint. Am J Public Health 1990;80:1240–1245.

74. U.S. Consumer Product Safety Commission. Consumer product safety alert: what you should know about lead-based paint in your home. Washington, DC: U.S. Consumer Product Safety Commission, 1990.

75. U.S. Environmental Protection Agency. Guides to pollution prevention: the paint manufacturing industry, EPA/625/7-90/005. Cincinnati: Center for Environmental Reasearch Information, 1990:5.

76. Burgess WA. Recognition of health hazards in industry: a review of materials and processes. New York: John Wiley & Sons, 1981:101–107.

77. Centers for Disease Control. Mercury exposure from interior latex paint—Michigan. MMWR 1990;39:125–126.

78. Hansen MK, Larsen M, Karl-Heinz C. Waterborne paints: a review of their chemistry and toxicology and the results of determinations made during their use. Scand J Work Environ Health 1987;13:473–485.

79. Dencker L. Disposition of metals in the embryo and fetus. In: Clarkson TW, Nordberg GF, Sager PR, eds. Reproductive and developmental toxicity of metals. New York: Plenum Press, 1983:607–631.

80. Lee IP. Effects of environmental metals on male reproduction. In: Clarkson TW, Nordberg GF, Sager PR, eds. Reproductive and developmental toxicity of metals. New York: Plenum Press, 1983:253–278.

81. Mattison DR. Ovarian toxicity: effects on sexual maturation, reproduction and menopause. In: Clarkson TW, Nordberg GF, Sager PR, eds. Reproductive and developmental toxicity of metals. New York: Plenum Press, 1983:317–342.

82. DeRosis F, Anastasio SP, Selvaggi L, Beltrame A, Moriani G. Female reproductive health in two lamp factories: effects of exposure to inorganic mercury vapour and stress factors. Br J Ind Med 1985;42:488–494.

83. Sikorski R, Juszkiewicz T, Paszkowski T, Szprengier-Juszkiewicz T. Women in dental surgeries: reproductive hazards in occupational exposure to metallic mercury. Int Arch Occup Environ Health 1987;59:551–557.

84. Lauwerys R, Roels H, Genet P, Toussaint G, Bouckaert A, DeCooman S. Fertility of male workers exposed to mercury vapor or to manganese dust: a questionnaire study. Am J Ind Med 1985;7:171–176.

85. Brodsky JB, Cohen EN, Witcher C, Brown BW, Wu ML. Occupational exposure to mercury in dentistry and pregnancy outcome. J Am Dent Assoc 1985;111:779–780.

86. Alcser KH, Brix KA, Fine LJ, Kallenbach LR, Wolfe RA. Occupational mercury exposure and male reproductive health. Am J Ind Med 1989;15:517–529.

87. Cordier S, Deplan F, Mandereau L, Hemon D. Paternal exposure to mercury and spontaneous abortions. Br J Ind Med 1991;48:375–381.

88. Heidam LZ. Spontaneous abortions among dental assistants, factory workers, painters, and gardening workers: a follow up study. J Epidemiol Comm Health 1984;38:149–155.

89. Olsen J. Risk of exposure to teratogens amongst laboratory staff and painters. Dan Med Bull 1983;30:24–28.

90. Daniell WE, Vaughn TL. Paternal employment in solvent related occupations and adverse pregnancy outcomes. Br J Ind Med 1988;45:193–197.

91. Fabia J, Thuy TD. Occupation of father at time of birth of children dying of malignant diseases. Br J Prevent Soc Med 1974;28:98–100.

92. Arundel SE, Kinnier-Wilson LM. Parental occupations and cancer: a review of the literature. J Epidemiol Comm Health 1986;40:30–36.

93. Scialli AR. Who should paint the nursery? Reprod Toxicol 1989;3:159–164.

94. Savitz DA, Chen J. Parental occupation and childhood cancer: review of epidemiologic studies. Environ Health Perspect 1990;88:325–337.

95. O'Leary LM, Hicks AM, Peters JM, London S. Parental occupational exposures and risk of childhood cancer: a review. Am J Ind Med 1991;20:17–35.

# Community Exposure to Toxic Substances

DAVID OZONOFF, ANN ASCHENGRAU

Perception and personal management of risk do not proceed by some neutral risk-benefit calculus, but inevitably involve community and cultural values. To most people, there is something intrinsically different about risks that are imposed from without and those that they choose, for whatever reasons, to accept for themselves. Such value considerations also account for the exquisite sensitivity of community residents to a suspected environmental threat to their health; here, the outrage that normally accompanies imposed risks is combined with a spontaneous impulse to protect dependents and offspring.

The perception of environmental threat usually arises in one of three forms (1):

(a) Exposure-driven situations. These situations occur when it is discovered or suspected that individuals have been exposed to an environmental hazard by virtue of their residence in a community. Here, the main concern is the consequence of the exposure for the health of these individuals or their families at some time in the future. They want to know, "What will happen to us?"

(b) Outcome-driven situations. An apparent cluster of disease occurrences often raises suspicion about environmental factors. A search for an environmental cause may be initiated, as the victims and their neighbors ask, "Why us?"

(c) Mixed situations. Here, a known or suspected exposure combines with a perception of unusual disease occurrence to prompt an investigation to confirm or refute a putative connection. People ask, "Are we sicker than our neighbors?"

These questions are clearly pertinent to the clinician in that they represent fundamental concerns of patients and their families. Of interest, these questions also correspond to the three basic types of epidemiological study design: the cohort study (exposure driven), the case-control study (outcome driven), and the cross-sectional design (mixed). Unfortunately, due to the nature of epidemiology and the particular difficulties inherent in performing community studies, scientists can rarely provide definitive and timely answers to citizens' concerns. In the clinical setting, it is as important to understand and to convey the limitations of science in this area as it is to delineate the technical facts about any one toxicant. In this chapter, we discuss and illustrate some of the methodological issues that influence our ability to understand the effects of environmental toxicants.

## MAGNITUDE OF THE PROBLEM

We are only now beginning to establish approximate bounds on the potential impact of the widespread environmental contamination of our communities. In doing so, we are handicapped by a lack of knowledge as to how much routine exposure to synthetic organic chemicals occurs. While market basket surveys of foodstuffs and adipose tissue samples have attempted to estimate this exposure, only a small portion of the mass of chemicals in tissue has been identified. One recent estimate suggests that "background" exposure is responsible for 1–2% of all cancer deaths (2). In other words, 10–20 people die daily of cancer in this country contracted as a result of breathing the air, drinking the water, and eating the food. This estimate does not account for identified exposures in a community or workplace that could put particular individuals at much higher risk.

Improper disposal of waste is one of the leading causes for contamination of our environment. The Office of Technology Assessment (OTA) estimates that more than 6 billion tons of waste (50,000 lb per capita) are disposed of annually in this country. This has produced more than 31,000 waste sites, of which so far more than 1200 have been assigned to the National Priority List for expedited clean-up because of their potential for exposing populations. The OTA also estimates that there may be more than 400,000 sites overall, most of them yet to be discovered (3).

This is a new situation. The development in the 1920s and 1930s of new methods in chemical engineering, such as catalytic crackling, made it possible to produce synthetic organic chemicals in high volume and in bewildering profusion. Many of these chemicals had never before existed on the face of the earth. This very fact was one of the keys to their usefulness, for no organism had evolved to use them for nutrients and, hence, to decompose them. The other side of this commercial utility, however, was environmental persistence, allowing these chemicals to build up slowly in the environment. Our environment is capable of withstanding truly prodigious perturbations, but there is much evidence that the activities of our industrial society have exceeded even this huge assimilative capacity.

Questions about possible health effects of exposure to toxic chemicals in the environment are being asked with increasing urgency. One expression of this growing concern has been the appearance of local community groups organized around specific issues such as a neighborhood waste site or a perceived birth defects cluster. These groups have enormous energy and motivation. They are emerging as the most important factor prompting public health and medical professionals to learn more about the effects of environmental contamination.

## ASSESSING ENVIRONMENTAL RISK

The complexity of the interaction between environmental factors and the health of an individual patient or community can seem overwhelming. A systematic approach is useful to organize the relevant information. In this section, we apply a model similar to that presented in Chapter 10 to illustrate salient points in the assessment of environmental risks. The main components of this approach include: (a) defining the conditions of exposure, i.e., who is exposed, to what agents, when, to how much, in what pattern, and by what means; (b) identifying the adverse effects, if any, that have been associated with the agents in question; (c) quantitating the relationship of exposure to each of the effects identified; and (d) evaluating the risk for each adverse effect, given the conditions of exposure. While it is unlikely that each step will be completed fully, this framework provides a way to analyze a disparate and confusing literature.

### Define the Conditions of Exposure

SOURCES OF EXPOSURE

Water

Water is one of the most common sources of exposure to environmental toxicants. As shown in Figure 27.1, most community drinking water is supplied by either surface water stored in reservoirs or groundwater that feeds into private wells or municipal systems. Improper dis-

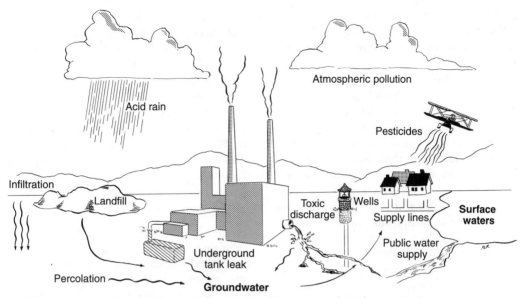

**Figure 27.1.** Primary sources of public water supply and contamination.

posal of waste materials, which may have occurred many decades in the past, leads to contaminated soil and water.

Groundwater contamination is an especially common problem in the U.S. While virtually any pollutant may be involved, a rather small set of chemicals is most often identified, reflecting both prevalence of use and the property of chemical stability that allows persistence in the environment. Thus, short-chain chlorinated hydrocarbons, such as trichloroethylene, tetrachloroethylene, and methylchloroform, are some of the most commonly found groundwater contaminants in the nation.

Chemicals in household water can be ingested or absorbed dermally when bathing or showering (4). In addition, volatile chemicals can be inhaled during showering, dishwashing, or toilet flushing, as these operations "air-strip" them from the water. This last route may contribute as much or more dose as ingestion; yet it is often neglected when an alternative source of drinking water, such as bottled water, is used to replace a contaminated source (5, 6). Ingested chemicals make a first pass through the liver; with dermal or inhalation exposure, the chemical immediately enters the systemic circulation.

Contaminants can be removed from water at the point of use using a variety of filters.

Different kinds of filters work for different kinds of contaminants. One of the most common is the granular activated charcoal filter that removes many volatile organics. These filters must be regularly changed, as they have a finite capacity, which, when exceeded, may release a sudden bolus of contaminant. Consumers should use such devices only for prescribed contaminants and with strict adherence to maintenance and operating instructions. These devices are not regulated by the government, but the U.S. Environmental Protection Agency (EPA) monitors the situation and is a good source of information.

Chemicals in water are measured either on a mass/volume basis, in terms of mg/liter, or as a mass/mass unit expressed as parts per billion (ppb) or parts per million (ppm). Inasmuch as 1 liter of water has a mass of 1000 g, 1 $\mu$g/liter is the same as 1 ppb, and 1 mg/liter equals 1 ppm.

## Air

Volatile chemicals can be present in the air of communities and can be inhaled by residents. Sources include waste or raw materials in open or leaking bulk containers; intentional releases (e.g., through a vent or stack of a factory or incinerator); so-called "fugitive emissions" (leaky facilities); and sudden releases such as spills, accidents, or fires. Contaminated soil can also constitute an air source of volatile chemicals.

Concentrations of chemicals in the air are very sensitive to meteorological conditions which, in turn, vary with season and even time of day. Certain states of the atmosphere, such as very light winds and surface temperatures relatively cooler than those aloft, can result in high concentrations over short periods of time.

The extent of exposure through the air is often unappreciated, due partly to confusion over units of measurement. Air contaminants are measured either on a mass/volume ($\mu g/m^3$) or a volume/volume basis (ppb). Unlike water units, however, there is no immediate equivalence between the two measures; in fact, the conversion factor differs for each substance because it depends on molecular weight.

The volume of air inspired by an individual is influenced by a number of factors including level of exertion and pregnancy. Assuming that an adult breathes approximately 1 $m^3$ of air per hour, continual presence in a neighborhood would result in inhalation of approximately 24 times the mass of chemical expressed in units of $\mu g/m^3$. This dose is often substantially more than that received through a contaminated water supply.

## Soil

Soil can act both as a reservoir and source of chemical pollution. In addition to contamination from improper disposal of wastes, landfills serve as specially designated areas where solid and toxic wastes are intentionally deposited between layers of soil. Percolation of rainwater through the soil forms a leachate that can pollute groundwater. The amount of waste generated in the U.S. is outstripping the capacity of existing landfills, and incineration is now promoted as a means of reducing the volume of waste. Unfortunately, incineration of toxic wastes can produce both hazardous air emissions and an ash laden with heavy metals and other contaminants that is deposited into landfills. Thus, the different sources of pollution are inextricably linked, and attempts to control one source may, in fact, contribute to another.

Community residents can be exposed to contaminated soil by direct contact (e.g., working or playing in it), by inhalation of particulate matter when soil is blown offsite, or by inadvertent ingestion of soil on hands or food. Soil can be an important source of exposure to heavy metals; for example, contamination of soil with lead contributes to childhood lead poisoning in the U.S. Soil contamination is expressed on a mass/mass basis, either in terms of mg or $\mu g$ of chemical/kg of soil, or ppm or ppb.

## Food Chain

Chemicals can translocate from air, soil, or water into the food chain. For example, polychlorinated biphenyls (PCBs) discharged into surface waters bind to sediment and are absorbed by bottom-feeding fish. These fish are eaten by fish predators higher on the food chain, consumption of which results in human exposure. This pathway is responsible for transplacental and breast milk exposure to infants born to women on the Great Lakes who ate contaminated fish during pregnancy (7).

The extent to which contaminants in soil translocate to fruits and vegetables varies with the chemical and the foodstuff. The processes involved are complex and poorly understood. Some organics may be directly incorporated into plant parts, but others are volatilized from the soil and absorbed by above-ground plant parts (8, 9).

Like soil contamination, chemical residues in food are expressed in terms of mass of chemical/mass of foodstuff ($\mu g/kg$, $\mu g/g$ or ppm, ppb). Many foodstuffs contain residues of a variety of chemicals, particularly persistent pesticides (10).

## ASCERTAINING EXPOSURE

A good exposure history is clearly important but is often difficult to obtain. As emphasized in Chapter 10, exposure to both parents should be assessed and attention paid to the dose and timing of exposure.

It is often possible to estimate the time when exposure began by using physical principles of contaminant transport within the exposure pathway. Air sources are usually the least problematic because exposures are roughly contemporaneous with the source itself. Recorded data may be helpful; for example, under the Community Right to Know Law (Chapter 12), inventories of toxic releases from industrial facilities are available. In many cases, neighborhood residents will report an odor. Although the presence of an odor is neither necessary nor sufficient proof that a hazard exists (many dangerous chemicals have high odor thresholds, while many relatively benign ones have low thresholds), odor detection does indicate that air-borne substances have reached residents. Odor thresholds for a variety of chemicals have been determined and can provide lower bound dose estimates if odors are detectable (11). Given characteristics of an air source (e.g., emission rate) and routinely collected meteorological data, health officials may be able to estimate the air concentrations expected over the long run using computer models.

The situation is more complex for water contamination. Clearly it is best to have actual measurements for the period of interest (e.g., during the pregnancy). However, most organic contaminants are not routinely monitored. Even if measurements were taken, the contaminant may not have been looked for or detected by the analytic method used. Contaminated water may, at times, present an off-taste or chemical odor. However, many natural waters periodically have off-tastes or odors from seasonal algal growths.

If a contaminant is detected in drinking water at a time later than the period of interest, it is difficult to determine how long it has been there and at what levels. If a source has been identified, estimates can be made of the amount of chemical that reached a particular wellhead by taking into account physical processes such as groundwater flow and contaminant transport. This complex undertaking requires information about the hydrogeological characteristics of the area around the source and the well. Estimating the extent or possibility of contamination from scanty hydrogeological measurements is risky. In our experience, such judgments are more likely to conclude falsely that hydrological connections between source and well are improbable than to conclude erroneously that they are. In the absence

of contemporaneous measurements, it is, therefore, unwarranted to rule out the possibility that exposure occurred unless evidence to the contrary is very convincing.

Even when it is determined that a substance has reached the wellhead, distribution of the chemical in the drinking water system may be uneven. Multiple wellheads are connected together in a municipal system, and only some of the wells may be contaminated. Here, some idea of who was exposed and to how much can be obtained by using a computer model of the distribution system.

While the use of sophisticated models to reconstruct exposure is beyond the reach of clinicians, it is important to be aware of these methods. It is often the clinician whose advice is first sought by the patient or by a local health officer. A call by a concerned clinician to the regional EPA may prompt investigation of suspected community or household contamination. In addition, these methods are sometimes important for research or legal purposes.

A patient's suspicions should be included as part of the medical history, even if the clinician is skeptical of them. Too little is known about this problem to be confident in ruling out particular environmental factors. The record in this field suggests that patients are extremely astute observers and often have solid insights. If the patient does not mention environmental factors in the history, the clinician should specifically inquire about them.

## Identify Adverse Effects

### OUTCOME-DRIVEN SITUATIONS

If the situation is what we call "outcome driven," the adverse effects will be given, often in the form of a "cluster" of reproductive problems. Geographically coherent patterns of cases, especially if they also occur over a short period of time (a "time-space" cluster), suggest environmental or communicable etiological factors.

Clinicians may be the first to note a cluster by virtue of treating patients in a particular geographic area, or they may be informed about one by their patients. In the latter case, the diagnoses must be verified, usually requiring the participation of state health officials.

Certain adverse reproductive outcomes, such as spontaneous abortions, are sufficiently frequent that a canvass of a neighborhood can expect to turn up a number of cases. As yet, there is no sensitive statistical test to determine if a cluster is "really" a cluster, i.e., it is not likely to have arisen by chance (12). Judgment is still needed.

While the investigation of a cluster can be difficult, the concept follows that of a classic case-control study. We try to understand what is different about the exposure history of the cases compared with those without the problem (the controls). To date, there has been limited success in the investigation of these disease clusters (13), but application of new techniques holds some promise for change. The investigation of a cluster presents an opportunity to develop new understandings of how adverse reproductive events arise and ways to prevent them. However, it is often difficult to engage health officials in the investigation of clusters given the technical difficulties and lack of resources (14). This apparent inattention generates considerable frustration among concerned community residents. Validation and advocacy from a local clinician may be decisive in assuring the assistance of the public health establishment.

## EXPOSURE-DRIVEN SITUATIONS

The problem here is to determine whether an exposure can cause adverse reproductive effects in a community setting. A first step is to determine what is already known about the effects of the agent in question. The literature reflects knowledge obtained from clinical experience, toxicological studies, and epidemiological studies. Each presents important partial views of the picture and complements the others.

The virtues and drawbacks of clinical histories ("case reports") are well known. Toxicological studies are experimental in nature, i.e., the investigator actively manipulates the independent variable (here, "exposure") while keeping other variables constant, usually by using two groups of otherwise identical animals. Epidemiological studies have the advantage of dealing with the species of interest (humans) under natural conditions; however, they are problematic because there are usually many differences (con-

founders) between the exposed and unexposed groups other than the exposure, which itself may be poorly characterized. In practice, we must combine the results of both kinds of studies, recognizing the limitations of each and interpreting the results with appropriate judgment.

## Quantitate the Relation Between Exposure and Effect

The quantitative relationship between the amount of exposure and the size of the effect is called the dose-response relationship. There are essentially two distinct kinds of response: an all-or-none or *dichotomous* response, such as cancer or a birth defect, and a severity or *continuous* response, such as birthweight. A continuous variable can always be converted to a dichotomous one by establishing a threshold, such as 2500 g for low birthweight. On the other hand, some responses, such as cancer, can only be expressed dichotomously.

Contaminants that are present in the environment at the ppb or even part per trillion (ppt) level may at first sight appear inconsequential. Indeed, a ppt of a substance in water does seem to be a de minimis amount for virtually any effect we can imagine. However, when a substance is detectable by our most sensitive analytical methods, it is already present in very large amounts from a molecular standpoint. Even a ppt in a liter of water represents an enormous number of molecules because of the truly huge size of Avogadro's number ($6 \times 10^{23}$), the factor that relates the number of molecules to their mass, given the molecular weight. Thus, an individual who drinks a liter of water with 1 ppt of trichloroethylene (TCE) ingests about $1 \times 10^{12}$ molecules of TCE daily. The biological result will depend upon what these molecules of TCE are able to do.

If the effect is to render a cell nonviable, the result may not be clinically serious. Usually, the death of a cell requires substantial numbers of molecules of a toxic substance. For many organ systems, a critical number of cells must be lost before biological function is overtly affected. For example, even the loss of 1000 liver cells is unlikely to have a clinically apparent effect.

The problem arises, however, when the body's own biological processes conspire to amplify the original injury. Thus, when one or several TCE molecules alter the DNA of a cell to produce a malignant phenotype, each cell division reproduces the original damage (the original TCE long gone) until a clone of cells with malignant behavior produces a tumor. In this case, even analytically borderline levels of a chemical may pose a threat.

Another natural amplifier is the nervous system. In fact, this system provides a nice example of how extremely low levels of chemicals can have large and visible biological effects. Thus, the human olfactory apparatus is capable of detecting very low levels of certain substances, one of the most well-known being hydrogen sulfide gas ($H_2S$), the source of "rotten-egg" odor. A concentration as low as 0.5 ppb of $H_2S$ in the air of a room is enough to make an adult leave the premises. What happens here is that a small signal produced by half a ppb of $H_2S$ in air is amplified by the central nervous system and entrains a coordinated and complex series of gross motor movements in the locomotory system.

Another amplifying system of particular relevance to this chapter is the process of reproduction itself, where an entire organism follows from a single biological event, conception. In some instances (e.g., transplacental carcinogenesis), interference with multipotent cells in utero can have large "downstream" effects. Here, we may need to be concerned about apparently small concentrations of chemicals in the environment. On the other hand, many other events (e.g., organ malformations resulting from cell loss) are the result of a direct (unamplified) toxic reaction. In these cases, substantial exposures may be necessary to produce clinically important effects.

The literature provides scant data for estimating true dose-response relationships for adverse reproductive effects in human populations. What we know at this time does not allow us to absolve analytically small concentrations of chemicals in the environment from producing some adverse reproductive or developmental effects.

## Evaluate the Risk for Adverse Effects

This step is commonly carried out as part of a "risk assessment," the process whereby plan-

ners and regulators try to put some bounds on the effects of an environmental change, for example, the building of an incinerator. Risk assessment methodology is also used by regulatory agencies to establish permissible contaminant levels in foods, water, and air. Under the 1986 Safe Drinking Water Act, for example, the EPA established Maximum Contaminant Levels (MCLs) for 85 pollutants in public water supplies, including synthetic organic chemicals, inorganic chemicals, radionuclides, and microbes. While these MCLs are legally enforceable, they are based on combined consideration of health effects data (including available data on reproductive, developmental, and mutagenic effects), treatment technologies, and cost. Nonenforceable Maximum Contaminant Level Goals (MCLGs) are strictly health based and represent concentrations of drinking water contaminants thought unlikely to result in adverse human health effects. Both MCLs and MCLGs for a number of important drinking water contaminants are listed in the Appendix at the end of the book. For some unregulated contaminants, the EPA issues Drinking Water Health Advisories that summarize available data on toxicokinetics and health effects and provide maximum recommended contaminant concentrations. More information regarding health advisories and regulations can be obtained by contacting the EPA's Safe Drinking Water Hotline (800–426–4791).

Data regarding mechanisms of action and detailed dose-response relationships are not available for most environmental toxicants, particularly in regards to reproductive and developmental effects. In the absence of these data, regulatory agencies usually apply an imprecise "uncertainty factor" approach when setting acceptable exposure limits for human populations. With this approach, the no-effect dose level in animal studies is divided by an uncertainty factor that reflects inadequacies in the study design, intra- and interspecies variability in sensitivity to the toxicant, and other considerations. Needless to say, any attempt to estimate risk by applying the meager information on adverse effects and dose-response relationships to the usually uncertain exposure data for a given situation is not likely to possess a high level of confidence. Such exercises may be useful, however, in refuting the proposition that no adverse effects are plausible. Unfortunately, risk assessments have often been used for the purpose of decision justification and should be viewed with a critical eye.

## COMMUNITY STUDIES OF ADVERSE REPRODUCTIVE OUTCOME ASSOCIATED WITH ENVIRONMENTAL CONTAMINATION

We discuss here three examples of environmental epidemiological studies of adverse reproductive outcome through illustration of the principal designs and review of results. These cases suggest just how difficult it can be to draw firm conclusions, even in flagrant contamination scenarios.

### Love Canal, New York

In the early 20th century, Love Canal was excavated as part of an ambitious project to link the Niagara River with Lake Ontario and to build a model industrial city with access to inexpensive water power (15). However, William T. Love never realized his dream project, primarily due to loss of financial backing. The partially built canal eventually became the site of chemical and municipal waste disposal. For approximately 25 yr, the Hooker Chemical Company of Niagara Falls used the site for the disposal of drummed wastes from their production of pesticides and other chemicals. During that time, about 20,000 tons of 250 different chemicals, including organic solvents and chlorinated hydrocarbons, were disposed of in the Canal. Dumping finally ended in 1953, and the Canal was covered with a clay cap.

In the late 1950s, the area surrounding the Canal underwent suburban residential development. The construction apparently disturbed the Canal's clay cap and, by the spring of 1978, chemical odors became quite noticeable in the homes adjacent to the Canal. Air, water, and soil sampling found numerous contaminants in the basements of the homes and at the site itself. These included human and animal carcinogens, mutagens, embryotoxins, and teratogens (16). Contaminants were found at low levels in the first two rings of homes around

the Canal but were initially not thought to extend much further.

In the summer of 1978, the New York State Health Commissioner declared a state-of-emergency and issued orders to develop engineering plans to limit the chemical seepage. He also ordered relocation of Love Canal residents and the purchase of their homes (15). Ninety-seven families (230 adults and 134 children) resided in the first ring of homes around the Canal at that time.

The first epidemiological study of reproductive events conducted by the Health Department examined the frequencies of miscarriages and birth defects among families living in the first ring of homes. Interviews were conducted with all women who had ever been pregnant. Reproductive histories for the periods before and during residence in the Canal area were compared. While based on small numbers, the crude rates of miscarriages and birth defects were higher for women during their years of residence near the Canal; the increases persisted even after controlling for birth order and maternal age. Maternal age was a particularly important variable to control because the women were obviously older during the pregnancies that occurred after moving.

Subsequently, the Health Department conducted studies among Love Canal residents beyond the first ring of homes (17). These investigations examined the possibility that natural drainage routes (swales) provided pathways of migration for the leachate, thereby exposing residents over a larger area than originally thought. The studies found that women who resided in homes transected by swales had higher crude frequencies of spontaneous abortion, congenital anomalies, and low birthweight compared to women living in nonswale areas.

An expanded study of low birthweight attempted to include all infants born to women who resided in the Love Canal area at any time from 1940–1978 (18). Birthweight data were obtained from birth certificates to lessen the possibility of recall bias, and data on potential confounders were obtained by interviewing the women. The current and historical location of the swales was determined from aerial photographs.

Investigators successfully interviewed approximately 93% of the identified women. Overall, 8.6% of children born in the study area had low birthweight; 12.1% occurred among children born to women in the swale areas and 6.5% among children born to women living directly adjacent to the Canal. Swale area residents also had a higher rate of low birthweight infants compared with women in the rest of the Canal area and in upstate New York. The low birthweight excess was seen from 1946–1958, which encompassed the peak years of dumping; no excess was observed in subsequent years. Other important characteristics of the mother, such as educational level, smoking, occupation, past medical conditions, or therapies, did not appear to explain the results.

In 1985, Goldman et al. (19) published the results of yet another investigation that reexamined the rates of low birthweight, prematurity, and birth defects among Love Canal neighborhood residents. Unlike the prior studies, this investigation included a contemporary comparison group from other Niagara Falls census tracts without known waste dumps. Data on reproductive outcomes were collected by interview, except for a small portion of birthweight data obtained from birth certificates.

A woman's residence during gestation and at birth determined whether or not the pregnancy was considered exposed. Two subgroups of exposed and unexposed children were examined: children who lived in single family homes (homeowners) and those who lived in government-subsidized housing (renters). Other potential confounders, including maternal age and smoking habits during pregnancy, were accounted for using special statistical techniques. The participation rate was 82% for eligible renters' children and 63% for eligible homeowners' children. Because the data were collected in 1980, the evacuated families who once lived closest to the Canal were not included.

No excess risk of prematurity was found. Overall, exposed children had a higher prevalence of low birthweight (12.3%) than unexposed children (8.6%). However, the excess was present only among the homeowners: 11.1% of exposed vs. 4.8% of unexposed homeowner children had low birthweight, while

13.8% of exposed renter children compared to 12.6% of unexposed children were low birthweight babies. After accounting for confounding variables, the adjusted relative risk of low birthweight was 3.05 among homeowners and 1.06 among renters. The reasons for this difference are not known, although it could conceivably relate to the way the structures were built or their locations.

Again, the low birthweight rate was associated with proximity to the swales. The prevalence was 17.5% among children whose families resided in "wet" Canal area homes compared with 9.6% among children whose families lived in "dry" homes. In contrast to the prior study, however, Goldman et al. (19) found that the low birthweight excess persisted during the years 1965–1978 after dumping had ceased.

The children of both exposed homeowners and renters had an increased risk of birth defects (adjusted RR = 1.95 and 2.87, respectively) including both congenital malformations and deformations. The numbers were too small to examine the risk of specific types of defects.

Because most of the outcome data were based on interviews, recall bias is a possible explanation for the results. The authors attempted to address this issue by comparing the prevalence of reported adverse pregnancy outcomes among mothers who moved into the Love Canal area after the study children were born with the prevalence among mothers who never lived in the area. The former were more likely to report congenital deformations but no more likely to report low birthweight, prematurity, or congenital malformations. This analysis suggests that recall bias was a possible explanation only for the increased risk of deformations.

Taken together, the Love Canal studies suggest that pregnant women who resided near the swales had an increased risk of low birthweight and congenital malformations. However, these findings are not concordant with results of environmental sampling conducted in 1978. Detectable contaminant levels were found only in the area encompassing the first two rings of homes around the Canal; only trace levels were found further away, including the swale areas. It is possible, however, that the sampling performed in 1978 did not reflect historical contaminant and exposure patterns.

While the epidemiological results from Love Canal may not be definitive, the incident became a powerful symbol of America's toxic waste problem and heightened the awareness of the public, government officials, and the scientific community. Unfortunately, the incident was not without great personal expense to the residents. Ultimately, approximately 2500 people left their homes, 240 homes and the elementary school were demolished, and more than 800 others have remained vacant since then. Although the dump was capped and a monitoring system installed, most of the chemicals remain buried beneath a 70-acre fenced-off mound. Recently, the New York State Love Canal Revitalization Agency put up several of the houses for sale but would not guarantee the safety of the houses in writing. It also announced that the neighborhood was being renamed "Black Creek Village" (20).

## Woburn, Massachusetts

Woburn, Massachusetts is a suburban community northwest of Boston with a long history of industrial activities including leather and chemical processing and the production of arsenical insecticides, textiles, paper, trinitrotoluene (TNT), and animal glue (21). In May of 1979, toxic wastes were discovered near two of the town's municipal wells, known as wells G and H. Testing for volatile organic compounds revealed high levels of the solvents trichloroethylene (267 ppb), tetrachloroethylene (21 ppb), and chloroform (12 ppb), prompting the wells' closure. The town's six other municipal wells met state and federal drinking water standards. This pattern of contamination was not surprising because wells G and H operated as a single source in east Woburn and tapped into a different aquifer than the other municipal wells.

At the same time, the mother of a young leukemia victim began to notice other mothers from the neighborhood when she took her child for chemotherapy. She alerted her pediatrician, who notified the Massachusetts Department of Public Health about the apparent cluster of leukemia cases in the town.

The Department reviewed mortality statistics for the prior 10 yr and found that the overall cancer mortality rate in Woburn was indeed higher than the rest of the state and adjacent communities.

A subsequent case-control study revealed that Woburn's childhood leukemia rate during 1969–1979 was 2.3 times higher than expected. Although 12 cases lived in one census tract south of Wells G and H and the contaminated site, the state studies did not address the relationship between contaminated water use and the occurrence of leukemia.

In 1981, a community action group contacted researchers from the Harvard School of Public Health. They decided to collaborate on a health survey that would specifically assess the relationship between use of wells G and H and adverse health outcomes. The resulting "Woburn Study" is one of the best known and most controversial investigations of community exposures. It consisted of two separate investigations, each with its own set of strengths and limitations.

Using state and hospital registry data, the leukemia portion of the study identified all cases of childhood leukemia diagnosed from 1964, the start date of pumping from wells G and H, until after the wells were closed in 1983. A second study investigated reproductive outcomes; information was collected on the frequency of adverse pregnancy outcomes (congenital anomalies, spontaneous abortion, perinatal death, low birthweight) and childhood disorders (lung and respiratory, kidney and other urinary, allergies and skin, neurological and sensory) during the period 1960–1982, using a telephone survey among a random sample of former and current members of Woburn households.

A detailed computer model of the water distribution system in the town was used to estimate the geographic and temporal distribution of water from contaminated wells G and H during their years of use. While wells G and H served only east Woburn, all town residents received a blend of water from several different wells. The specific blend depended on the time of year and the resident's location. The model partitioned the town into five zones representing increasing levels of exposure to water from wells G and H and estimated the annual percentage of each household's water supply that came from these wells.

The childhood leukemia study results confirmed that the rates in Woburn were significantly higher than expected on the basis of national rates (20 observed and 9.1 expected, $p < 0.001$). A positive association was also seen between availability of water from wells G and H and the leukemia incidence. However, at that time, the authors felt that use of wells G and H could not have accounted for the entire leukemia excess because the model indicated that 11 of the 20 cases were never supplied with water from these wells. Since then, a more refined model has indicated wider distribution of wells G and H contaminants than originally thought.

Due to budget constraints, the reproductive outcome telephone survey was conducted using volunteer interviewers mainly from Woburn and including family members of some of the leukemia cases. Interviews were completed with 5010 households (approximately 57% of the town's residences with listed telephone numbers). The survey collected information on all children born from 1960–1982 including vital status, birthweight, and the occurrence of congenital anomalies and childhood conditions, and on potential confounding variables, such as maternal age and smoking habits during pregnancy. In addition, the investigators attempted to verify the adverse pregnancy outcomes by reviewing medical records.

Significant associations were found for perinatal death after 1970 (RR = 10.0), eye/ear anomalies (RR = 14.9), and "environmentally related" anomalies (RR = 4.5), even after controlling for important confounders. The latter category comprised a heterogeneous grouping (e.g., central nervous system, chromosomal anomalies, and oral clefts) for which there was some evidence in the literature of positive associations with chemical exposures. Positive associations were also seen between exposure to water from wells G and H and the occurrence of lung/respiratory (RR = 1.3) and kidney/urinary tract disorders (RR = 1.7).

Publication of these results in 1986 (21) elicited numerous commentaries (22–26), many of which were critical of the study methodology. The low response rate, possible interviewer and respondent bias, the inclusion of conditions that are not traditionally classified as congenital anomalies (e.g., severe strabismus, cerebral palsy), and the ad hoc grouping of "environmentally related" malformations drew considerable criticism. On the other hand, several reviewers praised the investigators for undertaking a difficult study with little funding. They also acknowledged that the statistical methods used to analyze the results were innovative and represented the state-of-the-art in environmental epidemiology. In the end, the study raised as many questions as it answered, and additional long-term studies are now underway (27).

## Seveso, Italy

On July 10, 1976, an explosion at the ICMESA chemical plant in Meda, Italy, released a cloud of toxic chemicals over the surrounding countryside. The explosion was caused by a runaway reaction that occurred during the production of 2,4,5-trichlorophenol (TCP) (28). The cloud also contained other highly toxic chemicals, including 2,3,7,8-tetrachlorodibenzo-para-dioxin (TCDD).

Debris from the cloud fell south-southeast of the plant in an area including the towns of Meda and Seveso. Soil analyses were used to estimate the extent of contamination and, on this basis, the affected area was divided into three graded levels of exposure. The highest exposures appeared to have occurred in an 80-hectare area in Seveso immediately surrounding the plant, designated as Zone A. Zone A's average surface soil TCDD concentration was 192.8 $\mu g/m^2$. Zone B, a 269-hectare area further south and downwind of the plant, had an average concentration of 3 $\mu g/m^2$; and Zone R, a 1430-hectare area that surrounded Zones A and B, had an average concentration of 0.9 $\mu g/m^2$. A fourth zone, outside of the contaminated area but in the same local health district (Zone non-ABR), was designated as a control area. Examination of the frequency of animal mortality and chloracne, a human skin lesion associated with TCDD exposure, showed good correlation with the contaminant levels in the exposure zones.

While over 120,000 people lived in the municipalities affected by the explosion, only 730 people lived in Zone A (29). All Zone A residents were evacuated 2 weeks after the accident, but only children and pregnant women in Zones B and R were evacuated. Remaining residents were asked not to grow or to consume local agricultural products or to raise animals. Area residents were also advised to avoid conception.

Epidemiological investigations included immediate clinical follow-up as well as long-term morbidity studies among exposed residents. However, well-controlled systematic investigations of adverse pregnancy outcomes were not conducted at this time. Initial reports suggesting an increased frequency of spontaneous abortion were discounted, because there were no reliable baseline levels.

Rehder et al. (30) examined 34 fetuses from elective or spontaneous abortions among women who were exposed during the first trimester of pregnancy. They found no evidence of abnormalities that could be attributed to TCDD exposure; however, the findings were of limited value because the abortion procedure often left little intact fetal tissue for examination.

The establishment of a birth defects registry in October 1977 enabled a more extensive investigation of possible teratogenic effects of the explosion (28). The Seveso Congenital Malformation Registry monitored birth defects that occurred in all livebirths and stillbirths among women residents of Zones A, B, R, and non-ABR from January 1977 through December 1982. Thus, pregnant women who were in the area of the accident during the first trimester were included.

A surveillance system was set up in maternity hospitals, pediatric departments, and primary care pediatric services to ascertain malformations. All reported living cases were examined by the Registry's pediatric team, and, in the cases of death, medical records were reviewed. Infants were registered if they had one or more structural malformations or a recognized morphological syndrome or disease. Both major and mild defects were included.

Of 15,291 births, 742 malformations were registered over this period, resulting in a prevalence of 49.5/1000 births. Of the 26 births that

occurred to women who resided in Zone A, none had major malformations and only two had minor malformations (a hemangioma and a periurethral cyst). Thus, the prevalence of birth defects in Zone A was 76.9/1000. The corresponding prevalences in Zones B, R, and non-ABR were 57.5/1000, 45.1/1000, and 48.8/1000, respectively. While higher in Zones A and B, these prevalence proportions were not statistically different from those in Zones R and non-ABR, a common feature of analyses when numbers are small. The most frequent malformations seen in the contaminated areas were hemangiomas, congenital hip dislocation, and congenital heart defects.

Investigators also separately examined women from Zones A, B, and R who delivered during the first quarter of 1977 and so were most likely to have been exposed during the first trimester, the period of organogenesis. They found five malformed infants, all born to mothers in Zone R, the least contaminated but most populous of the three exposed zones.

While the study results generally indicated that pregnant women exposed to TCDD from the Seveso accident did not have an excess number of birth defects, there are reasons why a positive association may not have been detected. First, an increase in the number of aborted (spontaneous or induced) fetuses could have led to a decrease in the prevalence of defects seen at birth. While an increased frequency of spontaneous abortion was never confirmed, an observed decrease in the number of livebirths during the year following the accident suggested a larger than usual number of spontaneous or induced abortions. This cannot be specified further because induced abortion was illegal in Italy in 1976.

Second, while Seveso residents were one of the largest populations ever exposed to TCDD, the sample size was still small for a study of rare outcomes such as congenital malformations. In fact, the study was powerful enough to detect only very high (4.5-fold or higher) relative risks of all defects combined or specific types of defects among Zone A residents.

## Summary

These three cases illustrate the variety of actual and potential exposure routes (air, water, food chain, soil) to environmental contaminants; the various means used to estimate exposures (residence in a particular area, crude categorizations based on soil samples, computer models) and their problems; the influence and importance of information from the community; and the difficulties engendered when there is no established means of routine case ascertainment, when numbers are small, and when statistical techniques are not yet adapted to the problem of detecting unusual spatial patterns rather than comparing rates. However, they also show that persistence and creativity can result in incremental additions to our knowledge in this important area.

## RESOURCES

At the moment, it is difficult to find an appropriate referral for a patient you suspect to have an environmentally related problem. There is no subspecialty specific to environmental health; the closest substitute, occupational medicine, often proves inadequate because the workplace is sufficiently different from the community environment to make much of the knowledge nontransferable. A few individuals in various specialties have acquired experience in these matters, but they are rare. To date, these problems have been considered primarily from a public health, rather than from a clinical, perspective. The players principally involved are state and federal authorities, university research groups, environmental groups, and private consultants. Some of these resources are listed in Chapter 10 (Table 10.2).

Health problems related to environmental factors are normally investigated by units within state health departments. In addition, about half of the states have separate state environmental protection agencies with sanitary engineering, regulatory, and planning expertise. Jurisdictional responsibilities may be unclear, however, and it is not uncommon to have state agencies working at cross purposes. There is also a well-recognized reluctance on the part of state agencies to identify environmental problems (14). Understaffing and a high turnover in personnel hamper sustained efforts on difficult long-term studies.

On the federal level, the Agency for Toxic Substances and Disease Registry (ATSDR) within the U.S. Public Health Service is responsible for investigating health effects related to hazardous wastes. It receives its legislative mandate from the Superfund Law, the law that regulates the clean-up of hazardous waste sites. A specific request by a physician for an evaluation of a waste site automatically triggers a mandatory health assessment by ATSDR. Because ATSDR has an explicit policy of working with state health departments, it might fulfill a request through a state health department unit.

A number of university research groups work in the area of environmental epidemiology and toxicology and may provide advice and technical assistance. Additional information can be obtained from the International Society for Environmental Epidemiology and the Society of Toxicology. Private consulting companies may also be sources of information and analysis.

Within the last decade, a number of environmental and citizen groups have also developed independent technical units. They are an extremely important and valuable repository of expertise. Several have written useful handbooks (31). In addition, citizen groups can provide important emotional support for patients concerned about community contamination.

Unfortunately, there are few actions that individuals themselves can take to decrease exposures. For the most part, community residents are dependent on state and federal agencies to clean up the sources of contamination—a process that is often time-consuming and expensive. In addition to the identification and treatment of potential environmental health effects, providing support and advocacy for individuals in these frustrating circumstances are important aspects of patient care.

### REFERENCES

1. Ozonoff D, Wartenberg D. Toxic exposures in a community setting: the epidemiological approach. In: Groopman JD, Skipper P, eds. Molecular dosimetry and human cancer: analytical, epidemiological and social considerations. Boca Raton, FL: CRC Press, 1991:77–88.
2. Travis CC, Hester ST. Global chemical pollution. Environ Sci Technol 1991;25:815–818.
3. United State Congress, Office of Technology Assessment. Coming clean: superfund problems can be solved. OTA

report OTA-ITE-433. Washington, DC: U.S. Government Printing Office, 1989.

4. Brown HS, Bishop DR, Rowan CA. The role of skin absorption as a route of exposure for volatile organic compounds (VOCs) in drinking water. Am J Public Health 1984;74:479–484.

5. Andelman JB. Inhalation exposure in the home to volatile organic contaminants of drinking water. Sci Total Environ 1985;47:443–460.

6. McKone TE. Household exposure models. Toxicol Lett 1989;49:321–339.

7. Schwartz PM, Jacobson SW, Fein G, Jacobson JL, Price HA. Lake Michigan fish consumption as a source of polychlorinated biphenyls in human cord serum, maternal serum, and milk. Am J Public Health 1983;73:293–296.

8. Vaughan BE. State of research: environmental pathways and food chain transfer. Environ Health Perspect 1984;54:353–371.

9. Travis CC, Hattemer-Frey HA. Assessing the extent of human exposure to organics. In: Travis CC, ed. Carcinogen risk assessment. New York: Plenum Press, 1988:61–75.

10. U.S. Food and Drug Administration. Food and Drug Administration pesticide program. Residues in foods—1988. J Assoc Off Anal Chem 1989;72:133–152.

11. Amoore JE, Hautala E. Odor as an aid to chemical safety: odor thresholds compared with threshold limit values and volatilities for 214 industrial chemicals in air and water dilution. J Appl Toxicol 1983;3:272–290.

12. Wartenberg D, Greenberg M. Detecting disease clusters: the importance of statistical power. Am J Epidemiol 1990;132:S156–S166.

13. Rothman KJ. A sobering start for the cluster busters' conference. Am J Epidemiol 1990;132:S6–S15.

14. Ozonoff D, Boden L. Truth and consequences: health department responses to environmental problems. Science, Technology, and Human Values 1987;12:70–77.

15. New York State. Love Canal: public health time bomb. A special report to the governor and legislature. New York: Office of Public Health and Governor's Love Canal Inter-Agency Task Force, 1978.

16. Heath CW. Field epidemiologic studies of populations exposed to waste dumps. Environ Health Perspect 1983;48:3–7.

17. Vianna NJ. Adverse pregnancy outcomes: potential endpoints of human toxicity in the Love Canal. Preliminary results. In: Porter IH, ed. Embryonic and fetal death. New York: Academic Press, 1980.

18. Vianna NJ, Polan AK. Incidence of low birthweight among Love Canal residents. Science 1984;226:1217–1219.

19. Goldman LR, Paigen B, Magnant MM, Highland JH. Prematurity and birth defects in children living near the hazardous waste site, Love Canal. Haz Waste Haz Mat 1985;2:209–223.

20. Flippen A (Associated Press). Sale of Love Canal homes draws 2 dozen people. Boston Globe. August 16, 1990;29.

21. Lagakos SW, Wesson BJ, Zelen M. An analysis of contaminated well water and health effects in Woburn Massachusetts. J Am Stat Assoc 1986;81:583–596.

22. MacMahon B. Comment. J Am Stat Assoc 1986:81:597–599.

23. Prentice RL. Comment. J Am Stat Assoc 1986;81:600–601.

24. Rogan WJ. Comment. J Am Stat Assoc 1986;81:602–603.

25. Swan SW, Robins JM. Comment. J Am Stat Assoc 1986;81:604–609.

26. Whittemore AS. Comment. J Am Stat Assoc 1986;81:609–610.

27. Massachusetts Department of Public Health and Massachusetts Health Research Institute. Scientific protocol for the Woburn environmental and birth study, 1990.

28. Mastroiacovo P, Spagnolo A, Marni E, Meazza L, Bertollini R, Segni G. Birth defects in the Seveso area after TCDD contamination. JAMA 1988;259:1668–1672.

29. Pocchiari F, Silano V, Zampieri A. Human health effects from accidental release of tetrachlorodibenzo-p-dioxin (TCDD) at Seveso, Italy. Ann NY Acad Sci 1979;108:311–320.

30. Rehder H, Sanchioni F, Cefes G, Gropp A. Pathological-embryological investigations in cases of abortion related to the Seveso accident. J Swiss Med 1978;108:1817–1825.

31. Cohen G, O'Connor J. Fighting toxics: a manual for protecting your family, community and workplace. Washington, DC: Island Press, 1990.

....................................................

# Required and Recommended Exposure Limits for Some Chemicals Known or Suspected to Be Reproductive/Developmental Hazards[a]

| Chemical CAS No.[b] | OSHA PEL[c] | NIOSH REL[d] | ACGIH[e] | | EPA DW Regs[f] | | Some Reported Effects[g] |
|---|---|---|---|---|---|---|---|
| | | | TLV | BEI | MCL (mg/liter) | HA (mg/liter) | |
| **Metals** | | | | | | | |
| Arsenic, inorganic 7740–38–2 (metal) | 0.010 mg/m³ | C 0.002 mg/m³ | 0.2 mg/m³ | Urine (P): 50 μg/g creat; sample at end of work week | 0.05 (R) | | A: Embleth, terata H: SAB, LBW (smelter emissions); PTD/NNM with As poisoning (case report) M, Ca |
| Boron anhydride 1303–86–2 | 10 mg/m³ | Same | Same | | | Boron 0.9 (LT-C) 3 (LT-A) 0.6 (LF) (D,L) | Reacts with $H_2O$ to form boric acid A: (boric acid): RT (♂), terata H: ↓ libido, spermatotoxicity, ? terata (one report) |
| Cadmium, dusts and salts 7440–43–9 | 0.2 mg/m³ C 0.6 mg/m³ | Lowest feasible concentration | 0.05 mg/m³ 0.01 mg/m³ (P) ALARA | Urine: 10 μg/g creat, 5μg/g creat (P); blood: 10 μg/liter, 5 μg/liter (P) | 0.005 0.005 (MCLG) | | Accumulates in placenta A: RT (♂, ♀), embleth, fetotox, terata H: ↓ libido, spermatotoxicity (case reports) M, Ca (incl. prostate) |
| Chromium 7440–47–3 | 0.5 mg/m³ (Cr II & III cmps) 1 mg/m³ (metal) | 0.5 mg/m³ (metal, Cr II & III cmps) 0.001 mg/m³ (Cr VI cmps) | 0.5 mg/m³ (metal, Cr II & III cmps) 0.05 mg/m³ (Cr VI cmps) | Urine: 10 μg/g creat, increase during shift; 30 μg/g creat, end of shift at end of work week | 0.1 0.1 (MCLG) | | A: (Cr VI): RT (♂), embleth, terata H: No data Ca (Cr VI) |

| Substance | | | | | | | |
|---|---|---|---|---|---|---|---|
| Copper 7440–50–8 | | | | | | | |
| Dusts, mists | 1 mg/m³ | Same | Same | | 1.3 (action level—P) | | A: RT (♀), embleth, terata; H: ↓ fertility, SAB (Wilson's disease) |
| Fumes | 0.1 mg/m³ | Same | Same | | | | |
| Lead, inorganic 7439–92–1 | 0.05 mg/m³ (air) Suggests blood levels <0.03 mg/dl for prospective parents and fetus/newborn | 0.1 mg/m³ (air) <0.06 mg/dl (blood) | 0.15 mg/m³ | Urine: 150 µg/g creat; blood: 50 µg/dl; sampling time not critical | At tap 0.015 (action level) 0 (MCLG) | | Well-established human reproductive and developmental toxicant (♂); neurobehavioral deficits associated with blood lead levels as low as 0.01–0.015 mg/dl |
| Manganese 7439–96–5 | | | | | | | |
| Dusts, compounds | C 5 mg/m³ | 1 mg/m³ | C 5 mg/m³ | | | RFD 0.14 mg/kg/day (D) | A: RT (♂), postnatal growth deficits; H: ↓ libido, impotence with Mn toxicity |
| Fumes | 1 mg/m³ ST 3 mg/m³ | 1 mg/m³ ST 3 mg/m³ | 1 mg/m³ ST 3 mg/m³ | | | | |
| • Mercury 7439–97–6 | | | | | | | |
| Vapor Inorganic | 0.05 mg/m³ C 0.1 mg/m³ | Same | Same 0.1 mg/m³ | Urine (P): 35 µg/g creat, sample preshift; blood (P): 15 µg/liter, sample end of shift at end of work week | 0.002 0.002 (MCLG) | | Vapor/inorganic: A: RT (♂, ♀), terata, NNM; H: Menstrual dysfunction; ↓ libido, impotence with Hg toxicity; SAB (♂) |

| Chemical CAS No.[b] | OSHA PEL[c] | NIOSH REL[d] | ACGIH[e] | | EPA DW Regs[f] | | Some Reported Effects[g] |
|---|---|---|---|---|---|---|---|
| | | | TLV | BEI | MCL (mg/liter) | HA (mg/liter) | |
| Organic (alkyl) | 0.01 mg/m³ ST 0.03 mg/m³ | Same | Same | | | | Methylmercury: known human teratogen (microcephaly, mental retardation and cerebral palsy) |
| Nickel 7440–02–0 | 0.1 mg/m³ (soluble cmps) 1 mg/m³ (metal, insoluble cmps) | 0.015 mg/m³ | 0.1 mg/m³ (soluble cmps) 1 mg/m³ (metal, insoluble cmps) 0.05 mg/m³ (P) ALARA | | 0.1 (P) 0.1 (MCLG-P) | | A: RT ($\delta$, $\mathcal{P}$), embleth, fetotox, terata H: No data M, Ca |
| Selenium 7782–49–2 | 0.2 mg/m³ | Same | Same | | 0.05 0.05 (MCLG) | | A: RT ($\mathcal{P}$), fetotox, terata, NNM H: SAB (1 report) |

**Pesticides:[h] Rodenticides/Herbicides/Insecticides**

| Chemical CAS No.[b] | OSHA PEL[c] | NIOSH REL[d] | ACGIH[e] | | EPA DW Regs[f] | | Some Reported Effects[g] |
|---|---|---|---|---|---|---|---|
| | | | TLV | BEI | MCL (mg/liter) | HA (mg/liter) | |
| Acrolein (Aqualin) 107–02–8 | 0.1 ppm ST 0.3 ppm | Same | Same | | | | A: Embleth, fetotox, ± terata H: No data |
| Aldrin 309–00–2 | 0.25 mg/m³ | Same | Same | | | 0.0003 (LT-C) 0.0003 (LT-A) (D) | Metabolized to dieldrin A: Embleth, terata H: No data Ca No longer produced in U.S. |

| Agent | | | | | | |
|---|---|---|---|---|---|---|
| • Chlordecone (Kepone) 143–50–0 | | .001 mg/m³ | | | | A: RT (♂, ♀; estrogen agonist), embleth, fetotox, ± terata with maternal toxicity<br>H: Spermatotoxicity<br>Uses canceled 1977 |
| • Cyanazine 21725–46–2 | | | | (L) | 0.02 (LT-C)<br>0.07 (LT-A)<br>0.001 (LF) | A: Embleth, fetotox, terata with maternal toxicity<br>H: No data |
| DDT (dichloro-diphenyl-trichloroethane) 50–29–3 | | 0.5 mg/m³ | 1 mg/m³ | | | A: RT (♂, ♂; estrogen agonist), neurobehavioral deficits<br>H: Higher levels of DDT and metabolite DDE in abortuses and preterm infants and in semen of infertile men<br>Ca<br>Use canceled in U.S. |
| Dieldrin 60–57–1 | 0.25 mg/m³ | Same | Same | | 0.0005 (LT-C)<br>0.002 (LT-A) | A: Embryoleth, terata<br>H: No data<br>No longer produced in U.S. |
| • Dinoseb 88–85–7 | | | | 0.007 (P) | 0.007 (MCLG-P) | A: RT (♂), fetotox, terata<br>H: No data<br>Registration canceled 1986 |

| Chemical CAS No.[b] | OSHA PEL[c] | NIOSH REL[d] | ACGIH[e] | | EPA DW Regs[f] | | Some Reported Effects[g] |
|---|---|---|---|---|---|---|---|
| | | | TLV | BEI | MCL (mg/liter) | HA (mg/liter) | |
| Endrin 72–20–8 | 0.1 mg/m³ | Same | Same | | 0.002 (P) 0.002 (MCLG-P) | | A: Terata, neurobehavioral deficits, NNM; H: No data; Uses canceled in 1985 |
| Methyl parathion (metaphos) 298–00–0 | 0.2 mg/m³ | Same | Same | | | 0.03 (LT-C) 0.1 (LT-A) 0.002 (LF) | A: Embleth, fetotox, terata with maternal toxicity; behavioral deficits at subtoxic doses; H: Terata (case reports) |
| Picloram 1918–02–01 | 10 mg/m³ | | 10 mg/m³ | | 0.5 (P) 0.5 (MCLG-P) | | A: RT (♂), fetotox; H: No data |
| Toxaphene 8001–35–2 | 0.5 mg/m³ ST 1 mg/m³ | | Same | | 0.003 0 (MCLG) | | A: Neurobehavioral deficits; H: No data; Most uses canceled 1982 |
| Trichlorophenoxy-acetic acid (2,4,5-T) 93–76–5 | 10 mg/m³ | Same | Same | | (L) | 0.8 (LT-C) 1 (LT-A) 0.07 (LF) | Contaminated with highly-toxic 2,3,7,8-tetrachlorodibenzo-p-dioxin (TCDD); A: Fetotox, terata, neurobehavioral deficits; H: ± terata (♂), ± SAB (♂); all uses canceled 1985 |

| Substance | OSHA | ACGIH/NIOSH | | EPA (water) | Comments |
|---|---|---|---|---|---|
| • Warfarin 81–81–2 | 0.1 mg/m³ | Same | | | H: (medicinal use): Established human teratogen |
| **Fungicides/Fumigants/Sterilants** | | | | | |
| • Benomyl 17804–35–2 | 10 mg/m³ | Same | 10 mg/m³ | | A: Fetotox, terata<br>H: No data |
| °• 1,2-dibromo-3-chloro-propane (DBCP) 96–12–8 | 0.001 ppm | | | 0.0002<br>0 (MCLG) | Well-established male spermato-toxin with sterility in some workers, ± SAB (♂)<br>Ca<br>All uses banned 1986 |
| °• Ethylene di-bromide (EDB) 106–93–4 | 20 ppm<br>C30 ppm<br>Peak (5 min)<br>50 ppm | 0.045 ppm<br>C 0.13 ppm | ALARA | 0.00005<br>0 (MCLG) | A: RT (♂)<br>H: Spermatotoxic-ity, ± infertility<br>M, Ca<br>All uses canceled 1984 |
| °• Ethylene oxide 75–21–8 | 1 ppm<br>ST 5 ppm | <0.1 ppm<br>C5 ppm<br>(10 min/day) | 1 ppm<br>ALARA | | A: RT (♂, ♀), embleth, fetotox<br>H: SAB<br>M, Ca |
| °Ethylene thiourea 96–45–7 | | | | (L)<br>0.1 (LT-C)<br>0.4 (LT-A) | A: Embleth, feto-tox, terata<br>H: No data<br>M, Ca<br>No longer used in U.S. commerce but common degrada-tion product of eth-ylene bis-dithiocar-bamate fungicides |

| Chemical CAS No.[b] | OSHA PEL[c] | NIOSH REL[d] | ACGIH[e] | | EPA DW Regs[f] | | Some Reported Effects[g] |
|---|---|---|---|---|---|---|---|
| | | | TLV | BEI | MCL (mg/liter) | HA (mg/liter) | |
| • Hexachlorobenzene 118–74–1 | | | | | 0.001 (P) 0 (MCLG-P) | | A: RT (♀), fetotox, NNM H: Stillbirth, developmental abnormalities with postnatal exposure |
| Thiram 137–26–8 | 5 mg/m³ | Same | 1 mg/m³ | | | | A: RT (♀), terata H: No data |
| **Organic Solvents**[i] | | | | | | | |
| Benzene 71–43–2 | 1 ppm ST 5 ppm | 0.1 ppm ST 1 ppm | 10 ppm 0.1 ppm (P) ALARA | Urine phenol 50 creat; sample end of shift | 0.005 0 (MCLG) | | A: Fetotox, ± terata H: Menstrual dysfunction, ? SAB, maternal hemorrhage with toxicity M, Ca |
| °• Carbon disulfide 75–15–0 | 4 ppm ST 12 ppm | 1 ppm ST 10 ppm | 10 ppm | Urine TTCA[j] 5 mg/g creat; sample end of shift | | | A: RT (♂), terata H: ↓ libido, spermatotoxicity, menstrual dysfunction, SAB |
| Carbon tetrachloride 56–23–5 | 2 ppm | ST (60 min) 2 ppm | 5 ppm ALARA | | 0.005 0 (MCLG) | | A: RT (♂, ♀), fetotox, (high doses) H: No data, Ca |
| Dichloromethane (methylene chloride) 75–09–2 | 500 ppm 25 ppm (P) C 1000 ppm Peak (5 min in any 2 hr) 2000 ppm ST 125 ppm (P) | Lowest feasible concentration | 50 ppm ALARA | | 0.005 (P) 0 (MCLG-P) | | Metabolized to carbon monoxide A: RT (♂), fetotox, neurobehavioral deficits H: Spermatotoxicity (case reports), SAB M, Ca |

| | | | | |
|---|---|---|---|---|
| °Epichlorohydrin 106–89–8 | 2 ppm | Lowest feasible concentration | 2 ppm 0.1 ppm (P) ALARA | 0 (MCLG) | A: RT (♂) H: Inadequate data M, Ca |
| °• Ethylene glycol monoethyl ether (EGEE) 110–80–5 and its acetate (EGEEA) 111–15–9 | 200 ppm (EGEE) 100 ppm (EGEEA) | 0.5 ppm Urine ethoxyacetic acid 5 mg/g creat | 5 ppm | | A: RT (♂), terata H: spermatotoxicity, terata (case reports) |
| °• Ethylene glycol monomethyl ether (EGME) 109–86–4 and its acetate (EGMEA) 110–49–6 | 25 ppm | 0.1 ppm Urine methoxyacetic acid 0.8 mg/g creat | 5 ppm | | A: RT (♂), terata H: Inadequate data |
| Formamides Methylformamide (MMF) 123–39–7 Dimethylformamide (DMF) 68–12–2 | 10 ppm | Same | Same | Urine N-MMF 40 mg/g creat; sample end of shift | A: Embleth, terata MMF > DMF H: ? testicular Ca (DMF), SAB |

| Chemical CAS No.[b] | OSHA PEL[c] | NIOSH REL[d] | ACGIH[e] | | EPA DW Regs[f] | | Some Reported Effects[g] |
|---|---|---|---|---|---|---|---|
| | | | TLV | BEI | MCL (mg/liter) | HA (mg/liter) | |
| • Styrene 100–42–5 | 50 ppm ST 100 ppm | Same | Same | Urine mandelic acid 800 mg/g creat (end of shift), 300 mg/g creat (< next shift); urine phenyl-glyoxylic acid 240 mg/g creat (end of shift), 100 mg/g creat (< next shift); blood styrene 0.55 mg/ liter (end of shift), 0.02 mg/ liter (< next shift) | 0.1 | 0.1 (MCLG) | A: RT (♀), embleth, neurobehavioral deficits H: ± menstrual dysfunction, reduced birthweight |
| • Toluene 108–88–3 | 100 ppm ST 150 ppm | Same | Same 50 ppm TWA (P) | Urine hippuric acid 2.5 mg/g creat; urine o-creosol 1 mg/g creat (P); blood toluene 1 mg/ liter; sample end of shift | 1 | 1 (MCLG) | A: Fetotox H: Menstrual dysfunction, terata (high doses) |
| Xylenes 1330–20–7 95–47–6 108–38–3 106–42–3 (o-,m-,p-isomers) | 100 ppm ST 150 ppm | Same | Same | Urine methyl hippuric acid 1.5 mg/g creat (end of shift); 2 mg/min (last 4 hr of shift) | 10 | 10 (MCLG) | A: Embleth, fetotox, H: Terata, ± SAB with mixed organic solvent exposure (♂) |

**Other Chemicals**

| Chemical (CAS) | | | | | |
|---|---|---|---|---|---|
| Acrylonitrile 107–13–1 | 2 ppm C10 ppm | 1 ppm C10 ppm | 2 ppm ALARA | 0.001 (LT-C) 0.004 (LT-A) (D) | Asphyxiant A: ± RT (♂), terata H: No data |
| Benzo-a-pyrene 50–32–8 (coal tar pitch volatile) | 0.2 mg/m³ | 0.1 mg/m³ | ALARA | 0.0002 (P) 0 (MCLG-P) | Constituent of cigarette smoke A: RT (♂, ♀), embleth, fetotox, terata, sterility in offspring H: Smokers: ↓ fecundity and earlier age of menopause M, Ca |
| • Carbon monoxide 630–08–0 | 35 ppm C200 ppm | Same | 50 ppm ST 400 ppm 25 ppm (TWA-P) | Blood carboxyhgb <8%, 3.5% (P); sample end of shift | Asphyxiant A: RT, fetotox, NNM, brain damage H: Growth deficits, terata; fetal death, brain damage with severe CO poisoning |
| Chloroform 67–66–3 | 2 ppm | ST 2 ppm (60 min) | 10 ppm ALARA | 0.1 (L) | A: Embleth, fetotox, terata H: Inadequate data Ca |
| °Chloroprene 126–99–8 | 10 ppm | C 1 ppm | 10 ppm | | A: RT (♂), embleth, fetotox, ± terata H: ↓ libido, impotence, ↓ sperm motility, SAB (♂) M, Ca |

| Chemical CAS No.[b] | OSHA PEL[c] | NIOSH REL[d] | ACGIH[e] | | EPA DW Regs[f] | | Some Reported Effects[g] |
|---|---|---|---|---|---|---|---|
| | | | TLV | BEI | MCL (mg/liter) | HA (mg/liter) | |
| Cyanides KCN 151–50–8 NaCN 143–33–9 | 5 mg/m³ | C 5 mg/m³ | 5 mg/m³ | | | | Asphyxiant A: Terata H: Inadequate data |
| Di-n-butylphthalate 84–74–2 | 5 mg/m³ | Same | Same | | | RfD 0.1 mg/kg/day DWEL 4 mg/liter | A: RT (♂, ♀, high doses), embleth, fetotox, ± terata H: ↓ sperm density (1 report) |
| °Dinitrotoluene (DNT) 25321–14–6 | 1.5 mg/m³ | Same | Same 0.15 mg/m³ ALARA (P) | | (L) | 2,4-DNT: RfD 0.2 mg/kg/day (D) 2,6-DNT: RfD 0.1 mg/kg/day (D) | A: RT (♂, ♀) H: ± spermatotox-icity M, Ca |
| °Glycidyl ethers Allyl 106–92–3 | 5 ppm ST 10 ppm | Same | Same | | | | A: RT (♂) H: No data Ca (phenyl) |
| Butyl 2426–08–6 | 25 ppm | C5.6 ppm | 25 ppm | | | | |
| Phenyl 122–60–1 | 1 ppm | C1 ppm | 1 ppm | | | | |
| Methyl chloride 74–87–3 | 50 ppm ST 100 ppm | Lowest feasible concentration | 50 ppm ST 100 ppm | | (L) | 0.4 (LT-C) 1 (LT-A) 0.003 (LF) | A: RT (♂, high doses), ± terata H: No data M, Ca |

| Agent / CAS No. | OSHA PEL | NIOSH REL | ACGIH TLV | EPA (MCLG) | Effects |
|---|---|---|---|---|---|
| °● Polychlorinated biphenyls (PCBs) | | | | PCBs: 0.0005 0 (MCLG) | A: RT (♂, ♀; estrogen agonist), embleth, fetotox, NNM<br>H: Neonatal PCB syndrome (growth deficits, hyperpigmentation, conjunctivitis/exopthalmos), neurobehavioral deficits<br>Ca |
| 42% chlorine 53469-21-9 | 1 mg/m³ | 0.001 mg/m³ | 1 mg/m³ | | |
| 54% chlorine 11097-69-1 | 0.5 mg/m³ | 0.001 mg/m³ | 0.5 mg/m³ | | |
| Vinyl chloride 75-01-4 | 1 ppm C5 ppm | Lowest reliably detectable concentration | 5 ppm ALARA | 0.002 0 (MCLG) | A: Terata<br>H: ↓ libido, impotence, SAB (♂) M, Ca |
| °Waste anesthetic gases and vapors | | Halogenated agents C2 ppm; nitrous oxide 25 ppm | Halothane, nitrous oxide, 50 ppm; enflurane 75 ppm | | A: ± terata<br>H: SAB, ± terata (♂) |

[a]No comprehensive consensus list of potential human reproductive or developmental toxicants has yet been developed. This Appendix lists some occupational and environmental chemicals that warrant caution based on literature review and, in some cases, also on government agency warnings pertaining to reproductive hazards. The list is not meant to be inclusive and is subject to changes as new data accumulate. The exposure limits currently required or recommended by government agencies are not necessarily intended to protect specifically against adverse reproductive or developmental effects.

[b]CAS No. = Chemical Abstract Service registry number.

° = Designated as a potential human reproductive or developmental toxicant by NIOSH or OSHA.

● = Listed as a reproductive or developmental toxicant by the California EPA under provisions of the Safe Drinking Water and Toxic Enforcement Act of 1986 (Proposition 65).

[c]OSHA PEL = Occupational Safety and Health Administration Permissible Exposure Limit as found in Tables Z–1–A or Z–2 of the OSHA General Industry Air Contaminants Standard (29 CFR 1910.1000). PELs are enforceable time-weighted average (TWA) concentrations that must not be exceeded during any 8-hr workshift of a 40-hr workweek. C = Ceiling concentration that should not be exceeded during any part of a workday. ST = Short-term Exposure Limit (STEL) = 15-min TWA concentration (unless otherwise noted) that should not be exceeded during any part of a workday. ppm = parts per million; P = proposed.

[d]NIOSH REL = National Institute for Occupational Safety and Health Recommended Exposure Limit. RELs are time-weighted average concentrations for up to a 10-hr workday during a 40-hr workweek. Available data on reproductive and developmental effects are considered in REL determinations. RELs that differ from OSHA limits are nonenforceable. Data from U.S. Department of Health and Human Services, NIOSH. NIOSH pocket guide to chemical hazards. Washington, DC: U.S. Government Printing Office, 1990.

[e]ACGIH = American Conference of Governmental Industrial Hygienists. TLV = Threshold Limit Value = time-weighted average concentration for an 8-hr workday and a 40-hr workweek. BEI = Biological Exposure Indices = levels of chemicals or their metabolites most likely to be observed in biological specimens collected from workers with inhalation exposures at the TLV. BEIs apply to 8-hr exposures, 5 days/week. If biological measurements persistently exceed the BEI while air levels are within the TLV, consider other routes of exposure (dermal, ingestion) and/or nonoccupational exposure sources. ALARA = Keep exposures ''as low as reasonably achievable.'' ACGIH exposure limits that differ from OSHA limits are nonenforceable. Data from ACGIH. 1991–92 threshold limit values for chemical substances and physical agents and biological exposure indices. Cincinnati: ACGIH, 1991.

*EPA DW Regs = U.S. Environmental Protection Agency drinking water regulations and health advisories. MCL = Maximum Contaminant Level = Enforceable maximum permissible level of a contaminant in water that is delivered to any user of a public water system. MCLG = Maximum Contaminant Level Goal = Nonenforceable concentration of a drinking water contaminant that is protective of adverse human health effects and allows an adequate margin of safety. Available data on reproductive and developmental effects are considered in MCL and MCLG determinations. HA = Health Advisories = Nonenforceable concentrations of a drinking water contaminant that are not expected to cause adverse noncarcinogenic health effects over specific exposure durations; include a margin of safety to protect sensitive members of the population. LT = Longer-term HA = The concentration of a chemical in drinking water that is not expected to cause adverse noncarcinogenic effects up to approximately 7 yr (10% of an individual's lifetime) of exposure, with a margin of safety. LT-C (child) is based on a 10-kg child consuming 1 liter of water per day. LT-A (adult) is based on a 70-kg adult consuming 2 liters of water per day. Assumes all exposure to the chemical comes from drinking water. LF = Lifetime HA = The concentration of a chemical in drinking water that is not expected to cause adverse noncarcinogenic effects over a lifetime of exposure, with a margin of safety. Based on a 70-kg adult consuming 2 liters of water per day and adjusted for the amount of exposure from drinking water relative to other sources (e.g., food, air). Lifetime HAs are not recommended for suspect human carcinogens.

In some cases where data are inadequate to establish a HA value, a reference dose (RfD) and/or Drinking Water Equivalent Level (DWEL) are provided. The RfD is an estimate of a daily exposure to the human population (including sensitive subgroups) in mg/kg/day that is likely to be without appreciable risk of deleterious effects over a lifetime. The DWEL is an adjustment of the RfD for a 70-kg adult consuming 2 liters of water daily and represents a lifetime exposure concentration protective of adverse, noncarcinogenic health effects assuming all of the exposure comes from drinking water.

The status of the drinking water regulations and health advisories are final unless otherwise indicated. D = draft, L = listed for regulation, P = proposed, R = under review.

Data from U.S. EPA, Office of Water. Drinking water regulations and health advisories. Washington, DC: U.S. EPA, November 1991.

*A = experimental animals; H = humans. RT = reproductive toxicity, male (♂) or female (♀); emblteth = embryolethality; fetotox = fetotoxicity (e.g., growth deficits, delayed development); terata = teratogenesis; SAB = spontaneous abortion; LBW = low birthweight; PTD = preterm delivery; NNM = neonatal mortality; (♂) after a developmental outcome indicates a possible male-mediated effect.

M = mutagenic; Ca = potential human carcinogen
+/− = data very conflicting.

Data derived from numerous references cited in the chapters of this book plus the following:

U.S. Department of Health and Human Services, Agency for Toxic Substances and Disease Registry (ATSDR). Toxicological profiles for acrylonitrile, copper, di-n-butylphthalate, ethylene oxide, hexachlorobenzene, polycyclic aromatic hydrocarbons, total xylenes, toxaphene. Atlanta: ATSDR, 1990.

Barlow SM, Sullivan FM. Reproductive hazards of industrial chemicals. New York: Academic Press, 1982.

Jelovsek FR, Mattison DR, Chen JJ. Prediction of risk for human developmental toxicity: how important are animal studies for hazard identification? Obstet Gynecol 1989;74:624–636.

Mattison DR, Bogumil J, Chapin R, et al. Reproductive effects of pesticides. In: Baker SR, Wilkinson CF, eds. The effects of pesticides on human health. Volume XVIII. Advances in modern environmental toxicology. Princeton: Princeton Scientific Publications Co Inc, 1990:297–389.

Schardein JL. Chemically induced birth defects. New York: Marcel Dekker, Inc, 1985.

Shepard TH. Catalog of teratogenic agents. 6th ed. Baltimore: John Hopkins University Press, 1989.

U.S. Environmental Protection Agency. Drinking water health advisory: pesticides. Chelsea, MI: Lewis Publishers, Inc, 1989.

U.S. Department of Health and Human Services, National Institute for Occupational Safety and Health. Current intelligence bulletins. Cincinnati: NIOSH, various years of publication.

*Mixed pesticide exposure has been associated with fetal loss and malformations (particularly limb reduction defects) in some epidemiological studies. Pesticides that are no longer produced in the U.S. are included because they may still be found in drinking water sources due to environmental persistence.

*Occupational mixed organic solvent exposure has been associated with congenital malformations and, less consistently, with spontaneous abortion (including male-mediated effect) in some epidemiological studies.

*TTCA = 2-thiothiazolidine-4-carboxylic acid.

# Index

Page numbers followed by "f" denote figures; those followed by "t" denote tables.